Essentials of Obstetrics and Gynecology

second edition

NEVILLE F. HACKER, M.B.B.S.

Associate Professor of Obstetrics
and Gynecology
Director of Gynaecologic Oncology
University of New South Wales
Royal Hospital for Women
Sydney, New South Wales
Australia

J. GEORGE MOORE, M.D.

Professor and Chairman Emeritus
Department of Obstetrics and Gynecology
UCLA School of Medicine
Senior Physician
Los Angeles, California
UCLA Olive View Medical Center
Sylmar, California

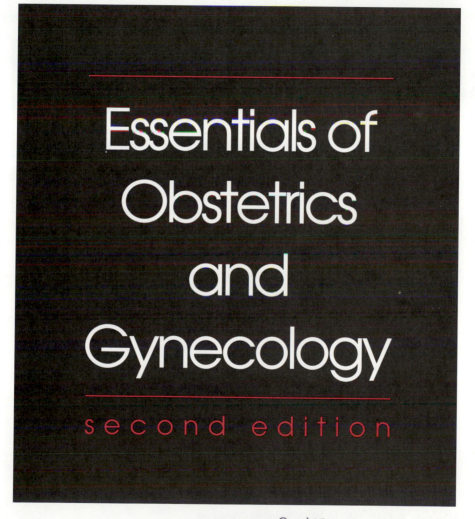

Essentials of Obstetrics and Gynecology

second edition

W. B. SAUNDERS COMPANY
Harcourt Brace Jovanovich, Inc.
Philadelphia   London   Toronto   Montreal   Sydney   Tokyo

W. B. Saunders Company
Harcourt Brace Jovanovich, Inc.

The Curtis Center
Independence Square West
Philadelphia, Pennsylvania 19106

Library of Congress Cataloging-in-Publication Data

Essentials of obstetrics and gynecology / [edited by] Neville F. Hacker, J. George
Moore.—2nd ed.
    p.   cm.
    Includes bibliographical references and index.
    ISBN 0-7216-3668-3
    1. Gynecology. 2. Obstetrics. I. Hacker, Neville F. II. Moore, J. George
    [DNLM: 1. Gynecology. 2. Obstetrics. WQ 100 E783]
  RG101.E87   1992
  618—dc20
  DNLM/DLC   92-8771

Editor: Joan T. Meyer
Designer: Ellen Bodner-Zanolle
Production Manager: Peter Faber
Manuscript Editors: Carol DiBerardino and Ellen Thomas
Illustration Specialist: Cecilia Roberts
Indexer: Dennis Dolan

Essentials of Obstetrics and Gynecology, 2nd edition   ISBN 10-7216-3668-3

Printed in the United States of America.

Last digit is the print number: 9   8   7   6   5   4   3   2

Contributors

EDITORS

NEVILLE F. HACKER, M.B.B.S.

Associate Professor of Obstetrics and Gynecology, Director of Gynecologic Oncology, University of New South Wales, Royal Hospital for Women, Sydney, New South Wales, Australia

> Breast Disease: A Gynecologic Perspective; Principles of Cancer Therapy; Vulvar and Vaginal Cancer

J. GEORGE MOORE, M.D.

Professor and Chairman Emeritus, Department of Obstetrics and Gynecology, UCLA School of Medicine, Los Angeles, CA; Senior Physician, Olive View Medical Center, Sylmar, CA

> Female Reproductive Anatomy; Obstetric and Gynecologic Evaluation; Surgical Conditions in Pregnancy; Benign Diseases of the Uterus; Benign Tumors of the Ovaries and Fallopian Tubes; Endometriosis and Adenomyosis; Ectopic Pregnancy; Contraception and Sterilization; Part 3: Gynecology

PART EDITORS

JONATHAN S. BEREK, M.D.

Professor and Vice-Chair, Chief of Gynecology, Director, Gynecologic Oncology, UCLA School of Medicine, Jonsson Comprehensive Cancer Center, Los Angeles, CA; Director, Rhonda Fleming Mann Clinic for Women's Comprehensive Care, UCLA Medical Center, Los Angeles, CA

> Ovarian Cancer; Gestational Trophoblastic Neoplasia; Part 5: Gynecologic Oncology

R. JEFFREY CHANG, M.D.

Professor and Chair, Department of Obstetrics and Gynecology, University of California, Davis School of Medicine; Davis, CA

> Virilism and Hirsutism; Part 4: Reproductive Endocrinology

CALVIN J. HOBEL, M.D.

Professor of Obstetrics, Gynecology and Pediatrics, UCLA School of Medicine, Los Angeles, CA; Miriam Jacobs Chair and Director of Maternal-Fetal Medicine, Cedars-Sinai Medical Center, Los Angeles, CA

> Prenatal Care; Normal Labor, Delivery, and the Puerperium; Resuscitation of the Newborn; Intrauterine Growth Retardation, Intrauterine Fetal Demise, and Post-Term Pregnancy; Operative Delivery; Part 2: Maternal-Fetal Medicine

OTHER CONTRIBUTORS

CAROL L. ARCHIE, M.D.

Assistant Professor, Division of Maternal-Fetal Medicine, Department of Obstetrics and Gynecology, UCLA School of Medicine, Los Angeles, CA

Licit and Illicit Drug Use in Pregnancy

RICHARD A. BASHORE, M.D.

Professor of Obstetrics and Gynecology, UCLA School of Medicine, Los Angeles, CA

Dystocia

MICHAEL J. BENNETT, M.B., Ch.B., M.D. (U.C.T.) F.C.O.G.(S.A.), F.R.C.O.G., F.R.A.C.O.G., D.D.U.

Professor and Head of School of Obstetrics and Gynaecology, University of New South Wales, Sydney, Australia; Clinical Director of Obstetrics and Gynaecology, Royal Hospital for Women, Sydney, Australia

Abortion

NARENDER N. BHATIA, M.D.

Attending Obstetrician Gynecologist, Associate Professor of Obstetrics and Gynecology, UCLA School of Medicine, Los Angeles, CA; Attending Physician, Harbor/UCLA Hospital, Torrance, CA

Pelvic Relaxation and Urinary Problems

JENNIFER BLAKE, M.D., F.R.C.S.(C)

Associate Professor, Obstetrics and Gynecology and Pediatrics, McMaster University: Chair, MD Programme, McMaster University, Hamilton, Ontario; Attending Physician, Chedore McMaster Hospital, Hamilton, Ontario, Canada

Pediatric Gynecology

CLIFFORD BOCHNER, M.D.

Attending Physician, Cedars-Sinai Medical Center, Los Angeles, CA

Anatomic Characteristics of the Fetal Head and Maternal Pelvis

J. ROBERT BRAGONIER, M.D., Ph.D.

Adjunct Professor of Obstetrics and Gynecology, UCLA School of Medicine; Director of Obstetrics and Gynecology, CIGNA Healthplans of California; Attending Physician, Cedars-Sinai Medical Center, AMI-South Bay Hospital, AMI-North Hollywood Medical Center, CIGNA Medical Center, Los Angeles, CA

Human Sexuality; Sexual Assault

CHARLES R. BRINKMAN, III, M.D.

Professor, Obstetrics and Gynecology, UCLA School of Medicine, Los Angeles, CA; Chairman Department of Obstetrics and Gynecology, Harbor/UCLA Medical Center, Torrance, CA

Obstetric and Gynecologic Evaluation; Hypertensive Disorders of Pregnancy

PHILIP G. BROOKS, M.D.

Clinical Professor of Obstetrics and Gynecology, USC School of Medicine; Attending Physician, Cedars-Sinai Hospital, Los Angeles, CA

Gynecologic Operative Techniques

RICHARD P. BUYALOS, JR., M.D.

Assistant Professor, Division of Reproductive Endocrinology, UCLA School of Medicine, Los Angeles, CA; UCLA Medical Center, Los Angeles, CA

Puberty and Precocious Puberty

MARY E. CARSTEN, Ph.D.

Professor of Obstetrics/Gynecology and Anesthesiology, UCLA School of Medicine, Los Angeles, CA

Endocrinology of Pregnancy and Parturition

KENNETH A. CONKLIN, M.D., Ph.D.

Associate Professor of Anesthesiology, Director, Obstetric Anesthesia, UCLA School of Medicine, Los Angeles, CA

Obstetric Analgesia and Anesthesia

JOHN A. EDEN, M.D., M.R.C.O.G., F.R.A.C.O.G.

Senior Lecturer in Reproductive Endocrinology, University of New South Wales, Sydney, Australia; Royal Hospital for Woman, Sydney; St. George Hospital, Kogarah, Sydney, Australia

Dysmenorrhea and Premenstrual Syndrome

LARRY C. FORD, M.D.

Clinical Associate Professor, Department of Obstetrics and Gynecology, University of California, Irvine, CA

Pelvic Inflammatory Disease

MICHELLE FOX, M.S.

Genetics Clinic Coordinator, UCLA Department of Pediatrics/Genetics, UCLA School of Medicine, Los Angeles, CA

Genetic Evaluation and Teratology

JOSEPH GAMBONE, D.O.

Assistant Professor, Department of Obstetrics and Gynecology, UCLA School of Medicine, Los Angeles, CA

Gynecologic Operative Techniques

ANN GARBER, M.S., Ph.D.

Assistant Clinical Professor, UCLA School of Medicine, Los Angeles, CA; Director, Genetic Counseling, Cedars-Sinai Medical Center, Los Angeles, CA

Genetic Evaluation and Teratology

ANNE D. M. GRAHAM, M.D., F.A.C.O.G.

Attending Physician, St. Mary's Hospital; Good Samaritan Medical Center; Consultant, Palm Beach Gardens Medical Center; Northwest Regional Hospital

Preterm Labor and Premature Rupture of Membranes

WILLIAM A. GROWDON, M.D.

Clinical Associate Professor of Obstetrics and Gynecology, UCLA School of Medicine, Los Angeles, CA; Associate Staff, Santa Monica Hospital Medical Center, Saint John's Hospital, Santa Monica, CA

Embryology and Congenital Anomalies of the Female Genital System

JOHN GUNNING, M.D.

Adjunct Professor of Obstetrics and Gynecology, UCLA School of Medicine; Los Angeles, CA; Chief of Gynecology, Harbor/UCLA Medical Center, Torrance, CA

Vaginal and Vulvar Infections

LEWIS A. HAMILTON, JR., M.D.

Associate Professor of Obstetrics and Gynecology, Charles R. Drew University of Medicine and Science, Los Angeles, CA; Director of Graduate Medical Education, King/Drew Medical Center, Los Angeles, CA

Intrauterine Growth Retardation, Intrauterine Fetal Demise, and Post-Term Pregnancy

HUNTER A. HAMMILL, M.D.

Associate Professor of Obstetrics and Gynecology, Baylor University School of Medicine, Houston, TX

Pelvic Inflammatory Disease

ROBERT H. HAYASHI, M.D.

J. Robert Willson Professor of Obstetrics, Director, Maternal-Fetal Medicine, Department of Obstetrics and Gynecology, University of Michigan, Ann Arbor, MI; University of Michigan Hospitals, Ann Arbor, MI

Postpartum Hemorrhage and Puerperal Sepsis

JAMES M. HEAPS, M.D.

Clinical Assistant Professor, Department of Obstetrics and Gynecology, Division of Gynecologic Oncology, UCLA School of Medicine, Los Angeles, CA

Uterine Corpus Cancer

SAMIR KHALIFÉ, M.D.

Assistant Professor, Department of Obstetrics and Gynecology, McGill University, Montreal, Canada; Director, Division of Ultrasonography, Royal Victoria Hospital, Montreal, Canada

Medical Complications of Pregnancy

OSCAR A. KLETZKY, M.D.

Professor and Chief, Division of Reproductive Endocrinology, Department of Obstetrics and Gynecology, UCLA School of Medicine, Los Angeles, CA; Division Chief, Division of Reproductive Endocrinology, Department of Obstetrics and Gynecology, Harbor/UCLA Medical Center, Los Angeles, CA

Amenorrhea and Abnormal Uterine Bleeding

THOMAS B. LEBHERZ, M.D.

Professor Emeritus of Obstetrics and Gynecology, UCLA School of Medicine, Los Angeles, CA

Benign Lesions of the Vulva, Vagina, and Cervix

RONALD S. LEUCHTER, M.D.

Associate Professor of Obstetrics and Gynecology, UCLA School of Medicine, Los Angeles, Cedars-Sinai Hospital, Los Angeles, CA

Gynecologic Operative Techniques; Uterine Corpus Cancer

JOHN K. H. LU, Ph.D.

Professor of Obstetrics and Gynecology and Anatomy, UCLA School of Medicine, Los Angeles, CA

The Menstrual Cycle, Ovulation, Fertilization, Implantation, and the Placenta

DONALD E. MARSDEN, B. MED. SC. (HONS.), M.B., B.S., F.R.C.O.G., F.R.A.C.O.G., C.G.O.

Head, Department of Obstetrics and Gynaecology, Sub Dean, Faculty of Medicine, University of Tasmania, Hobart, Australia;

Director, Women and Children's Health; Gynaecologic Oncologist, Royal Hobart Hospital, Hobart, Australia

An Approach to Ethical Decision Making in Obstetrics and Gynecology

ARNOLD L. MEDEARIS, M.D.

Clinical Assistant Professor Obstetrics and Gynecology, UCLA School of Medicine, Los Angeles, CA; Attending Physician, Cedars-Sinai Hospital, Los Angeles, CA

Immunology of Pregnancy; Fetal Malpresentations; Multiple Gestation

DAVID R. MELDRUM, M.D.

Clinical Professor, Department of Obstetrics and Gynecology, UCLA School of Medicine, Los Angeles, CA; Staff Physician, AMI South Bay Hospital, Redondo Beach, CA

Infertility

JOHN P. NEWNHAM, M.D. (W.AUST), M.R.C.O.G., F.R.A.C.O.G., D.D.U.

Associate Professor, The University of Western Australia; Maternal-Fetal Medicine Specialist, King Edward Memorial Hospital, Bagot Road, Subiaco, Western Australia

Operative Delivery

BAHIJ NUWAYHID, M.D., Ph.D.

Professor, Obstetrics, Gynecology, Physiology, McGill University, Montreal, Quebec, Canada; Director of Maternal-Fetal Medicine Program, McGill University; Director of Obstetric Royal Victoria Hospital, Montreal, Quebec, Canada

Medical Complications of Pregnancy

ALDO PALMIERI, M.D.

Assistant Professor of Obstetrics and Gynecology, UCLA School of Medicine, Los Angeles, CA; Assistant Professor, UCLA School of Medicine, Los Angeles, CA; Physician Specialist, Olive View Medical Center, Sylmar, CA

Ectopic Pregnancy

GROESBECK P. PARHAM, M.D.

Assistant Professor of Obstetrics and Gynecology, Drew University of Medicine and Science, Los Angeles, CA; Chief, Gynecologic Oncology, Martin Luther King, Jr. Hospital, Los Angeles, CA

Cervical Dysplasia and Cancer

ANDREA J. RAPKIN, M.D.

Associate Professor, Obstetrics and Gynecology, UCLA School of Medicine, Los Angeles, CA

Chronic Pelvic Pain

ANTHONY E. READING, Ph.D.

Assistant Professor of Psychiatry, UCLA School of Medicine, Los Angeles, CA

Human Sexuality; Sexual Assault

JEAN M. RICCI, M.D.

Department of Obstetrics and Gynecology, Marshfield Clinic, Marshfield, WI

Antepartum Hemorrhage; AIDS and Infectious Diseases in Pregnancy

MICHAEL G. ROSS, M.D., M.P.H.

Associate Professor of Obstetrics and Gynecology and Public Health, UCLA School of Medicine and UCLA School of Public Health, Los Angeles, CA; Attending Physician, Harbor/UCLA Medical Center, Torrance, CA

Normal Labor, Delivery, and the Puerperium

EDWARD W. SAVAGE, JR., M.D.

Professor of Obstetrics and Gynecology, Charles R. Drew Postgraduate Medical School; Adjunct Professor of Obstetrics and Gynecology, UCLA School of Medicine, Los Angeles, CA; Chief, Division of Gynecology, King/Drew Medical Center, Los Angeles, CA

Cervical Dysplasia and Cancer

JAMES R. SHIELDS, M.D.

Department of Maternal-Fetal Medicine, AMI-Tarzana Regional Medical Center, Tarzana, CA

Fetal Malpresentations; Multiple Gestation

KLAUS J. STAISCH, M.D.

Associate Professor of Obstetrics and Gynecology, Washington University School of Medicine; Obstetrician-Gynecologist-in-Chief, St. Louis Regional Medical Center, St. Louis, MO; Barnes Hospital; St. Louis Regional Medical Center, St. Louis, MO

Identification and Management of Fetal Distress During Labor

ERIC S. SURREY, M.D.

Assistant Professor of Obstetrics and Gynecology, UCLA School of Medicine, Los Angeles, CA; Division of Reproductive Endocrinology, Cedars-Sinai Hospital, Los Angeles, CA

The Menstrual Cycle, Ovulation, Fertilization, Implantation, and the Placenta

KHALIL TABSH, M.D.

Professor of Obstetrics and Gynecology, UCLA School of Medicine, Los Angeles, CA; Chief of Obstetrics, UCLA Medical Center, Los Angeles, CA

Genetic Evaluation and Teratology; Rhesus Isoimmunization

NANCY THEROUX, R.N., M.S.N.

Assistant Clinical Professor, UCLA School of Nursing, Los Angeles, CA; Perinatal Clinical Nurse Specialist, UCLA Medical Center, Los Angeles, CA

Rhesus Isoimmunization

PAUL J. TOOT, M.D.

Associate Professor of Obstetrics and Gynecology, UCLA School of Medicine, Los An-geles, CA; Physician Specialist, Olive View Medical Center, Sylmar, CA

The Menstrual Cycle, Ovulation, Fertilization, Implantation, and the Placenta

NATHAN WASSERSTRUM, M.D., Ph.D.

Assistant Professor, Department of Obstetrics and Gynecology, Division of Maternal-Fetal Medicine; Assistant Professor, Department of Medicine, Baylor College of Medicine, Houston, TX; Attending Physician, Ben Taub General Hospital, Houston, TX

Maternal Physiology

BARRY G. WREN, M.D., M.B.B.S., M.H.P.Ed., F.R.A.C.O.G., F.R.C.O.G.

Director, Centre for the Management of the Menopause, Royal Hospital for Women, Sydney, New South Wales, Australia; Consultant Gynecologist, Royal Hospital for Women, Sydney, New South Wales, Australia

The Menopause

Preface to the Second Edition

The second edition of *Essentials of Obstetrics and Gynecology* has been entirely updated with the addition of a section on Aids, Ethics, Drug Abuse, and Pediatric Gynecology. The chapters on Ectopic Pregnancy and Operative Techniques have been completely rewritten to reflect advances in diagnostic procedures and surgical techniques such as pelviscopy and hysteroscopy.

The revised edition consists of over 700 pages and includes over 190 illustrations. The bibliography has been updated and the index substantially enlarged. As a result, the second edition is suited to the needs of core residents as well as students. Because many of the original contributors have moved on to other posts, the text no longer necessarily reflects the view of the Department of Obstetrics and Gynecology at the University of California, Los Angeles.

Shortly after the first edition appeared, Dr. Hacker moved to the post of Director of Gynecologic Oncology at the University of New South Wales in Sydney, Australia. On two occasions, Dr. Moore worked with Dr. Hacker at the Royal Hospital for Women in Paddington, Sydney. As a consequence, several of the new contributors have been recruited from colleagues in Australia and Canada.

With these changes, along with the Spanish edition, the second edition of *Essentials of Obstetrics and Gynecology* is no longer a parochial text but has taken the form of an international source book.

J. GEORGE MOORE
NEVILLE F. HACKER

Preface to the First Edition

A generation ago most schools of medicine in the United States presented courses in theoretical obstetrics and gynecology extending over a period of 18 months, supplemented by practical clerkships of 8 to 16 weeks in the third and fourth years. Most students procured as source textbooks a fairly complete compendium of obstetrics and another in gynecology. These texts not only served the students in medical school but were of great value during their housestaff training and were added to their reference library as they entered practice.

During the decade of the 1960's, theoretical obstetrics and gynecology in many institutions were condensed into a general course known as "An Introduction to Clinical Medicine" or "The Pathophysiology of Disease." Practical work in the clinics and wards was condensed into core clerkships, and in obstetrics and gynecology the "core" was generally restricted to six or eight weeks with electives available in subspecialty areas (high-risk obstetrics, gynecologic oncology, reproductive endocrinology, acting internships, and outpatient gynecology). This condensation of experience into the "core" of obstetrics and gynecology during the clinical years left students with a difficult choice in selecting a textbook that would not overwhelm them with information yet would still stimulate their interest in the subject. Understandably it became increasingly difficult to hold the student responsible for a critical body of knowledge.

Textbooks prescribed for the core clerkships often do not have sufficient depth and sometimes do not possess key references or practical information. On the other hand, the classic texts of obstetrics and gynecology or gynecologic surgery are generally considered by students to be too expensive or too comprehensive for them to absorb during the clerkship. This book is a response to their dilemma. The chapters have all been written by members of the Obstetrics and Gynecology Faculty at the University of California, Los Angeles (UCLA) Medical Center and its affiliated hospitals — Harbor (LA County) General Hospital, Cedars-Sinai Medical Center, Martin Luther King, Jr. General Hospital, and Kern County Medical Center. Some authors have changed their institutional affiliation prior to the publication of the book. It is hoped that the book will serve the needs of the student, be useful during housestaff training, and be a helpful text in the medical practitioner's library. Fundamental principles and practice of obstetrics and gynecology are presented succinctly, but we have endeavored to cover all important aspects of the subject in sufficient detail to allow a reasonable understanding of the pathophysiology and a safe approach to clinical management.

The text is divided into five sections: an introductory section, obstetrics, reproductive endocrinology, gynecology, and gynecologic oncology. Special emphasis is given to family planning and important aspects of women's health. The basic operations of obstetrics and gynecology are included to allow a reasonable understanding of the technical procedures. Neville F. Hacker and J. George Moore have been responsible for the overall organization of the book. The most difficult tasks have been to maintain uniformity of style and to keep the text within 550 pages without sacrificing essential information. Calvin Hobel, John Marshall, J. George Moore, and Jonathan Berek have organized their particular sections. Neville F. Hacker has been largely responsible for the final editing of all the sections.

This book would not have been possible without the special help of the following individuals to whom we are most grateful:

Gwynne Gloege, the very talented principal medical illustrator at UCLA, who was responsible for the overall uniformity and high quality of the illustrations; Yao-shi Fu, M.D., and Roberta Nieberg, M.D., from the Department of Pathology, who provided illustrations and advice regarding gynecologic pathology; Norman Chang, who was responsible for the photography; and Linda Olt, who provided invaluable editorial assistance and also prepared the index. At W. B. Saunders, we are particularly grateful to Dana Dreibelbis, the Executive Editor who provided the initial inspiration and subsequent guidance for this project. Finally, this project would never have been completed without the untiring efforts, skill, and ever cheerful countenance of Cheri Buonaguidi, the Obstetrics and Gynecology student coordinator at UCLA. She carefully read and accurately typed each version of the manuscript and worked with each of the contributors until all chapters were completed.

J. GEORGE MOORE, M.D.
NEVILLE F. HACKER, M.D.

Contents

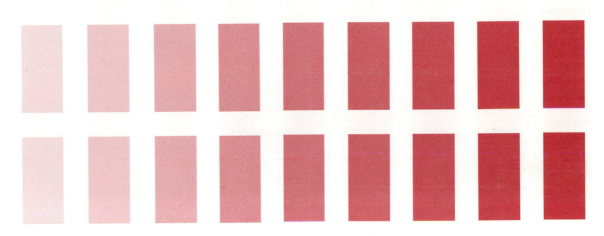

Part 4
Reproductive Endocrinology
R. JEFFREY CHANG

Part 5
Gynecologic Oncology
JONATHAN S. BEREK

Part 1

Introduction

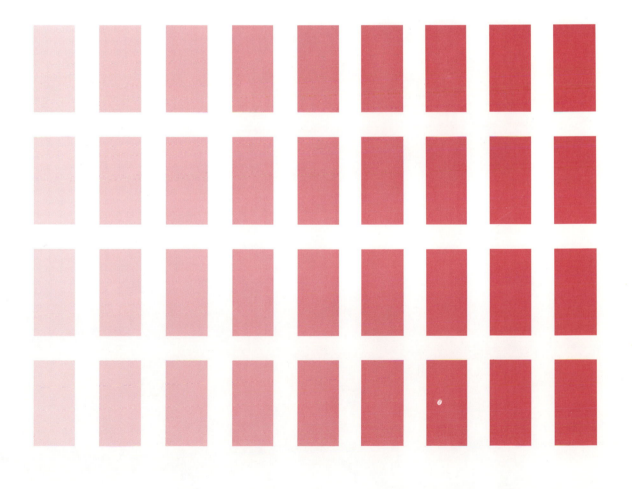

One

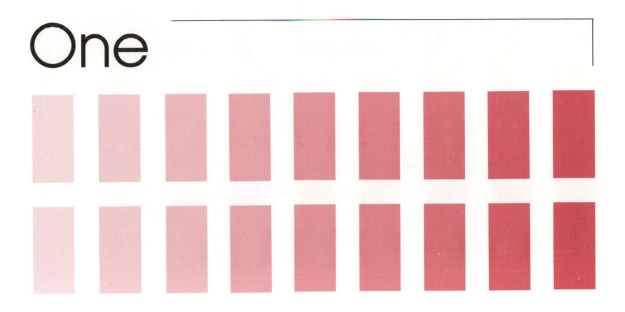

Female Reproductive Anatomy

J. GEORGE MOORE

The scope of obstetrics and gynecology assumes a reasonable background in reproductive anatomy, physiology, and endocrinology. A physician cannot effectively practice obstetrics and gynecology without understanding the physiologic processes that transpire in a woman's life as she passes through infancy, adolescence, reproductive maturity, and the menopause. As the various clinical problems are addressed, it is important to consider those anatomic and physiologic changes that normally take place at key points in a woman's life cycle. Virtually all organ systems are involved, and much of gynecology involves monitoring normal physiologic changes.

Most of this text deals with the disruptive deviations from normal female anatomy and physiology, whether they be congenital, functional, traumatic, inflammatory, neoplastic, or even iatrogenic. As the etiology and pathogenesis of clinical problems are considered, each must be studied in the context of normal anatomy and physiology. This chapter discusses those aspects of female reproductive anatomy that are essential to obstetrics and gynecology.

PERINEUM

The perineum represents the inferior boundary of the pelvis. It is bounded superiorly by the levator ani muscles and inferiorly by the skin between the thighs (Fig. 1–1). Anteriorly, the perineum extends to the symphysis pubis and the inferior borders of the pubic bones. Posteriorly, it is limited by the ischial tuberosities, the sacrotuberous ligaments, and the coccyx. The superficial and deep transverse perineal muscles cross the

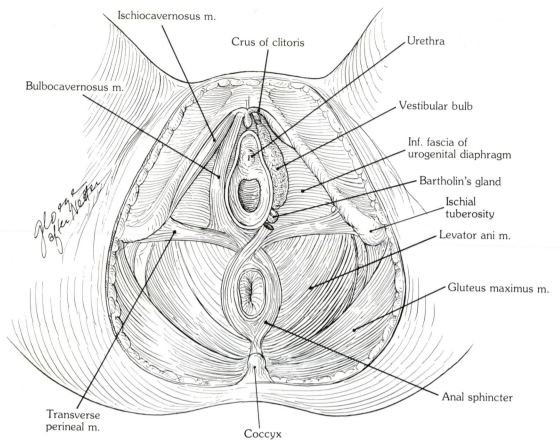

Ischiocavernosus m.

Crus of clitoris

Urethra

Bulbocavernosus m.

Vestibular bulb

Inf. fascia of urogenital diaphragm

Bartholin's gland

Ischial tuberosity

Levator ani m.

Gluteus maximus m.

Anal sphincter

Transverse perineal m.

Coccyx

Figure 1–1. The perineum, showing superficial structures on the left and deep structures on the right.

pelvic outlet between the two ischial tuberosities and divide the space into the urogenital triangle anteriorly and the anal triangle posteriorly.

The urogenital diaphragm is a fibromuscular sheet that stretches across the pubic arch. It is pierced by the vagina, urethra, the artery of the bulb, the internal pudendal vessels, and the dorsal nerve of the clitoris. Its inferior surface is covered by the crura of the clitoris, the vestibular bulbs, the greater vestibular (Bartholin's) glands, and the superficial perineal muscles. Bartholin's glands are situated just posterior to the vestibular bulbs, and their ducts empty into the introitus just below the labia minora. They are often the site of gonococcal infections and painful abscesses.

EXTERNAL GENITALIA

The external genitalia are referred to collectively as the vulva. As shown in Figure 1–2, the vulva includes the mons veneris, labia majora, labia minora, clitoris, vulvovaginal (Bartholin's) glands, fourchette, and perineum. The most prominent features of the vulva, the labia majora, are large, hair-covered folds of skin that contain sebaceous glands and lie on either side of the introitus. The labia minora lie medially and contain no hair but have a rich supply of venous sinuses, sebaceous glands, and nerves. The labia minora may vary from scarcely noticeable structures to leaf-like flaps measuring up to 3 cm in length. Anteriorly, each splits into two folds. The posterior pair of folds attach to the inferior surface of the clitoris where they unite to form the frenulum of the clitoris. The anterior pair unite like a hood over the clitoris, forming the prepuce. Posteriorly, the labia minora extend almost to the fourchette.

The clitoris lies just in front of the urethra and consists of the glans, the body, and the crura. Only the glans of the clitoris is visible externally. The body, composed of a pair of

Figure 1-2. Female external genitalia.

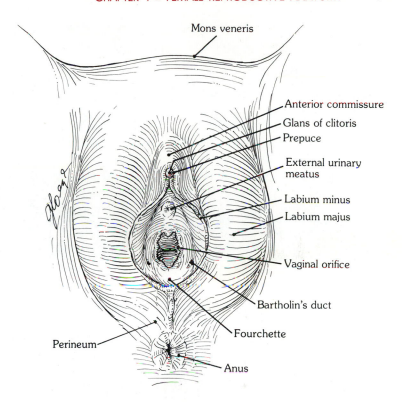

Mons veneris

Anterior commissure

Glans of clitoris

Prepuce

External urinary meatus

Labium minus

Labium majus

Vaginal orifice

Bartholin's duct

Fourchette

Perineum

Anus

corpora cavernosa, extends superiorly for a distance of several centimeters and divides into two crura, which are attached to the undersurface of either pubic ramus. Each crus is covered by the corresponding ischiocavernosus muscle. The vestibular bulbs (equivalent to the corpus spongiosum of the penis) extend posteriorly from the glans on either side of the lower vagina. Each bulb is attached to the inferior surface of the perineal membrane and covered by the bulbocavernosus muscle. These muscles aid in constricting the venous supply to the erectile vestibular bulbs and also act as the sphincter vaginae.

As the labia minora are spread, the vaginal introitus, guarded by the hymenal ring, is seen. Usually, the hymen is represented only by a circle of carunculae myrtiformes around the vaginal introitus. The hymen may take many forms, however, such as a cribriform plate with many small openings or a completely imperforate diaphragm.

The vestibule of the vagina is that portion of the introitus extending inferiorly from the hymenal ring between the labia minora. The fourchette represents the posterior portion of the vestibule just above the perineal body. Most of the vulva is innervated by the

branches of the pudendal nerve. Anterior to the urethra, the vulva is innervated by the ilioinguinal and genitofemoral nerves.

VAGINA

The vagina is a flattened tube extending from the hymenal ring at the introitus up to the fornices that surround the cervix (Fig. 1-3). Its epithelium is stratified squamous in type, is normally devoid of mucous glands and hair follicles, and is nonkeratinized. Deep to the vaginal epithelium are the muscular coats of the vagina, which consist of an inner circular and an outer longitudinal smooth muscle layer. Remnants of the mesonephric ducts may sometimes be demonstrated along the vaginal wall in the subepithelial layers and may give rise to Gartner's duct cysts. The vagina averages about 8 cm in length, although its size varies considerably with age, parity, and the status of ovarian function. An important anatomic feature is the immediate proximity of the posterior fornix of the vagina to the pouch of Douglas, which allows easy access to the peritoneal

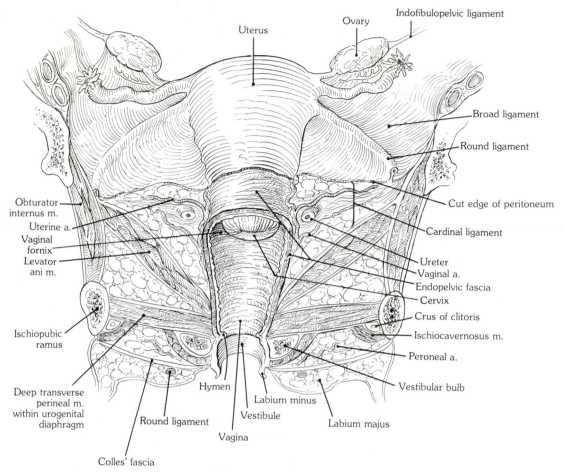

Figure 1–3. Coronal section of the pelvis at the level of the uterine isthmus and ischial spines, showing the ligaments supporting the uterus.

cavity from the vagina, by either culdocentesis or colpotomy.

UTERUS

The uterus consists of the cervix, isthmus, and the uterine corpus, which are joined by the isthmus (Fig. 1–4). The uterine isthmus represents a transitional area wherein the endocervical epithelium gradually changes into the endometrial lining. In late pregnancy, this area elongates and is referred to as the lower uterine segment.

The cervix is generally 2 to 3 cm in length. The portion that protrudes into the vagina and is surrounded by the fornices is covered with a nonkeratinizing squamous epithelium. At about the external cervical os, the squamous epithelium covering the exocervix changes to a simple columnar epithelium, the site of transition being referred to as the squamocolumnar junction. The cervical canal is lined by an irregular, arborized, simple columnar epithelium, which extends into the stroma as cervical "glands" or crypts.

The uterine corpus is a thick, pear-shaped organ, somewhat flattened anteroposteriorly, that consists of largely interlacing, smooth muscle fibers. The endometrial lining of the uterine corpus may vary from 2 to 10 mm in thickness, depending on the stage of the menstrual cycle. Most of the surface of the uterus is covered by the peritoneal mesothelium.

Four paired sets of ligaments are attached to the uterus (Fig. 1–4). Each round ligament inserts on the anterior surface of the

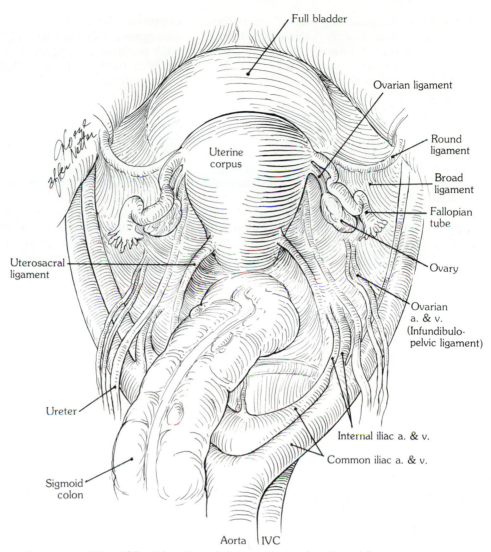

Figure 1–4. View of the internal genital organs in the female pelvis.

uterus just in front of the fallopian tube, passes to the pelvic side wall in a fold of the broad ligament, traverses the inguinal canal, and ends in the labium majus. The round ligaments are of little supportive value but help to keep the uterus anteverted. The uterosacral ligaments are condensations of the endopelvic fascia that arise from the sacral fascia and insert into the posteroinferior portion of the uterus at about the level of the isthmus. These ligaments contain sympathetic and parasympathetic nerve fibers that supply the uterus. They provide important support for the uterus and are also significant in

precluding the development of an enterocele. The cardinal ligaments (Mackenrodt's) are the other important supporting structures of the uterus that prevent prolapse. They extend from the pelvic fascia on the lateral pelvic walls and insert into the lateral portion of the cervix and vagina, reaching superiorly to the level of the isthmus. The pubocervical ligaments pass anteriorly around the bladder to the posterior surface of the pubic symphysis.

In addition, there are four peritoneal folds. Anteriorly, the vesicouterine fold is reflected from the level of the uterine isthmus onto the bladder. Posteriorly, the rectouterine fold passes from the posterior wall of the uterus, to the upper fourth of the vagina, and thence onto the rectum. It forms a cul-de-sac called the pouch of Douglas. Laterally, the two broad ligaments each pass from the side of the uterus to the lateral wall of the pelvis. Between the two leaves of each broad ligament are contained the fallopian tube, the round ligament, and the ovarian ligament, in addition to nerves, blood vessels, and lymphatics. The fold of broad ligament containing the fallopian tube is called the mesosalpinx. Between the end of the tube and ovary and the pelvic side wall, adjacent to the common iliac vessels, is the infundibulopelvic ligament, which contains the vessels and nerves for the ovary.

FALLOPIAN TUBES

The oviducts are bilateral muscular tubes (about 10 cm in length) with lumina that connect the uterine cavity with the peritoneal cavity. They are enclosed in the medial four fifths of the superior aspect of the broad ligament. The tubes are lined by a ciliated, columnar epithelium that is thrown into branching folds. That segment of the tube within the wall of the uterus is referred to as the interstitial portion. The medial portion of each tube is superior to the round ligament, is anterior to the ovarian ligament, and is relatively fixed in position. This nonmobile portion of the tube has a fairly narrow lumen and is referred to as the isthmus. As the tube proceeds laterally, it is located anterior to the ovary; it then passes around the lateral portion of the ovary and down toward the cul-de-sac (Fig. 1–5). The ampullary and fimbriated portions of the tube are suspended from the broad ligament by the mesosalpinx and are quite mobile. The mobility of the fimbriated end of the tube plays an important role in fertility.

OVARIES

The ovaries are oval, flattened, compressible organs, approximately 3 by 2 cm in size. They are situated on the superior surface of the broad ligament and are suspended between the ovarian ligament medially and the suspensory ligament of the ovary or infundibulopelvic ligament laterally and superiorly. Each occupies a position in the ovarian fossa (of Waldeyer), which is a shallow depression on the lateral pelvic wall just posterior to the external iliac vessels and anterior to the ureter and hypogastric vessels. In endometriosis and salpingo-oophoritis, the ovaries may be densely adherent to the ureter. Generally, the serosal covering and the tunica albuginea of the ovary are quite thin, and developing follicles and corpora lutea are readily visible.

The blood supply to the ovaries is provided by the long ovarian arteries, which arise from the abdominal aorta immediately below the renal arteries. These vessels course downward and cross laterally over the ureter at the level of the pelvic brim, passing branches to the ureter and the fallopian tube. The ovary also receives substantial blood supply from the uterine artery. The venous drainage from the right ovary is directly into the inferior vena cava, whereas that of the left ovary is into the left renal vein (Fig. 1–5).

URETERS

The ureters extend 25 to 30 cm from the renal pelves to their insertion into the bladder at the trigone. Each descends immediately under the peritoneum, crossing the pelvic brim beneath the ovarian vessels just anterior to the bifurcation of the common iliac artery. In the true pelvis, the ureter initially courses inferiorly, just anterior to the hypogastric vessels, and stays closely attached to the peritoneum. It then passes forward along the side of the cervix and beneath the uterine artery toward the trigone of the bladder.

LYMPHATIC DRAINAGE

The lymphatic drainage of the vulva and lower vagina is principally to the inguinofemoral lymph nodes and then to the external iliac chains (see Fig. 56–3). The lymphatic drainage of the cervix takes place through the parametria (cardinal ligaments) to the pelvic nodes (the hypogastric, obturator, and external iliac groups) and then to the common iliac and para-aortic chains. The

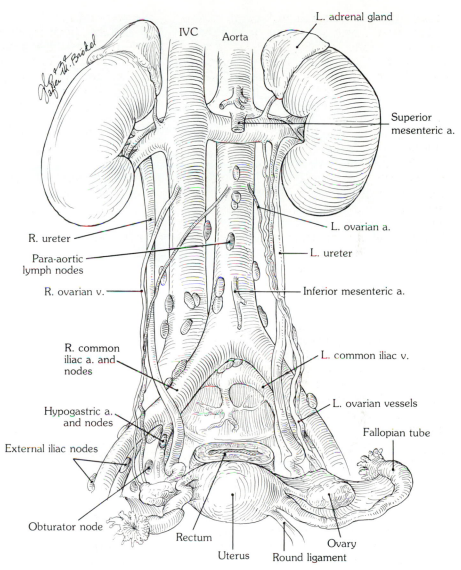

Figure 1–5. Lymphatic drainage of the internal genital organs.

lymphatic drainage from the endometrium is through the broad ligament and infundibulopelvic ligament to the pelvic and para-aortic chains. The lymphatics of the ovaries pass via the infundibulopelvic ligaments to the pelvic and para-aortic nodes (Fig. 1–5).

LOWER ABDOMINAL WALL

Because most intra-abdominal gynecologic operations are performed through lower abdominal incisions, it is important to review the anatomy of the lower abdominal wall

with special reference to the muscles and fasciae. After transecting the skin, subcutaneous fat, superficial fascia (of Camper), and deep fascia (of Scarpa), the anterior rectus sheath is encountered (Fig. 1–6). The rectus sheath is a strong fibrous compartment formed by the aponeuroses of the three lateral abdominal wall muscles. The aponeuroses meet in the midline to form the linea alba and partially encase the two rectus abdominis muscles. The composition of the rectus sheath differs in its upper and lower portions. Above the midpoint between the umbilicus

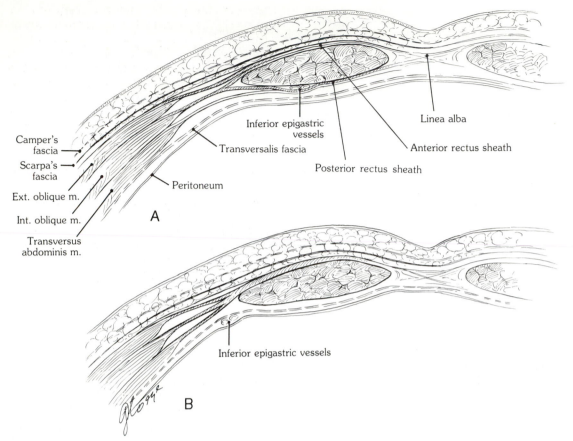

Camper's fascia
Scarpa's fascia
Ext. oblique m.
Int. oblique m.
Transversus abdominis m.
Inferior epigastric vessels
Transversalis fascia
Peritoneum
Posterior rectus sheath
Linea alba
Anterior rectus sheath

A

Inferior epigastric vessels

B

Figure 1–6. Transverse section through the anterior abdominal wall *(A)* just below the umbilicus and *(B)* just above the pubic symphysis. Note the absence of the posterior rectus sheath in *B*.

and the symphysis pubis, the rectus muscle is encased anteriorly by the aponeurosis of the external oblique and the anterior lamina of the internal oblique aponeurosis and posteriorly by the aponeurosis of the transversus abdominis and the posterior lamina of the internal oblique aponeurosis. In the lower fourth of the abdomen, the posterior aponeurotic layer of the sheath terminates in a free crescentic margin, the semilunar fold of Douglas.

Each rectus abdominis muscle, encased in the rectus sheath on either side of the midline, extends from the superior aspect of the symphysis pubis to the anterior surface of the fifth, sixth, and seventh costal cartilages. A variable number of tendinous intersections (three to five) crosses each muscle at irregular intervals, and a transverse rectus surgical in-

cision forms a new fibrous intersection during healing. The muscle is not attached to the posterior sheath and, following separation from the anterior sheath, can be retracted laterally, as in the Pfannenstiel incision. Each rectus muscle has a firm aponeurosis at its attachment to the symphysis pubis, and this tendinous aponeurosis can be transected if necessary to improve exposure, as in the Cherny incision, and resutured securely during closure of the abdominal wall.

The inferior epigastric arteries arise from the external iliac arteries and proceed superiorly just lateral to the rectus muscles between the transversalis fascia and the peritoneum. They enter the rectus sheaths at the level of the semilunar line and continue their course superiorly just posterior to the rectus muscles. In a transverse rectus muscle–cutting

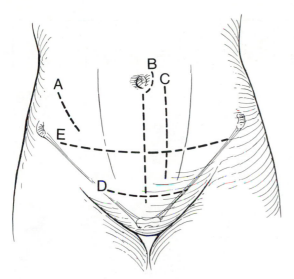

Figure 1–7. Abdominal wall incisions: *(A)* McBurney's, *(B)* lower midline, *(C)* left lower paramedian, *(D)* Pfannenstiel or Cherny, and *(E)* transverse, Maylard or Bordenhower.

does not always give sufficient exposure for extensive operations, it has cosmetic advantages in that it is generally 2 cm above the symphysis pubis, and the scar is later covered by the pubic hair. Because the rectus abdominis muscles are not cut, eviscerations and wound hernias are extremely uncommon. For extensive pelvic procedures (e.g., radical hysterectomy and pelvic lymphadenectomy), a transverse muscle–cutting incision (Maylard) at a slightly higher level in the lower abdomen gives sufficient exposure. In addition, the skin incision falls within the lines of Langer, so a good cosmetic result can be expected. When it is anticipated that upper abdominal exploration will be necessary, such as in a patient with suspected ovarian cancer, a midline incision through the linea alba or a paramedian vertical incision is indicated.

incision, the epigastric arteries can be retracted laterally or ligated to allow a wide peritoneal incision.

ABDOMINAL WALL INCISIONS

The most commonly used lower abdominal incision in gynecologic surgery is the Pfannenstiel incision (Fig. 1–7). Although it

SUGGESTED READING

Clemente CD: Regional Atlas of the Human Body. Philadelphia, Lea & Febiger, 1975.

Grant JCB: An Atlas of Human Anatomy. 7th ed. Baltimore, Williams & Wilkins, 1978.

Maylard EA: Directions of abdominal incisions. Br J Med 2:895, 1907.

Smout CFV, Jacoby F, Lillie EW: Gynecological and Obstetrical Anatomy. Baltimore, Williams & Wilkins, 1969.

Ulfelder H: Mechanism of pelvic support in women. Am J Obstet Gynecol 72:856, 1956.

Two

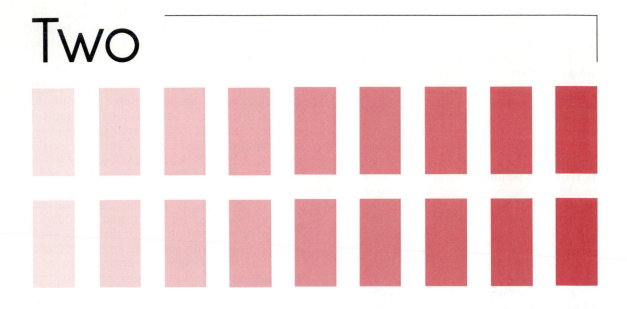

Obstetric and Gynecologic Evaluation

CHARLES R. BRINKMAN III AND J. GEORGE MOORE

As in most areas of medicine, a careful history and physical examination form the basis for patient evaluation and clinical management in obstetrics and gynecology. This chapter outlines the essential details of the clinical evaluation of the obstetric and gynecologic patient and discusses some pertinent ethical considerations and obstetric statistics.

OBSTETRIC HISTORY

A complete history must be recorded at the time of the prepregnancy evaluation or at the initial antenatal visit. Several detailed standardized forms are available for recording the pertinent aspects of the antenatal history, but this does not negate the need for a detailed chronologic history taken personally by the physician who will be caring for the patient throughout pregnancy. While taking the history, major opportunities arise to provide counseling and explanations that serve to establish close rapport and to allay apprehensions.

Previous Pregnancies

Each prior pregnancy should be reviewed in chronologic order and the following information recorded:

1. *Date of delivery* (or pregnancy termination).
2. *Location of delivery* (or pregnancy termination). Recording the city, name of hos-

pital, and name of the attending physician may become important later if further details are required.

3. *Duration of gestation* (recorded in weeks). When correlated with birth weight, this information allows an assessment of fetal growth patterns. The gestational age of any spontaneous abortion is of etiologic significance.

4. *Type of delivery* (or method of terminating pregnancy). This information is important for planning the method of delivery in the present pregnancy. A difficult forceps delivery or a cesarean section may require a personal review of the labor and delivery records.

5. *Duration of labor* (recorded in hours). This may alert the physician to the possibility of an unusually long or short labor.

6. *Type of anesthesia.* Any complications of anesthesia should be noted.

7. *Maternal complications.* Urinary tract infections, vaginal bleeding, hypertension, and postpartum complications may be repetitive; such knowledge is helpful in anticipating problems with the present pregnancy.

8. *Newborn weight* (in grams or pounds and ounces). This information may give indications of gestational diabetes, fetal growth problems, shoulder dystocia, or cephalopelvic discordance.

9. *Newborn gender.* This may provide insight into patient and family expectations and may indicate certain genetic risk factors.

10. *Fetal and neonatal complications.* Certain questions should be asked to elicit any problems and to determine the need to obtain further information. Inquiry should be made as to whether the baby had any problems after it was born, whether the baby breathed and cried right away, and whether the baby left the hospital with the mother. In addition to providing an assessment of risks, answers to questions such as these may allow insight into the mother's attitude during this pregnancy.

Menstrual History

A good menstrual history is essential because it is the determinant for establishing the expected date of confinement (EDC). Nägele's rule for establishing the EDC is to subtract 3 months and add 7 days to the first day of the last normal menstrual period (LMP). For example:

LMP—July 20, 1991
EDC—April 27, 1992

This calculation depends on a normal 28-day cycle, and adjustments must be made for longer or shorter cycles. Any bleeding or spotting since the last normal menstrual period should be reviewed in detail. Many abnormalities may be associated with bleeding in the first and second trimester, such as threatened abortion, ectopic pregnancy, placenta previa, and cervical neoplasia.

Contraceptive History

This information is important for risk assessment. Oral contraceptives taken during early pregnancy have been associated with birth defects, and retained intrauterine devices can cause early pregnancy loss and premature delivery. Discussion of contraception also allows the physician to gain insight into whether the pregnancy was planned and desired.

Medical History

The importance of a good medical history cannot be overemphasized. In addition to common disorders such as diabetes mellitus, hypertension, and renal disease, which are known to affect pregnancy outcome, all serious conditions should be recorded. An episode of hepatitis would dictate laboratory evaluation for a carrier state. An unexplained period of proteinuria would require investigations to rule out undiagnosed renal disease or a collagen vascular disease such as systemic lupus erythematosus.

Surgical History

Each surgical procedure should be recorded chronologically, including age, hospital, surgeon, and complications. Trauma must also be listed, since a fractured pelvis may result in diminished pelvic capacity.

Social History

The social history not only plays a role in risk assessment, but also provides insight into the patient's personal qualities. Habits such as smoking, alcohol use, and drug abuse are important factors that must be recorded and managed appropriately (see Chapter 17). The patient's contact or exposure to domesticated animals, particularly cats, with their associated risk of toxoplasmosis, is an important item to uncover.

The patient's type of work and lifestyle may affect the pregnancy. Exposure to solvents or insulators (PCP) in the workplace may lead to teratogenesis. A woman who does heavy manual labor may not be able to continue working throughout the entire pregnancy, whereas one with a more sedentary position may continue to work until the onset of labor.

OBSTETRIC PHYSICAL EXAMINATION

General Physical Examination

This procedure must be systematic and thorough and performed as early as possible in the prenatal period. A cursory or perfunctory examination is not sufficient, since this may be the first complete examination the woman has had since childhood. A complete physical examination provides an opportunity to detect previously unrecognized abnormalities. Normal baseline levels must also be established, particularly those of weight, blood pressure, funduscopic appearance, and cardiac status.

Pelvic Examination

The initial pelvic examination should be done early in the prenatal period and should include (1) inspection of the external genitalia, vagina, and cervix; (2) collection of cytologic specimens from the ectocervix and endocervical canal; and (3) palpation of the cervix, uterus, and adnexa.

Palpation of the uterus is important. Uterine abnormalities may be detected and the approximate duration of gestation determined. The initial estimate of gestational age by uterine size becomes less accurate as pregnancy progresses. Rectal and rectovaginal examinations are also important aspects of this initial pelvic evaluation.

Clinical Pelvimetry

This assessment is carried out following the bimanual pelvic examination and before the rectal examination. It is important that clinical pelvimetry be carried out systematically. The details of clinical pelvimetry are described in Chapter 10.

DIAGNOSIS OF PREGNANCY

The diagnosis of pregnancy and its location may be quite challenging during the early weeks of amenorrhea. For the most part, pregnancy is diagnosed on clinical grounds without the necessity of resorting to laboratory or imaging methods. Unless there is some specific clinical or social reason making early diagnosis desirable, cost-effective practice would dictate a purely clinical diagnosis, although office ultrasonography is used increasingly as a routine.

Symptoms of Pregnancy

The most common symptoms in the early months of pregnancy are amenorrhea, urinary frequency, breast engorgement, nausea, tiredness, and easy fatigability. Amenorrhea in a previously normally menstruating, sexually active woman should be considered to be caused by pregnancy until proved otherwise. Urinary frequency is most likely caused by the pressure of the enlarged uterus on the bladder. Morning urgency on awakening is common in early pregnancy. Breast engorgement, which many women are aware of in the luteal phase, continues and becomes exaggerated in early pregnancy.

Signs of Pregnancy

The signs of pregnancy may be divided into presumptive, probable, and positive.

Presumptive Signs. The presumptive signs are primarily those associated with skin and mucous membrane changes. Discoloration and cyanosis of the vulva, vagina, and cervix are related to the generalized engorgement of the pelvic organs and are, therefore, nonspecific. The dark discoloration of the vulva and vaginal walls is known as Chadwick's sign. Pigmentation of the skin and abdominal striae are nonspecific and unreliable signs. The most common sites for pigmentation are the midline of the lower abdomen and over the bridge of the nose and under the eyes. The former is called the linea nigra, while the latter is called chloasma or the mask of pregnancy. Chloasma is also a fairly uncommon side effect of oral contraceptives.

Probable Signs. The probable signs of pregnancy are those mainly related to the detectable physical changes in the uterus. During early pregnancy, the uterus changes its size, shape, and consistency. Early uterine enlargement tends to be in the anteroposterior diameter so that the uterus becomes globular. Uterine consistency becomes softer, and it may not be possible to palpate the connection between the cervix and fundus. This change is referred to as Hegar's sign. The cervix also begins to soften early in pregnancy. Later, ballottement of the fetus or a fetal part and mapping of a fetal outline by palpation are also probable signs of pregnancy. Finally, the palpatory presence of uterine contractions is a probable sign of pregnancy, although other causes of uterine enlargement can result in uterine contractions.

Positive Signs. The positive signs of pregnancy include the detection of a fetal heart beat and the recognition of fetal movements. Modern Doppler techniques for detecting the fetal heart beat may be successful as early as 10 weeks and are nearly always positive by 12 weeks. Fetal heart tones can usually be detected with a stethoscope between 16 and 20 weeks. The multiparous woman generally recognizes fetal movements between 15 and 17 weeks, whereas the primigravida usually does not recognize fetal movements until 18 to 20 weeks. An experienced observer may palpate fetal movements with increasing reliability after 20 to 24 weeks.

Laboratory Tests for Pregnancy

Pregnancy Tests. Tests to detect pregnancy have revolutionized early diagnosis. Although they are considered a probable sign of pregnancy, the accuracy of these tests is good. All commonly used methods depend on the detection of chorionic gonadotropin or its beta subunit. Depending on the specific sensitivity of the test, pregnancy may be suspected even prior to a missed period. The available tests and their sensitivities are discussed in Chapter 39.

Diagnostic Ultrasonography. The imaging technique of ultrasonography has made a significant contribution to the diagnosis and evaluation of pregnancy. Using real-time ultrasonography, an intrauterine gestational sac can be identified at 5 weeks (twenty-first postovulatory day) and a fetal image can be detected by 6 to 7 weeks. A beating heart is noted at 8 weeks. Radiographic imaging depends on detection of the fetal skeleton, which is usually not seen until 16 weeks.

GYNECOLOGIC HISTORY

A full history is equally as important in evaluating the gynecologic patient as in evaluating a patient in general medicine or surgery. The history taking must be systematic to avoid omissions, and it should be conducted with sensitivity and without haste.

Following the introductory amenities, recording the referral source, age, place of birth, education, and present occupation conveniently sets the tone for a friendly and nonadversarial interview.

Present Illness

The patient is asked to state her main complaint and to relate her present illness sequentially in her own words. Pertinent negative information should be recorded, and, as far as possible, questions should be reserved until after the patient has described the course of her illness. Generally, the history provides substantial clues to the diagnosis, so it is important to evaluate fully the more common symptoms encountered in gynecologic patients.

Abnormal Vaginal Bleeding. Vaginal bleeding before the age of 9 and after the age of 52 is cause for concern and requires investigation. These are the limits of normal menstruation, and although the occasional woman may menstruate regularly and normally up to the age of 57 or 58 years, it is important to ensure that she is not bleeding from uterine cancer or from exogenous estrogens. Prolongation of menses beyond 7 days or bleeding between menses, except for a brief *kleine regnung* at ovulation, may connote abnormal ovarian function, uterine myomata, or endometriosis.

Abdominal Pain. Many gynecologic problems are associated with abdominal pain. The common gynecologic causes of acute lower abdominal pain are salpingo-oophoritis with peritoneal inflammation, torsion and infarction of an ovarian cyst, or rupture of an ectopic pregnancy. Patterns of pain radiation should be recorded and may provide an important diagnostic clue. Chronic lower abdominal pain is generally associated with endometriosis, chronic pelvic inflammatory disease, or large pelvic tumors.

Amenorrhea. The most common causes of amenorrhea are pregnancy and the normal menopause. It is abnormal for a young woman to reach the age of 17 without menstruating (primary amenorrhea). Pregnancy should be suspected in a woman between 15 and 45 years of age who fails to menstruate within 35 days from the first day of her last menstruation. In a patient with amenorrhea who is not pregnant, enquiry should be made about menopausal or climacteric symptoms such as hot flashes, vaginal dryness, or depression.

Other Symptoms. Other pertinent symptoms of concern in a gynecologic patient's present illness include dysmenorrhea, premenstrual tension, fluid retention, leukorrhea, constipation, dyschezia, dyspareunia, and abdominal distention. Lower back and sacral pain may indicate uterine prolapse, enterocele, or rectocele.

Menstrual History

The menstrual history should include the age at menarche (average is 12 to 13 years), interval between periods (21 to 35 days with a median of 28 days), duration of menses (average is 5 days), and character of the flow (scant, normal, heavy, with or without clots). Any intermenstrual bleeding (metrorrhagia) should be noted. The date of onset of the LMP, and the date of the previous menstrual period (PMP), should be recorded. Inquiry should be made regarding menstrual cramps (dysmenorrhea); if present, the age of onset, severity, and character of the cramps should be recorded, together with an estimate of the disability incurred. Midcycle pain (*mittelschmerz*) and a midcycle increase in vaginal secretions are indicative of ovulatory cycles. In postmenopausal patients, inquiry should be made regarding age at the time of cessation of menses.

Contraceptive History

The type and duration of each contraceptive method must be recorded, along with any attendant complications. These may include amenorrhea or thromboembolic disease with oral contraceptives; dysmenorrhea, heavy bleeding (menorrhagia), or pelvic infection with the intrauterine device; or contraceptive failure with the diaphragm.

Obstetric History

Each pregnancy, delivery, and any associated complications are listed.

Marital History

The date and duration of each marriage should be recorded, along with the purported reason for termination. The health and relationship of the husband or consort(s) may provide insight into the present complaints. Enquiry should be made regarding any pain (dyspareunia), bleeding, or dysuria associated with sexual intercourse. Sexual satisfaction must be tactfully evaluated.

Past History

As in the obstetric history, any significant past medical or surgical history should be recorded, as should the patient's family history. A list of medications used (estrogens, diuretics) is important.

Systemic Review

A review of all other organ systems should be undertaken. Habits (tobacco, alcohol, drug abuse), medications, usual weight with recent changes, and loss of height (osteoporosis) are important parts of the system review.

GYNECOLOGIC PHYSICAL EXAMINATION

General Physical Examination

A complete physical examination must be performed on each new patient and repeated at least annually. The initial examination should include the patient's height, weight, and arm span (in adolescent patients or those with endocrine problems) and should be carried out with the patient completely disrobed but suitably draped. The examination should be systematic and should include the points that follow.

Vital Signs. Temperature, pulse rate, respiratory rate, and blood pressure should be recorded.

General Appearance. The patient's body build, posture, state of nutrition, demeanor, and state of well-being should be recorded. A well-described general appearance should allow the patient to be identified on the ward after the description in the chart has been read.

Head and Neck. The evaluation should include the ears, throat, tonsils, cervical lymph nodes, thyroid gland, and fundi. Evidence of supraclavicular lymphadenopathy, oral lesions, webbing of the neck, or goiter may be pertinent to the gynecologic assessment.

Breasts. The breast examination, discussed in Chapter 41, is particularly important in gynecologic patients.

Heart and Lungs. A complete examination of the heart and lungs is of importance, particularly in a patient requiring surgery. The presence of a pleural effusion may be indicative of a disseminated malignancy, particularly ovarian cancer.

Abdomen. Examination of the abdomen is critical in the evaluation of the gynecologic patient. The contour, whether flat, scaphoid, or protuberant, should be noted. The latter appearance may suggest ascites. The presence and distribution of hair, especially in the area of the escutcheon, should be recorded, as should the presence of striae or operative scars.

Abdominal tenderness must be determined by placing one hand flat against the abdomen in the nonpainful areas initially, then gently and gradually exerting pressure with the fingers of the other hand (Fig. 2–1). Rebound tenderness (a sign of peritoneal irritation), muscle guarding, and abdominal rigidity should be gently elicited, again first in the nontender areas. A "doughy" abdomen, in which the guarding increases gradually as the pressure of palpation is increased, is often seen with a hemoperitoneum.

It is important to palpate any abdominal mass. The size should be specifically noted. Other characteristics may be even more important, however, in suggesting the diagnosis, such as whether the mass is cystic or solid, smooth or nodular, or fixed or mobile, and whether it is associated with ascites. In determining the reason for abdominal distention (tumor, ascites, or distended bowel), it is important to percuss carefully the areas of tympany (gaseous distention) and dullness. A large tumor is generally dull on top with loops of bowel displaced to the flanks. Dullness that shifts as the patient turns onto her side (shifting dullness) is suggestive of ascites.

The presence and character of the peristaltic waves are important. High-pitched, tinkling bowel sounds suggest the recent onset of a bowel obstruction, whereas the absence of peristalsis may connote ileus, peritonitis, or a long-standing bowel obstruction.

Back. Abnormal curvature of the vertebral column (dorsal kyphosis or scoliosis) is an important observation in evaluating osteoporosis in a postmenopausal woman. Costovertebral angle tenderness suggests pyelonephritis, whereas psoas muscle spasm may occur with gynecologic infections. A sciatic radiation of pain may suggest orthopedic problems or a recurrent pelvic malignancy impinging on the sciatic nerve.

Extremities. The presence or absence of varicosities, edema, pedal pulsations, and cu-

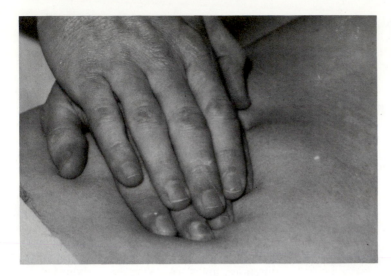

Figure 2–1. Palpation of the abdomen by placing the left palm flat against the abdominal wall and then gently exerting pressure with the fingers of the right hand.

taneous lesions is important in evaluating and managing the gynecologic patient.

Pelvic Examination

In a gynecologic patient, pelvic examination may represent the most important part of the assessment. It must be conducted systematically and with careful sensitivity, especially if it is the patient's first such examination. The procedure should be unhurried, performed with smooth and gentle movements, and accompanied by reasonable explanations.

Vulva. The character and distribution of hair, the degree of development or atrophy of the labia, and the character of the hymen (imperforate or cribriform) and introitus (virginal, nulliparous, or multiparous) should be noted. Any clitoromegaly should be noted, as should cysts, tumors, or inflammation of Bartholin's gland. The urethra and Skene's glands should be inspected for any purulent exudates. The labia should be inspected for any inflammatory, dystrophic, or neoplastic lesions, as described in Chapters 31 and 56. Perineal relaxation and scarring should be noted because they may cause dyspareunia and defects in rectal sphincter tone.

Speculum Examination. The vagina and cervix are inspected with an appropriately sized bivalve speculum (Fig. 2–2), which should be warmed and lubricated with warm water only so as not to interfere with the examination of cervical cytology or any vaginal exudate (see Chapter 35). After gently spreading the labia to expose the introitus, the speculum should be inserted with the blades entering the introitus transversely then directed posteriorly in the axis of the vagina with pressure exerted against the relatively insensitive perineum to avoid contacting the sensitive urethra. As the anterior blade reaches the cervix, the speculum is opened to bring the cervix into view. As the vaginal epithelium is inspected, it is important to rotate the speculum through 90 degrees, so that lesions on the anterior or posterior walls of the vagina ordinarily covered by the blades of the speculum will not be overlooked. Vaginal wall relaxation should be evaluated using either a Sims' speculum or the posterior blade of a bivalve speculum (see Chapter 37). The patient is asked to bear down (Valsalva's maneuver) or to cough to demonstrate any stress incontinence. If the patient's complaint involves urinary stress or urgency, this portion of the examination should be carried out before emptying the bladder.

The cervix should be inspected to determine its size, shape, and color. The nulliparous patient generally has a conical, unscarred cervix with a circular, centrally placed os; the multiparous cervix is generally bulbous with a transverse configuration of the os (Fig. 2–3). Any purulent cervical discharge should be cultured. Plugged, distended cervical glands (nabothian follicles) may be seen on the ectocervix. In premenopausal women,

Figure 2–2. *A,* Pediatric speculum; *B,* Pederson speculum; and *C,* Graves speculum. The Pederson speculum is narrower and more appropriate for examining a nulliparous patient.

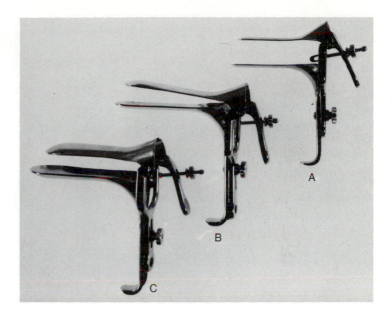

the squamocolumnar junction of the cervix is usually visible around the cervical os, particularly in patients of low parity. Postmenopausally, the junction is invariably retracted within the endocervical canal. A cervical cytologic smear (Papanicolaou) should be taken before the speculum is withdrawn. The exocervix is gently scraped with a wooden spatulum and the endocervix sampled with a cytobrush.

Bimanual Examination. The bimanual pelvic examination provides information about the uterus and adnexa (fallopian tubes and ovaries). During this portion of the examination, the urinary bladder should be emptied;

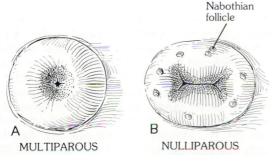

MULTIPAROUS   NULLIPAROUS

Figure 2–3. Cervix of a nulliparous patient (*A*) and cervix of a multiparous patient (*B*). Note the circular os in the nulliparous cervix and the transverse os, owing to lacerations at childbirth, in the multiparous cervix.

if it is not, the internal genitalia will be difficult to delineate, and the procedure is more apt to be uncomfortable for the patient. Occasionally, because of pain-evoked guarding, the bimanual examination must be carried out under anesthesia. The labia are separated, and the gloved, lubricated index finger is inserted into the vagina, avoiding the sensitive urethral meatus. Pressure is exerted posteriorly against the perineum and puborectalis muscle, which causes the introitus to gape somewhat, thereby allowing the middle finger to be inserted as well. Intromission of the two fingers into the depth of the vagina may be facilitated by having the patient bear down slightly.

The cervix is palpated for consistency, contour, size, and tenderness to motion. If the vaginal fornices are absent, as may occur in postmenopausal women, it is not possible to appreciate the size of the cervix on bimanual examination. This can be determined only on rectovaginal or rectal examination.

The uterus is evaluated by placing the abdominal hand flat on the abdomen with the fingers pressing gently just above the symphysis pubis. With the vaginal fingers supinated in either the anterior or the posterior vaginal fornix, the uterine corpus is pressed gently against the abdominal hand (Fig. 2–4). As the uterus is felt between the examining fingers of both hands, the size, configura-

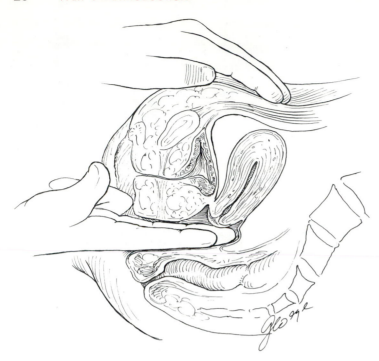

Figure 2–4. Bimanual evaluation of the uterus by gently pressing the uterus with the vaginal fingers against the abdominal hand.

tion, consistency, and mobility of the organ are appreciated. If the muscles of the abdominal wall are not compliant or if the uterus is retroverted, the outline, consistency, and mobility must be determined by ballottement with the vaginal fingers in the fornices; in these circumstances, however, it is impossible to discern uterine size accurately.

By shifting the abdominal hand to either side of the midline and gently elevating the lateral fornix up to the abdominal hand, it may be possible to outline an adnexal mass (Fig. 2–5). The left adnexa are best appreciated with the fingers of the left hand in the vagina (Fig. 2–6). The examiner should stand sideways, facing the patient's left, with the left hip maintaining pressure against the left elbow, thereby providing better tactile sensation because of the relaxed musculature in the forearm and examining hand. The pouch of Douglas is also carefully assessed for nodularity or tenderness, as may occur with endometriosis, pelvic inflammatory disease, or metastatic carcinoma.

It is usually impossible to feel the normal tube, and conditions must be optimal to appreciate the normal ovary. The ovary has the size and consistency of a shelled oyster and may be felt with the vaginal fingers as they are passed across the undersurface of the abdominal hand. The ovaries are very tender to compression, and the patient is uncomfortably aware of any ovarian compression or movement during the examination.

It may be impossible to differentiate between an ovarian or tubal mass or even a lateral uterine mass. Generally, left adnexal masses are more difficult to evaluate than those on the right because of the position of the sigmoid colon on the left side of the pelvis.

Rectal Examination

The anus should be inspected for lesions, hemorrhoids, or inflammation. Rectal sphincter tone should be recorded and any mucosal lesions noted. A guaiac test should be performed to determine the presence of occult blood. Colorectal cancer is the third most common cancer among women in the United States, and a baseline barium enema, colonoscopy, or both should be considered at age 50, particularly if there are any significant risk factors.

A rectovaginal examination is helpful in evaluating masses in the cul-de-sac, the rectovaginal septum, or adnexa. It is essential in evaluating the parametrium in patients with

Figure 2–5. Bimanual examination of the right adnexa.

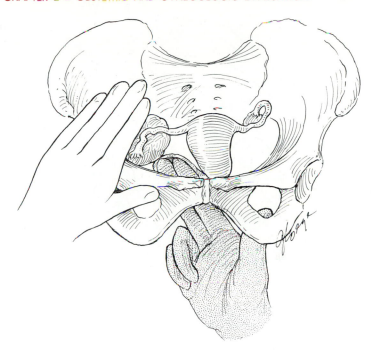

cervical cancer (Fig. 2–7). Following hysterectomy or in postmenopausal patients with obliteration of the vaginal fornices, rectal examination is very helpful in evaluating the adnexa. Rectal examination may also be essential in differentiating between a rectocele and an enterocele. The rectovaginal bimanual examination may be necessary in a virginal or nulliparous patient in whom two fingers cannot be accommodated adequately in the vagina. In an infant or child, the bimanual evaluation is done with the rectal finger

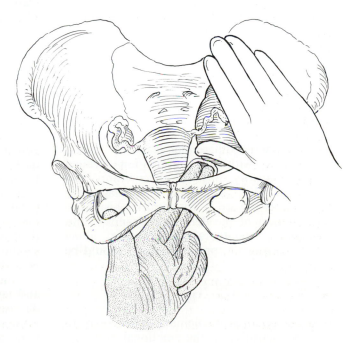

Figure 2–6. Bimanual examination of the left adnexa. Note that the fingers of the hand are in the vagina.

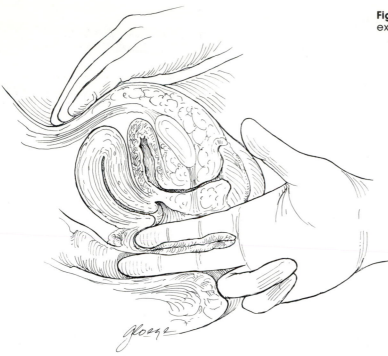

Figure 2–7. Rectovaginal bimanual examination.

pressed against the suprapubic fingers, under anesthesia if necessary.

Laboratory Evaluation

Following the history and physical examination, appropriate laboratory tests should be ordered. Tests normally include a urinalysis, complete blood count, erythrocyte sedimentation rate, and blood chemistry. Special tests, such as tumor markers and hormone assays, are obtained when indicated.

Assessment

A reasonable differential diagnosis should be possible with the information gleaned from the history, physical examination, and laboratory tests. The plan of management should aim toward a chemical or histologic confirmation of the definitive diagnosis, and the appropriate therapeutic options, along with the rationale for each option, should be recorded.

APPROACH TO THE PATIENT

In few areas of medicine is it necessary to be more sensitive to the emotional and psychological needs of the patient than in the fields of obstetrics and gynecology. By their very nature, the history and physical examination may cause embarrassment to some patients. The members of the medical care team are individually and collectively responsible for ensuring that each patient's privacy and modesty are respected while providing the highest level of medical care. This objective is particularly challenging, but not impossible, on a teaching service.

The clinician should strive to meet the highest expectations of the patients in dress, manner, and attitude. While a casual and familiar approach may be acceptable to many younger patients, it may offend others and be quite inappropriate for many older patients. Different circumstances with the same patient may dictate different levels of formality. Cleanliness and good grooming are mandatory when dealing with patients in the outpatient or hospital setting. The manner of dress should avoid extremes and should at all times be neat and clean.

Patients should be addressed courteously and respectfully. Great care must be taken in discussing medical conditions, since the discussions are easily misinterpreted by the patient, and the emotional impact can be devastating. A bedside discussion with the patient must be carried out with more care and sensitivity than coffee room repartee with medical colleagues. Medical slang must be avoided. No matter how trivial the problem, it is important to the patient, and there is no place for a casual approach or frivolous attitude on the part of the physician.

Entrance to the patient's room should be announced by a knock and spoken identification. An appropriate salutation using the patient's surname and a personal introduction with the stated reason for the visit are minimal requirements before any questions are asked or an examination is begun. It is advisable that the general physical and pelvic examinations be carried out in the presence of a chaperone.

OBSTETRIC STATISTICS

Vital statistics are provided by the National Center for Health Statistics. Despite the approximate 3-year delay in compiling yearly birth and death reports, the statistics facilitate an understanding of the impact of human reproduction on a population.

Births

The *birth rate* is the number of live births per 1000 population. It is a reasonable index of the need for obstetric services. During 1988, 3,913,000 live births were registered in the United States. This figure represents a 5 per cent increase over the 3,680,537 registered in 1982. The birth rate was 6.4 live births per 1000 population in 1988.

The *fertility rate* is the number of live births per 1000 females in the population between the ages of 15 and 44 years. The fertility rate of 67.3 in 1988 was higher than in previous years, and the largest increase occurred in women in their late thirties and early forties. This trend continues the generally observed pattern of the last decade, that is, the shift in childbearing to women in somewhat older age groups. In contrast, the number of deliveries by teenagers has decreased. Over the years, the *sex ratio* at birth has varied very little with 1051 to 1055 male births per 1000 female births.

Table 2–1. UNITED STATES MATERNAL DEATHS 1979–1986

TIME OF DEATH	PER CENT
After live birth	51.6
With ectopic pregnancy	13.0
After stillbirth	9.9
With abortion	4.7
Undelivered	5.5
After hydatidiform mole	0.5
Unknown	14.8

From Atrash HK, Koonin LM, Lawson HW, et al.: Maternal mortality in the United States, 1979–1986. Obstet Gynecol 76:1055, 1990.

Maternal Mortality

A *maternal death* is the death of any woman from any cause whatsoever while she is pregnant or within 90 days of the termination of her pregnancy. The *maternal mortality rate* is the number of maternal deaths per 100,000 live births. The maternal mortality rate has decreased dramatically over the past 50 years. In 1940, the rate was 376, and this dropped to 83.3 in 1950, 37 in 1960, and 9 in 1980. The provisional figure for 1989 is 6.5 per 100,000 live births.

In 1988, 330 women were reported as dying from the complications of pregnancy and childbirth. More than half of maternal deaths occurred after live births as opposed to 9.9 per cent after stillbirths and 13 per cent after ectopic pregnancies (Table 2–1). In 1988, the rate for blacks was 3.3 times that for whites, and it was higher in all age groups (Fig. 2–8). The maternal mortality rate increases with age and is highest for women over 40 years of age. Unmarried white women have 2.7 times the rate for married white women, whereas the age-adjusted maternal mortality rate for unmarried black women is only 1.2 times that for married black women. The maternal mortality is higher for primigravidas and decreases with increasing live birth order. Figure 2–9 indicates that pulmonary embolism, pregnancy-induced hypertension, and hemorrhage have remained the predominant causes of maternal mortality over the past decade. These causes as listed are a bit misleading because the serious threats of congenital cardiac

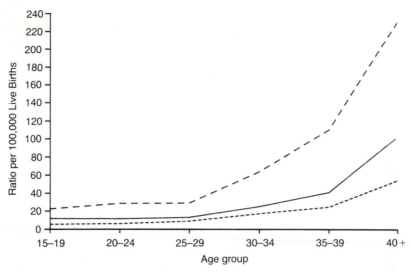

Figure 2–8. Maternal mortality rates by age and race, 1980 through 1985. From the Maternal Mortality Collaborative. (Dashed line = black and other, solid line = total, and dotted line = white.) (From Rochat RW, Koonin LN, Atrash HK, et al: Maternal mortality in the US: Report of the Maternal Mortality Collaborative. Obstet Gynecol 72:91, 1988. Reprinted with permission from The American College of Obstetricians and Gynecologists.)

anomalies, pulmonary hypertension (Eisenmenger's syndrome), and systemic lupus are not emphasized.

The *reproductive mortality rate* is a more expanded figure and represents the deaths per 100,000 women aged 15 to 44 years from pregnancy-related and contraception-related causes. This rate is slightly over one per 100,000.

Infant Mortality

In 1988, there were 38,910 deaths of infants under 1 year of age. The infant mortality rate of 10 infant deaths per 1000 live births was the lowest ever recorded in the United States. The rate was 8.5 for white infants and 17.6 for blacks. The neonatal death rate (under 28 days) was 6.3 per 1000 live births. It is perhaps significant that among the Hispanic populations (Mexican, Puerto Rican, and Cuban) the infant mortality is less than that of the non-Hispanic white population. As expected, the infant mortality in 1988 was higher for males than for females (19:16).

The *perinatal mortality rate* is the number of stillbirths and neonatal deaths per 1000 live births. As with maternal mortality, the perinatal mortality rate has dropped dramatically over the past 30 years from 39.7 per 1000 live births in 1950 to 14.7 per 1000 live births in 1985. The drop in mortality has been most dramatic in the past 15 years, the result, it is thought, of improvements in social services, obstetric care, and neonatal intensive care. The major cause of perinatal mortality is prematurity, and improvements in prenatal care are progressively reducing the incidence of this occurrence.

GLOSSARY

The following section is a listing of some frequently used terms in obstetrics.

Gravidity. The total number of pregnancies in a given patient.

Parity. The number of pregnancies a patient has carried to viability (20 weeks or more). It should be noted that both gravidity and parity refer to the number of *pregnancies*, not fetuses or infants delivered. A multiple gestation is counted as one pregnancy. Therefore, a woman who is currently pregnant and has had one previous singleton pregnancy and one previous twin gestation would be G_3P_2. A woman who is currently pregnant and has had one abortion and one ectopic pregnancy would be G_3P_0.

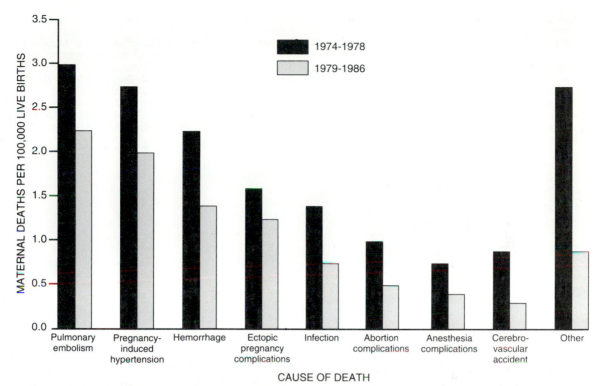

Figure 2–9. Cause-specific maternal mortality ratios in the United States, 1974–1978 (after Kaunitz et al, 1985) and 1979–1986 (after Atrash et al, 1990).
   Adapted from Kaunitz AM, Hughes JM, Grimes DA, et al: Causes of Maternal mortality in the United States. Obstet Gynecol 65:605, 1985; and Atrash HK, Koonin LM, Lawson HW, et al; Maternal mortality in the United States, 1979–1986. Obstet Gynecol 76:1055, 1990.

A system used to express more information involves including under parity the number of term pregnancies, premature deliveries, abortions, and living children. Using this system, a woman who is G_5P_{2112} would be currently pregnant for the fifth time, and have had two term pregnancies, one premature delivery, and one abortion. She would currently have two living children.

Term Delivery. Delivery of an infant after 37 weeks of gestation (252 days after conception). Deliveries occurring after 42 weeks are post-term or postdate deliveries.

Premature delivery. Delivery of an infant weighing between 500 and 2500 gm after 20 weeks and prior to 37 weeks gestation.

Abortus. Fetus or embryo weighing less than 500 gm delivered before 20 weeks gestation. The fetus should not have a crown–rump length of more than 16.5 cm.

Fetal death. Death occurring in utero at or before birth and after 20 weeks gestation. It is synonymous with stillbirth.

Neonatal death. An infant death occurring after delivery and prior to 29 days of age. (An early neonatal death occurs before 7 days; a late neonatal death occurs between 7 and 29 days).

Perinatal death. Fetal or infant death occurring after 20 weeks gestation and before 29 neonatal days.

Fetal death (stillbirth) rate. The number of fetal deaths per 1000 births.

Neonatal death rate. The number of neonatal deaths per 1000 live births.

Infant death rate. The number of infant deaths per 1000 live births up to the first year of life.

SUGGESTED READING

Atrash HK, Koonin LM, Lawson HW, et al: Maternal mortality in the United States, 1979–1986. Obstet Gynecol 76:1055, 1990.

Guidelines for Perinatal Care. Elk Grove Village, IL, American Academy of Pediatrics, and Washington, DC, American College of Obstetricians and Gynecologists, 1983.

Kaunitz AM, Hughes JM, Grimes DA, et al: Causes of maternal mortality in the United States. Obstet Gynecol 65:605, 1985.

National Center for Health Statistics: Monthly Vital Statistics Report: Advance Report of Final Mortality Statistics, 1990, Vol 39, No 7 (suppl), November 28, 1990.

O'Sullivan JB, Mahan CM, Charles D, Dandrow RV: Screening criteria for high-risk gestational dia-betic patients. Am J Obstet Gynecol 116:895, 1973.

Rochat RW, Koonin LN, Atrash HK, et al: Maternal mortality in the US: Report of the Maternal Mortality Collaborative. Obstet Gynecol 72:91, 1988.

Rosenberg MJ, Rosenthal SM: Reproductive mortality in US: Recent trends and methodologic considerations. Am J Public Health 77:833, 1987.

Sachs BP, Layde PM, Rubin GL, et al: Reproductive mortality in the United States. JAMA 247(20):2789, 1982.

Three

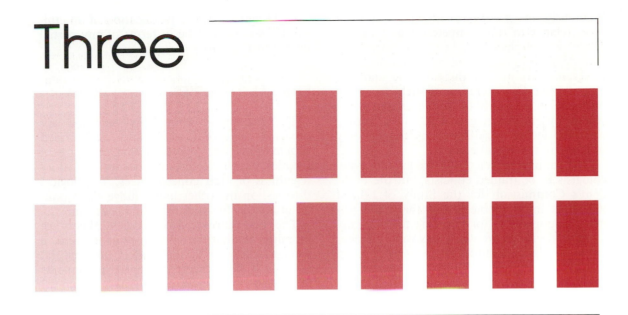

An Approach to Ethical Decision Making in Obstetrics and Gynecology

DONALD E. MARSDEN

Science and technology have greatly increased the range and effectiveness of possible medical interventions. As skills and knowledge grow, so does our responsibility to reflect on how and when advances should be used and in whose interests. New technologies are generally expensive, making demands on the public purse greater, thereby raising the issues of who should have access to which facilities and services and who should pay for them. As the world becomes "smaller," questions relating to the inequality of resources in different countries assume greater importance, as do cultural differences in moral standards.

Ethical considerations affect all branches of medicine, but obstetrics and gynecology has many high-profile areas widely discussed in the community at large. Such areas include in vitro fertilization and the related techniques, abortion, the use of aborted tissue for research or treatment, surrogacy, contraception for minors, sterilization of the mentally handicapped, and many other issues. Feminists raise issues regarding the rights of women to control their social and biological destinies in accordance with their own principles and question the whole structure of medical ethics.

These highly publicized areas of concern notwithstanding, most of the ethical problems in the practice of medicine come up in cases in which the medical condition or desired procedure itself presents no moral problem.

Previously, the main areas of ethical concern have related to the competence and beneficence of the physician, but they now must include patient goals, values, ambitions, and preferences as well as those of the community at large. Consideration of such issues can only enrich the study of obstetrics and gynecology by emphasizing that scientific knowledge and technical skills are meaningful only in a social and moral context.

One cannot expect obstetricians and gynecologists to be trained ethicists, but the President's Commission for the Study of Ethical Problems in Medicine stated that "the primary responsibility for ensuring that morally justified decisions are made lies with the physician." Many institutions are setting up committees to help with the more difficult decisions, but all medical practitioners must understand the principles of ethical decision making.

WHAT IS ETHICS?

The term *ethics* is derived from an ancient Greek word meaning "pertaining to custom or habit." *Morality* was the Latin equivalent. In general parlance, morality often refers to concepts of right and wrong, and ethics or moral philosophy to the systematic study of moral behavior. Socrates described moral philosophy as the discussion of "how we ought to live," and all humans have concepts of how they ought to live, based on their life experiences and personal beliefs. These values form the basis for their everyday decision making. The study of moral philosophy makes this process more rational and consistent, but there are many situations in which the carefully developed personal beliefs of the parties involved are in conflict, and a formalized process is demanded. To help this process, Rachels defined a minimum conception of morality:

. . . morality is, at the very least, the effort to guide one's conduct by reason—that is to do what there are the best reasons for doing—while giving equal weight to the interests of each individual who will be affected by one's conduct.

If ethical decision making is feasible and decisions justifiable, a degree of universality must be possible. All schools of ethical thought agree that the justification of an ethical decision cannot be in terms of any partial or sectional group.

ETHICAL THEORIES

The two most commonly accepted approaches to moral philosophy are termed *deontological* and *teleological*. Deontological theories state that certain acts are obligatory regardless of their consequences. Teleological theories, on the other hand, judge the morality of actions by their nonmoral outcome.

The best known deontological theory of morality is that based on religion, and a similar approach is that based on "natural law." One of the most influential proponents of the deontological view was Immanuel Kant, who aimed to demonstrate that moral laws exist that are as rigorously logical as the laws of science and are capable of universal application. He believed human reason was autonomous and capable of formulating such laws and was the supreme principle of morality. He asserted that one must never use another human being as a means to one's own ends. Kant's final formulation was the so-called categorical imperative that states: "Act only on the maxim through which you can at the same time will that it should become universal law."

The most common teleological theory is utilitarianism, which is generally considered to have two forms. *Act utilitarianism* is the belief that a person ought to act in a particular situation in the way that produces the greatest balance of good over evil for everyone concerned. *Rule utilitarianism* has as its principle that one ought to act according to the rule that, if generally followed, would produce the greatest balance of good over evil, everyone considered. Although the differences and relative merits of these two forms of utilitarianism have been debated, both depend on the concepts of good and evil and our ability to calculate the balance of each.

Ross recognized that neither Kantian deontology nor classic utilitarianism provided solutions when faced with the conflict of apparently equally pressing duties. He proposed a series of prima facie duties, derived not from a single principle such as that of utility or the categorical imperative, but from the many morally significant relationships in which we are all involved. These relationships are those such as husband and wife, debtor and creditor, student and teacher, parent and child, citizen and state, and so on. When prima facie duties conflict, the best that can be expected is that one should make a reflective, considered decision as to which of the competing duties has priority. Ross identified seven prima facie duties: fidelity, reparation, gratitude, beneficence, nonmaleficence, justice, and self-improvement, each derived from relationships of undoubted moral significance. This approach, developed to respond to the promptings of "ordinary moral consciousness," has an immediate intuitive appeal, but it does not really address the issue of deciding between prima facie duties of apparently equal importance: In such cases, one must presumably use either deontological or teleological reasoning.

None of these moral theories are without problems in certain situations. It is not possible in the scope of this chapter to explore any one of them in detail. A number of excellent texts that do so, however, are listed in the Suggested Reading.

ETHICAL PRINCIPLES AND RELATED CONCEPTS

Although there is considerable debate about the theoretical basis of morality, in the day-to-day consideration of ethical dilemmas, a number of principles and the concepts derived from them are commonly accepted and taken into account.

Autonomy

The right of individuals to self-determination is a basic concept of biomedical ethics and is supported by proponents of both the deontological and the utilitarian schools of thought, although for slightly different reasons. To exercise autonomy, an individual must be capable of effective deliberation and be neither coerced into a particular course of action nor limited in choices by external constraints. Being capable of effective delib-

eration implies not only a certain level of intellectual capacity, but also the ability to exercise that capacity. Strong emotions such as fear or grief, physical conditions such as tiredness or illness, and medications such as tranquilizers or opiates may limit this ability, as may ignorance. Social, economic, or geographic factors may limit autonomy by reducing the range of options available.

Although autonomy is considered a basic moral principle, there are many situations in which it is thought reasonable to limit its exercise. It is generally considered permissible to restrict autonomy to prevent harm to others, to prevent offense to others, or to prevent a person from harming himself or acting immorally. Most would accept limiting autonomy to prevent murder, rape, or theft, but to what extent it should be constrained to prevent offense to others is more problematic.

The exercise of autonomy may put considerable strain on those providing health care, as in the case of a woman with a ruptured ectopic pregnancy who refuses a life-saving blood transfusion for religious reasons and dies despite the best efforts of the medical team. A more complex question was raised when a court ordered that a cesarean section be performed on a dying woman, against her expressed wishes, in what proved to be a futile attempt to save her 26-week fetus. Whether the decision was legally justifiable or not, the morality of the act must be subject to considerable debate.

Nonmaleficence

The injunction "first, do no harm" has been included in codes of medical ethics from ancient times. Although few would dispute the basic concept, in our day-to-day medical practice we accept the infliction of varying degrees of harm to achieve a desired outcome. For example, we are not prevented from performing a life-saving operation by the fact that it will inevitably result in some pain and a degree of disability. Although radical hysterectomy and lymphadenectomy are associated with significant morbidity and some risk of mortality, all would consider that the risks and consequences of the operation are more than outweighed by the potential benefits in properly selected patients.

Beneficence

It is a very ancient belief that we have a duty to promote the welfare of others when in a position to do so, and the duties of beneficence and nonmaleficence were both part of the Hippocratic Oath. Although it is clear that both principles are linked, many would see that of nonmaleficence as the more pressing responsibility and beneficence as an ideal rather than a duty. A wealthy person could save many starving people in a Third World country by giving half his or her income in aid, but few would consider the person morally bound to do so. A physician prevented by conscience from participating in an abortion would generally be expected to provide life-saving care for a woman suffering complications following such a procedure.

Paternalism

There are situations in which some health care professionals and administrators believe that personal autonomy may be legitimately curtailed in the best interests of the individual. Medical paternalism implies that the physician knows best what is in the patient's interests, making the duty of beneficence on the part of the physician more pressing than that of preserving the autonomy of the patient. When one may legitimately intervene to prevent others from following a course of action believed to be detrimental to their well-being is a major issue in medical ethics. Paternalism has long been accepted as a reasonable approach to medical decision making and has been a normal part of the physician's role for centuries. Feinberg, however, distinguishes "weak paternalism," applied in situations in which there is legitimate doubt as to whether the true autonomy of the patient is being hampered by such factors as disease, mental incompetence, or inappropriate information, from "strong paternalism," in which liberty is being limited, even though the person has made an informed, voluntary choice. Obviously, the practice of weak paternalism is easier to justify.

Justice

The principle of justice relates to the way in which the benefits and burdens of society are distributed. The general principle that equals should be treated equally was espoused by Aristotle and is widely accepted today, but it does require that one can define what are relevant differences between individuals and groups. Some believe all rational persons to have equal rights; others emphasize need, effort, contribution, and merit; while still others seek criteria that maximize both individual and social utility. In most Western societies, considerations such as race, sex, and religion are not considered morally legitimate criteria for the distribution of benefits, although they too may be taken into account to right what are perceived to be historical wrongs in programs of reverse discrimination. When there is a scarcity of resources, issues of justice become even more acute because there are often competing claims from parties who appear equal by all relevant criteria, and the selection criteria themselves become a moral issue.

An example is the United States Supreme Court ruling in *Rust v. Sullivan,* which bans discussion of abortion in federally funded health clinics and may, to quote *Time* magazine, lead to "the further exaggeration of a two-tiered health-care system: one that provides affluent women with the full range of options and offers poor women either skewed information or a range of services severely constrained by funding limitations."

Informed Consent

The concept of informed consent is derived from respect for the autonomy of the patient, and there is general agreement that consent must be genuinely voluntary. Varying degrees of paternalism are inevitably involved in determining those risks or complications that are of sufficient magnitude to warrant disclosure. There is a natural desire to avoid unnecessary stress for the patient, and the competence of the patient to comprehend what is being disclosed must also be taken into account. Variations of emphasis in explanation can easily be coercive. This is an area in which legal and ethical requirements interface and sometimes appear to be in conflict, but as the President's Commission stated, it is essentially an ethical imperative. It depends on mutual respect and participation, and it is essential that the physician recognize the right of the patient to reject any or all treatments and that the patient recognize the physician's right to provide services of acceptable standard in accordance with his or her own moral beliefs.

Veracity and Fidelity

The right of the patient to complete and honest information about his or her condition is derived from the concept of autonomy. Although some would consider it legitimate to limit the information given in order to "protect" the patient, this type of paternalism would generally be considered to infringe on the rights of the patient. From a practical point of view, a failure of disclosure may well damage the bond of trust that must exist between a physician and a patient if the outcome is to be optimal, and from this perspective, veracity is mandated not only to preserve autonomy but also to promote beneficence. It is common to hear experienced physicians qualifying their support for honesty with riders such as "telling the patient when she asks" or "when she is ready to know," and although the motive for such an approach may be laudable, it may equally be based on less clearly articulated factors such as the reluctance of the physician to discuss such emotive issues or even on occasion a failure to accept the rights of the patient. A common clinical scenario is that of relatives wishing to prevent anxiety and stress for their loved ones by asking the physician to withhold or distort information. For example, it may be suggested that an elderly woman with advanced ovarian cancer not be told the actual diagnosis lest her last days be spoiled by the worry such a revelation would bring.

Fidelity or the obligation to keep promises is different from veracity in that by making a promise, one creates an expectation in another person that the promise will be honored. This obligation is based on a respect for personal autonomy and trust. In undertaking to provide medical care for a patient, a duty of fidelity is created. In its simplest form, this

obligates a physician to provide an appropriate standard of care and withdraw from a case only after giving sufficient notice to the patient to allow an alternative physician to be obtained. Again, the principles of autonomy and beneficence are both involved.

Confidentiality

Confidentiality is a cornerstone of the relationship between physician and patient. This duty arises from considerations of autonomy but also helps promote beneficence, as is the case with honesty. In obstetrics and gynecology, conflicts can arise, as in the case of a woman with a sexually transmitted disease who refuses to have a sexual partner informed or in the case of a school-aged girl seeking contraceptive advice or abortion.

There are many other situations in which conflicting responsibilities make confidentiality a difficult issue. There are many factors to consider, but the position of Beauchamp and Childress is helpful:

Anyone who thinks that a disclosure of confidential information is morally justified or even mandatory in some circumstances bears a burden of proof. While this approach requires balancing various duties, it also establishes a structure of moral reasoning and justification. It is not enough to determine which act will respect the most duties or maximize the good, for the strong presumption against revealing confidences establishes the direction and burden of deliberation and justification.

PHYSICIAN-PATIENT RELATIONSHIP

Veach describes four models for the relationship between physician and patient. In the *engineering* model, the physician is a technician or applied scientist who, after presenting the facts, carries out, without regard for his or her own views or moral scruples, the wishes of the patient. The *priestly* model, based on beneficence and paternalism, places decision making firmly in the hands of the physician. Veach believes this time-honored model of medical practice is inherently wrong in that it equates technical expertise with moral authority, overvalues nonmaleficence, compromises autonomy and dignity, and betrays the duties of veracity and fidelity. The *collegial* model, in which the physician and the patient are equal partners in decision-making processes, interacting in a spirit of trust and confidence, is seen as a "mere pipedream" because of the inevitable conflicts of class as well as economic, educational, ethnic, and social values. The relationship Veach favors is the *contractual* model, in which physician and patient enter a mutually agreed-upon contract to pursue particular goals, recognizing that their interests are not entirely mutual. Under the contract, the patient is justified in believing that the physician will make the day-to-day decisions according to agreed-upon frames of reference. The contract is not static, but recognizes that changes in circumstances inevitably lead to the need for further modifications of the relationship.

MATERNAL-FETAL RELATIONSHIPS

Caring for a pregnant woman is a unique relationship because the management of the mother inevitably affects her baby. Until recently, the only way by which an obstetrician could produce a healthy baby was by maintaining optimal maternal health, but as the fetus becomes more accessible to diagnostic and therapeutic interventions, new problems emerge. Procedures performed on the fetus violate the personal integrity and autonomy of the mother. The obstetrician with a dual responsibility to mother and fetus faces potential conflicts of interest. Provided that clear and accurate information is supplied by appropriate consultants, most conflicts can be resolved owing to the willingness of most women to undergo even considerable self-sacrifice to benefit their fetus. When a woman refuses consent for a procedure that presents her with considerable risk, her autonomy will generally be respected. There may be cases, however, in which a mother refuses an intervention that is likely to be efficacious, carries little risk, and can be expected to prevent substantial harm to the fetus. Such cases have, on occasions, ended in court-ordered intervention. Although many will disagree, Nelson and Milliken, in a carefully reasoned argument, conclude that while the decision to carry a pregnancy confers significant ethical responsibilities on the mother:

. . . we do not believe that this ethical obligation should be legally enforced. The attempt to do so would not itself be ethical, practically effective or advantageous for society or the individual . . . society will, in the end, gain far more by allowing each pregnant woman to live as seems good to her rather than by compelling each to live as seems good to the rest of us.

In surrogacy, a totally different relationship exists between the mother, her fetus, and third parties. The pregnant woman has no intention of keeping the child, and others have a strong vested interest in the "quality" of what may easily be seen as a "product." The mother may be under threat of liability for damages if the baby is harmed as a result of her actions, or she may be forced to behave in a way prescribed by contract. Legal questions aside, the ethical implications of these relationships are immense.

RELATIONSHIPS WITH OTHER HEALTH PROFESSIONALS

Modern medical practice inevitably involves more people in the provision of health care. Traditionally, the physician has been the final arbitrator and decision maker, but this has often imposed extreme strain on other health care providers. Rejection of the "Nuremberg defense" of obedience to the orders of a superior and increasing recognition of professional rights has led to a situation in which all those involved in health care claim a right to participate in decision making. Physicians have not been as aware of the sensitivities of the nursing profession as they could have been. For example, the decision, no matter how it is made, either to operate or not to operate on a newborn with severe spina bifida and hydrocephalus inevitably leaves nurses with a range of responsibilities to the infant, the parents, and the physician that may be in direct conflict with their own personal values. They may rightly request to be party to the decision-making process, and although the exact models whereby such a goal may be achieved are debatable, physicians must be aware of the legitimate moral concerns of nurses and other health care providers.

RELATIONSHIPS WITH OTHER PARTIES

Health care takes place in an increasingly complex environment. Hospitals, health insurance companies, and governments all claim an interest in what services are made available or paid for, and this may prevent individual patients from receiving what their physician may consider optimal care. This poses moral problems for physicians on a case-by-case basis but also for society as a whole.

The interface of medicine and the law raises major ethical issues because legality and morality are not always synonymous. In particular, "defensive medicine" forced on physicians by a fear of legal consequences may easily compromise care. Professional liability insurance premiums for obstetricians are testimony to the relevance of legal issues to obstetric practice. As Jennings states, defensive medicine is not necessarily good medicine:

The "strangle-hold" of professional liability is affecting every major decision that is made by the practicing obstetrician and gynecologist and under these conditions, the "tunnel vision" that ensues obscures the ability to clearly see answers to ethical questions.

There is also a growing tendency for others such as "pro life" and civil rights groups to seek to intervene in individual cases in which once the relationship was between those directly involved. The case of Baby Jane Doe in 1983 is one example: Although the baby was born with spina bifida, hydrocephaly, and microencephaly, her parents declined to permit surgery. A lawyer representing right-to-life groups petitioned the New York State Supreme Court to overturn the parents' decision, and his request was granted, only to be reversed on appeal by a higher court that described the first suit as "offensive." The Federal Government then intervened against the parents' decision on the grounds of discrimination against a handicapped child, but that suit too was dismissed.

PROCESS FOR ETHICAL DECISION MAKING

Know Your Own Biases

Before approaching any ethical argument, one must have a clear idea of the personal values and viewpoints one has in this area. This insight is something one gains over time with continuing reflection, reading, and above all debate regarding ethical issues. "Why do I feel this way about this subject?" is a critical question that one must always strive to answer.

Identify Those Legitimately Involved

Although ultimately the mother should make the decisions, we must be aware that many decisions have impact on the ethical concerns of others who also have rights, including the fetus and its father. Consideration should be given to whether the patient is capable of making the necessary decisions. Not every person has the capacity to understand the complex issues involved. This is not the same as to say that the person is incompetent to make a decision. Competence is a legal decision, capacity an educational one. In cases in which the appropriate decision maker is unable, for one reason or another, to make a decision, it is necessary to find a surrogate decision maker. Often in the past, this has been the physician, or a nominee of the physician. Although the physician must certainly be involved in offering advice and assistance, he or she has no innate right to make the decisions. The process can be helped by reference to the patient's expressed views regarding similar situations in the past. The following approach is based on that proposed by the American College of Obstetricians and Gynecologists:

Clarify the Facts and Identify the Options. Many problems are clarified if the facts are clearly defined. Objectivity and the free use of expert consultation are critical to this process. In many situations, the facts are unfortunately disputed. It is usually helpful to identify all major options to ensure that no significant choice remains unconsidered.

Evaluate the Options, Identify Conflicts, and Set Priorities. Once the range of options is placed before the decision makers, one can seek common ground and identify areas of disagreement. It is important that the ethical consequences of the possible actions and their likely outcomes are taken into account. Some options may be immediately excluded, but others may merit further consideration and modification. The principles underlying each option should be considered and an attempt made to rate their relative importance to the decision maker. Those who have read and reflected on ethical matters may frequently be helped by reference to similar cases.

Find the Most Justifiable Options. The ultimate goal is to arrive at a rational resolution of the problem that is justifiable in terms of recognized ethical principles. Such an end can usually be achieved if free and open communication based on the best facts available has been used throughout, with a sincere desire to resolve the conflict. The physician can facilitate this process by a calm, unbiased, and understanding attitude that respects the hopes, fears, and uncertainties of the patient. Jennings sums up this process admirably:

It is important to take the time to listen to the patients' complaints, evaluate their priorities, show respect for their opinions and then finally give advice . . . human beings . . . are endowed with the ability to interpret sincerity from others and in most patients this is acutely sensitized. There is no substitute for honesty and integrity. . . . It is from the strength of the doctor-patient relationship that the solutions to our most difficult ethical questions come.

Re-evaluate the Decision After It Is Acted On. This is a crucial point, as one must constantly seek a deeper understanding of ethical matters if one is to improve one's skills in this area.

CONCLUSIONS

All branches of medicine, but especially obstetrics and gynecology, will face an increasing number of ethical problems in the future, and it is essential that we prepare ourselves to deal with them, partly because, as Park says, "it is the ethics of our practice that transform us from mere dispensers of health care to the caring and responsive physicians to whom patients come with confidence and trust," and partly because if we do not respond to this challenge, other less qualified elements of our society will respond for us, to the detriment of both physicians and patients.

SUGGESTED READING

American Academy of Pediatrics Committee on Bioethics: Fetal therapy: Ethical considerations. Pediatrics 81:898, 1988.

American College of Obstetricians and Gynecologists: Ethical decision making in obstetrics and gynecology. ACOG Technical Bulletin 136, November, 1989.

American College of Obstetricians and Gynecologists: Patient choice: Maternal-fetal conflict. Washington, DC, ACOG Committee Opinion 55, 1987.

Beauchamp TL, Childress JF: Principles of Biomedical Ethics. 3rd ed. New York, Oxford University Press, 1989.

Beauchamp TL, Walters L: Contemporary Issues in Bioethics. 3rd ed. Belmont, CA, Wadsworth Publishing, 1989.

Callahan D: Modernizing mortality: Medical progress and the good society. Hastings Center Report, p 28, January/February, 1990.

Edwards RB, Graber GC: Bio-Ethics. New York, Harcourt Brace Jovanovich, 1988.

Jennings JC: Ethics in obstetrics and gynecology: A practitioner's review and opinion. Obstet Gynecol Surv 44:656, 1989.

Mappes TA, Zembaty JS: Biomedical Ethics. 2nd ed. New York, McGraw-Hill, 1986.

Nelson LJ, Milliken N: Compelled medical treatment of pregnant women: Life, liberty and law in conflict. JAMA 259:1060, 1988.

Park RC: Old bedfellows: Ethics and obstetrics and gynecology. Obstet Gynecol 73:1, 1989.

Part 2

Maternal-Fetal Medicine

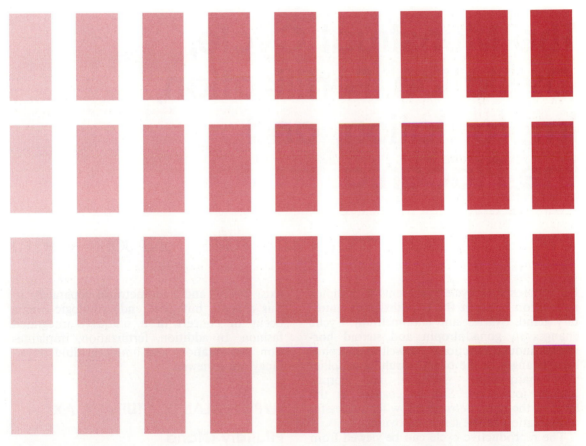

CALVIN J. HOBEL — SUBEDITOR

Four

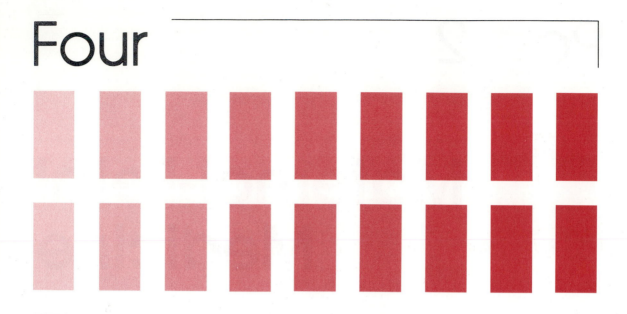

The Menstrual Cycle, Ovulation, Fertilization, Implantation, and the Placenta

PAUL J. TOOT, ERIC S. SURREY, and JOHN K. H. LU

Each menstrual cycle represents a complex interaction between the hypothalamus, pituitary gland, ovaries, and endometrium. Cyclic changes in gonadotropin and steroid hormones induce functional as well as morphologic changes in the ovary, resulting in follicular maturation, ovulation, and corpus luteum formation. Similar changes at the level of the endometrium allow for successful implantation of the fertilized ovum.

The reproductive cycle can be viewed from the perspectives of each of the aforementioned organ systems. We approach the cyclic changes within the hypothalamic-pituitary axis, ovary, and endometrium separately in this chapter, but these endocrinologic events occur in concert in a uniquely integrated fashion. In addition, fertilization, implantation, placentation, and amniotic fluid physiology are reviewed.

HYPOTHALAMIC-PITUITARY AXIS

Pituitary Gland

The pituitary gland lies below the hypothalamus at the base of the brain within a

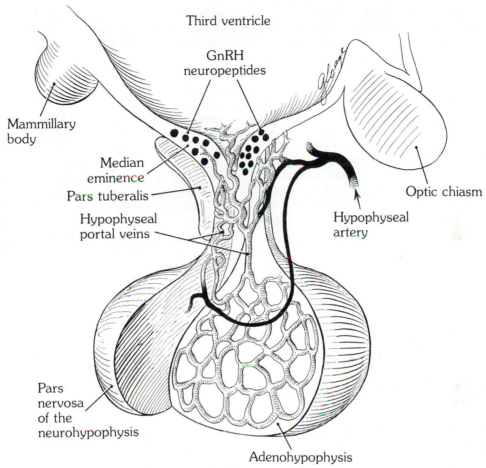

Figure 4-1. Pituitary and hypothalamus.

bony cavity (sella turcica) and is separated from the cranial cavity by a condensation of dura mater overlying the sella turcica (diaphragma sellae). The pituitary gland is divided into two major portions (Fig. 4-1). The neurohypophysis, consisting of the posterior lobe (pars nervosa) and the neural stalk (infundibulum), is derived from neural tissue and is in direct continuity with the hypothalamus and central nervous system. The adenohypophysis, consisting of the pars distalis (anterior lobe), pars intermedia (intermediate lobe), and pars tuberalis, which surrounds the neural stalk, is derived from ectoderm.

The arterial blood supply to the neural stalk (hypophyseal-pituitary portal system) represents a major avenue of transport for hypothalamic secretions to the anterior pituitary.

The neurohypophysis serves primarily to transport oxytoxcin and vasopressin (antidiuretic hormone) along neuronal projections from the supraoptic and paraventricular nuclei of the hypothalamus to their release into the circulation.

The anterior pituitary contains different cell types that produce six protein hormones: follicle-stimulating hormone (FSH), luteinizing hormone (LH), thyroid-stimulating hormone (TSH), prolactin, growth hormone (GH), and adrenocorticotropic hormone (ACTH).

The gonadotropins, FSH and LH, are synthesized and stored in cells called gonadotrophs, whereas TSH is produced by thyrotrophs. FSH, LH, and TSH are glycoproteins, consisting of alpha and beta subunits. The alpha subunits of FSH, LH, and TSH are identical. The same alpha subunit is also present in human chorionic gonadotropin (hCG). The beta subunits are individual for each hormone. The half-life for circulating LH is about 30 minutes, while that of FSH is several hours. The difference in half-life may account for the differential secretion patterns of these two gonadotropins.

Prolactin is secreted by lactotrophs. Unlike the case with other peptide hormones produced by the adenohypophysis, pituitary release of prolactin is under chronic inhibition by the hypothalamus. The half-life for circulating prolactin is about 20 to 30 minutes. In addition to its lactogenic effect, prolactin may directly or indirectly influence hypothalamic, pituitary, and ovarian functions in relation to the ovulatory cycle, particularly in the pathologic state of chronic hyperprolactinemia (see Chapter 48).

Gonadotropin Secretory Patterns

A normal ovulatory cycle can be divided into a follicular and a luteal phase (Fig. 4–2). The follicular phase begins with the onset of menses and culminates in the preovulatory surge of LH. The luteal phase begins with the onset of the preovulatory LH surge and ends with the first day of menses.

Decreasing levels of estradiol and progesterone from the regressing corpus luteum of the preceding cycle initiate a rise in FSH, which stimulates follicular growth and estradiol secretion. LH levels begin to increase in a slow fashion several days after FSH. As ovarian estradiol levels begin to rise, a negative feedback mechanism is initiated that enhances gonadotropin secretion, culminating in a surge of LH and FSH, with ovulation occurring 30 to 38 hours after the onset of this midcycle LH surge.

During the luteal phase, both LH and FSH are significantly suppressed through the negative feedback effect of elevated circulating estradiol and progesterone levels. This inhibition persists until progesterone and estradiol levels decline near the end of the luteal phase as a result of corpus luteal regression should pregnancy fail to occur. The net effect is a rise in serum FSH, which initiates follicular growth for the subsequent cycle. The dura-

tion of the corpus luteum's functional regression is such that menstruation generally occurs 14 days after the LH surge.

Hypothalamus

Five different small peptides or biogenic amines that affect the reproductive cycle have been isolated from the hypothalamus. All exert specific effects on the hormonal secretion of the anterior pituitary gland. They are gonadotropin-releasing hormone (GnRH), thyrotropin-releasing hormone (TRH), somatotropin release–inhibiting factor (SRIF) or somatostatin, corticotropin-releasing factor (CRF), and prolactin release–inhibiting factor (PIF). Only GnRH and PIF are discussed here.

GnRH is a decapeptide, synthesized primarily in the arcuate nucleus, that is responsible for the synthesis and release of both LH and FSH. Because it usually causes the release of more LH than FSH, it is commonly called LH-releasing hormone (LH-RH) or LH-releasing factor (LRF). Both FSH and LH appear to be present in two different forms within the pituitary gonadotrophs. One is a releasable form and the other a storage form. GnRH reaches the anterior pituitary via the hypophyseal portal vessels and stimulates the synthesis of both FSH and LH, which are stored within gonadotrophs. Subsequently, GnRH activates and transforms these molecules into releasable forms. GnRH can also induce immediate release of both LH and FSH into the circulation.

GnRH is secreted in a pulsatile fashion throughout the menstrual cycle. The frequency and amplitude of these pulses vary through each phase of the menstrual cycle. The frequency of GnRH release, as assessed indirectly by measurement of LH pulses, varies from approximately every 90 minutes in the early follicular phase to every 60 to 70 minutes in the immediate preovulatory period. During the luteal phase, pulse frequency decreases while pulse amplitude increases. A considerable variation among individuals has been identified.

Administration of exogenous pulsatile GnRH has been used to induce ovulation in selected women who are anovulatory as a result of hypothalamic amenorrhea. It is in-

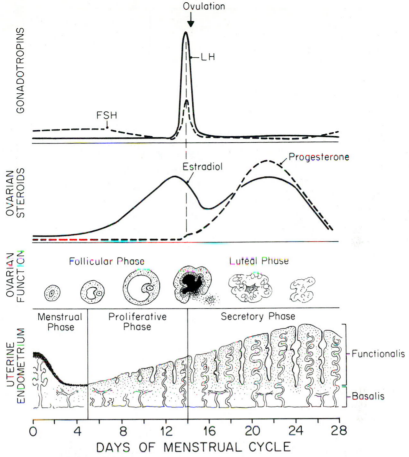

Figure 4–2. Hormone levels during a normal menstrual cycle.

teresting to note that continuous infusion of GnRH results in a reversible inhibition of gonadotropin secretion through a process of "down-regulation" or desensitization of pituitary gonadotrophs (Fig. 4–3). This represents the basic mechanism of action for the new GnRH agonists that have been successfully used in the therapy of such ovarian hormone-dependent disorders as endometriosis, leiomyomata, hirsutism, and precocious puberty.

Several mechanisms control the secretion of GnRH. Estradiol appears to enhance hypothalamic release of GnRH and may help induce the midcycle LH surge by increasing GnRH release or by enhancing pituitary responsiveness to the decapeptide. Gonadotropins have an inhibitory effect on GnRH release. Catecholamines may play a major regulatory role as well. Dopamine is synthe-

sized in the arcuate and periventricular nuclei and may have a direct effect on GnRH secretion via the tuberoinfundibular tract that projects onto the median eminence. Serotonin also appears to inhibit, whereas norepinephrine stimulates, GnRH pulsatile release. Endogenous opioids suppress release of GnRH from the hypothalamus in a manner that may be partially regulated by ovarian steroids.

The hypothalamus produces PIF, which exerts chronic inhibition of prolactin release from the lactotrophs. A number of pharmacologic agents (e.g., chlorpromazine [Thorazine]) that affect dopaminergic mechanisms influence prolactin release. Dopamine itself is secreted by hypothalamic neurons into the hypophyseal portal vessels and inhibits prolactin release directly within the adenohypophysis. Based on these observations, it has

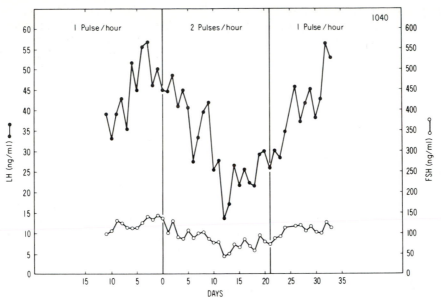

Figure 4–3. Gonadotropin secretion in a rhesus monkey with a lesion at the level of the arcuate nucleus. Pulsatile administration of GnRH results in normal gonadotropin release. Continuous GnRH administration inhibits this release in a reversible manner once GnRH pulses were resumed. (From Knobil E: The neuroendocrine control of the menstrual cycle. Recent Prog Horm Res 36:77, 1980.)

been proposed that hypothalamic dopamine may be the PIF. In addition to the regulation of prolactin release by PIF, the hypothalamus may also produce prolactin-releasing factors (PRF) that can elicit large and rapid increases in prolactin release under different conditions, such as breast stimulation during nursing. Neither PIF nor PRF has been well characterized biochemically. TRH serves to stimulate prolactin release as well. This phenomenon explains the association between primary hypothyroidism (with secondary TRH elevation) and hyperprolactinemia. The precursor protein for GnRH (GAP) has been identified to be both a potent inhibitor of prolactin secretion and a stimulator of gonadotropin release. These findings suggest that this GnRH-associated peptide may be the physiologic PIF and could explain the inverse relationship between gonadotropin and prolactin secretion seen in many reproductive states.

OVARIAN CYCLE

Estrogens

During early follicular development, circulating estradiol levels are relatively low.

About 1 week before ovulation, levels begin to increase, at first slowly, then rapidly. The levels generally reach a maximum 1 day before the LH peak. After this peak and before ovulation, there is a marked and precipitous fall. During the luteal phase, estradiol rises to a maximum 5 to 7 days after ovulation and returns to baseline shortly before menstruation. Estrone secretion by the ovary is considerably less than that of estradiol, but follows a similar pattern. Most of the estrone is derived from the conversion of androstenedione through the action of the enzyme aromatase (aromatization).

Progestins

During follicular development, the ovary secretes only very small amounts of progesterone and 17-hydroxyprogesterone. The bulk of the progesterone comes from the peripheral conversion of adrenal pregnenolone and pregnenolone sulfate. Just before ovulation, the unruptured but luteinizing graafian follicle begins to produce increasing amounts of progesterone. At about this time, there is also a marked increase in 17-hydroxyprogesterone. The elevation of basal body temperature is temporally related to the central effect of progesterone. As with estradiol, secretion of progestins by the corpus luteum reaches a maximum 5 to 7 days after ovulation and returns to baseline shortly before menstruation.

Androgens

Both the ovary and the adrenals secrete small amounts of testosterone, but most of the testosterone is derived from the metabolism of androstenedione, which is also secreted by both the ovary and the adrenal gland. Near midcycle, there is an increase in plasma androstenedione, reflecting enhanced secretion from the follicle. During the luteal phase, there is a second rise in androstenedione, reflecting enhanced secretion by the corpus luteum. The adrenal gland also secretes androstenedione in a diurnal pattern similar to that of cortisol. The ovary secretes small amounts of dihydrotestosterone (DHT), but the bulk of DHT is derived from the conversion of androstenedione and testosterone. The majority of both dehydroepiandrosterone (DHEA) and DHEA sulfate (DHEA-S) is secreted by the adrenal glands, although small amounts of DHEA are secreted by the ovary.

Serum-Binding Proteins

Circulating estrogens and androgens are mostly bound to specific sex hormone–binding globulins (SHBG) or to serum albumin. The remaining fraction of sex hormones is unbound (free), and this is the biologically active fraction. It is unclear whether steroids bound to serum proteins are accessible for tissue uptake and utilization. The synthesis of SHBG in the liver is increased by estrogens and thyroid hormones but decreased by testosterone.

Prolactin

Serum prolactin levels do not change strikingly during the normal menstrual cycle. Both the serum level of prolactin as well as prolactin release in response to TRH, however, are somewhat more elevated during the luteal phase than during the midfollicular phase of the cycle. This suggests that high amounts of circulating estradiol and progesterone may enhance prolactin release. Prolactin release does exhibit a diurnal pattern, with the highest levels occurring during nocturnal sleep.

Prolactin may participate in the control of ovarian steroidogenesis. Prolactin concentrations in follicular fluid change markedly during follicular growth. The highest prolactin concentrations are seen in small follicles during the early follicular phase. Prolactin concentrations in the follicular fluid may be inversely related to the production of progesterone. In addition, hyperprolactinemia may alter gonadotropin secretion. Despite these observations, the physiologic significance of prolactin during the normal menstrual cycle has not been established.

Follicular Development

Primordial follicles undergo sequential development, differentiation, and maturation until a mature graafian follicle is produced. The follicle then ruptures, releasing the ovum. Subsequent luteinization of the ruptured follicle produces the corpus luteum.

At approximately 8 to 10 weeks of fetal development, oocytes become progressively surrounded by precursor granulosa cells, which then separate themselves from the underlying stroma and oocyte by a basal lamina. This oocyte is called a primordial follicle. In response to gonadotropin and ovarian steroids, the follicular cells become cuboidal and the stromal cells around the follicle become prominent. This process, which takes place between 20 and 24 weeks of gestation, results in a primary follicle. As granulosa cells proliferate, a clear gelatinous material surrounds the ovum, forming the zona pellucida. This larger unit is called a secondary follicle.

In the adult ovary, a graafian follicle forms as the innermost three or four layers of rapidly multiplying granulosa cells become cuboidal and adherent to the ovum (cumulus oophorus). In addition, a fluid-filled antrum forms among the granulosa cells. As the liquor continues to accumulate, the antrum enlarges and the centrally located primary oocyte migrates eccentrically to the wall of the follicle. The granulosa cells of the cumulus oophorus, which are in close contact with the zona pellucida, become elongated and form the corona radiata. The corona radiata is shed with the oocyte at ovulation. Surrounding the granulosa cells is a thin basement membrane. Outside this membrane the connective tissue cells organize themselves into two coats: the theca interna and externa.

During each cycle, a cohort of follicles is selected for development. Among these many developing follicles, usually only one continues its differentiation and maturation into a graafian follicle that ovulates. The remaining follicles undergo atresia. On the basis of antral fluid steroid levels, growing follicles can be identified as either estrogen-predominant or androgen-predominant. Follicles greater than 8 mm in diameter are usually estrogen-predominant, whereas smaller follicles are usually androgen-predominant. Mature preovulatory follicles reach mean diameters of approximately 18 to 25 mm. Furthermore, in larger estrogen-predominant follicles, antral fluid FSH concentrations continue to rise while blood FSH levels are declining. In contrast, in smaller androgen-predominant follicles, antral fluid FSH values decrease while blood FSH levels decline; thus, the intrafollicular steroid milieu appears to play an important role in determining whether a follicle undergoes maturation or atresia.

Follicular maturation is dependent on the sequential development of receptors for FSH, estradiol, and LH. FSH receptors are present in granulosa cells. Under FSH stimulation, the granulosa cells proliferate and the number of FSH receptors per follicle increases markedly. Thus, the growing primary follicle becomes increasingly more sensitive to stimulation by FSH and, as a result, estradiol levels increase. Estrogens, particularly estradiol, enhance the induction of FSH receptors and act synergistically with FSH to increase LH receptors.

During early stages of folliculogenesis, LH receptors are present only on theca interna cells. LH stimulation induces steroidogenesis and increases the synthesis of androgens by these cells. In nondominant follicles, high local androgen levels may enhance follicular atresia. However, in that follicle destined to achieve ovulation, FSH induces aromatase enzyme receptor formation within the granu-

losa cells. As a result, androgens produced in the theca interna of the dominant follicle diffuse into the granulosa cells and are aromatized into estrogens. FSH also enhances the induction of LH receptors on the granulosa cells of the follicle that is destined to ovulate. These are essential for the appropriate response to the LH surge, leading to the final stages of maturation, ovulation, and the luteal phase production of progesterone. Thus, the presence of greater numbers of FSH receptors and granulosa cells and increased induction of aromatase enzyme and its receptors may differentiate between the follicle of the initial cohort that will develop normally and those that will undergo atresia.

Growth factors such as insulin, insulin-like growth factor I (IFGI), fibroblast growth factor (FGF), and epidermal growth factor (EGF) may also play significant mitogenic roles in folliculogenesis.

Ovulation

During the late follicular phase, the maturing follicle secretes large amounts of estrogen, and the rapidly increasing blood estradiol levels stimulate the hypothalamus and the pituitary to initiate both the LH and FSH midcycle surges. The preovulatory LH surge initiates a sequence of structural and biochemical changes that culminate in ovulation. Before ovulation, there are general dissolution of the entire follicular wall and localized disintegration of that portion of the wall that is on the surface of the ovary, both presumably caused by proteolytic enzymes. With degeneration of the cells on the surface, a stigma forms, and the follicular basement membrane finally bulges through the stigma. When this ruptures, the oocyte and corona radiata are expelled into the peritoneal cavity, and ovulation occurs.

Ovulation is now known from ultrasonic studies to be a gradual phenomenon, with the collapse of the follicle taking from several minutes to as long as an hour or more. The oocyte adheres to the surface of the ovary, allowing an extended period during which the muscular contractions of the tube may bring it in contact with the tubal epithelium. Probably both muscular contractions and tubal ciliary movement contribute to the transportation of the oocyte into and along the tube. Ciliary activity is not essential since at least some women with immotile cilia become pregnant.

At birth, primary oocytes are in the prophase of the first meiotic division. They continue in this phase until the next maturation division occurs in conjunction with ovulation. A few hours preceding ovulation, the chromatin is resolved into distinct chromosomes, and meiotic division takes place with unequal distribution of the cytoplasm to form a secondary oocyte and the first polar body. Each element contains 23 chromosomes, each in the form of two monads. The second maturation spindle forms immediately and remains at the surface. No further development takes place until after ovulation and fertilization have occurred. At that time, and before the union of the male and female pronuclei, another division occurs to reduce the chromosomal component of the egg pronucleus to 23 single chromosomes (22 plus X), each composed of one monad. The ovum and a second polar body are thus formed. The first polar body may also divide.

Luteinization and Corpus Luteum Function

After ovulation and under the influence of LH, the granulosa cells of the ruptured follicle undergo luteinization. These luteinized granulosa cells, plus the surrounding theca cells, capillaries, and connective tissue, form the corpus luteum, which produces copious amounts of progesterone and some estradiol. The normal functional life span of the corpus luteum is about 14 days. After this time, it regresses, and unless pregnancy occurs, menstruation ensues and the corpus luteum is gradually replaced by an avascular scar called a corpus albicans. The events occurring in the ovary during a complete cycle are shown in Figure 4–4.

HISTOPHYSIOLOGY OF THE ENDOMETRIUM

The endometrium is uniquely responsive to the circulating progestins, androgens, and es-

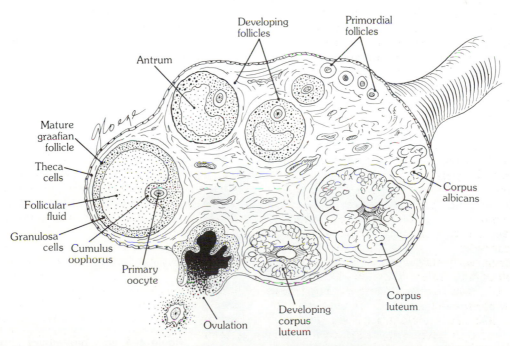

Figure 4–4. Schematic representation of the sequence of events occurring in the ovary during a complete follicular cycle. (Adapted from Yen SC, Jaffe R (eds): Reproductive Endocrinology. Philadelphia, WB Saunders, 1978, p 64.)

trogens. It is this responsiveness that gives rise to menstruation and makes implantation and pregnancy possible.

Functionally, the endometrium is divided into two zones: (1) the upper portion, or *functionalis,* that undergoes cyclic changes in morphology and function during the menstrual cycle and is sloughed off at menstruation; (2) the lower portion, or *basalis,* that remains relatively unchanged during each menstrual cycle and, after menstruation, provides stem cells for the renewal of the functionalis. Basal arteries are regular blood vessels found in the basalis, whereas spiral arteries are specially coiled blood vessels seen in the functionalis.

The cyclic changes in histophysiology of the endometrium can be divided into three stages: the menstrual phase, the proliferative or estrogenic phase, and the secretory or progestational phase.

Menstrual Phase

Because it is the only portion of the cycle that is visible externally, the first day of menstruation is taken as day one of the menstrual cycle. The first four days of the cycle are defined as the menstrual phase. During this phase, there is disruption and disintegration of the endometrial glands and stroma, leukocyte infiltration, and red blood cell extravasation. In addition to this slough-

ing of the functionalis, there is a compression of the basalis due to the loss of ground substances. In spite of these degenerative changes, early evidence of renewed tissue growth is usually present at this time within the basalis of the endometrium.

Proliferative Phase

The proliferative phase is characterized by endometrial proliferation or growth secondary to estrogen stimulation. Because the bases of the endometrial glands lie deep within the basalis, these epithelial cells are not destroyed during menstruation. As menstruation ends each month, they provide the source of stem cells that divide and migrate through the stroma to form a new epithelial lining of the endometrium and new endometrial glands.

During this phase of the cycle, the large increase in estrogen secretion causes marked cellular proliferation of the epithelial lining, the endometrial glands, and the connective tissues of the stroma (Fig. 4–5). Numerous mitoses are present in these tissues. There is an increase in the length of the spiral arteries, which traverse almost the entire thickness of the endometrium. By the end of the proliferative phase, cellular proliferation and endometrial growth have reached a maximum, the spiral arteries are elongated and convoluted, and the endometrial glands are straight, with narrow lumens containing some glycogen.

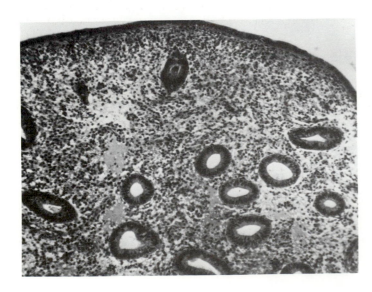

Figure 4–5. Early proliferative phase endometrium. Note the regular, tubular glands lined by pseudostratified columnar cells.

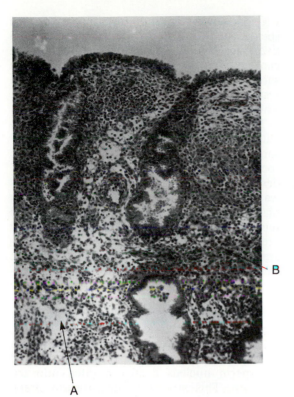

Figure 4-6. Late secretory phase endometrium. Note the tortuous, saw-toothed appearance of the endometrial glands with secretions in the lumen. Edema is seen on the left (*A*) and decidua (*B*) on the right.

True secretory function in the glands must await progesterone secretion by the corpus luteum.

Secretory Phase

Following ovulation, progesterone secretion by the corpus luteum stimulates the glandular cells to secrete glycogen, mucus, and other substances. The glands become tortuous, and the lumens are dilated and filled with the secretion. The stroma becomes edematous. Mitoses are rare. The spiral arteries continue to extend into the superficial layer of the endometrium and become convoluted (Fig. 4-6).

The marked changes that occur in endometrial histology during the secretory phase permit relatively precise timing (dating) of secretory endometrium.

If pregnancy does not occur by day 23, the corpus luteum begins to regress, secretion of progesterone and estradiol declines, and the endometrium undergoes involution. About one day prior to the onset of menstruation, there is marked constriction of the spiral arterioles causing ischemia of the endometrium followed by leukocyte infiltration and red blood cell extravasation. It is postulated that this occurs secondary to prostaglandins produced by the endometrium. The resulting necrosis causes menstruation or sloughing of the endometrium. Thus, menstruation, which clinically marks the beginning of the menstrual cycle, is actually the terminal event that enables the uterus to prepare itself to receive another conceptus.

SPERMATOGENESIS, SPERM CAPACITATION, AND FERTILIZATION

Fertilization, or conception, is the union of male and female pronuclear elements. Conception takes place in the fallopian tube, after which the fertilized ovum continues to the uterus where implantation occurs and development begins.

Spermatogenesis requires about 74 days. Together with transportation, a total of about 3 months elapses before sperm are ejaculated. The sperm achieve motility during their transport through the epididymis, but sperm capacitation, which renders them capable of fertilization, does not occur until they are removed from the seminal plasma after ejaculation.

Estrogen levels are high at the time of ovulation, resulting in an increased amount, decreased viscosity, and changed electrolyte content of the cervical mucus. These are the most favorable characteristics for sperm penetration. The average ejaculate contains 2 to 5 ml of semen; 200 to 300 million sperm may be deposited in the vagina, 60 to 90 per cent of which are morphologically normal. Fewer than 200 sperm achieve proximity to the egg. Only one sperm fertilizes the single egg released at ovulation.

The major loss of sperm occurs in the vagina following coitus, with expulsion of semen from the introitus playing an important role. In addition, there are digestion of sperm by vaginal enzymes, destruction of some by the vaginal acidity, phagocytosis of sperm along the reproductive tract, and further loss from passage through the fallopian tube into the peritoneal cavity.

Those sperm that do migrate from the alkaline environment of the semen to the alkaline environment of the cervical mucus exuding from the cervical os are directed along channels of lower viscosity mucus into the cervical crypts where they are stored for later ascent. Two waves of passage to the tubes may occur. Uterine contractions, probably facilitated by prostaglandin in the seminal plasma, propel sperm to the tubes within 5 minutes. Some evidence indicates that these sperm may not be as capable of fertilization as those that arrive later largely under their own power. It is of interest, however, that the seminal concentration of prostaglandins has been found to be lower in males of infertile couples. Sperm may be found within the peritoneal cavity for long periods, but it is conjectural whether they are capable of fertilization. Ova are usually fertilized within 12 hours of ovulation.

Capacitation is the physiologic change sperm must undergo in the female reproductive tract before fertilization. Human sperm can acquire the ability to fertilize after a short incubation in defined media without residence in the female reproductive tract. Therefore, in vitro fertilization is possible.

The acrosome reaction is one of the principal components of capacitation. The acrosome, a modified lysosome, lies over the sperm head as a kind of "chemical drill-bit" designed to enable the sperm to burrow its way into the oocyte (Fig. 4–7). The overlying plasma membrane and the outer acrosomal membrane become unstable and eventually break down, releasing hyaluronidase, a neuraminidase, and corona-dispersing enzyme. Acrosin, bound to the remaining inner acrosomal membrane, may play a role in the final penetration of the zona pellucida. The latter contains species-specific receptors for the plasma membrane. After traversing the zona, the postacrosomal region of the sperm head fuses with the oocyte membrane, and the sperm nucleus is incorporated into the ooplasm. This process triggers release of the contents of the cortical granules that lie at

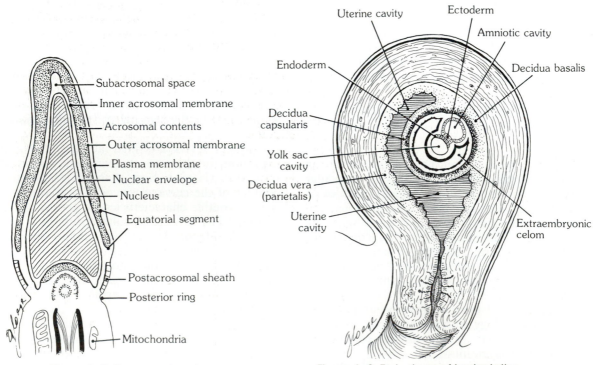

Figure 4–7. The sperm head.

Figure 4–8. Early stage of implantation.

the periphery of the oocyte. This cortical reaction results in changes in the oocyte membrane and zona pellucida that prevent the entrance of further sperm into the oocyte.

The process of capacitation may be inhibited by a factor in the semen, thus preserving maximum enzyme release to allow effective penetration of the corona and zona pellucida surrounding the oocyte. The cellular investments of the oocyte may further activate the sperm, thus facilitating penetration to the oocyte membrane. The corona is not required for normal fertilization to occur, since its removal has no effect on the rate or quality of fertilization in vitro. The major function of these surrounding granulosa cells and their intercellular matrix may be to serve as a sticky mass that causes adherence to the ovarian surface and the mucosa of the tubal epithelium.

Following penetration of the oocyte, the sperm nucleus decondenses to form the male pronucleus, which approaches and finally fuses with the female pronucleus at syngamy to form the zygote. Fertilization restores the diploid number of chromosomes and determines the sex of the zygote.

CLEAVAGE, MORULA, BLASTOCYST

Following fertilization, cleavage occurs. This consists of a rapid succession of mitotic divisions that produce a mulberry-like mass known as a morula. Fluid is secreted by the outer cells of the morula, and a single fluid-filled cavity develops, known as the blastocyst cavity. An inner-cell mass can be defined, attached eccentrically to the outer layer of flattened cells; the latter becomes trophoblast. The embryo at this stage of development is called a blastocyst, and the zona pellucida disappears at about this time.

IMPLANTATION

The fertilized ovum reaches the endometrial cavity about three days after ovulation.

Hormones influence egg transport. Estrogen causes "locking" of the egg in the tube, and progesterone reverses this action. Prostaglandins have diverse effects. Prostaglandin E relaxes the tubal isthmus, whereas prostaglandin F stimulates tubal motility. It is unknown whether abnormalities of egg transport play a role in infertility, but in animal studies, acceleration of ovum transport causes a failure of implantation.

Upon reaching the uterine cavity, the embryo undergoes further development for 2 to 3 days before implanting. The zona is shed, and the blastocyst then adheres to the endometrium, a process probably dependent on changes in the surface characteristics of the embryo, such as electrical charge and glycoprotein content. A variety of proteolytic enzymes may play a role in separating the endometrial cells and digesting the intercellular matrix.

Initially, the wall of the blastocyst facing the uterine lumen consists of a single layer of flattened cells. The thicker opposite wall has two zones: the trophoblast and the inner cell mass (embryonic disc). The latter differentiates at 7.5 days into a thick plate of primitive "dorsal" ectoderm and an underlying layer of "ventral" endoderm. Between the embryonic disc and trophoblast appear small cells that enclose a space that becomes the amniotic cavity.

Under the influence of progesterone, decidual changes occur in the endometrium of the pregnant uterus. The endometrial stromal cells enlarge and form polygonal or round decidual cells. The nuclei become round and vesicular, and the cytoplasm becomes clear, slightly basophilic, and surrounded by a translucent membrane. During pregnancy, the decidua thickens to a depth of 5 to 10 mm. The decidua basalis is the decidua directly beneath the site of implantation. The decidua capsularis is the portion overlying the developing ovum and separating it from the rest of the uterine cavity. The decidua vera (parietalis) is the remaining lining of the uterine cavity (Fig. 4–8). The space between the decidua capsularis and decidua vera is obliterated by the fourth month with fusion of the capsularis and vera.

The decidua basalis enters into the formation of the basal plate of the placenta. The spongy zone of the decidua basalis consists mainly of arteries and dilated veins. The decidua basalis is invaded extensively by trophoblastic giant cells, which first appear as early as the time of implantation. Minute levels of hCG appear in the maternal serum at this time. Nitabuch's layer is a zone of fibrinoid degeneration where the trophoblast meets the decidua. When the decidua is defective, as in placenta accreta, Nitabuch's layer is absent.

When the free blastocyst contacts the endometrium after 4 to 6 days, the syncytiotrophoblast, a syncytium of cells, differentiates from the cytotrophoblast. At about 9 days, lacunae, irregular fluid-filled spaces, appear within the thickened trophoblastic syncytium. This is soon followed by the appearance of maternal blood within the lacunae, as maternal tissue is destroyed and the walls of the mother's capillaries are eroded.

As the blastocyst burrows deeper into the endometrium, the trophoblastic strands branch to form the solid, primitive villi traversing the lacunae. The villi, which are first distinguished about the twelfth day after fertilization, are the essential structures of the definitive placenta. Located originally over the entire surface of the ovum, the villi later disappear except over the most deeply implanted portion, the future placental site.

Embryonic mesenchyme first appears as isolated cells within the cavity of the blastocyst. When the cavity is completely lined with mesoderm, it is termed the *extraembryonic celom.* Its membrane, the chorion, is composed of trophoblast and mesenchyme. When the solid trophoblast is invaded by a mesenchymal core, presumably derived from cytotrophoblast, secondary villi are formed.

Maternal venous sinuses are tapped about 15 days after fertilization. By the seventeenth day, both fetal and maternal blood vessels are functional, and a placental circulation is established. The fetal circulation is completed when the blood vessels of the embryo are connected with chorionic blood vessels that are formed from cytotrophoblast. Proliferation of cellular trophoblasts at the tips of the villi produces cytotrophoblastic columns that progressively extend through the peripheral syncytium. Cytotrophoblastic extensions from columns of adjacent villi join together to form the cytotrophoblastic shell, which attaches the villi to the decidua. By the nineteenth day of development, the cytotrophoblastic shell is thick. Villi contain a central core of chorionic mesoderm, where blood vessels are developing, and an external covering of syncytiotrophoblasts or syncytium.

By 3 weeks, the relationship of the chorion to the decidua is evident. The greater part of the chorion, denuded of villi, is designated the smooth chorion or *chorion laeve.* Until near the end of the third month, the chorion laeve remains separated from the amnion by the extraembryonic celomic cavity. Thereafter, amnion and chorion are in intimate contact. The villi adjacent to the decidua basalis enlarge and branch (chorion frondosum) and progressively assume the form of the fully developed human placenta (Fig. 4-9). By 4.5 months, the chorion laeve contacts and fuses with the decidua vera, thus obliterating most of the uterine cavity.

VARIATIONS IN THE PLACENTA

Placental implantation variations include bipartite or tripartite placentas, in which vessels cross between incompletely divided lobes; duplex or triplex placentas, in which blood vessels do not cross between the completely divided lobes; and placenta succenturiata, in which blood vessels course through the membranes to connect the distant accessory lobe(s) to the main placenta. Eccentric insertion of the umbilical cord results in a battledore placenta, which is of little clinical significance. With velamentous insertion of the cord, blood vessels course unprotected for long distances through the membranes to insert into the margin of the placenta. In both placenta succenturiata and velamentous insertion, the blood vessels course through the membranes and may pass over the internal cervical os, where they are in a position to be compressed by the presenting fetal part or torn at the time of membrane rupture. Either of these events may be a disaster for the fetus.

In placenta circumvallata (Fig. 4-10), there is a large central circular depression on the fetal surface of the placenta surrounded by an elevated ridge. Amnion and chorion are folded back on themselves, forming a double layer of fetal membranes at this site. Developmentally, the regression of villi, which originally surrounded the whole chorion, progresses too far, and the placental plate becomes too small. Secondary proliferation of villi occurs after the membranes are attached to the edge of the original placenta. The incidence of abortion in early pregnancy and bleeding in late pregnancy is somewhat increased with placenta circumvallata.

Figure 4–9. Relationship of the chorion to the placenta.

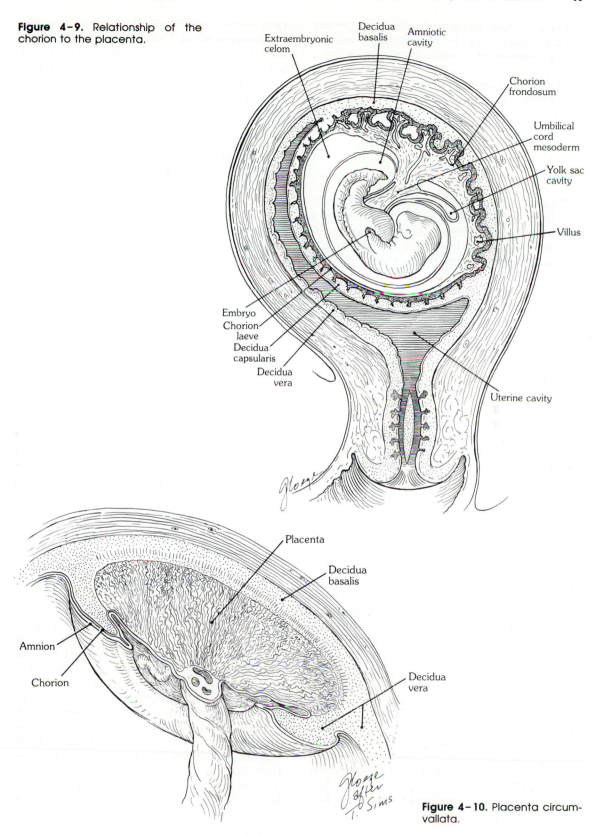

Extraembryonic celom

Decidua basalis

Amniotic cavity

Chorion frondosum

Umbilical cord mesoderm

Yolk sac cavity

Villus

Embryo

Chorion laeve

Decidua capsularis

Decidua vera

Uterine cavity

Placenta

Decidua basalis

Amnion

Chorion

Decidua vera

Figure 4–10. Placenta circumvallata.

Placenta membranacea results from persistence of the villi of the chorion laeve as well as the chorion frondosum, producing a large, thin placenta that entirely surrounds the fetal membranes. Separation and expulsion may be incomplete during the third stage of labor, increasing the incidence of postpartum hemorrhage.

AMNIOTIC FLUID

Throughout normal pregnancy, the amniotic fluid compartment allows the fetus room for growth, movement, and development. Without amniotic fluid, the uterus would contract and compress the fetus. In cases of leakage of amniotic fluid early in the first trimester, the fetus may develop structural abnormalities including facial distortion, limb reduction, and abdominal wall defects secondary to uterine compression.

Toward midpregnancy (20 weeks), the amniotic fluid becomes increasingly important for fetal pulmonary development. The latter requires a fluid-filled respiratory tract and the ability of the fetus to "breathe" in utero, moving amniotic fluid into and out of the lungs. The absence of adequate amniotic fluid during midpregnancy is associated with pulmonary hypoplasia at birth, often incompatible with life.

The amniotic fluid also has a protective role for the fetus. It contains antibacterial activity and acts to inhibit the growth of potentially pathogenic bacteria. During labor and delivery, the amniotic fluid continues to serve as a protective medium for the fetus, aiding dilatation of the cervix. The premature infant, with its fragile head, may benefit most from delivery with the amniotic membranes intact (en caul). In addition, the amniotic fluid may serve as a means of communication for the fetus. Fetal maturity and readiness for delivery may be signaled to the maternal uterus via fetal urinary hormones excreted into the amniotic fluid.

Volume and Composition

Amniotic fluid volume and composition are regulated by a complex system of fluid exchange between maternal and fetal fluid compartments. The amniotic fluid may represent an extension of the fetal extracellular fluid compartment. In the first trimester, the volume of amniotic fluid is minimal (5 to 25 ml), arising from transudation of fetal plasma through the nonkeratinized fetal skin or umbilical cord, or of maternal plasma through the vascularized uterine decidua. This fluid is iso-osmotic with fetal and maternal plasma, although essentially devoid of protein. Beginning in the second trimester, the amniotic fluid becomes a dynamic model of fluid exchange. At term, the human fetus is estimated to excrete 600 to 700 ml of hypotonic urine into the amniotic cavity per day, accounting for the hypo-osmolality of the amniotic fluid. The fetal respiratory tract actively secretes up to 250 ml per day into the amniotic fluid. Fetal swallowing at term removes 500 ml of fluid per day, and the remainder is reabsorbed by a flow of water across the chorioamnion in response to the osmotic gradient created by the hypo-osmotic amniotic fluid and the iso-osmotic maternal plasma. Consequently, the volume of amniotic fluid at term (700 to 1000 ml) is continually exchanged every 24 hours. The amniotic fluid index (AFI) at term is an important determinant of fetal well-being (see Chapter 8).

Abnormalities of the amniotic fluid may occur as a result of changes in fetal renal function, swallowing, lung fluid production, or transchorionic water flow. The fetus may autonomously regulate the fetal sites of amniotic fluid secretion and resorption through hormones including vasopressin, cortisol, and catecholamines.

Oligohydramnios

Oligohydramnios refers to a marked deficiency in the volume of amniotic fluid. A diminished volume of amniotic fluid may produce fetal hypoxia as a result of umbilical cord compression secondary to fetal movements or uterine contractions. Furthermore, the passage of fetal meconium into a reduced volume of amniotic fluid results in a thick, particulate suspension that may cause fetal respiratory compromise.

It is essential to classify oligohydramnios according to its etiology. Oligohydramnios is associated with intrauterine growth retardation in 60 per cent of cases. When associated with ultrasonic evidence of asymmetric growth retardation, fetal compromise is very likely. Those cases secondary to spontaneous rupture of fetal membranes may not be associated with prior fetal distress. Oligohydramnios may occur as a result of fetal stress in utero; the secretion of fetal stress hormones (catecholamines, vasopressin) may inhibit lung fluid resorption via fetal swallowing. Finally, there are cases associated with a variety of fetal malformations, such as Potter's syndrome (renal agenesis), in which detailed ultrasonic and genetic evaluations are necessary.

Polyhydramnios

Polyhydramnios refers to an excessive amount of amniotic fluid, usually exceeding 2 liters. The fluid usually accumulates slowly, although acute hydramnios may occasionally occur, particularly with a twin gestation. The complications of polyhydramnios include an increased risk of premature labor (owing to overdistention of the uterus), maternal respiratory discomfort, umbilical cord prolapse at the time of rupture of the membranes, and fetal malpresentation.

The etiology of polyhydramnios may be discussed in terms of the sites of fluid secretion and resorption. Fetal anomalies in which decreased swallowing or gastrointestinal absorption occurs (e.g., anencephaly, duodenal atresia, tracheoesophageal fistula) are often associated with polyhydramnios. Occasionally, anomalies of the pulmonary system (e.g., cystic adenomatoid malformation of the lung) may be associated with increased fluid production. Abnormalities of transchorionic water flow may result in the accumulation of excess fluid, as sometimes occurs in diabetic pregnancies. In addition, polyhydramnios occurs in most pregnancies marked by immune or nonimmune hydrops. The fetus and placenta become edematous in this condition, as a result of fetal congestive heart failure, hypoproteinemia, or severe anemia. Transudation of placental fluid as well as increased fetal production of fluid may account for the polyhydramnios.

If polyhydramnios is suspected, a definitive diagnosis may be made by ultrasonography. A complete ultrasonic fetal evaluation should be performed to exclude hydrops or malformations. Maternal testing should include screening for diabetes, a Rhesus antibody titer, glucose-6-phosphate dehydrogenase determination, hemoglobin electrophoresis, and viral (TORCH) titers when appropriate.

Although it is possible to drain the excessive amniotic fluid via amniocentesis, the reaccumulation of up to 1 liter per day limits this approach. Beta-agonist tocolytic agents to decrease uterine activity may be of value, and the patient should be advised to rest as much as possible. In the acute form, induction of labor may be necessary to relieve severe maternal distress.

SUGGESTED READING

Benirschke K: The endometrium. In Yen SSC, Jaffe RB (eds): Reproductive Endocrinology. 2nd ed. Philadelphia, WB Saunders, 1986, p 385.

Daughaday WH: The anterior pituitary. In Wilson JD, Foster DW (eds): Williams Textbook of Endocrinology. 7th ed. Philadelphia, WB Saunders, 1985, p 568.

Erikson GF, Garzo VG, Magoffin DA: Insulin-like growth factor (IGF-1) regulates aromatase activity in human granulosa luteal cells. J Clin Endocrinol Metab 69:716, 1989.

Knobil E: The neuroendocrine control of the menstrual cycle. Rec Prog Horm Res 36:53, 1980.

McNatty KP: Cyclic changes in antral fluid hormone concentrations in humans. J Clin Endocrinol Metab 7:577, 1978.

McNatty NP, Makris A, DeGrazier C, et al: The production of progesterone, androgens, and estrogens by granulosa cells, thecal tissue, and stromal tissue from human ovaries in vitro. J Clin Endocrinol Metab 49:678, 1979.

Moore RY: Neuroendocrine mechanisms: Cells and systems. In Yen SSC, Jaffe RB (eds): Reproductive Endocrinology. 2nd ed. Philadelphia, WB Saunders, 1986, p 3.

Pitkin RM: Acute polyhydramnios recurrent in successive pregnancies: Management with multiple amniocenteses. Obstet Gynecol 48(suppl):42s, 1976.

Ross GT, Schreiber JR: The ovary. In Yen SSC, Jaffe RB (eds): Reproductive Endocrinology. 2nd ed. Philadelphia, WB Saunders, 1986, p 119.

Seed AE: Current concepts of amniotic fluid dynamics. Am J Obstet Gynecol 138:575, 1980.

Speroff L, Glass RH, Kase NG: Clinical Gynecologic Endocrinology and Fertility. 4th ed. Baltimore, Williams & Wilkins, 1989.

Yen SSC: The human menstrual cycle. In Yen SSC, Jaffe RB (eds): Reproductive Endocrinology. 2nd ed. Philadelphia, WB Saunders, 1986, p 200.

Five

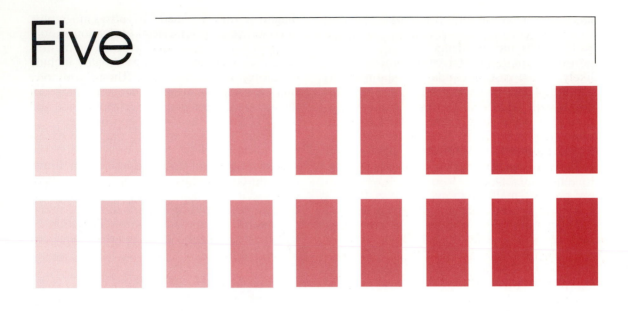

Endocrinology of Pregnancy and Parturition

MARY E. CARSTEN

Women undergo major endocrinologic and metabolic changes in order to establish, maintain, and terminate pregnancy. The aim of these changes is the delivery of an infant that can survive outside the uterus. The maturation of the fetus and the adaptation of the mother are regulated by a variety of hormones. This chapter deals with the properties, functions, and interactions of the most important of these hormones as they relate to pregnancy and parturition.

FETOPLACENTAL UNIT

The concept of the fetoplacental unit is based on observations of interactions of hormones of fetal and maternal origin. The feto-placental unit largely controls the endocrine events of the pregnancy.

Components of the Unit

Although there is input from the fetus, the placenta, and the mother, the fetus appears to play the most active and controlling role in its growth and maturation and probably also in the events that lead to parturition.

Fetal Adrenal Gland. The adrenal gland is the major endocrine component of the fetus. In midpregnancy, it is larger than the fetal kidney. The fetal adrenal cortex consists of an outer, definitive or adult zone and an inner, fetal zone. The definitive zone later develops into the three components of the adult adrenal cortex: the zona fasciculata, the zona glomerulosa, and the zona reticularis. During fetal life, the definitive zone secretes primarily glucocorticoids and mineralocorticoids. The fetal zone, at term, constitutes 80 per cent of the fetal gland and primarily secretes androgens during fetal life. It involutes following delivery and completely disappears by the end of the first year of life. The fetal adrenal medulla synthesizes and stores catecholamines. It is poorly developed, and its role during fetal growth and maturation is not known.

Placenta. The placenta produces both steroid and peptide hormones in amounts that vary with gestational age. Precursors for progesterone synthesis come from the maternal circulation. Because of the lack of the enzyme 17α-hydroxylase, the human placenta cannot directly convert progesterone to estrogen but must use androgens, largely from the fetal adrenal, as its source of precursor for estrogen production.

Peptide Hormones

Human Chorionic Gonadotropin (hCG). This hormone is secreted by trophoblastic cells of the placenta and maintains pregnancy. It is a glycoprotein with a molecular weight of 40,000 to 45,000 and consists of two subunits: alpha (α) and beta (β). The α subunit is shared with luteinizing hormone (LH) and thyroid-stimulating hormone (TSH). The specificity of hCG is related to its β subunit, and a radioimmunoassay, specific for the β subunit, allows positive identification of hCG. The presence of hCG at times other than pregnancy signals the presence of an hCG-producing tumor, usually a hydatidiform mole, choriocarcinoma, or embryonal carcinoma.

During pregnancy, hCG begins to rise 8 days after ovulation (9 days after the midcycle LH peak). This provides the basis for virtually all immunologic or chemical pregnancy tests. With continuing pregnancy, hCG values peak at 60 to 90 days and then decline to a moderate, more constant level. For the first 6 to 8 weeks of pregnancy, hCG maintains the corpus luteum and thereby ensures continued progesterone output until progesterone production shifts to the placenta.

Titers of hCG are usually abnormally low in patients with an ectopic pregnancy or threatened abortion and abnormally high in those with trophoblastic disease. This hormone may also regulate steroid biosynthesis in the placenta and the fetal adrenal gland and stimulate testosterone production in the fetal testicle. Although immune suppression has been ascribed to hCG, this function cannot be verified using pure preparations.

Human Placental Lactogen (hPL). HPL originates in the placenta. It is a single chain polypeptide with a molecular weight of 22,300 and resembles pituitary growth hormone and human prolactin in structure. Maternal serum concentrations parallel placental weight, rising throughout gestation to maximum levels in the last 4 weeks. At term, HPL accounts for 10 per cent of all placental protein production. Low values are found with threatened abortion and intrauterine fetal growth retardation. HPL antagonizes the cellular action of insulin and decreases glucose utilization. Therefore, it may play a role in shifting glucose availability toward the fetus.

Prolactin. Prolactin is a peptide from the anterior pituitary with a molecular weight of about 20,000. Normal nonpregnant levels are approximately 10 ng/ml. During pregnancy, maternal prolactin levels rise in response to increasing maternal estrogen output that stimulates the anterior pituitary lactotrophs. Although the decidua is a secondary source of prolactin production, this contributes little to the plasma pool. Amniotic fluid levels exceed those in the circulation. The main effect of prolactin is stimulation of milk production. In the second half of pregnancy, prolactin secreted by the fetal pituitary may be an important stimulus of fetal adrenal growth. Prolactin may also play a role in fluid and electrolyte shifts across the fetal membranes.

Steroid Hormones

Progesterone. Progesterone is the most important human progestogen. In the luteal phase, it induces secretory changes in the endometrium; in pregnancy, higher levels induce decidual changes. Up to the sixth or seventh week of pregnancy, the major source

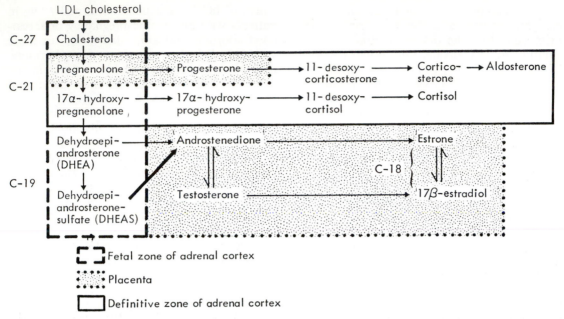

Figure 5–1. Main pathways of steroid hormone biosynthesis. Adrenal DHEA is largely transported as its sulfate, DHEA-S, which can also be formed from steroid sulfates starting with cholesterol sulfate.

of progesterone is the ovary. Thereafter, the placenta begins to play the major role. Progesterone production by the corpus luteum is essential for continuation of pregnancy up to 7 weeks. If the corpus luteum of pregnancy is removed before 7 weeks and continuation of the pregnancy is desired, progesterone should be given to prevent spontaneous abortion. Circulating progesterone is mostly bound to carrier proteins (albumin, orosomucoid, transcortin); less than 10 per cent is free. Probably only the free progesterone is physiologically active.

The myometrium receives progesterone directly from the venous blood draining the placenta. Progesterone prevents uterine contractions. Progesterone may also induce some immune tolerance for the products of conception.

The fetus inactivates progesterone by transformation to corticosteroids or by hydroxylation or conjugation to inert excretory products. However, the placenta can convert these inert materials back to progesterone. Steroid biochemical pathways are shown in Figure 5–1.

Estrogens. Both fetus and placenta are involved in the biosynthesis of estrone, estradiol, and estriol. Cholesterol is converted to pregnenolone and pregnenolone sulfate in the placenta. These precursors are converted to dehydroepiandrosterone sulfate (DHEA-S) largely in the fetal and to a lesser extent in the maternal adrenals. The DHEA-S is further metabolized by the placenta to estrone (E_1) and, via testosterone, to estradiol (E_2). Estriol (E_3), the most abundant estrogen in human pregnancy, is synthesized in the placenta from 16α-hydroxy-DHEA-S, which is produced in the fetal liver from adrenal DHEA-S. Placental sulfatase is required to deconjugate 16α-hydroxy-DHEA-S prior to conversion to E_3 (Fig. 5–2). Steroid sulfatase activity in the placenta is high except in rare cases of sulfatase deficiency.

A sudden decline of estriol in the maternal circulation may indicate fetal compromise. Anencephalic fetuses lack a hypothalamus and have hypoplastic anterior pituitary and adrenal glands; thus, estriol production is only about 10 per cent of normal. Although estriol determinations have been used as a means of monitoring fetal well-being, present use is limited, and estriol measurements have generally been replaced by biophysical assessments.

Androgens. During pregnancy, androgens originate mainly in the fetal zone of the fetal

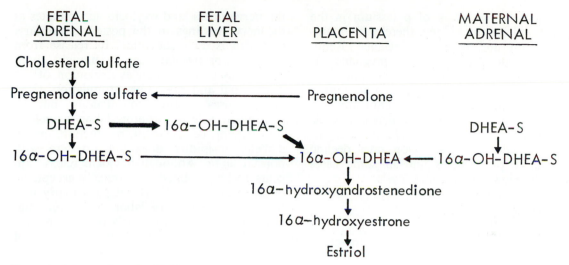

Figure 5–2. Formation of estriol in the fetal placental unit.

adrenal cortex. Androgen secretion is stimulated by adrenocorticotropic hormone (ACTH) and hCG, the latter being effective primarily in the first half of pregnancy when it is present in high concentration. The fetal adrenal favors production of DHEA over testosterone and androstenedione, and it sulfurylates almost all steroids. Fetal androgens enter the placental circulation and serve as precursors for estradiol and estriol (see Fig. 5–1).

The fetal testis also secretes androgens, particularly testosterone. Testosterone is converted within target cells to dihydrotestosterone, which is required for the development of the male external genitalia. The main trophic stimulus appears to be hCG.

Glucocorticoids. Cortisol is derived from circulating cholesterol (see Fig. 5–1). Maternal plasma cortisol concentrations rise throughout pregnancy, and the diurnal rhythm of cortisol secretion persists. The plasma level of transcortin rises in pregnancy, probably stimulated by estrogen, and the plasma free cortisol concentration doubles.

Both the fetal adrenal and the placenta participate in cortisol metabolism. The fetal adrenal is stimulated by ACTH, originating from the fetal pituitary, to produce both cortisol and DHEA-S. In contrast to DHEA-S, which is produced in the fetal zone, cortisol originates in the definitive zone (see Fig. 5–1). Cortisol plays an important function in the maturation of the lungs. It promotes dif-

ferentiation of type II alveolar cells and the biosynthesis and release of surfactant into the alveoli. Surfactant decreases the force required to inflate the lungs. Insufficiency of surfactant leads to respiratory distress in the premature infant, which can cause death.

CHANGES IN MATERNAL METABOLISM

Maternal metabolism adapts to pregnancy through endocrine regulation. The changes in insulin and thyroid hormone metabolism are discussed in Chapter 6.

Angiotensin-Aldosterone

Aldosterone is a mineralocorticoid synthesized in the zona glomerulosa of the adrenal cortex. The main source in pregnancy is the maternal adrenal. The fetal adrenal and the placenta do not participate significantly in aldosterone production, although the fetal adrenal is capable of synthesizing aldosterone. Aldosterone secretion is regulated by the renin-angiotensin system. Increased renin formed in the kidney converts angiotensinogen (renin substrate) to angiotensin I, which is further metabolized to angiotensin II; this, in turn, stimulates aldosterone secretion. Aldosterone stimulates the absorption of sodium and the secretion of potassium in the distal tubule of the kidney, thereby maintaining sodium and potassium balance. Renin substrate concentration rises in pregnancy. It is thought that the high concentrations of progesterone and estrogen present during pregnancy stimulate renin and renin substrate formation, thus giving rise to increased levels of angiotensin II and greater aldosterone production. Aldosterone secretion rates decline in toxemic pregnancies and in some cases may fall below nonpregnant levels.

Calcium Metabolism

Although calcium absorption is increased in pregnancy, total maternal serum calcium declines. The fall in total calcium parallels that of serum albumin, since approximately half of the total calcium is bound to albumin. Ionic calcium, the physiologically important calcium fraction, remains essentially constant throughout pregnancy because of increased maternal production of parathyroid hormone. In late pregnancy, coinciding with maximal calcification of the fetal skeleton, increased serum parathyroid hormone enhances both intestinal absorption of calcium and bone resorption. The latter counteracts the inhibition of bone resorption caused by increased circulating estrogen. Urinary calcium excretion is decreased.

Calcium ions are actively transported across the placenta, and fetal serum levels of total as well as ionized calcium are higher than maternal levels in late pregnancy. High fetal ionic calcium suppresses fetal parathyroid hormone production and parathyroid hormone does not cross the placenta. Furthermore, calcitonin production is stimulated, thus providing the fetus with ample calcium for calcification of the skeleton. In the first 24 to 48 hours postpartum, the total serum calcium concentration in the neonate usually falls, while the phosphorus concentration rises. Both adjust to adult levels within 1 week.

Other Hormones and Transmitters

Oxytocin. The oxytocin prohormone originates in the supraoptic and paraventricular nuclei of the hypothalamus. It migrates down the nerve fibers, and oxytocin accumulates at the nerve endings in the posterior pituitary. Oxytocin is an octapeptide. Its release from the posterior pituitary can be brought about by various stimuli, such as distention of the birth canal and mammary stimulation. Oxytocin causes uterine contractions, but its physiologic role in initiating labor is unclear. Impairment of oxytocin production, as in diabetes insipidus, does not interfere with normal labor. Although oxytocin release appears to be inhibited by clinically acceptable levels of ethanol, this is not particularly useful for suppression of labor. Moreover, maternal serum oxytocin levels do not rise before labor but only during the first stage of labor. Toward the end of pregnancy, the number of myometrial oxytocin receptors as well as myometrial sensitivity to oxytocin increases. Administered oxytocin can induce labor only at or near term.

Prostaglandins and Leukotrienes. Prostaglandins are a family of ubiquitous, biologically active lipids that have many functions. They are not true hormones: They are not synthesized in one gland and transported via the circulating blood to a target organ. Rather, they are synthesized at or near their site of action. Prostaglandin E_2 (PGE_2) and prostaglandin $F_{2\alpha}$ ($PGF_{2\alpha}$) are synthesized in the endometrium and myometrium and cause contraction of the uterus. They can also cause contraction of other smooth muscles, such as those of the intestinal tract. Hence, when used pharmacologically, prostaglandins may give rise to undesirable side effects such as nausea, vomiting, and diarrhea. The amniotic fluid concentrations of PGE_2 and $PGF_{2\alpha}$ rise throughout pregnancy and increase further during spontaneous labor. Levels are lower in women who require oxytocin for induction of labor than in women going into spontaneous labor. Administration of PGE_2 or $PGF_{2\alpha}$ by various routes induces labor or abortion at any stage of gestation. A synthetic prostaglandin, prostaglandin $F_{2\alpha}$ 15-methylester, can be used clinically to terminate a second-trimester pregnancy.

Since prostaglandins are thought to play a major role in the initiation and control of labor, their synthesis is reviewed in that context. Prostaglandin synthesis begins with the formation of arachidonic acid, an obligatory precursor of the prostaglandins of the "2"

Figure 5–3. Diagram of prostaglandin and leukotriene biosynthesis.

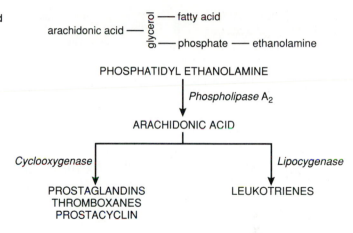

series (PGE_2, $PGF_{2\alpha}$). Arachidonic acid is stored in esterified form as glycerophospholipid in the trophoblastic membranes. The initial step is the hydrolysis of glycerophospholipids, which is catalyzed by phospholipase A_2 or C. Phospholipase A_2 preferentially acts on chorionic phosphatidyl ethanolamine to release arachidonic acid (Fig. 5–3). Free arachidonic acid does not accumulate. Labor appears to be accompanied by a cascade of events in the chorion, amnion, and decidua that releases arachidonic acid from its stored form and converts it to active prostaglandins. 17β-Estradiol stimulates several enzymes active in the synthesis of prostaglandins from arachidonic acid.

Increased phospholipase A_2 activity may lead to premature labor. Endocervical, intrauterine, or urinary tract infections are often associated with premature labor. Many of the organisms producing these infections have phospholipase A_2 activity, which could produce free arachidonic acid, followed by prostaglandin synthesis, which could trigger labor.

Prostaglandin synthetase inhibitors can prolong gestation. Nonsteroidal anti-inflammatory drugs inhibit phospholipase A_2, whereas aspirin-like drugs inhibit cyclooxygenase. Since PGE_2 keeps the ductus arteriosus open, fetal death may occur after ingestion of aspirin in large amount.

An additional pathway for arachidonic acid metabolism is the conversion of arachidonic acid to leukotrienes (Fig. 5–3). Both prostaglandins and leukotrienes induce decidualization, which means they initiate changes in the endometrium to facilitate implantation of the fertilized ovum.

Although $PGF_{2\alpha}$ is most potent in uterine contractile activity, PGE_2 is the most potent prostaglandin in ripening the cervix by inducing changes in the connective tissue. Hence, PGE_2 and its synthetic derivatives are clinically useful for cervical ripening before induction of labor or abortion.

Biochemical Basis of Contraction

Contraction of the myometrium is brought about by the sliding of actin and myosin filaments and requires adenosine triphosphate (ATP) and calcium. A rise in the intracellular calcium concentration occurs as calcium is released from intracellular compartments or enters from the extracellular fluid through both voltage-operated and receptor-operated channels that briefly open.

Unlike skeletal muscle contraction, which requires innervation, smooth muscle contraction is triggered primarily by hormonal stimuli. Receptors for oxytocin and for prostaglandins have been found in the myometrial cell membrane. Receptors for prostaglandins, which are synthesized inside the cell, are also found in the sarcoplasmic reticulum, an intracellular calcium storage area.

The binding of oxytocin to its receptor activates a phospholipase C, which hydrolyzes phosphatidylinositol 4,5-bisphosphate, a lipid present in the cell membrane, to inositol trisphosphate and diacylglycerol (Fig. 5–4). The inositol trisphosphate induces release of calcium from the sarcoplasmic reticulum. Subsequently, more calcium enters from the

arachidonic acid ── glycerol ── fatty acid

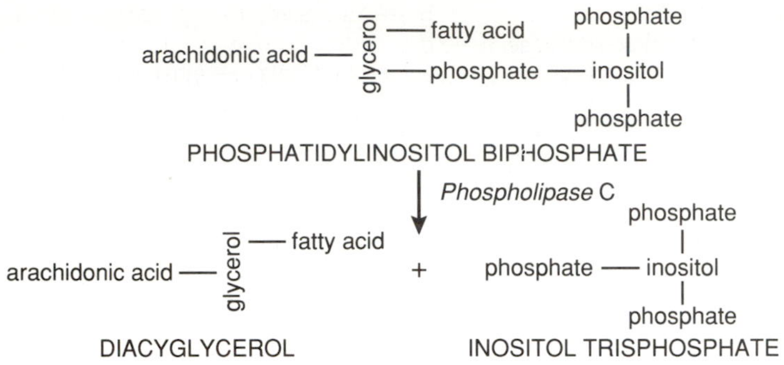

glycerol ── phosphate ── inositol ── phosphate / phosphate

PHOSPHATIDYLINOSITOL BIPHOSPHATE

↓ *Phospholipase* C

arachidonic acid ── glycerol ── fatty acid

DIACYGLYCEROL

+ phosphate ── inositol ── phosphate / phosphate

INOSITOL TRISPHOSPHATE

Figure 5–4. Diagram of inositol trisphosphate formation.

extracellular space. The high calcium concentration thus created enables the myofibrils of the myometrium to contract. Prostaglandins, on the other hand, seem to release calcium directly from the sarcoplasmic reticulum.

Unlike in the heart, where the bundle of His is present, no anatomic structures for synchronization of contractions have been found in the uterus. Instead, contraction spreads as current flows from cell to cell through areas of low resistance. Such areas are associated with gap junctions, which become especially prominent at parturition. Estradiol and prostaglandins promote the appearance of gap junctions, whereas progesterone opposes this action of estradiol.

PARTURITION

Hormonal Control of Gestational Length and Initiation of Labor

Gestational length is under hormonal control and in most species under the hormonal control of the fetus. Each species, however, has not only a unique gestational length but also unique mechanisms for controlling the length of gestation. Thus, although animal models provide important insight, they do not provide specific information concerning the control of the human gestational length or the mechanisms controlling initiation of labor in the human. Nevertheless, animal models are well worth examining.

Animal Models. Most studies have been conducted in the sheep. In the sheep, the fetus appears to control the onset of labor. The fetal hypothalamus stimulates the fetal pituitary to secrete ACTH, which brings about a surge of cortisol from the fetal adrenal. The cortisol surge induces the placental enzyme 17α-hydroxylase and formation of androgens, which are estrogen precursors (see Fig. 5–1), simultaneously decreasing progesterone formation. The rise in the estrogen to progesterone ratio leads to (1) greater secretion of prostaglandins; (2) formation of myometrial gap junctions, which provide areas of low resistance to current flow and increase coordinated uterine contractions; (3) cervical ripening; and (4) the onset of labor. Administered ACTH, glucocorticoids, or dexamethasone can also initiate parturition. Removal of the fetal pituitary or adrenal, both of which are required for the cortisol surge, results in prolonged pregnancy.

In a breed of Guernsey cows with a genetic defect resulting in fetal pituitary and adrenal malfunction, pregnancy is prolonged, and normal vaginal delivery does not occur. In the rabbit, parturition directly follows a decline in progesterone production secondary to a decline in corpus luteal function. Abortion can be prevented by administration of progesterone.

The Human. In the human, hormonal effects are important in determining gestational length and in initiating labor. Undoubtedly fetal-maternal interaction occurs throughout pregnancy, but the event initiating parturition is not known. Some clinical experience supports a hypothesis similar to that postulated for the sheep, whereas some does not. Fetal anencephaly and adrenal hypoplasia frequently cause prolonged pregnancy, which supports the hypothesis. However, infusion of ACTH, glucocorticoids, or dexamethasone does not cause premature labor in the human. A fall in maternal serum progesterone is not present with the onset of labor. Progesterone injection has not been found helpful in the treatment of premature labor, but injected progesterone may not reach the myometrial cells in a sufficiently high concentration to inhibit contractions. A precipitous increase in estradiol has not been demonstrated before the onset of labor, and 17α-hydroxylase activity is absent in the human placenta. Administration of estradiol will not induce labor, although it seems likely that the changes in the estrogen to progesterone ratio play a facilitative role in initiating the onset of human parturition.

Estrogen is known to stimulate prostaglandin biosynthesis in the fetal membranes and the decidua, the formation of gap junctions in the myometrium, and the synthesis of oxytocin receptors. But neither the concentration of circulating oxytocin nor of prostaglandins rises before the onset of labor. In fact, the oxytocin concentration rises only in the first stage of labor. In the cervix, however, increased prostaglandin E_2 induces changes that lead to cervical ripening.

Largely unknown is the role of relaxin in human parturition. Relaxin is a peptide hormone originating from the ovary. Relaxin is present in the maternal circulation throughout pregnancy. There is some support for its implication in cervical ripening.

Although all these observations are correct, we may have to modify our interpretation. As already mentioned for oxytocin, circulating hormone levels do not change before the onset of labor, but the number of receptors in the myometrium changes. Up-regulation and down-regulation of oxytocin receptors are steroid hormone–dependent and are pronounced during pregnancy and during the menstrual cycle. The sensitivity of the myometrium to oxytocin parallels oxytocin receptor concentration. This opens up a broader picture of possible changes in the number of receptors and hormone sensitivity for multiple hormones.

There is a broadening interest in multiple peptides, found in the nerve endings of the urogenital tract. Some play a role in controlling uterine blood flow, whereas some also affect the mechanical activity of myometrial smooth muscle cells; examples are vasoactive intestinal peptide (VIP) and neuropeptide Y (NPY). The complete physiologic action of many peptides is still unknown, but hormone-like effects have been observed, so that they have systemic (endocrine) and local (paracrine) action. Thus, there is a strong possibility of new compounds exhibiting synergism or antagonism to known hormones, and they may participate in the cascade of events leading to the onset of labor.

Furthermore, we may have to look for hormonal changes in pregnancy-related tissues, such as the decidua and the fetal membranes. In the amnion, prostaglandin synthesis is accelerated at term and in labor, and the concentration of prostaglandins increases during labor. Human fetal membranes contain leukotrienes and platelet activating factor. Platelet activating factor is a glycerophospholipid. In late gestation, the concentration of platelet activating factor in maternal plasma rises. Like prostaglandins, platelet activating factor can initiate uterine contractions. Another source of prostaglandins and platelet activating factor may be the fetal lung. Increasing amounts of prostaglandins and platelet activating factor along with surfactant are synthesized as the fetal lung matures. The concept of a role for the fetal lung in the initiation of parturition seems particularly attractive because the fetal lung is the last major organ to mature.

Knowledge of what initiates parturition is important for solving the riddle of premature labor. At this point, it is known that in preterm labor, myometrial oxytocin receptors rise prematurely, and the concentration of platelet activating factor increases in the amniotic fluid. Future research along these lines should increase our knowledge in this important area, and, it is hoped, improve our ability to prevent premature labor and delivery, which are currently the leading causes of perinatal mortality.

SUGGESTED READING

Albrecht ED, Pepe GJ: Placental steroid hormone biosynthesis in primate pregnancy. Endocrine Rev 11:124, 1990.

Angle MJ, Johnston JM: Fetal tissues and autacoid biosynthesis in relation to the initiation of parturition and implantation. In Carsten ME, Miller JD (eds): Uterine Function: Molecular and Cellular Aspects. New York, Plenum Press, 1990, p 471.

Burghardt RC, Fletcher WH: Physiological roles of gap junctional communication in reproduction. In Carsten ME, Miller JD (eds): Uterine Function: Molecular and Cellular Aspects. New York, Plenum Press, 1990, p 277.

Carsten ME, Miller JD: Calcium control mechanisms in the myometrial cell and the role of the phosphoinositide cycle. In Carsten ME, Miller JD (eds): Uterine Function: Molecular and Cellular Aspects. New York, Plenum Press, 1990, p 121.

Carsten ME, Miller JD: A new look at uterine muscle contraction. Am J Obstet Gynecol 157:1303, 1987.

Chaudhuri G: Biosynthesis and function of eicosanoids in the uterus. In Carsten ME, Miller JD (eds): Uterine Function: Molecular and Cellular Aspects. New York, Plenum Press, 1990, p 423.

Jaffe RB: Endocrine physiology of the fetus and fetoplacental unit. In Yen SSC, Jaffe RB (eds): Reproductive Endocrinology: Physiology, Pathology and Clinical Management. Philadelphia, WB Saunders, 1986, p 737.

Kamm KE, Stull JT: The function of myosin and myosin light chain kinase phosphorylation in smooth muscle. Annu Rev Pharmacol Toxicol 25:593, 1985.

Ottesen B, Fahrenkrug J: Regulatory peptides and uterine function. In Carsten ME, Miller JD (eds): Uterine Function: Molecular and Cellular Aspects. New York, Plenum Press, 1990, p 393.

Pitkin RM: Calcium metabolism in pregnancy and the perinatal period: A review. Am J Obstet Gynecol 151:99, 1985.

Soloff MS: Endocrine control of parturition. In Wynn RM, Jollie WP (eds): Biology of the Uterus. New York, Plenum Medical Book Company, 1989, p 559.

Six

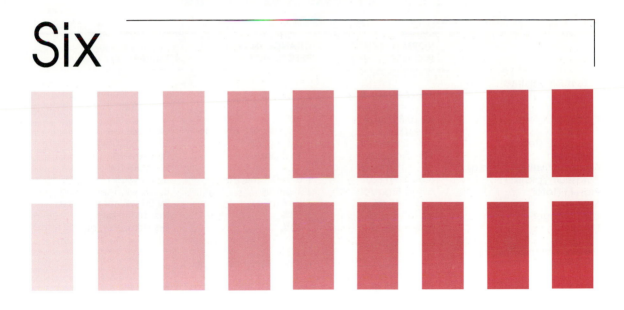

Maternal Physiology

NATHAN WASSERSTRUM

Maternal adjustments in pregnancy are designed to support the requirements of fetal homeostasis and growth without unduly jeopardizing maternal well-being. This is accomplished by adapting maternal systems to deliver energy and growth substrates to the fetus and to remove inappropriate heat and waste products. In addition, the sheer physical presence of the enlarging uterus impinges on diverse maternal functions, including circulation, respiration, and renal function. The limits of the fetal role in maintaining fetal homeostasis are clear. Although breathing movements and urine production occur in utero, the fetal lung and kidney appear to play no role in fetal respiration and excretion. The fetus is capable, however, of redistributing its cardiac output and oxygen delivery among different organs in response to physiologic demands.

NORMAL VALUES IN PREGNANCY

The normal values for several hematologic, biochemical, and physiologic indices during pregnancy differ markedly from the nonpregnant range and may also vary according to the duration of the pregnancy. These alterations are shown in Table 6–1.

CARDIOVASCULAR SYSTEM

Cardiac Output

The hemodynamic changes associated with pregnancy are summarized in Table 6–2. The plasma volume rises as early as the sixth week of pregnancy and plateaus at approximately 50 per cent above nonpregnant levels

Table 6-1. COMMON LABORATORY VALUES IN PREGNANCY

TEST	NORMAL RANGE (NONPREGNANT)	CHANGE IN PREGNANCY	TIMING
Serum Chemistries			
Albumin	3.5–4.8 gm/dl	↓ 1 gm/dl	Most by 20 wk, then gradual
Calcium (total)	9–10.3 mg/dl	↓ 10%	Gradual fall
Chloride	95–105 mEq/L	No significant change	Gradual rise
Creatinine (female)	0.6–1.1 mg/dl	↓ 0.3 mg/dl	Most by 20 wk
Fibrinogen	1.5–3.6 gm/L	↑ 1–2 gm/L	Progressive
Glucose, fasting (plasma)	65–105 mg/dl	↓ 10%	Gradual fall
Potassium (plasma)	3.5–4.5 mEq/L	↓ 0.2–0.3 mEq/L	By 20 wk
Protein (total)	6.5–8.5 gm/dl	↓ 1 gm/dl	By 20 wk, then stable
Sodium	135–145 mEq/L	↓ 2–4 mEq/L	By 20 wk, then stable
Urea nitrogen	12–30 mg/dl	↓ 50%	First trimester
Uric acid	3.5–8 mg/dl	↓ 33%	First trimester, rise at term
Urinary Chemistries			
Creatinine	15–25 mg/kg/day (1–1.4 gm/day)	No significant change	
Protein	Up to 150 mg/day	Up to 250–300 mg/day	By 20 wk
Creatinine clearance	90–130 ml/min per 1.73 m²	↑ 40–50%	By 16 wk
Serum Enzymatic Activities			
Amylase	23–84 IU/L	↑ 50–100%	Controversial
Transaminase			
Glutamic pyruvic (SGPT)	5–35 mU/ml	No significant change	
Glutamic oxaloacetic (SGOT)	5–40 mU/ml	No significant change	
Hematocrit (female)	36–46%	↓ 4–7%	Bottoms at 30–34 wk
Hemoglobin (female)	12–16 gm/dl	↓ 1.5–2 gm/dl	Bottoms at 30–34 wk
Leukocyte count	4.8–10.8 × 10³/mm³	↑ 3.5 × 10³/mm³	Gradual
Platelet count	150–400 × 10³/mm³	Slight decrease	
Serum Hormone Values			
Cortisol (plasma)	8–21 µg/dl	↑ 20 µg/dl	
Prolactin (female)	25 ng/ml	↑ 50–400 ng/ml	Gradual, peaks at term
Thyroxine, total (T_4)	5–11 µg/dl	↑ 5 µg/dl	Early sustained
Triiodothyronine, total (T_3)	125–245 ng/dl	↑ 50%	Early sustained

Adapted and reproduced with permission from Main DM, Main EK: Obstetrics and Gynecology, A Pocket Reference. Chicago, Year Book, 1984, p 7.

Table 6-2. CARDIOVASCULAR CHANGES IN PREGNANCY

PARAMETER	AMOUNT OF CHANGE	TIMING
Arterial blood pressures		
Systolic	↓ 4–6 mm Hg	All bottom at 20–24 wks, then rise gradually to prepregnancy values at term
Diastolic	↓ 8–15 mm Hg	
Mean	↓ 6–10 mm Hg	
Heart rate	↑ 12–18 BPM	Early 2nd trimester, then stable
Stroke volume	↑ 10–30%	Early 2nd trimester, then stable
Cardiac output	↑ 33–45%	Peaks in early 2nd trimester, then stable until term

Adapted and reproduced with permission from Main DM, Main EK: Obstetrics and Gynecology, A Pocket Reference. Chicago, Year Book, 1984, p 18.

by about 32 to 34 weeks' gestation, after which there is little further change. The red blood cell mass appears to continue to rise throughout pregnancy. Hence, if iron stores are adequate, the hematocrit tends to rise from the second to the third trimester. Cardiac output rises by the tenth week of gestation; it reaches about 40 per cent above nonpregnant levels by 20 to 24 weeks, after which there is little change. Cardiac output reaches its peak while blood volume is still rising and reflects increases in both stroke volume and heart rate.

Intravascular Pressures

Systolic pressure falls only slightly during pregnancy, whereas diastolic pressure decreases more markedly, beginning in the first trimester, reaching its nadir in midpregnancy, then returning toward nonpregnant levels by term. These changes reflect the elevated cardiac output and reduced peripheral resistance that characterize pregnancy; toward the end of pregnancy, vasoconstrictor tone normally increases, and with it the blood pressure. The normal rise of blood pressure toward prepregnant levels as term approaches must be recognized, and the implications for the diagnosis of pre-eclampsia appreciated (see Chapter 15).

Blood pressure, as measured with a sphygmomanometer cuff around the brachial artery, varies with posture. In late pregnancy, it is probably highest when the gravida is sitting, somewhat lower when she is lying down (a minority show a dramatic fall due to vena caval compression), and lower still when she lies on one side.

When elevations in blood pressure are clinically detected during pregnancy, it is customary to repeat the measurement with the patient on her side. This practice usually introduces a systematic error. In the lateral position, the blood pressure cuff around the brachial artery is raised about 10 cm above the heart. This leads to a hydrostatic fall in measured pressure, yielding a reading about 7 mm Hg lower than if the cuff were at heart level, as occurs during sitting or supine measurements.

Mechanical Circulatory Effects of the Gravid Uterus

As pregnancy progresses, the enlarging uterus displaces and compresses various abdominal structures, including the iliac veins and inferior vena cava (and probably also the aorta), with marked effects. The supine position accentuates this venous compression, producing a fall in venous return and hence cardiac output. In most gravidas, a compensatory rise in peripheral resistance minimizes the fall in blood pressure. In up to 10 per cent of gravidas, however, there is a significant fall in blood pressure accompanied by symptoms of nausea, dizziness, and even syncope. This "supine hypotensive syndrome" is relieved by changing position to the side. It is noteworthy (and of some diagnostic value) that the expected baroreflexive tachycardia, which normally occurs in response to other maneuvers that reduce cardiac output and blood pressure, does not accompany caval compression. In fact, bradycardia is often associated with the syndrome.

The venous compression by the gravid uterus elevates pressure in veins draining the legs and pelvic organs, thereby exacerbating varicose veins in the legs and vulva and causing hemorrhoids. As expected, venous pressure is unaltered in the arm, where drainage is not compromised by the uterus. The rise in venous pressure is the major cause of the lower extremity edema that characterizes pregnancy. The hypoalbuminemia associated with pregnancy also shifts the balance of the other major factor in the Starling equation—colloid osmotic pressure—in favor of fluid transfer from the intravascular to the extracellular space. Because of venous compression, the rate of blood flow in the lower veins is also markedly reduced, predisposing to thrombosis. The various effects of caval compression are somewhat mitigated by the development of a paravertebral collateral circulation that permits blood from the lower body to bypass the occluded inferior vena cava.

During late pregnancy, the uterus can also partially compress the aorta and its branches; this is thought to account for the observation in some patients of lower pressure in the femoral artery compared with the brachial artery. This aortic compression can be accentuated during uterine contractions and may be a cause of fetal distress when a patient is in the supine position. This phenomenon has been referred to as the "Poseiro effect." Clinically, it can be suspected when the femoral pulse is not palpable.

Regional Blood Flow

Blood flow to most regions of the body increases and plateaus relatively early in pregnancy. Notable exceptions occur in the uterus, kidney, and skin, in each of which blood flow increases with gestational age. Two of the major increases (those to the kidney and to the skin) serve purposes of elimination: the kidneys of waste material, the skin of heat. Both processes require plasma rather than whole blood, which gives point to the disproportionate increase of plasma over red blood cells in the blood expansion.

Control of Cardiovascular Changes

The precise mechanisms accounting for the cardiovascular changes in pregnancy remain to be proved. It has been suggested that the rise in cardiac output and fall in peripheral resistance during pregnancy might be explained in terms of the circulatory response to an arteriovenous shunt, represented by the uteroplacental circulation. The elevations in cardiac output and uterine blood flow follow different time courses in pregnancy, however, the former reaching its maximum in the second trimester, the latter increasing to term.

Oxygen-Carrying Capacity of Blood

As already indicated, plasma volume expands proportionately more than red blood cell volume, leading to a fall in hematocrit. The optimum hematocrit is 35 for the white gravida and 33 for the black gravida. Hematocrits below 27 to 29, or above 39 to 41, are associated with progressively less favorable outcomes. In spite of the relatively low "optimal" hematocrit, the arteriovenous oxygen difference in pregnancy is below nonpregnant levels. This supports the concept that the hemoglobin concentration in pregnancy is more than sufficient to meet oxygen-carrying requirements.

Although the epidemiologic data are inadequate, it appears that a high proportion of women in the reproductive age group enter pregnancy without sufficient stores of iron to meet the increased needs of pregnancy.

RESPIRATORY SYSTEM

The major respiratory changes in pregnancy are due to three factors: the mechanical effects of the enlarging uterus, the increased total body oxygen consumption, and the respiratory stimulant effects of progesterone.

Respiratory Mechanics in Pregnancy

The changes in lung volume and capacities associated with pregnancy are detailed in Table 6–3. As pregnancy progresses, the enlarging uterus elevates the resting position of the diaphragm. This results in a less negative intrathoracic pressure and a decreased resting lung volume, that is, a decreased functional residual capacity (FRC). The enlarging uterus produces no impairment in diaphragmatic or thoracic muscle motion. Hence, the vital capacity (VC) remains unchanged. These characteristics—reduced FRC with unimpaired VC—are analogous to those seen in pneumoperitoneum and contrast with those seen in severe obesity or abdominal binding, in which the elevated diaphragm is accompanied by decreased excursions of the respiratory muscles. Reductions in both the expiratory reserve volume and the residual volume contribute to the reduced FRC.

Oxygen Consumption and Ventilation

Total body oxygen consumption increases about 15 to 20 per cent in pregnancy. Approximately half of this increase is accounted

Table 6-3. LUNG VOLUMES AND CAPACITIES IN PREGNANCY

TEST	DEFINITION	CHANGE IN PREGNANCY
Respiratory rate	—	No significant change
Tidal volume	The volume of air inspired and expired at each breath	Progressive rise throughout pregnancy of 0.1–0.2 L
Expiratory reserve volume	The maximum volume of air that can be additionally expired after a normal expiration	Lowered by about 15% (0.55 L in late pregnancy compared with 0.65 L postpartum)
Residual volume	The volume of air remaining in the lungs after a maximum expiration	Falls considerably (0.77 L in late pregnancy compared with 0.96 L postpartum)
Vital capacity	The maximum volume of air that can be forcibly inspired after a maximum expiration	Unchanged, except for possibly a small terminal diminution
Inspiratory capacity	The maximum volume of air that can be inspired from resting expiratory level	Increased by about 5%
Functional residual capacity	The volume of air in lungs at resting expiratory level	Lowered by about 18%
Minute ventilation	The volume of air inspired or expired in 1 minute	Increased by about 40% as a result of the increased tidal volume and unchanged respiratory rate

Adapted and reproduced with permission from Main DM, Main EK: Obstetrics and Gynecology, A Pocket Reference. Chicago, Year Book, 1984, p 14.

for by the uterus and its contents. The remainder is accounted for mainly by increased maternal renal and cardiac work; smaller increments are due to work of the respiratory muscles and the breasts.

In general, a rise in oxygen consumption is accompanied by cardiorespiratory responses that facilitate oxygen delivery (i.e., by increases in cardiac output and alveolar ventilation). To the extent that elevations in cardiac output and alveolar ventilation keep pace with the rise in oxygen consumption, the arteriovenous oxygen difference and the arterial partial pressure of carbon dioxide (Pco_2), respectively, remain unchanged. In pregnancy, the elevations in both cardiac output and alveolar ventilation are greater than those required to meet the increased oxygen consumption. Hence, despite the rise in total body oxygen consumption, the arteriovenous oxygen difference and arterial Pco_2 both fall. The fall in Pco_2, by definition, indicates hyperventilation.

The rise in minute ventilation reflects an approximate 40 per cent increase in tidal volume at term; the respiratory rate does not change during pregnancy.

When injected into normal nonpregnant subjects, progesterone increases ventilation. The respiratory center becomes more sensitive to CO_2 (i.e., the curve describing the ventilatory response to increasing CO_2 has a steeper slope). Such increased respiratory center sensitivity to CO_2 characterizes pregnancy and probably accounts for the hyperventilation of pregnancy.

Alveolar-Arterial Gradient and Arterial Blood Gases

As already noted, pregnancy is characterized by hyperventilation (the arterial Pco_2 falls to a level of 27 to 32 mm Hg) and its associated respiratory alkalosis. Renal compensatory bicarbonate excretion leads to a final pH between 7.40 and 7.45. During labor (without conduction anesthesia), the hyperventilation associated with each contraction produces a further transient fall in Pco_2. By the end of the first stage of labor, when cervical dilatation is complete, a decrease in arterial Pco_2 persists, even between contractions.

In general, when alveolar P_{CO_2} falls during hyperventilation, alveolar P_{O_2} shows a corresponding rise, leading to a rise in arterial P_{O_2}. This occurs in pregnancy, and in the first trimester, the mean arterial P_{O_2} may be 106 to 108 mm Hg. There is a slight downward trend in arterial P_{O_2} as gestation proceeds. This reflects, at least in part, an increased alveolar-arterial gradient, possibly resulting from the decrease in FRC discussed previously, which leads to ventilation-perfusion mismatch.

Dyspnea of Pregnancy

In general, airway resistance is unchanged or even decreased in pregnancy. Despite this absence of obstructive or restrictive effects, dyspnea is a common symptom in pregnancy. Gravidae with dyspnea of pregnancy show no changes in pulmonary function tests, compared with those without the symptom. However, these women tend to demonstrate a relatively higher nonpregnant P_{CO_2}. It has therefore been suggested that with pregnancy, the marked change in P_{CO_2} to unusually low levels results in the sensation of dyspnea.

RENAL PHYSIOLOGY

Anatomic Changes in the Urinary Tract

The urinary collecting system, including the calyces, renal pelves, and ureters, undergoes marked dilatation in pregnancy, as is readily seen on intravenous urograms. The dilatation is generally more prominent on the right side, begins in the first trimester, is present in 90 per cent of women at term, and may persist until the twelfth to sixteenth postpartum week. This occurrence probably reflects the influence of both humoral and physical factors. Progesterone appears to produce smooth muscle relaxation in various organs, including the ureter. As the uterus enlarges, partial obstruction of the ureter occurs at the pelvic brim in both the supine and the upright positions. Because of the relatively greater effect on the right side,

some have ascribed a role to the dilated ovarian venous plexus. Ovarian venous drainage is asymmetric, with the right vein emptying into the inferior vena cava and the left into the ipsilateral renal vein.

Renal Blood Flow and Glomerular Filtration Rate

Renal plasma flow and the glomerular filtration rate (GFR) increase early in pregnancy, plateau at about 40 per cent above nonpregnant levels by midgestation, and then remain unchanged to term. The mechanism of these increases is unclear. A facile explanation based on the marked volume expansion associated with pregnancy is insufficient. As was true for cardiac output, renal blood flow and GFR (clinically measured as the creatinine clearance) reach their peak relatively early in pregnancy, before the greatest increase in intravascular and extracellular volume occurs. The elevated GFR is reflected in lower serum levels of creatinine and urea nitrogen, as noted in Table 6–1.

Fluid Volumes

The maternal extracellular volume, which consists of intravascular and interstitial components, increases throughout pregnancy, leading in effect to a state of physiologic extracellular hypervolemia. The intravascular volume, which consists of plasma and red cell components, increases approximately 50 per cent during pregnancy. The plasma component increases approximately twice as much as the red cell mass (leading to a fall in hematocrit beginning early in pregnancy), and the two components follow different time courses, as discussed earlier. Maternal interstitial volume shows its greatest increase in the last trimester.

The magnitude of the rise in maternal plasma volume correlates with the size of the fetus; it is particularly marked in multiple gestation. Multiparae with poor reproductive histories show smaller increments in plasma volume and GFR when compared with those with a history of normal pregnancies and normal-sized babies.

Although the changes in volume of the different body compartments and in the various humoral and physical factors known to affect volume can be described, volume regulation in pregnancy is poorly understood.

Renin-Angiotensin System in Pregnancy

The elements of the renin-angiotensin system are markedly altered in pregnancy. Plasma concentrations of renin, renin substrate, angiotensin I, and angiotensin II are increased. Renin levels remain elevated throughout pregnancy. It is possible that at least a portion of the elevated renin measured in the peripheral blood of pregnant women may represent a different, high-molecular-weight form or an inactive form of the enzyme.

The uterus, like the kidney, can produce renin, and extremely high concentrations of renin occur in the amniotic fluid. The role played by this renin is not yet clear.

HOMEOSTASIS OF MATERNAL ENERGY SUBSTRATES

The metabolic regulation of energy substrates, including glucose, amino acids, fatty acids, and ketone bodies, is complex and interrelated.

Insulin Effects and Glucose Metabolism

In pregnancy, the insulin response to glucose stimulation is augmented. By the tenth week of normal pregnancy and continuing to term, fasting concentrations of insulin are elevated and those of glucose reduced. Until midgestation, these changes are accompanied by improved intravenous glucose tolerance (although oral glucose tolerance remains unchanged). Glycogen synthesis and storage by the liver increases, and gluconeogenesis is inhibited. Thus, during the first half of pregnancy, the anabolic actions of insulin are potentiated.

After early pregnancy, insulin resistance emerges, so glucose tolerance is impaired. The fall in serum glucose for a given dose of insulin is reduced, compared with earlier pregnancy. There is prolonged elevation of circulating glucose after meals, although fasting glucose remains reduced, as in early pregnancy.

A variety of humoral factors have been suggested to account for the anti-insulin environment of the latter part of pregnancy. Perhaps the most important is human placental lactogen (hPL), which antagonizes the peripheral effects of insulin. It is secreted by the placenta into the maternal circulation in amounts parallel to placental growth. Free levels of cortisol are also increased. In addition, progesterone may exert some anti-insulin effects.

Other potential diabetogenic factors that probably do not play important roles in producing glucose intolerance in pregnancy should be considered. Although basal levels of glucagon are elevated in pregnancy, secretion of glucagon is suppressed normally by a glucose challenge. Growth hormone is not elevated, and the pituitary response to hypoglycemia is diminished. Finally, the half-life of intravenous insulin is unchanged during pregnancy; therefore, accelerated metabolic degradation probably does not play a role in glucose intolerance.

Lipid Metabolism

The potentiated anabolic effects of insulin that characterize early pregnancy lead to the inhibition of lipolysis. During the second half of pregnancy, however, probably as a result of rising hPL, lipolysis is augmented, and the plasma concentration of free fatty acids after an overnight fast is elevated. Teleologically, the free fatty acids act as substrates for maternal energy metabolism, whereas glucose and amino acids cross the placenta to the fetus. In the humoral milieu of the second half of the pregnancy, the increased free fatty acids lead to ketone body (β-hydroxybutyrate and acetoacetate) formation. Pregnancy is thus associated with an increased risk of ketoacidosis, especially after prolonged fasting.

In the context of maternal lipid metabolism, mention must be made of the most

Table 6-4. MATERNAL-FETAL TRANSFER DURING PREGNANCY

FUNCTION	SUBSTANCE	PLACENTAL TRANSFER
Glucose homeostasis	Glucose	Excellent—"facilitated diffusion"
	Amino acids	Excellent—active transport
	Free fatty acids (FFA)	Very limited—essential FFA only
	Ketones	Excellent—diffusion
	Insulin	No transfer
	Glucagon	No transfer
Thyroid function	Thyroxine (T_4)	Very poor—diffusion
	Triiodothyronine (T_3)	Poor—diffusion
	Thyrotropin-releasing hormone (TRH)	Good
	Thyroid-stimulating immunoglobulin (TSI)	Good
	Thyroid-stimulating hormone (TSH)	Negligible transfer
	Propylthiouracil	Excellent
Adrenal hormones	Cortisol	Excellent transfer and active placental conversion of cortisol to cortisone
	ACTH	No transfer
Parathyroid function	Calcium	Active transfer against gradient
	Magnesium	Active transfer against gradient
	Phosphorus	Active transfer against gradient
	Parathyroid hormone	Not transferred
Immunoglobulins	IgA	Minimal passive transfer
	IgG	Good—both passive and active transport from 7 weeks' gestation
	IgM	No transfer

Adapted and reproduced with permission from Main DM, Main EK: Obstetrics and Gynecology, A Pocket Reference. Chicago, Year Book, 1984, p 37.

dramatic lipid change in pregnancy, the rise in fasting triglyceride concentration.

PLACENTAL TRANSFER OF NUTRIENTS

The transfer of substances across the placenta occurs by several mechanisms, including simple diffusion, facilitated diffusion, and active transport. Several physiochemical factors, such as molecular size, degree of ionization, and lipid solubility, affect the rate of diffusion. Substances with molecular weights greater than 1000, such as polypeptides and proteins, cross the placenta slowly, if at all.

Amino acids are actively transported across the placenta, making fetal levels higher than maternal. Glucose is transported by facilitated diffusion, leading to rapid equilibrium with only a small maternal-fetal gradient. Free fatty acids diffuse passively across the placenta, and fetal levels are lower than maternal levels. Glucose is the main energy sub-

strate of the fetus. Recent studies suggest, however, that amino acids and lactate may contribute up to 25 per cent of fetal oxygen consumption. The degree and mechanism of placental transfer of these and other substances are summarized in Table 6-4.

OTHER ENDOCRINE CHANGES

Thyroid

The thyroid gland normally shows moderate enlargement during pregnancy. This is not due to elevation of thyroid-stimulating hormone, which remains unchanged.

Circulating thyroid hormone exists in two primary active forms: thyroxine (T_4) and tri-iodothyronine (T_3). The former circulates in higher concentrations, is more highly protein-bound, and is less metabolically potent than T_3, for which it may serve as a prohormone. Circulating T_4 is bound to carrier proteins, approximately 85 per cent to thyroxine-binding globulin (TBG) and most of the re-

Table 6–5. ANALYSIS OF WEIGHT GAIN IN PREGNANCY

TISSUES AND FLUIDS	INCREASE IN WEIGHT (gm) UP TO:			
	10 weeks	20 weeks	30 weeks	40 weeks
Fetus	5	300	1500	3400
Placenta	20	170	430	650
Amniotic fluid	30	350	750	800
Uterus	140	320	600	970
Mammary gland	45	180	360	405
Blood	100	600	1300	1250
Interstitial fluid (no edema or leg edema)	0	30	80	1680
Maternal stores	310	2050	3480	3345
Total weight gained	650	4000	8500	12,500

Adapted with permission from Hytten F, Chamberlain G (eds): Clinical Physiology in Obstetrics. Oxford, Blackwell Scientific, 1980, p 221.

mainder to another protein, thyroxine-binding prealbumin. It is believed that only the unbound fraction of the circulating hormone is biologically active. TBG is increased during pregnancy because the high estrogen levels induce increased hepatic synthesis. The body responds by raising total circulating levels of T_4 and T_3. The net effect is that the free, biologically active concentration of each hormone is unchanged from that in the nonpregnant state. Therefore, clinically, the free T_4 index, which corrects the total circulating T_4 for the amount of binding protein, is an appropriate measure of thyroid function, with the same normal range as in the nonpregnant state. Thyroid hormones do not cross the placenta.

Adrenal

Adrenocorticotropic hormone (ACTH) and plasma cortisol are both elevated from 3 months' gestation to delivery. Although less so than thyroid hormones, circulating cortisol is also bound, primarily by a specific plasma protein, corticosteroid-binding globulin (CBG) or transcortin. Unlike the thyroid hormones, the mean unbound level of cortisol is elevated in pregnancy; there is also some loss of the diurnal variation that characterizes its concentration in nonpregnant women. It is not clear to what extent this elevated cortisol is responsible for some of the "pseudo-Cushingoid" features of pregnancy, such as striae gravidarum and impaired glucose tolerance.

WEIGHT GAIN IN PREGNANCY

The average weight gain in pregnancy uncomplicated by generalized edema is 12.5 kg (28 lb). The components of this weight gain are indicated in Table 6–5. The products of conception constitute only about 40 per cent of the total maternal weight gain.

PLACENTAL TRANSFER OF OXYGEN AND CARBON DIOXIDE

Fetal Oxygenation

The uteroplacental circulation subserves fetal gas exchange. Figure 6–1 demonstrates the normal blood gases on the maternal and fetal sides of the placenta. The umbilical vein of the fetus, like the pulmonary vein of the adult, carries the circulation's most highly oxygenated blood. The umbilical venous Po_2 of about 28 mm Hg is relatively low by adult standards. The fetus normally lives at these low oxygen tensions. The delivery system produces a large fall in oxygen tension from the uterine artery to the umbilical vein — analogous in the adult to the fall in oxygen tension from inspired air ($PIo_2 = 150$) to the pulmonary veins ($Po_2 = 100$). This relatively

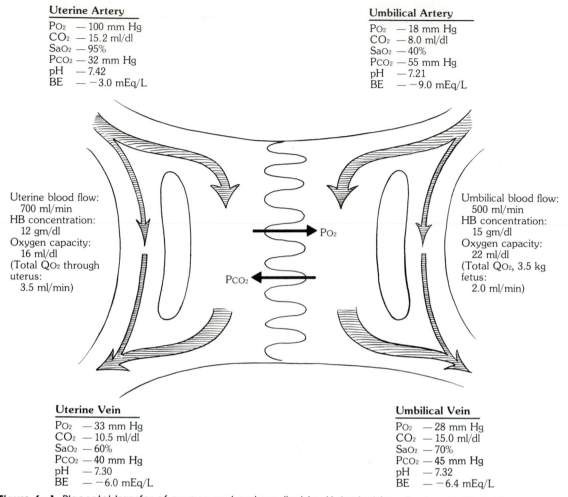

Uterine Artery

PO₂ — 100 mm Hg
CO₂ — 15.2 ml/dl
SaO₂ — 95%
PCO₂ — 32 mm Hg
pH — 7.42
BE — −3.0 mEq/L

Umbilical Artery

PO₂ — 18 mm Hg
CO₂ — 8.0 ml/dl
SaO₂ — 40%
PCO₂ — 55 mm Hg
pH — 7.21
BE — −9.0 mEq/L

Uterine blood flow:
  700 ml/min
HB concentration:
  12 gm/dl
Oxygen capacity:
  16 ml/dl
(Total QO₂ through
uterus:
  3.5 ml/min)

Umbilical blood flow:
  500 ml/min
HB concentration:
  15 gm/dl
Oxygen capacity:
  22 ml/dl
(Total QO₂, 3.5 kg
fetus:
  2.0 ml/min)

Uterine Vein

PO₂ — 33 mm Hg
CO₂ — 10.5 ml/dl
SaO₂ — 60%
PCO₂ — 40 mm Hg
pH — 7.30
BE — −6.0 mEq/L

Umbilical Vein

PO₂ — 28 mm Hg
CO₂ — 15.0 ml/dl
SaO₂ — 70%
PCO₂ — 45 mm Hg
pH — 7.32
BE — −6.4 mEq/L

Figure 6–1. Placental transfer of oxygen and carbon dioxide. (Adapted from Bonica JJ: Obstetric Analgesia and Anesthesia, 2nd ed. Amsterdam, World Federation of Societies of Anesthesiologists, 1980, p 29.)

low fetal tension is essential for survival in utero because a high PO₂ initiates adjustments, such as closure of the ductus arteriosus, which normally occur in the neonate but would be harmful in utero.

The placenta receives 60 per cent of the combined ventricular output, whereas the postnatal lung receives 100 per cent of the cardiac output. Unlike the lung, which consumes little of the oxygen it transfers, a significant percentage of the oxygen derived from maternal blood at term is consumed by placental tissue. The degree of functional shunting of placental blood past exchange sites is normally approximately tenfold greater than in the lung. The cause of this functional shunting is probably a mismatch between maternal and fetal blood flow at the exchange sites, analogous to the ventilation-perfusion inequalities that may occur in the lung.

Fetal and Maternal Hemoglobin Dissociation Curves

Most of the oxygen in blood is carried by hemoglobin in red blood cells. The maximum amount of oxygen carried per gram of hemoglobin, that is, the amount carried at 100 per cent saturation, is fixed at 1.34 ml.

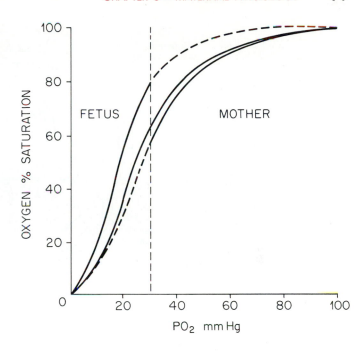

Figure 6-2. The oxygen dissociation curve for fetal blood compared with maternal blood. The central continuous curve is for normal adult blood. A vertical line at an oxygen partial pressure of 30 mm Hg divides the curves. The fetal curve normally operates below that level and the maternal curve above it. (From Hytten F, Chamberlain G (eds): Clinical Physiology in Obstetrics. 2nd ed. Oxford, Blackwell Scientific Publications, 1991, p 418.)

The affinity of hemoglobin for oxygen, however, which is the per cent saturation at a given oxygen tension, depends on chemical conditions. As is illustrated in Figure 6-2, when compared with that in nonpregnant adults, the binding of oxygen by hemoglobin is much greater in the fetus. In contrast, maternal affinity is lower. The shape of the fetal oxygen dissociation curve permits larger amounts of oxygen to be transported per unit of blood at relatively low oxygen tensions. Furthermore, the difference between maternal and fetal hemoglobin dissociation curves permits transplacental transfer of large volumes of oxygen. Thus, transplacental equilibration of maternal blood with a Po_2 of 30 mm Hg and saturation of 55 per cent will result in fetal blood with a Po_2 of 30 mm Hg but a saturation of almost 80 per cent.

The decrease in the affinity of hemoglobin for oxygen produced by a fall in pH is referred to as the Bohr effect. Because of the unique situation in the placenta, a double Bohr effect facilitates oxygen transfer from mother to fetus. When CO_2 and fixed acids are transferred from fetus to mother, the associated rise in fetal pH increases the fetal red blood cell affinity for oxygen uptake; the concomitant reduced maternal blood pH decreases oxygen affinity and promotes its unloading from maternal red cells.

FETAL CIRCULATION

Several anatomic and physiologic factors must be noted in considering the fetal circulation (Fig. 6-3 and Table 6-6).

The normal adult circulation is a series circuit. The blood circulates serially through the right heart, to the lungs, then through the left heart, to the systemic circulation, finally returning to the right heart. In the fetus, such a series circulation does not exist. Instead, output of the right ventricle is about double that of the left ventricle, blood from both ventricles circulates to the lower body, and only a small fraction of right ventricular output goes to the lungs.

The fetal circulation is characterized by channels (ductus venosus, foramen ovale, and ductus arteriosus) and preferential streaming, which function to maximize the delivery of more highly oxygenated blood to the upper body and brain, less highly oxygenated blood to the lower body, and very low blood flow to the nonfunctional lungs. The umbilical vein, carrying oxygenated (80 per cent saturated) blood from the placenta to the fetal body, enters the portal system. A portion of this umbilical-portal blood passes through the hepatic microcirculation, where oxygen is extracted, and thence through the hepatic veins into the inferior vena cava. The remainder

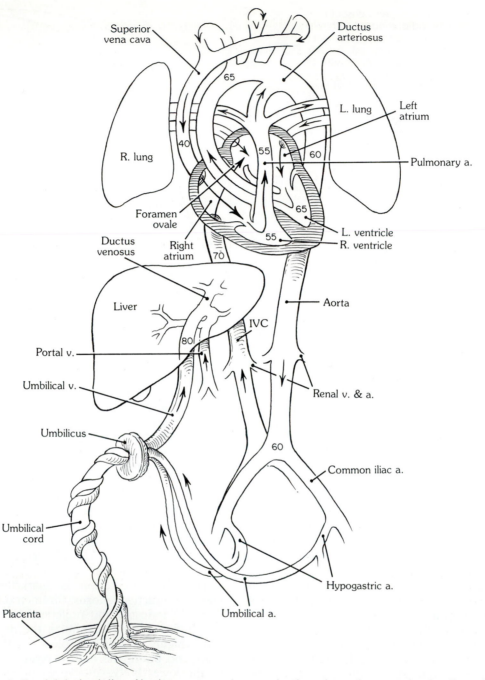

Figure 6-3. The fetal circulation. Numbers represent approximate values of per cent saturation of blood with oxygen in utero. (Adapted from Parer JJ: Fetal circulation. In Sciarra JJ (ed): Obstetrics and Gynecology. Vol 3, Maternal and Fetal Medicine. Hagerstown, MD, Harper & Row, 1984, p 2.)

Table 6-6. COMPONENTS OF THE FETAL CIRCULATION		
FETAL STRUCTURE	**FROM/TO**	**ADULT REMNANT**
Umbilical vein	Umbilicus/ductus venosus	Ligamentum teres hepatis
Ductus venosus	Umbilical vein/inferior vena cava (bypasses liver)	Ligamentum venosum
Foramen ovale	Right atrium/left atrium	Closed atrial wall
Ductus arteriosus	Pulmonary artery/descending aorta	Ligamentum arteriosum
Umbilical artery	Common iliac artery/umbilicus	Superior vesical arteries
		Lateral vesicoumbilical ligaments

Adapted and reproduced with permission from Main DM, Main EK: Obstetrics and Gynecology, A Pocket Reference. Chicago, Year Book, 1984, p 34.

enters the ductus venosus, which bypasses the liver and directly enters the inferior vena cava. The inferior vena cava also receives the unsaturated (25 per cent saturated) venous return from the lower body. As it enters the heart, the inferior vena cava carries the most highly oxygenated blood (70 per cent saturated) to reach the heart.

Before it mixes with the unsaturated blood returning via the superior vena cava (25 per cent saturated), approximately one third of inferior vena caval blood preferentially streams across the foramen ovale into the left atrium. There it mixes with the relatively meager pulmonary venous return, goes to the left ventricle, and thence to the aorta. The proximal aorta, carrying the most highly saturated blood leaving the heart (65 per cent saturated), gives off branches that supply the brain and upper body. In its descending portion, the aorta is joined by the ductus arteriosus branch of the pulmonary artery, carrying relatively less saturated blood (55 per cent saturated). The saturation of the descending aortic blood supplying the lower body (60 per cent saturated) is thus lower than that supplying the brain and upper body.

The role of the ductus arteriosus must be emphasized. As already noted, one third of the highly saturated inferior caval blood flows through the foramen ovale directly into the left atrium. The remaining two thirds enters the right atrium and right ventricle. Unsaturated superior vena caval blood is directed toward the tricuspid valve, leading to a relatively lower saturation of right compared with left ventricular blood; in normal fetuses, essentially no superior vena caval blood tra-

verses the foramen ovale into the left atrium. Right ventricular output enters the pulmonary trunk, from which its major portion bypasses the lungs by flowing through the ductus arteriosus to the descending aorta. Although the descending aorta supplies branches to the lower fetal body, the major portion of descending aortic flow goes to the umbilical arteries, which return deoxygenated blood to the placenta.

SUGGESTED READING

Brody SA, Ueland K (eds): Endocrine Disorders in Pregnancy. Norwalk, CT, Appleton & Lange, 1989.

Garn SM, Ridella SA, Petzold AS, et al: Maternal hematologic levels and pregnancy outcomes. Semin Perinatol 5:155, 1981.

Heymann MA: Fetal cardiovascular physiology. In Creasy RK, Resnick R (eds): Maternal-Fetal Medicine. 2nd ed. Philadelphia, WB Saunders, 1989, p 288.

Hytten FR, Chamberlain G (eds): Clinical Physiology in Obstetrics. 2nd ed. Oxford, Blackwell Scientific Publications, 1991.

Lindheimer MD, Katz AI: The kidney in pregnancy. In Brenner BM, Rector FC Jr (eds): The Kidney. 3rd ed. Philadelphia, WB Saunders, 1986.

Longo LL: Some physiological implications of altered uteroplacental blood flow. In Moawad AH, Lindheimer MD (eds): Uterine and Placental Blood Flow. New York, Masson Publishing USA, 1982, p 93.

Metcalfe J, McAnulty JH, Ueland K: Burwell and Metcalfe's Heart Disease in Pregnancy: Physiology and Management. Boston, Little, Brown, 1986.

Prowse CM, Gaensler EA: Respiratory and acid base changes during pregnancy. Anesthesiology 26:381, 1965.

Seven

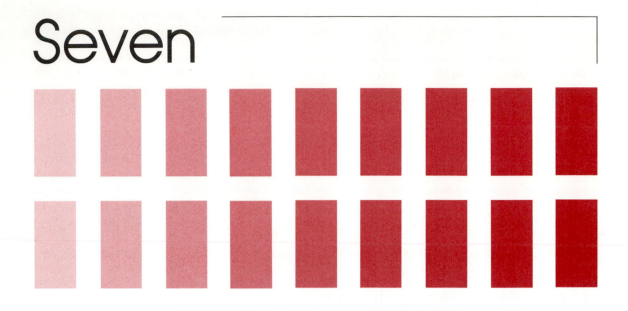

Immunology of Pregnancy

ARNOLD L. MEDEARIS

Pregnancy represents one of the most significant areas of study for the immunobiologist. The reasons for the success of gestation in both normal and abnormal pregnancies remain unclear because the fetus is antigenically dissimilar to the mother. The immunologic response of the mother to her fetus is an are of increasing interest.

The importance of immunology to obstetrics is often not appreciated. The identification of the Rhesus factor and the development of a preventive program using immunosuppression of the maternal response to fetal cell leakage at the time of delivery are two of the major successes in the field of perinatology.

Briefly addressed in this chapter are four areas in which an initial understanding of immunology is important. These are (1) the immunobiology of the maternal-fetal interaction, (2) the immunologic response during normal pregnancy, (3) the role of immunology in pregnancy-associated conditions, and (4) the maternal and fetal effects of autoimmune diseases in pregnancy.

IMMUNOBIOLOGY OF THE MATERNAL-FETAL INTERACTION

The maintenance of the antigenically dissimilar fetus in the uterus of the mother is of primary importance in obstetrics. Most of the attention in this field has come from the study of organ transplantation. The presence of the fetus is analogous to the grafting of tissues or organs between two individuals of the same species who are genetically dissimilar. Since all humans (except identical twins) are considered to be genetically dissimilar (allogeneic), such transplants are referred to as allografts. There are a number of mechanisms that have been proposed to account for the tolerance and subsequent success of the fetal allograft.

The primary sites of modulation of the maternal response to the fetus are the uterus, regional lymphatics, and placental surface. The uterus has been considered to be an immunologically privileged site, similar to the anterior chamber of the eye, the adrenal gland, and the cheek pouch of the hamster. These sites appear to have decreased or altered afferent lymphatic systems that allow them to modify the host response to an allograft, and it appears that a similar mechanism may apply in the uterus during pregnancy.

The T cells, which primarily mediate the cellular response to foreign tissue by acting either to help or to suppress the immune response, are also locally altered in pregnancy. Cytotoxic T lymphocytes at the maternal-fetal interface have limited ability to mount an immune response to the trophoblast antigens. Pregnancy-related suppressor T cells capable of decreasing the maternal lymphocyte response have been described. These cells, in conjunction with placental interventions, can lead to an altered local immunologic environment.

The separate vascular compartments found in the hemomonochorial placentation of the human effectively remove the fetus from direct contact with the maternal immunologic defense system. This allows the placenta to function as an interface between two distinct systems. Tight trophoblastic intercellular junctions and a fibrinous covering of the trophoblast lead to control of the cellular and molecular fetomaternal transport. Although the trophoblast has been shown to possess class I human leukocyte antigens (HLA), the placenta lacks the class II major histocompatibility antigens that are necessary for the maternal lymphocytes to initiate an effective immunologic response.

The placenta produces a number of pregnancy-associated plasma proteins and steroids that may alter the maternal immune response. These include alpha-2 globulins, pregnancy-specific beta-1 glycoprotein (SP1), human placental lactogen (hPL), and human chorionic gonadotropin (hCG) as well as the sex steroids estrogen and progesterone. All of these substances have been shown to suppress nonspecifically the local immune response in pregnancy.

In addition, the placenta functions as an immunoabsorbent to decrease the response against the fetus. Antibodies that are generated by the maternal immune response against paternal antigens in the placental surface (masking antibodies) and local immune complexes (blocking antibodies) may be trapped in the placenta. These complexes can modify or block the immune response, or both, by facilitating enhancing antibodies and cellular suppression.

These mechanisms, which are summarized in Table 7–1, are thought to account for the maternal tolerance and the lack of host rejection seen in the majority of pregnancies.

IMMUNOLOGIC RESPONSE DURING NORMAL PREGNANCY

The mother's immunologic defense system remains intact during pregnancy. While allowing the fetal allograft to exist, the mother must still be able to protect herself and her fetus from infection and antigenically foreign substances. The nonspecific mechanisms of the immunologic system (including phagocytosis and the inflammatory response) are not affected by pregnancy. The specific mechanisms of the immune response (humoral and cellular) are also not significantly affected. There is no significant change in the leukocyte count. The percentage of B or T lymphocytes is not altered, nor is there any consistent alteration in their performance during pregnancy.

Immunoglobulin levels do not change in pregnancy. The levels of specific maternal IgG antibodies are of particular importance because of their ability to cross the placenta. Maternal IgG is the major component of the fetal immunoglobulin in utero and the early neonatal period. IgG is the only immunoglobulin that is transported across the placenta. Significant passive immunity can be transferred in this manner to the fetus and aids in protecting it from infection during the perinatal period. IgM, because of its larger molecular size, is unable to cross the placenta. The other immunoglobulins—IgA, IgD, and IgE—are also confined to the maternal compartment and do not present any direct harm or benefit to the fetus.

Table 7–1. PROPOSED MECHANISMS FOR THE SUCCESS OF THE FETAL ALLOGRAFT

MATERNAL		FETAL	
Systemic	Uterus and Local Lymphatic System	Placenta	Systemic
None (Normal cell-mediated immunity)	Privileged immunologic site Localized, nonspecific suppression induces tolerance and generates suppressor T cells	Separation of the maternal-fetal circulations, including tight local barriers Lack of expression of the class II major histocompatibility antigen (HLA) at the maternal-fetal interface Limited immune response of cytotoxic T lymphocytes to trophoblast	Unidentified humoral and cellular immunosuppressive elements

The fetal immune system develops early. Lymphocytes are present by the seventh week, and antigen recognition is demonstrable by the twelfth week. All of the immunoglobulin classes except IgA have fetal components present by week 12. Production of the various immunoglobulins is progessive throughout gestation. The newborn fetus at term has developed a sufficient defense system to combat bacterial and viral challenges.

ROLE OF IMMUNOLOGY IN PREGNANCY-ASSOCIATED CONDITIONS

The major pregnancy-associated immunologic disease process is hemolytic disease of the newborn. Rhesus factor incompatibility, which is the most important of these conditions, is discussed in Chapter 27.

Hemolytic disease secondary to non-Rhesus sensitization and the destruction of lymphocytes or platelets secondary to sensitization against specific surface antigens have the same pathogenesis. Fetal cellular antigens leak into the maternal circulation, primarily at birth, and initiate an immune response. The reaction to these foreign antigens is by the humoral component (B cells) of the immune system. Antibody production is initiated, and IgM immunoglobulins, IgG immunoglobulins, or both are produced. Many times no response or only a weak response can be measured. IgG, if present in low concentration, does not cause any appreciable fetal compromise. High levels of IgG, however, can lead to a destructive response if the fetal antigen against which it is directed is present in the current pregnancy or a subsequent one. Antibodies to white cells and platelets are not routinely evaluated. Fetal lymphopenia or thrombocytopenia may occur secondary to maternal sensitization, but these are diagnosed infrequently.

An exception to the above-mentioned mechanism is found in ABO incompatibility, in which naturally occurring antibodies can be found prior to any fetal cellular leakage. These antibodies are generally IgM and not clinically significant. In group O individuals, however, both IgG and IgM antibodies may occur naturally, and the IgG antibodies may cross the placenta. ABO incompatibility occurs largely in mothers of blood group O with infants of blood group A or B. The hemolytic effect is less severe than Rhesus hemolytic disease, and hydrops fetalis does not occur.

Blood transfusions can also sensitize the mother to fetal red cell antigens. If the patient has a history of receiving a red cell transfusion and is sensitized to one of the irregular antigens, it is important to confirm the antigen status of the father, if possible, to determine whether the fetus is at risk for hemolytic disease. For example, if the patient has antibodies to Kell and the father is Kell-negative, the fetus could not inherit the Kell antigen and would therefore not be at risk.

There is evidence to support an important role for immunologic factors in the development of pre-eclampsia. No consistent abnormality has been demonstrated, however, in the immune system of pre-eclamptic patients studied by current techniques, and no definitive description or explanation of the immune anomaly has been presented. Although pre-eclampsia may represent a form of late fetal rejection, the evidence is not yet compelling.

AUTOIMMUNE DISEASE IN PREGNANCY

An autoimmune disease is one in which antibodies are developed against the host's own tissues. A number of autoimmune diseases can significantly affect either the maternal or the fetal outcome in pregnancy. These include rheumatoid arthritis, systemic lupus erythematosus (SLE), idiopathic thrombocytopenic purpura (ITP), isoimmune thrombocytopenia, Graves' disease, and myasthenia gravis. A summary of the interactions of primary immunologic disorders and pregnancy is shown in Table 7–2. In general, the severity of maternal disease depends on the end organ primarily involved. The fetus is affected if an IgG antibody is produced against a vital organ (e.g., anticardiolipin against the cardiac conducting system).

Rheumatoid Arthritis

Rheumatoid arthritis is a chronic systemic disease that affects individuals between the ages of 20 and 60 years, most commonly females. It is manifested primarily in the joints, but extra-articular manifestations may also be present, including subcutaneous nodules on the extensor surfaces of the forearms and involvement of the cardiac, pulmonary, ocular, nervous, and lymphatic systems. As a result of the deposition of immune complexes in the blood vessels, vasculitis may be present. The kidneys are usually spared.

Investigations. Laboratory findings include a normocytic, normochromic anemia; leuko-

penia; elevated platelet count; high sedimentation rate; and hypergammaglobulinemia. The rheumatoid factor may be present in about 80 per cent of the affected individuals, whereas the antinuclear antibody test is positive in about 20 per cent.

Treatment. Drug treatment is recommended for those individuals who are symptomatic or in whom the clinical picture worsens.

Salicylates. Salicylates are the mainstay of drug treatment in rheumatoid arthritis. They intefere with platelet aggregation, although bleeding is rare. The drugs have been used during pregnancy and are known to cross the placental barrier. Maternal side effects include prolonged gestation and greater blood loss during delivery and in the immediate postpartum period. Reports of fetal and neonatal side effects are mainly related to clotting defects. As prostaglandin inhibitors, they pose the potential risks of affecting premature closure of the ductus arteriosus in the fetus and causing pulmonary hypertension in the neonate. Although parents should be aware of the potential maternal and fetal-neonatal risks, clinical experience suggests that salicylates are relatively safe when taken during pregnancy.

Nonsteroidal Anti-inflammatory Agents. These drugs are used when salicylates fail to relieve the inflammatory response. Several preparations are available, among which are indomethacin, ibuprofen, and naproxen. None of these drugs has been studied in depth during pregnancy, although it is known that they cross the placenta and reach the fetus. As antiprostaglandins, they pose risks to the fetus and neonate similar to those of salicylates.

Disease-Suppressive Medications. Such agents include gold, antimalarials, and penicillamine. *Gold* toxicity includes skin rashes, bone marrow suppression, and nephrotoxicity and hepatotoxicity. Gold is protein-bound, crosses the placenta very poorly, and has no reported fetal and neonatal side effects. *Antimalarials* compare favorably with gold. Side effects are mainly gastrointestinal and ocular. Because they cross the placenta readily, they are not recommended during pregnancy. *Penicillamine* compares favorably with gold and has the same drug toxicity problems as

Table 7–2. AUTOIMMUNE DISEASE IN PREGNANCY

DISEASE	EFFECT OF DISEASE ON PREGNANCY Mother	Fetus	EFFECT OF PREGNANCY ON DISEASE	ANTIBODIES THAT CROSS PLACENTA
Rheumatoid arthritis	No significant effect	No significant effect Teratogenic effects of medication	Improved commonly	None
Idiopathic thrombo-cytopenic purpura (ITP)	Ante-, intra-, and postpartum hem-orrhage	Fetal hemorrhage (particularly intra-cranial bleeding)	None	Platelet antibodies
Thrombotic thrombo-cytopenic purpura	No significant effect	Similar to ITP	None	Platelet antibodies
Graves' disease	No significant effect	Intrauterine growth retardation Neonatal thyrotoxi-cosis	Improved during pregnancy Exacerbation post-partum	Long-acting thyroid stimulator (LATS)
Myasthenia gravis	No significant effect	Transient neonatal myasthenia	Variable during pregnancy Moderate exacer-bation postpar-tum	Anti-acetylcholin-esterase
Systemic lupus ery-thematosus	Increased incidence of uterine infec-tion Increased incidence of pre-eclampsia	Abortion (spontane-ous) Prematurity Intrauterine growth retardation Stillbirth Congenital heart block Endomyocardial fibrosis	Exacerbation of disease Deterioration of renal condition Anemia, leuko-penia, and throm-bocytopenia	Various tissues and membranes

gold salts. Because it crosses the placenta, the potential risks to the fetus are enormous. It should not be used during pregnancy.

Cytotoxic Agents. Cyclophosphamide and azathioprine have been used in several controlled trials in patients with rheumatoid arthritis. Their main side effect is bone marrow toxicity. They should be avoided during pregnancy.

Corticosteroids. Although steroids are the best available anti-inflammatory agents, their use should be limited to severe cases in which other drug regimens have failed. Aside from their maternal and fetal side effects, systemic steroids may mask the inflammatory response to the joints and allow bone destruction to proceed unabated. Intra-articular steroids are useful, have limited systemic side effects, and may even be used in pregnant women with

minimal concern about fetal and neonatal well-being.

Prognosis. Prognosis during pregnancy is usually good, with the majority of the patients (75 per cent) showing improvement.

Systemic Lupus Erythematosus

SLE is a chronic connective tissue disease that is characterized by multiple system involvement. The disease tends to affect young women in the second to fourth decades, although it may occur at any age. The incidence of SLE has increased dramatically over the past 2 decades, the present estimate being one case per 1000 population.

Manifestations. The clinical and laboratory manifestations are variable. This prompted

Table 7–3. AMERICAN RHEUMATISM ASSOCIATION CRITERIA FOR DIAGNOSIS OF SYSTEMIC LUPUS ERYTHEMATOSUS

1. Malar rash (butterfly distribution)
2. Discoid rash
3. Photosensitivity
4. Oral ulcers (generally painless)
5. Arthritis (usually polyarthritis and peripheral)
6. Serositis (pleuritis or pericarditis)
7. Renal involvement (persistent proteinuria or cellular casts)
8. Neurologic involvement (seizure or psychosis)
9. Hematologic involvement (hemolytic anemia, leukopenia, lymphopenia, or thrombocytopenia)
10. Immunologic evidence of disorder (positive lupus erythematosus cell, anti-DNA ab, anti-SM ab, or false-positive serologic test for syphilis)
11. Antinuclear antibody

Note: Four or more of these 11 criteria should be present, either serially or simultaneously, to confirm the diagnosis of SLE.

From Tan EM, Cohen AS, Fries JF, et al: The 1982 revised criteria for the classification of systemic lupus erythematosus. Arthritis Rheum 25:1271, 1982.

the American Rheumatism Association to list 11 criteria that include the most common findings in SLE patients (Table 7–3). The presence of any four or more of these manifestations correlates very highly with the clinical presence of lupus.

Once the diagnosis of SLE is made, it is imperative to follow the disease activity. The hallmark of this connective tissue disorder is the presence of various circulating antibodies, including anti-DNA, anti-RNA, antiplatelet, and many others. The presence of anti-DNA and depressed complement levels (C3) are frequently connected with disease activity and specifically with lupus nephritis. In a small number of patients (most probably those who are free of lupus nephritis), there is no correlation between the serologic findings and the activity of the disease.

Association with Pregnancy. Patients with SLE should be counseled against pregnancy during the active phase of the disease. Additionally, they should be informed about the potential maternal, fetal, and neonatal complications. Pregnancy counseling should cover the following areas.

Flare-ups. In patients with mild disease or those who enter the pregnancy with the disease quiescent, no major flare-ups are encountered during pregnancy or the postpartum period.

Genetic Penetrance. First-degree relatives of patients with SLE have about a 12 per cent incidence of the disease, compared with an incidence of 0.001 per cent in the general population.

Pregnancy Outcome. Although fertility rates are not affected in patients with SLE, the abortion and stillbirth rates are much higher than normal. Arteriolitis (decidual vasculitis) affecting the uterine vessels has been implicated. Even if the pregnancy continues, the poor blood supply to the uteroplacental circulation may result in a growth-retarded fetus. Studies suggest a good fetal outcome if renal functions are preserved.

Neonatal Status. A number of offspring have been found with congenital heart block, endomyocardial fibrosis, skin rashes, and circulating antibodies. The association between maternal SLE and fetal-neonatal cardiac conditions is strong, and it is believed that the presence of maternal antibodies (anticardiolipins) to the fetal heart may play a role in their development.

Treatment. The management of SLE in pregnancy does not differ from accepted management practices in the nonpregnant individual. The presence of anti-DNA antibodies and depressed complement levels are suggestive of active disease or impending flare-up. Systemic steroids are the mainstay of treatment, and the daily dose should be adjusted according to the individual needs. Cytotoxic or antimalarial drugs that pose great risk to the fetus should be avoided. If circulating lupus anticoagulant is present, low-dose steroids, salicylates, and low-dose heparin have been reported possibly to be of help. Fetal studies (nonstress test, contraction stress test, obstetric sonograms) are indicated when fetal viability has been reached. The perinatal mortality rate, however, remains extremely high when compared with other groups of patients receiving antepartum surveillance.

The management of labor and delivery follows obstetric indications. Mothers who are using systemic steroids or who have received such medications for a period of several months are at risk of manifesting adrenal insufficiency and should receive intravenous hydrocortisone sodium succinate (Solu-Cortef), 100 mg every 8 hours, or an equivalent dose of corticosteroids, during labor and for 48 to 72 hours after delivery. Patients who were receiving steroids during pregnancy can then revert to their previous dose. If the patient was not on systemic steroids during pregnancy, the steroids commenced during labor may be tapered gradually over a period of several weeks. Breast feeding is not contraindicated during the period of steroid treatment.

Contraceptive Counseling. Contraceptive counseling is essential for patients with SLE. Oral contraceptives are known to induce lupus-like manifestations in healthy women and might worsen the symptoms in patients with SLE. Intrauterine devices may lead to recurrent pelvic infections, especially if steroids or cytotoxic agents are in use by the patient. The risk of heavy vaginal bleeding is increased if thrombocytopenia or a circulating anticoagulant is present. For these reasons, oral contraceptives and intrauterine devices should be avoided. Barrier methods are the safest, although the risk of pregnancy is higher. In patients who have completed their family or in whom the disease is far advanced or debilitating, permanent sterilization is recommended.

Idiopathic Thrombocytopenic Purpura

Although the exact etiology is not known, this entity is associated with SLE, lymphoma, viral infection, and thyroid disease. Available information suggests that platelet production is normal or increased, but peripheral platelet destruction exceeds bone marrow production. An IgG immunoglobulin has been isolated from the plasma of these patients. When this immunoglobulin attaches itself to the platelets, it causes structural damage. Subsequently, these platelets are sequestered in the reticuloendothelial system.

Treatment. Every effort should be made to uncover the underlying etiologic factors and to treat them accordingly. Low platelet counts per se should not be treated. Only when associated petechiae and hemorrhages

are present is treatment recommended. Corticosteroids, in a dose equivalent to 60 to 80 mg per day of prednisone, are given initially, maintained for 2 to 3 weeks, then tapered slowly. Within 2 weeks of commencing corticosteroid treatment, the platelet count increases, although it may remain below control levels. Even in the absence of changes in the platelet level, hemostasis is improved. Splenectomy should be considered for patients who fail to respond to corticosteroid treatment. Platelet transfusions are not usually recommended except in life-threatening situations, since platelets are destroyed quickly in the peripheral circulation.

The treatment of ITP during pregnancy follows the same guidelines already outlined. Because the platelet-associated IgG immunoglobulin crosses the placenta, fetal thrombocytopenia might develop. About 50 per cent of fetal mortality in patients with ITP is attributed to hemorrhage. There is poor correlation between maternal and fetal platelet counts, and a decision to perform a cesarean section should not be based solely on maternal platelet levels. Serious neonatal hemorrhage is unlikely to occur if the neonatal platelet count exceeds $50,000/mm^3$.

Three approaches might be employed for management of labor and delivery in the pregnant patient with ITP.

1. Cesarean section may be performed at or near term and prior to the onset of labor.
2. The onset of spontaneous labor may be awaited. When cervical dilatation allows fetal blood sampling, a fetal platelet count is obtained. If the count is less than $50,000/mm^3$, a cesarean section is done; otherwise, vaginal delivery is allowed.
3. Percutaneous umbilical blood sampling has been used to assess the fetal platelet count antepartum or in early labor before significant cervical dilatation. Labor management is similar to that used when platelet counts are assessed by fetal scalp sampling.

Thrombotic Thrombocytopenic Purpura

Thrombotic thrombocytopenic purpura is a syndrome that includes thrombocytopenic purpura, hemolysis, fragmentation of red blood cells, fever, and neurologic and renal manifestations. The maternal mortality rate is about 80 per cent. In the treatment of thrombotic thrombocytopenic purpura, advances in the initial therapy include exchange transfusions, infusion of fresh frozen plasma, and administration of antiplatelet medication. Splenectomy for maternal indications may be recommended if newer therapeutic approaches are inadequate.

Antiphospholipid Antibodies (Lupus Anticoagulant and Anticardiolipin)

Subclinical autoimmune disease and circulating antibodies to negatively charged phospholids (lupus anticoagulant and anticardiolipin) have been implicated as a cause of recurrent abortion, early fetal loss, severe intrauterine growth retardation, preterm birth, and arterial and venous thrombosis. When these conditions are present and unexplained in a patient, it may be helpful to obtain an antinuclear antibody titer, although patients with immunologic problems represent a small proportion of the total number of patients with these complications of pregnancy. Lupus anticoagulant can be screened for with an activated prothrombin time; a sensitive and specific radioimmunoassay is available for the detection of anticardiolipin. Women with a history of recurrent pregnancy loss may benefit from screening for antiphospholipid antibodies, although no therapy or management has been shown to improve outcome consistently in this group.

Miscellaneous Disorders

The immunologic disorders caused by receptor antibodies, Graves' disease and myasthenia gravis have primary fetal effects. Graves' disease, which is discussed in Chapter 18, can cause neonatal thyrotoxicosis owing to the transplacental passage of long-acting thyroid stimulator. The fetus of the mother with myasthenia gravis can experience transient symptoms of muscle weakness during the neonatal period similar to those experienced by the mother. Both of these conditions are exacerbated postpartum.

SUGGESTED READING

Adelsberg BR: Immunology of pregnancy. Mt Sinai J Med 52:5, 1985.

Beer AE, Billingham RE: The Immunobiology of Mammalian Reproduction. Englewood Cliffs, NJ, Prentice-Hall, 1976.

Bernales R, Bellanti J: Fetal and neonatal immunology. In Quilligan EJ, Kretchmer N (eds): Fetal and Maternal Medicine. New York, Wiley, 1980, p 267.

Cauchi M: Obstetric and Perinatal Immunology. London, Edward Arnold, 1981.

Dhindsa DS, Schumacher GFB: Immunological Aspects of Infertility and Fertility Regulation. Amsterdam, Elsevier, 1980.

Jones WR: Immunological aspects of reproduction. Clin Obstet Gynecol 6(3):383, 1979.

Jones WR, Storey B, Norton G, et al: Pregnancy complicated by acute idiopathic thrombocytopenic purpura. J Obstet Gynaecol Br Commonwealth 81:330, 1974.

Lockshin MD, Gibosky A, Peebles CL, et al: Neonatal lupus erythematosus with heart block: Family study of a patient with anti SS-A and SS-B antibodies. Arthritis Rheum 26:210, 1983.

Oliver TK, Kirschbaum TH, Scott JR (eds): Immunology of Reproduction. In Seminars in Perinatology. New York, Grune & Stratton, 1977

Scott JS, Maddison PG, Taylor PV, et al: Connective tissue disease, antibodies in ribonucleoprotein, and congenital heart block. N Engl J Med 309:209, 1983.

Wegmann TG, Gill TJ: Immunology of Reproduction. London, Oxford University Press, 1983.

Eight

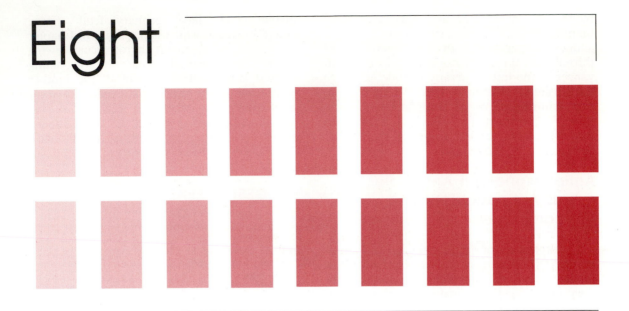

Prenatal Care

CALVIN J. HOBEL

The objective of prenatal care is to assure that every wanted pregnancy is given the maximal chance to culminate in the delivery of a healthy baby, without impairing the health of the mother. It is known that prenatal care is associated with improved reproductive outcome, but it is not certain which components of the total process are responsible. The purpose of this chapter is to describe the components of modern prenatal care.

PREPREGNANCY HEALTH CARE

The concept of prepregnancy health care has been established, and ideally, prenatal care should be a continuation of such a physician-supervised program for women. For example, prepregnancy counseling provides the woman and her husband or the future father of the child with information about the potential risks of a pregnancy (see Chapter 9). Prepregnancy management of the diabetic to assure optimal control of blood glucose levels during the early weeks of pregnancy has the potential of preventing birth defects.

SPECIFIC OBJECTIVES OF PRENATAL CARE

The precise content of prenatal care has been defined by the American College of Obstetricians and Gynecologists. The specific objectives are to prevent and manage those conditions that cause poor pregnancy outcomes. These conditions include premature labor and delivery, intrauterine growth retardation, birth defects, hypertension, diabetes mellitus, perinatal infections, and post-term pregnancy.

COMPONENTS OF PRENATAL CARE

Access to prenatal care is very important. Community education is important, for reaching patients who choose not to seek prenatal care. The majority of prenatal care services are provided outside the hospital setting. Established links among the private physician's office, the community clinic, and the hospital are important to allow access to ancillary services for high-risk patients. This linkage is also important for the timely transfer of antenatal information and the patient's risk status in order to assure appropriate intrapartum and newborn care.

The First Visit

At the first prenatal visit, a thorough history must be taken and physical examination performed, as outlined in Chapter 2. A complete assessment of risk must also be undertaken. This may be done in an organized fashion using a standardized form. One such system is the Problem Oriented Prenatal Risk Assessment System (POPRAS).

In assessing risk at the first and subsequent visits, historical facts must be considered (subjective information), together with the findings on physical examination and the results of laboratory and other special tests (objective information). Problems, risk factors, or both can be listed as "active," "inactive," or "potential." Once problems are identified, a specific plan of action should be established for each problem.

ROUTINE TESTS DURING PREGNANCY

In ordering laboratory tests, it is appropriate to strike a balance between the benefits of the information obtained and the cost of the test. Certain laboratory evaluations, which have either become traditional or are legislatively mandated, may be questioned from the standpoint of cost-effectiveness. Therefore, appropriate individualization should be exercised for each prenatal patient. Table 8–1 lists the commonly performed evaluations.

Table 8–1. PRENATAL LABORATORY TESTS AND INVESTIGATIONS
ROUTINE Cervical cytology Complete blood count (CBC) Urinalysis (UA) and screen for bacilluria Blood group, Rh factor, and antibody screen Serology test for syphilis Rubella antibody titer.

COMMONLY PERFORMED
Blood glucose screen
Serum alpha-fetoprotein (AFP)
Ultrasonography
Tuberculin skin testing
Hepatitis B surface antigen (HBsAG) titer
Urine culture
Cervical culture for
    Neisseria gonorrhoeae
    Group B streptococci
    Chlamydia trachomatis
    Mycoplasma hominis

OTHER TESTS Toxoplasmosis antibody test Hemoglobin electrophoresis

Cervical Cytology

This test should be carried out on every newly pregnant woman unless a normal Papanicolaou smear has been obtained within the past 6 months.

Blood Count

Hematologic investigations can, for all practical purposes, be restricted to the determination of either the hemoglobin concentration or the packed red cell volume (hematocrit). A white cell count and differential are not cost-effective but may identify the rare case of leukemia that occurs during pregnancy if there is any clinical suspicion. Anemic women of Mediterranean extraction should be evaluated with a hemoglobin electrophoresis to detect thalassemia.

Urinalysis

A "clean-catch" midstream urine specimen should be obtained and subjected to the fol-

Table 8–2. SCREENING TESTS FOR DIABETES MELLITUS	
Fasting	<100 mg/dl
1 hour after 50-gm glucose load	<135 mg/dl
2 hours after 100-gm glucose load	<140 mg/dl

lowing tests: (1) analysis for the presence of glucose, ketones, and, protein, (2) microscopic examination of the sediment; and (3) either quantitative culture or a biochemical screen for the presence of bacilluria. This last evaluation is probably cost-effective when balanced against the incidence and associated morbidity of urinary tract infections in pregnancy.

Blood Group, Rhesus Factor, and Antibody Screen

Every pregnant woman should have a blood group, Rhesus (Rh) factor, and antibody screen performed at the first prenatal visit. If discovered on a positive screen, the antibody present can be identified and the patient appropriately managed (see Chapter 27).

Test for Syphilis

A serologic test for syphilis is mandated by law in virtually all states. Early diagnosis and treatment of syphilis reduce perinatal morbidity.

Rubella Antibody Screen

A rubella antibody screen should be done on each prenatal patient who is known to be susceptible (nonimmune) or whose status is unknown. Following delivery, nonimmune women should be offered the rubella vaccine.

Glucose Screen

Glucose screening for gestational diabetes is best carried out between 24 and 28 weeks, when insulin requirements are maximal. Several screening methods are acceptable, as outlined in Table 8–2. Any patient with one

or more of the risk factors listed in Table 8–3 should be screened at the first visit if the visit is prior to 24 weeks.

Serum Alpha-fetoprotein Test

Each pregnant woman should be counseled regarding the availability of the maternal serum alpha-fetoprotein test. This test, which may predict an open neural tube defect, is best carried out between 16 and 20 weeks. Further evaluation of patients with elevated levels is discussed in Chapter 9.

Ultrasonography

Ultrasonic dating of the pregnancy and an ultrasonic fetal survey to detect gross abnormalities have been recommended in some clinics as a routine part of early prenatal care. Routine ultrasonography is most cost-effective in patients in whom the date of the last menstrual period is uncertain and in patients with a family history of congenital anomalies. Considerable individualization should be exercised in making the decision to order this evaluation. If ultrasonography is performed, it is most informative between 16 and 20 weeks.

Tuberculin Skin Testing

All prenatal patients who have no history of tuberculosis should be skin-tested with 0.1 ml of purified protein derivative (PPD) containing 5 tuberculin units. If the test is negative, no further work-up is necessary. If

Table 8–3. RISK FACTORS FOR DIABETES MELLITUS
Age 25 years or older
Obesity
Family history of diabetes mellitus
Previous infant weighing greater than 4000 gm
Previous stillborn infant
Previous congenitally deformed infant
Previous polyhydramnios
History of recurrent abortions

the test is positive and the patient asymptomatic, a chest x-ray study should be obtained. If this is negative, no further work-up is necessary and no treatment should be given antepartum. If active disease is suspected, the patient should be hospitalized and have her sputum, gastric aspirates, and morning urine cultured and tested with acid-fast stains. If tuberculosis is definitively diagnosed, treatment with isoniazid (INH) should begin postpartum and be continued for 6 months to 1 year depending on local health department recommendations.

Hepatitis B Surface Antigen (HBsAG)

The American College of Obstetricians and Gynecologists recommends that this test be performed on all antenatal patients. If the mother is a carrier of the antigen, the infant has a 70 to 90 per cent risk of acquiring hepatitis B virus (HBV) infection and an 85 to 90 per cent risk of becoming a chronic HBV carrier. Treatment of the newborn of a positive mother with hepatitis B immune globin (HBIG) and hepatitis B (HB) vaccine is 85 to 90 per cent effective in preventing the development of the HBV chronic carrier state.

Other Tests

Because of increasing concern for the role of infections as a cause of perinatal morbidity, some clinics routinely culture the urine and cervix at the first prenatal visit. Gonococcal cervicitis is associated with midtrimester loss and must be treated with appropriate antibiotics. A cervical culture identifying group B streptococci and treatment near term may be very helpful in reducing the risk of neonatal infection. A toxoplasmosis antibody test for all cat owners is appropriate. Nonimmune patients should be advised to avoid contact with cats and, particularly, cat excrement. All black women who have not previously been screened for the sickle trait should be screened with a hemoglobin electrophoresis.

SUBSEQUENT PRENATAL CARE

Careful surveillance of the obstetric patient is directed toward the identification of developing problems that may affect the fetus adversely.

Weight Gain

The pregnant patient should be weighed at each visit. A total weight gain of 26 to 28 pounds is ideal for most pregnancies. Excessive weight gain is not harmful, although it may be associated with gestational diabetes. Sudden weight gain in the third trimester is a warning sign of impending pre-eclampsia. Inadequate weight gain or weight gain of less than 10 pounds at 28 weeks is associated with the risk of premature labor or intrauterine fetal growth retardation. Deviation from normal may require counseling or referral to a dietitian.

Urinalysis

At each visit, a urine sample should be checked for sugar and protein. Urine samples obtained in the clinic are usually 2 to 3 hours postprandial and, therefore, may contain sugar. If glycosuria is identified, a repeat sample should be obtained in the fasting state to rule out glycosuria, which is a possible first sign of diabetes. Proteinuria may be a sign of renal disease or pre-eclampsia.

Blood Pressure

Blood pressure should be monitored at each visit to allow early detection of pre-eclampsia. Both the systolic and the diastolic pressures are normally lowest at the end of the second and the beginning of the third trimester.

Gestational Age Estimate and Fundal Height Measurements

At each visit, the gestational age must be assessed and recorded. From 22 weeks until term, the fundal height, measured in centimeters from the symphysis pubis to the top of the fundus, is equivalent to the gestational age in weeks. A discrepancy of greater than 2 to 3 cm suggests a size/dates problem. This may be the first indication of a multiple gestation (size at least 3 cm more than dates) or of intrauterine growth retardation (size at least 3 cm less than dates). An ultrasonic examination is indicated for further evaluation of a size/dates discrepancy.

Examination of the Abdomen

Beginning at 28 weeks, systematic examination of the abdomen is carried out to identify the attitude, lie, presentation, and position of the fetus. The fetal heart should also be auscultated.

The attitude refers to the relationship of parts of the fetus to each other. Normally, the fetus conforms to the shape of the uterus and the attitude is one of complete flexion. The fetus is folded, with its back convex, head flexed, and thighs over the abdomen. The arms are crossed over the thorax leaving a protected space for the umbilical cord between the face and the knees. With a deflexed attitude, as in a brow presentation, the head is extended and the spinal curvature reduced.

The lie of the fetus is the relationship of the long axis of the fetus to the long axis of the mother. The lie can be either longitudinal, transverse, or oblique.

The presenting part is the portion of the fetus that descends first through the birth canal. When the lie is longitudinal, the presenting part is either the head (cephalic presentation) or breech (breech presentation). When the lie is transverse, the presenting part can be the shoulder.

The position refers to the relationship of some definite part of the fetus (the denominator) to the maternal pelvis. For example, in vertex presentations, the denominator is the occiput, whereas in breech presentations, the denominator is the sacrum.

Leopold Maneuvers. The fetal location within the uterus is determined by the maneuvers of Leopold. The first maneuver is carried out with the physician facing the patient's head and standing to one side as she lies supine on the examining table. The ex-

aminer's hands palpate the fundal area and distinguish which part of the fetus occupies the fundus. The head is round and hard, whereas the breech is irregular and soft.

The second maneuver is accomplished when the hands are placed on either side of the abdomen to determine on which side the fetal back lies. The back is linear and firm, whereas the extremities have multiple parts. The location of the back can help determine the position of the fetus.

The third maneuver is done with a single examining hand placed just above the symphysis to determine the presenting part. The presenting part is grasped between the thumb and third finger. The unengaged vertex is round, firm, and ballotable, whereas the breech is irregular and nodular.

The fourth maneuver is done with the examiner facing the patient's feet and placing both hands on either side of the lower abdomen just above the inlet. This maneuver determines head flexion or extension. When pressure is executed in the direction of the inlet, one hand usually descends further than the other. When the head is flexed, the cephalic prominence (brow) preventing descent of one hand is on the same side as the small parts, whereas when the head is extended, the occiput is felt prominently on the same side as the back.

The Leopold maneuvers should be carried out at each visit during the third trimester to identify an abnormal lie, presentation, or position of the fetus.

SPECIAL CONCERNS DURING PREGNANCY

Exercise

Exercise is a very important part of maintaining health. Exercise is beneficial during pregnancy because it helps to maintain a feeling of well-being. The amount of exercise should be maintained at approximately the same level as before pregnancy. A patient who does not exercise should not be advised to begin an aggressive program during pregnancy. A mild exercise program, however, designed to improve strength and flexibility of muscles should be encouraged. Muscle strength and flexibility are thought to improve posture and muscle tone and reduce common discomforts of pregnancy. Aggressive exercise, such as prolonged jogging and skiing, should be avoided because posture changes brought about by the developing fetus can affect balance.

Work

Limiting the amount of work during pregnancy is recommended to avoid fatigue. Heavy forms of housework or heavy employment outside the home should be discouraged. For women who do work, rest periods are recommended to reduce the likelihood of fatigue. Stressful work during pregnancy is associated with a greater risk of preterm delivery and poor fetal growth.

Travel and Change in Residence

In general, travel by car, train, or airplane is not harmful during pregnancy. Fatigue must be avoided, however, by taking frequent rest periods. Of greatest concern is the stress associated with travel or a change in residence, which is thought to be associated with preterm labor.

Sexual Intercourse

Sexual intercourse may continue throughout pregnancy except in patients at risk for abortion or premature labor or in patients with placenta previa. Breast stimulation can induce uterine activity and should also be discouraged in high risk patients. Labor may follow coitus near term, probably because of the effect of prostaglandins in seminal fluid.

Bathing

Tub bathing or showers are permitted during pregnancy. Care must be taken to avoid slipping on the wet surface of the bath or shower because of the mother's altered center of gravity.

ASSESSMENT OF FETAL WELL-BEING

The assessment of fetal health is challenging, since the fetus is not easily seen or heard. During the past 20 years, electronic advances have provided new technology that has made the fetus more accessible and allowed visualization of the fetus and the recording of intrauterine fetal events. A combination of the nonstress test, contraction stress test, and real-time ultrasonic assessment is used to assess fetal well-being.

Figure 8–1 presents an algorithm that may be used to follow a high-risk pregnancy. Table 8–4 indicates the recommended frequency for biophysical profile testing for various high-risk conditions.

Nonstress Test

The first assessment of fetal well-being is the nonstress test. With the mother resting in the lateral supine position, a continuous fetal heart rate tracing is obtained using external Doppler equipment. The mother reports each fetal movement, and the effects of the fetal movements on heart rate are determined. A normal fetus responds to fetal movement with an acceleration in fetal heart rate of 15 beats or more per minute above the baseline for at least 15 seconds (Fig. 8–2). If at least two such accelerations occur in a 20-minute interval, the fetus is regarded as being healthy, and the test is said to be reactive. A nonreactive nonstress test is shown in Figure 8–3.

Ultrasonic Assessment

The next step in prenatal assessment is to determine the adequacy of amniotic fluid volume by real-time ultrasonography. Reduced fluid (oligohydramnios) suggests fetal compromise. Oligohydramnios can be defined by the following: (1) the largest vertical pocket of fluid is less than or equal to 2 cm or (2) the amniotic fluid index (AFI) is less than 5. The AFI represents the total of the linear measurements in centimeters of the largest amniotic fluid pockets noted on ultra-

ANTENATAL TESTING GUIDELINES

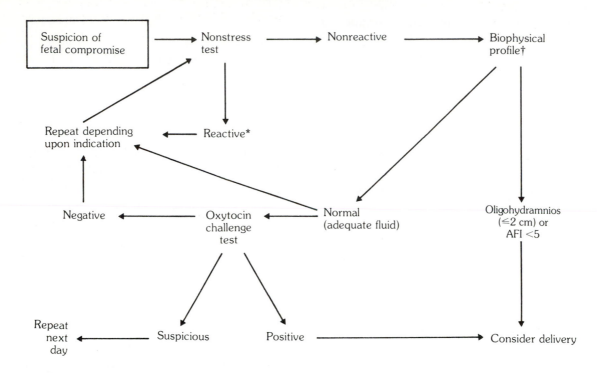

*All pregnancies complicated by IUGR or postdatism should have a complete biophysical profile that includes an ultrasonic evaluation.

†Ultrasonic assessment: (A) fetal movements, 3 per 10 minutes; (B) fetal breathing, 30 per 10 minutes; (C) amniotic fluid, >2 cm in vertical dimension (largest pocket) or amniotic fluid index (AFI) (N = 5–20).

Figure 8–1. Algorithm for the antenatal evaluation of a high-risk pregnancy.

sonic inspection of each of the four quadrants of the gestational sac. When there is reduced amniotic fluid, the fetus is more likely to become compromised as a result of umbilical cord compression. Fetal breathing (chest wall movements) and fetal movements (stretching and rotational movements) are also used to assess the fetus. A fetus who has at least 30 breathing movements in 10 minutes or three body movements in 10 minutes is considered healthy. A combination of a reactive nonstress test, adequate amniotic fluid, and adequate fetal breathing and fetal movement is frequently referred to as a *normal biophysical profile.*

Contraction Stress Test

The contraction stress test is a test for uteroplacental dysfunction, a common condi-

tion in the high-risk pregnancy. A dilute infusion of oxytocin is given to establish at least three uterine contractions in 10 minutes. If late decelerations are observed with each contraction, the test is positive. If only one deceleration is observed, the test is suspicious. When the test is positive, the baby should usually be delivered.

SPECIAL PROGRAMS FOR HIGH-RISK PREGNANCIES

For any high-risk pregnancy, it is essential to establish gestational age as early as possible, preferably during the first trimester. If gestational age is questionable according to either the history or physical examination, an ultrasonogram should be obtained for measurement of the biparietal diameter, head and

Table 8-4. RECOMMENDED FREQUENCY FOR BIOPHYSICAL PROFILE TESTING	
HIGH-RISK CONDITION	**FREQUENCY**
Intrauterine growth retardation (IUGR)	
Mild	Weekly
Moderate*	Twice weekly
Diabetes mellitus	
Class A	Weekly, 37 to 40 weeks
	Twice weekly, beyond 40 weeks
Class B and worse	Twice weekly, beginning at 34 weeks
Post-term pregnancy	Twice weekly, beginning at 42 weeks
Other	
Maternal or physician concern	Weekly
Decreased fetal movements	Weekly
Other high-risk conditions	Weekly

* For severe IUGR, delivery is usually indicated.

abdominal circumferences, and femur length. These measurements establish gestational age as accurately as possible and provide baseline values for future comparison.

For the purpose of illustration, four special problems are discussed that lend themselves to identification, assessment, intervention, and prevention of perinatal morbidity or mortality. These are preterm labor, intrauterine growth retardation, diabetes mellitus, and post-term pregnancy.

Low-Birth-Weight Infants

In modern obstetrics, low birth weight is the leading cause of poor pregnancy outcome. Low-birth-weight infants can be either preterm (less than 37 weeks' gestational age) or growth retarded (small for gestational age). Table 8-5 lists those factors that identify patients at risk for preterm labor and intrauterine growth retardation. Following identification of patients at risk, a special prenatal care program should be instituted to reduce the incidence of the problem.

Preterm Labor

Patients at risk for preterm labor need additional assessments at each prenatal visit. Uterine activity, which is always abnormal prior to 30 weeks, should be monitored and a pelvic examination performed to identify early effacement, cervical dilatation, or both. In addition, these patients should be taught the symptoms and signs of preterm labor and

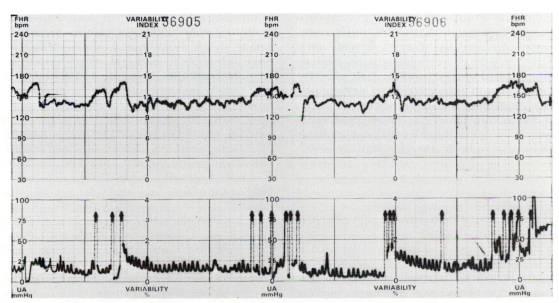

Figure 8-2. Reactive nonstress test. Note the fetal heart rate accelerations with fetal movements.

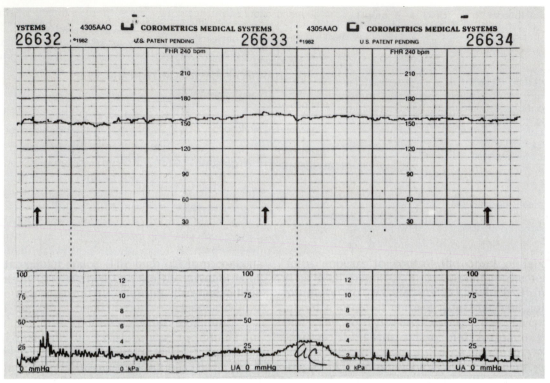

Figure 8-3. Nonreactive nonstress test. Note the lack of beat to beat variability and the lack of acceleration of the fetal heart rate with fetal movements *(arrows)*.

advised to go to the hospital immediately should labor start. They should also be advised to avoid manual labor, sexual intercourse, breast stimulation, long trips, and smoking. As much rest as possible is recommended. Patients with evidence of uterine activity, early cervical changes, or both may require more extensive interventions, such as prolonged bed rest, work leave, and oral tocolytics (uterine relaxants). Most women can be taught self-palpation; uterine activity can also be monitored in the home by visiting nurses or by special devices that can transmit data by telephone to the physician or hospital.

Intrauterine Growth Retardation (IUGR)

One of the first clinical signs suggesting an abnormality of fetal growth is a discrepancy between uterine size and gestational age as determined by the last menstrual period (size/dates discrepancy). When the fundus fails to increase in size, an ultrasonogram should be obtained to facilitate the diagnosis of IUGR. One of the earliest sonographic findings of poor fetal growth is an abdominal circumference below the tenth percentile. When IUGR is diagnosed, serial testing for fetal well-being is indicated (see Table 8-4). Implementation of the interventions listed in Table 8-6 is known to help improve fetal growth, and the abdominal circumference may return to normal (fiftieth percentile). In cases of severe IUGR, all fetal measurements (abdomen, head, and femur) can be reduced. Oligohydramnios (amniotic fluid pocket 2 cm × 2 cm or less on ultrasonography) indicates fetal compromise and warrants induction of labor.

Diabetes

Greater attention is being placed on the early recognition of patients at risk for glu-

Table 8-5. PRENATAL IDENTIFICATION OF HIGH-RISK PREGNANCIES

PRENATAL RISK CONDITION	HISTORICAL RISK FACTORS	DEVELOPING RISK FACTORS
Preterm labor	Previous history of induced abortion, preterm delivery, or neonatal death Habitual abortion Uterine/cervix anomaly History of genitourinary infections Renal disease Smoking Psychiatric hospitalization Low socioeconomic status Maternal age <20 or >35 years Single parent Heavy work Long travel	Size/dates discrepancy Severe anemia Threatened abortion Incompetent cervix Surgery Multiple pregnancy Bleeding after 20 weeks Pre-eclampsia Polyhydramnios Urinary tract infection Preterm effacement and/or dilatation of the cervix Engagement of fetal head before 36 wks
Intrauterine growth retardation	Previous low-birth-weight infant Race (black) Height ≤62 inches Weight ≤100 pounds Narcotic abuse Cigarettes ≥1 pack/day Chronic hypertension	Pregnancy-induced hypertension Threatened abortion Congenital malformations
Diabetes mellitus	Age greater than 25 years Previous macrosomic infant Previous perinatal death Family history of diabetes	Size greater than dates Abnormal screen or glucose tolerance test Multiple pregnancy Polyhydramnios Glycosuria
Post-term	Patient under 19 years of age Previous post-term pregnancy	Threatened abortion Congenital malformations

cose intolerance (see Table 8-3). Once this problem is diagnosed, special interventions are necessary (see Table 8-6), and later in pregnancy antenatal testing is required (see Table 8-4). Early in pregnancy, the fetus is at increased risk for malformations and poor fetal growth, whereas late in pregnancy the fetus is at risk for excessive growth and sudden intrauterine fetal death.

Post-Term Pregnancy

The post-term pregnancy (greater than 42 weeks) has been the most common late pregnancy problem associated with fetal and newborn morbidity and mortality. There are limited prenatal historical and developing problems for early identification of this problem (see Table 8-5). To prevent poor outcome, a systematic approach should be undertaken for the assessment of fetal well-being using a combination of fetal heart rate monitoring, real-time ultrasonic assessment of amniotic fluid volume, fetal breath-

ing patterns, and fetal movements (see Chapter 25). The post-term pregnancy requiring this special assessment is usually one without other medical problems and with a cervix not favorable for induction of labor.

PREVENTIVE HEALTH CARE

Management prior to and during pregnancy presents an opportunity for patient education and the practice of preventive medicine. Most women do not have regular contact with a team of health care professionals at any other time in their lives. Childbirth preparation classes for both the patient and her husband are very educational, particularly during the first pregnancy. The presence and encouragement of the baby's father can be most helpful during labor and delivery. These classes provide an important opportunity for both parents to enhance bonding to the infant before birth.

Although prenatal and obstetric information is of primary importance, other topics

Table 8–6. PRENATAL INTERVENTIONS FOR SELECTED HIGH-RISK CONDITIONS

PRENATAL RISK CONDITION	SELECTED ASSESSMENT	SELECTED INTERVENTIONS
Preterm labor	Uterine activity Cervical length and dilatation	Patient education Bed rest (3 times daily) Work leave Oral tocolytics
Intrauterine growth retardation	Uterine activity Fetal assessment	Patient education Bed rest Early management of medical problems Nutritional counseling Stop smoking
Diabetes mellitus	Home glucose monitoring Fetal assessment	Patient education Dietary management Insulin
Post-term	Fetal assessment	Induction of labor if abnormal fetal assessment profile or ripe cervix

that may have lifelong relevance can be introduced and emphasized during prenatal care. The pregnancy itself is frequently a strong motivator for women to eliminate potentially harmful habits or dietary patterns and to become more aware of their general health. Therefore, a systematic approach to the dissemination of preventive health care information will generally be well received by the pregnant woman at this time.

SUGGESTED READING

A report of the Public Health Service Expert Panel on the content of prenatal care: Caring for our future: The content of prenatal care. Washington, DC, Public Health Service Department of Health and Human Services, 1989.

Bragonier JR, Cushner IM, Hobel CJ: Social and personal factors in the etiology of preterm birth. In Fuchs F, Stubblefield PG (eds): Preterm Birth, Causes, Prevention, and Management. New York, Macmillan, 1984, p 64.

Cefalo RC, Moos MK (eds): Preconceptional Health Promotion, A Practical Guide. Rockville, Md, Aspen Publishing, 1988.

Collings CA, Curet LB, Mullin JP: Maternal and fetal responses to a maternal aerobic exercise program. Am J Obstet Gynecol 145:702, 1983.

Committee Reports, Nutrition During Pregnancy: Part I, Weight Gain, Part II, Nutrition Supplements: Institute of Medicine. Washington, DC, National Academy Press, 1990.

Evertson LR, Paul RH: Antepartum fetal heart rate testing: The nonstress test. Obstet Gynecol 132:895, 1978.

Freeman RK, Anderson G, Dorchester W: A prospective multi-institutional study of antepartum fetal heart rate monitoring. II. Contraction stress test versus nonstress test for primary surveillance. Am J Obstet Gynecol 143:778, 1982.

Fuhrmann K, Reiher H, Semmler K, et al: Prevention of congenital malformations in infants of insulin-dependent diabetic mothers. Diabetes Care 6:219, 1983.

Hobel CJ: Routine antenatal laboratory tests. In Queenan J, Hobbins J (eds): Protocols for High-Risk Pregnancies. Oradell, NJ, Medical Economics Co Inc, 1982, p 19.

Hobel CJ: Identification of the patient at high-risk. In Bolognese RJ, Schwarz RH (eds): Perinatal Medicine: Management of the High-Risk Fetus and Neonate. Baltimore, Williams & Wilkins, 1978.

Iams JD, Johnson FF, O'Shaughnessy RW: A prospective random trial of home uterine activity monitoring in pregnancies at risk of preterm labor II. Am J Obstet Gynecol 159:595, 1988.

Main DM, Gabbe SG, Richardson D, Strong S: Can preterm deliveries be prevented? Am J Obstet Gynecol 151:892, 1985.

Manning FA, Platt LA, Sipo L: Antepartum fetal evaluation: Development of a fetal biophysical profile. Am J Obstet Gynecol 136:787, 1980.

Merkatz IR, Thompson JE (eds): New Perspectives on Prenatal Care. New York, Elsevier, 1990.

National Institute of Health: Consensus development conference on diet and exercise in noninsulin-dependent diabetes mellitus. Diabetes Care 10:639, 1987.

Phelan JP, Smith CV, Broussard P, Small M: Amniotic fluid volume assessment with four-quadrant technique at 36–42 weeks gestation. J Reprod Med 32:540, 1987.

Tafari N, Naeye RL, Cobezie A: Effects of maternal undernutrition and heavy physical work during pregnancy on birth weight. Br J Obstet Gynaecol 87:222, 1980.

Nine

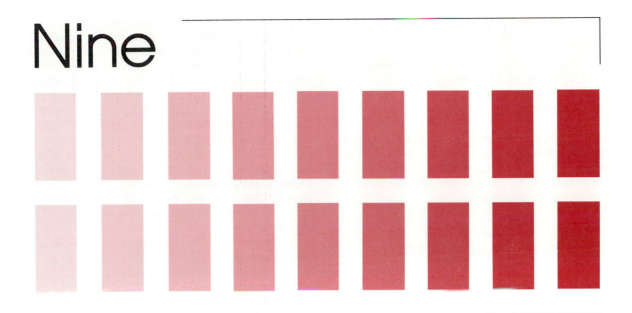

Genetic Evaluation and Teratology

ANN GARBER, MICHELLE FOX, AND KHALIL TABSH

A comprehensive approach to the pregnant patient includes identification of women with an increased risk for carrying a malformed fetus based on genetic or teratogenic risk factors. Physicians must be cognizant of current genetic screening and diagnostic issues and the effects of an increasing number of medications and other environmental hazards on the developing fetus. A growing number of fetal abnormalities are now prenatally diagnosable as a result of expanding technology in the areas of ultrasonography and molecular diagnosis.

PATIENTS REQUIRING GENETIC COUNSELING

As a result of technologic advances, genetic counseling has become increasingly important. The most significant screening tool available to every physician is the personal and family history. Ideally, couples should be questioned about their health history before they decide to have children, so that genetic disease in the patient or her family may be identified before pregnancy. Women with ongoing exposure to certain environmental agents also need to be appropriately counseled before pregnancy, so that teratogenic risks can be minimized.

The major reason couples are referred for prenatal diagnosis is age. Women over 34 years of age have an increased risk of giving birth to children with chromosomal abnormalities. Other major indications for prenatal diagnosis include:

1. A previous child or family history of birth defects, mental retardation, chromosomal abnormality, or known genetic disorder.

2. Multiple fetal losses.

3. A baby who has died in the neonatal period.

4. Maternal conditions predisposing the fetus to congenital abnormalities.

5. A current pregnancy history of teratogenic exposure.

It is crucial to establish an accurate diagnosis of the affected family member by obtaining medical records, autopsy reports, and laboratory data or by having the family member examined by a geneticist.

CONGENITAL AND HEREDITARY DISORDERS

Chromosome Disorders

Chromosome abnormalities occur in 0.5 per cent of live births, but the incidence associated with spontaneous abortions is much higher and estimated to be approximately 50 per cent. The most common chromosomal abnormalities among liveborn infants are sex chromosomal aneuploidies (i.e., Turner's syndrome, Klinefelter's syndrome), balanced robertsonian translocations (translocations between groups D and D or D and G), and autosomal trisomies such as Down's syndrome.

Women over 34 years of age are at increased risk of giving birth to children with autosomal trisomies (i.e., trisomy 21, 13, or 18) (Figs. 9–1 and 9–2). The overall incidence of Down's syndrome is one per 800 live births. It increases to about one per 300 live births for women who are 35 to 39 years of age and to about one in 80 for those 40 to 45 years of age (Table 9–1). The incidence of Down's syndrome diagnosed at the time of amniocentesis is considerably higher. In women 35 to 39 years of age, the rate is about one in 125; in those 40 to 45, it is about one in 20. The discrepancy between the rate of occurrence at delivery and that at amniocentesis is believed to be due in part to fetal loss in the late second and third trimesters.

Ninety-five per cent of cases of Down's syndrome are due to meiotic nondisjunction leading to 47 chromosomes with an extra copy of chromosome 21, whereas 4 per cent of Down's syndrome cases are due to an unbalanced translocation. Parents of a child with translocation Down's syndrome should be karyotyped to exclude the possibility of a familial balanced translocation. The most common translocations causing Down's syndrome are rearrangements between chromosome 21 and chromosomes 14, 15, 21, or 22. The remaining 1 per cent of individuals with Down's syndrome are mosaics, having two populations of cells, one with 46 chromosomes (a normal karyotype) and one with 47 chromosomes.

A couple who has had a previous child with trisomy 21 (Down's syndrome) or another meiotic nondisjunctional type of chromosomal abnormality is believed to be at a small increased risk (about 1 per cent) of giving birth to another child with a chromosomal abnormality and should be referred for amniocentesis.

Approximately one in 500 individuals carries a balanced translocation. Blood chromosomal studies should be performed on a couple following three or more spontaneous abortions because in approximately 3 to 5 per cent of such couples, one member is a balanced translocation carrier. The recurrence risk for spontaneous abortion, abnormal offspring, or both is greatly increased among balanced translocation carriers and can be estimated according to the type of translocation present. These couples should be alerted to the advisability of prenatal diagnosis because of their increased risk for liveborn children with unbalanced translocations.

Single Gene Disorders

Single gene disorders are relatively uncommon, but they can result in significant medical and psychosocial problems. These disorders follow the laws of mendelian inheritance and may be passed from generation to generation such as with autosomal dominant disorders; they may affect siblings without a history of other affected family members, such as in autosomal recessive disorders; or they may be x-linked recessive with males

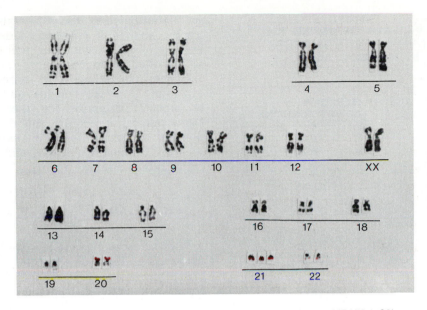

Figure 9–1. Karyotype of a patient with Down's syndrome (47,XX + 21).

being affected and healthy females transmitting the abnormal gene.

Autosomal Dominant Disorders

In autosomal dominant disorders, only one abnormal gene is necessary for disease manifestation. The affected individual has a 50 per cent chance of passing the gene and the disorder on to each of his or her offspring. Unaffected offspring cannot pass on the gene or the disorder. The occurrence and transmission of the genes are usually not influenced by gender; males and females are equally affected.

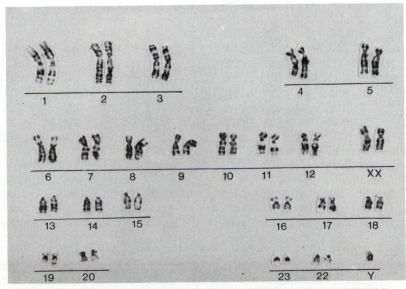

Figure 9–2. Karyotype of a patient with Klinefelter's syndrome (47,XXY).

Table 9-1. RISK OF HAVING AN INFANT WITH DOWN'S SYNDROME BY MATERNAL AGE

MATERNAL AGE (years)	FREQUENCY OF DOWN'S SYNDROME
30	1/885
31	1/826
32	1/725
33	1/592
34	1/465
35	1/365
36	1/287
37	1/225
38	1/176
39	1/139
40	1/109
41	1/85
42	1/67
43	1/53
44	1/41
45	1/32
46	1/25
47	1/20
48	1/16
49	1/12

From Hook EB, Chambers GM: Estimated rates of Down's syndrome in live births by one year maternal age intervals in a New York State study—implications of the risk figures for genetic counselling and cost-benefit analysis of prenatal diagnosis programs. Birth Defects: Orig Art Ser 13(3A):123, 1977.

A spontaneous mutation of genetic material in the germ cells of clinically normal parents can also result in an affected offspring. A hallmark of autosomal dominant disease is the variable expressivity. It is important to determine whether a child is affected by a spontaneous mutation or is the product of a parent with minimal expression of the same gene. A careful history and physical examination of family members, in addition to possible biochemical, radiologic, or histologic testing, may be necessary to determine the parents' genetic status.

Some of the common autosomal dominant disorders include tuberous sclerosis, neurofibromatosis, achondroplasia, craniofacial synostosis, adult-form polycystic kidney disease, and several types of muscular dystrophy. Until more recently, most of these disorders could not be diagnosed prenatally. Now many autosomal dominant genes have been mapped, including those for neurofibromato-

sis, Huntington's disease, myotonic dystrophy, and adult polycystic kidney disease. Using molecular techniques, prenatal diagnosis can often be undertaken.

Genetic counseling is an essential step in explaining the risks, benefits, and limitations of prenatal diagnosis for these disorders. Many ethical issues are raised in offering prenatal diagnosis for late-onset disorders such as Huntington's disease and adult polycystic kidney disease.

Autosomal Recessive Disorders

With autosomal recessive disorders, two affected genes must be present for manifestation of the disease. Usually there is no family history of another affected individual. If there is a family history, siblings of either sex are equally as likely to be affected. Consanguineous couples are at an increased risk for having a child who is homozygous for a deleterious recessive gene, with subsequent pregnancies being at a 25 per cent risk for producing a similarly affected child.

Many autosomal recessive disorders may be diagnosed prenatally. Biochemical genetic disorders (e.g., Tay-Sachs disease) can be diagnosed by enzymatic assay, whereas others (sickle cell anemia, beta-thalassemia, and cystic fibrosis) are diagnosable by DNA analysis from amniocytes or chorionic villi.

Genetic Screening for Autosomal Recessive Disorders

Carrier screening programs for autosomal recessive disorders have traditionally focused on high-risk populations, in which the frequency of heterozygotes is greater than in the general population. Tay-Sachs screening among the Eastern European Jewish and French Canadian populations has proved to be particularly successful in the recognition of couples with a 25 per cent risk for offspring affected with this fatal disease. With comprehensive genetic counseling, many couples, aware of their positive carrier status, elect to use chorionic villus sampling (CVS) or amniocentesis or explore other reproductive options. Frequently, couples will be identified in which only one member of the

Table 9-2. SELECTED AUTOSOMAL RECESSIVE DISEASES IN DEFINED ETHNIC GROUPS

DISEASE	ETHNIC GROUP	CARRIER FREQUENCY
Sickle cell disease	Blacks	1/10
Cystic fibrosis	Whites	1/25
Tay-Sachs disease	Jews, French Canadians	1/30
Thalassemia	Mediterraneans Southeast Asians	1/25

couple is a carrier. These individuals may respond with significant anxiety to such results and benefit by careful counseling to help them understand their risk situation. Table 9-2 lists selected autosomal recessive disorders for which genetic screening has been initiated.

The most common gene carried by North American whites is the cystic fibrosis gene (carrier frequency: 1/25). Until more recently, carrier detection was not possible. Now with the use of recombinant DNA technology, the cystic fibrosis gene has been mapped to chromosome number 7, and a gene deletion (delta-F508) has been found in approximately 70 per cent of carriers. Genetic counseling is essential when offering cystic fibrosis carrier detection to ensure that patients understand that up to 30 per cent of carriers (and maybe more depending on ethnic group) may go undetected with current technology. In families in which the affected family member is alive, a combination of linkage analysis and deletion studies provides the most accurate information and may make prenatal diagnosis possible.

Sex-Linked Disorders

Sex-linked disorders, caused by recessive genes located on the X chromosome, primarily affect males, whereas unaffected (or mildly affected) females carry the deleterious gene. There is no male to male transmission of X-linked disorders. Until more recently, the female carrier of an X-linked recessive gene was faced with aborting any male fetus she carried because the affected male could not be distinguished from the normal male. Using recombinant DNA technology, many sex-linked disorders such as Duchenne's muscular dystrophy (DMD) or fragile-X syndrome can now be diagnosed by CVS or amniocentesis.

X-linked disorders can occur because of new mutations of genetic material as a sporadic event or from the inheritance of the X-linked recessive gene from the carrier mother. In some cases, it may be difficult to distinguish between the two situations. Fifty per cent of the males born to carrier females will be affected with the X-linked disorder. Similarly, 50 per cent of carrier females' daughters will also be carriers.

The DMD gene has been mapped and isolated, and the protein produced by this gene has been identified (dystrophin). In 60 to 65 per cent of DMD families, a deletion on the short arm of the X chromosome (Xp21) has been detected. The finding of a deletion in the dystrophin gene confirms the diagnosis of DMD and can identify carrier status in females. In addition, prenatal diagnosis can be offered for carrier females. In families without an identifiable deletion, linkage analysis studies requiring the study of multiple family members can be offered. The discovery of the dystrophin gene has enabled scientists to study the basic mechanism of the disorder and develop a therapeutic intervention.

Fragile-X syndrome is an X-linked disorder that is the second most common form of mental retardation after Down's syndrome, with an incidence of about one in 1000 males. Mental impairment is variable in heterozygous females, with as many as 70 per cent of carriers demonstrating mild to severe retardation. Prenatal diagnosis is possible using a combination of cytogenetic studies to detect the fragile site on the long arm of the X chromosome and molecular analysis.

Multifactorial Disorders

In single gene disorders, there is a known and predictable pattern of inheritance. The majority of birth defects, however, are inherited in a multifactorial fashion, which means

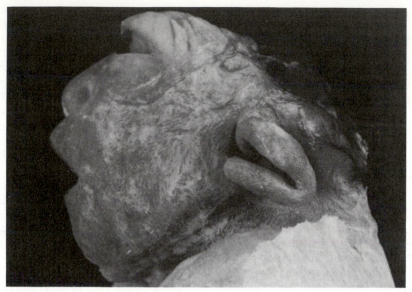

Figure 9–3. Infant with anencephaly. Note the absence of development of the vault of the skull caused by congenital absence of the forebrain.

that both genes and the environment play a role. Common multifactorial disorders include cleft lip or palate, neural tube defects (spina bifida or anencephaly), congenital heart defects, and pyloric stenosis.

Neural tube defects occur in about one per 1000 births in the United States. In Northern Ireland, Wales, and Scotland, the incidence of neural tube defects is 6 to 8 per 1000 births. Both anencephaly (congenital absence of the forebrain) (Fig. 9–3) and spina bifida (open spine) are believed to occur prior to 30 days' gestation because of failure of the neural tube to close. Newborns with anencephaly are stillborn or die within the first few days of life. Newborns with spina bifida have a variable course, depending on the site of the lesion and whether it is a meningocele (herniation of the meninges through an open spinal defect with the cord remaining in its usual position) or a myelocele (herniation of the spinal cord). Infants with a myelocele are at risk for muscle paralysis or weakness below the level of the lesion and incontinence of bowel and bladder. In approximately 75 per cent of cases, hydrocephalus is also present.

With multifactorial disorders in general and in neural tube defects in particular, the couple who has given birth to one affected child has an increased risk of approximately 3 per cent of giving birth to another similarly affected child.

Maternal Serum Alpha-Fetoprotein Screening

Alpha-fetoprotein (AFP) levels are frequently elevated in blood samples of women carrying fetuses affected with neural tube defects. Approximately 80 to 85 per cent of all open neural tube defects can be detected by maternal serum AFP (MSAFP). In addition to open neural tube defects, ventral wall defects (gastroschisis or omphalocele) can cause elevations of MSAFP. MSAFP screening takes place optimally in the sixteenth to eighteenth week of gestation. If the MSAFP level is elevated, ultrasonography is done to rule out multiple gestation, fetal demise, or inaccurate gestational age (all of which can give false-positive results). If none of these factors contributes to the elevated serum AFP level, an amniocentesis is recommended to determine the amniotic fluid AFP level and measure acetylcholinesterase (AChE). AChE is a protein that is present only if there is an open neural tube defect. For reasons still unclear, patients who have normal amniotic fluid AFP levels following an elevated

MSAFP level are considered at increased risk for third-trimester complications.

An association between low MSAFP and Down's syndrome has been noted. Prior to MSAFP screening, only maternal age was used to screen for Down's syndrome. Using MSAFP screening, it is estimated that 20 per cent of fetal Down's syndrome can be detected in mothers under 35 years of age. The first step following a low MSAFP result is ultrasonography to rule out a dating discrepancy or fetal demise which may account for a low MSAFP level. Following the ultrasonography, an amniocentesis is performed to establish the fetal karyotype. The sensitivity of MSAFP screening for trisomy 21 is improved further when maternal serum human chorionic gonadotropin and unconjugated estriol concentrations are also considered. Although positive-low MSAFP will detect about 20 per cent of Down's syndrome pregnancies, the combination of low MSAFP, low unconjugated estriol, and elevated human chorionic gonadotropin will detect at least 60 per cent of Down's syndrome pregnancies. Prenatal screening using all three chemical markers has the potential for replacing maternal age as the primary variable for determining which women should undergo amniocentesis. At the present time, many patients do not schedule their first prenatal visit until after 20 weeks of pregnancy and are thus unable to take advantage of screening. Studies have shown that abnormal MSAFP results are associated with a significant increase in parental anxiety. Genetic counseling is an essential component of screening programs to provide education and alleviate anxiety for patients with abnormal test results.

DIAGNOSTIC PROCEDURES

Recombinant DNA technology coupled with first-trimester fetal tissue sampling has enhanced the growth and development of prenatal diagnosis. Genetic counseling must be included as an integral part of prenatal diagnosis so that patients are well informed of the risks, benefits, and limitations of the procedures and laboratory testing. Counseling must include the fact that other chromosomal abnormalities in addition to Down's syndrome can be diagnosed. Many couples are faced with difficult decisions regarding the fetal diagnosis of Turner's syndrome (45,XO) or Klinefelter's syndrome (47,XXY), both of which are characterized by growth and learning problems but are not commonly associated with severe mental retardation.

Patients must be reminded that prenatal diagnosis is not a guarantee of a normal, healthy baby. Every female undertaking a pregnancy has a 3 to 4 per cent risk of delivering a baby with structural congenital anomalies, a genetic disorder, or both.

Amniocentesis

Amniocentesis, the withdrawal of amniotic fluid from the amniotic sac, is the most widely used prenatal diagnostic test. It was originally used in the 1950s to analyze amniotic fluid for evidence of Rh sensitization during the third trimester of pregnancy. Techniques for culturing amniotic cells became available in the 1960s and led to the first prenatal diagnosis of Down's syndrome in 1967.

Patients should be informed about the two types of fetal abnormalities that are routinely evaluated with this technique: chromosomal disorders and neural tube defects. Amniotic fluid AFP values are done routinely, even though the problem of neural tube defects is not age-related.

Amniocentesis is an outpatient procedure performed 16 to 20 weeks after the first day of the last menstrual period. Guided by ultrasonography, a 20- or 21-gauge needle with a stylet is introduced through the abdominal wall under sterile conditions. The stylet is removed and 20 ml of amniotic fluid is aspirated. The initial 2 ml of amniotic fluid may be discarded to lessen the chance of maternal contamination. Chromosomal analysis of cultured amniotic cells takes approximately 10 to 14 days. Most reports indicate a 99 to 99.6 per cent accuracy rate for chromosomal results.

Early Amniocentesis

Early amniocentesis is defined as an amniocentesis performed at less than 15 weeks gestation. It is often offered to patients in whom CVS cannot be performed. Chromosome analysis and AFP measurement can be done at the time of early amniocentesis. The risks associated with early amniocentesis may be slightly increased when compared with amniocentesis at 16 weeks.

Chorionic Villus Sampling

CVS is usually performed between 9 and 12 weeks gestation. The procedure can be done by a transabdominal or transcervical approach depending on anatomic and clinical considerations. Direct study of the dividing cells can identify a chromosomal abnormality in 48 hours. Indirect study or culturing the cells provides confirmatory results in approximately 10 to 14 days. Biochemical genetic disorders can also be diagnosed by this method. Enzyme determination for Tay-Sachs disease, for example, can be obtained in less than 24 hours. Using recombinant DNA technology and the polymerase chain reaction, DNA analysis using a direct or indirect method can also be readily applied to CVS tissue.

The risk of miscarriage associated with CVS is about 1 per cent above the background risk of miscarriage in the first trimester. Many women over 35 are choosing CVS rather than amniocentesis because of the advantages of first-trimester termination in the event of an abnormality. AFP cannot be measured by CVS, and maternal serum screening is routinely recommended for all patients using this prenatal diagnostic technique.

Placental Biopsy

The technique of transabdominal CVS can be applied to later pregnancies for the purpose of rapid fetal karyotyping. Using the direct method, a cytogenetic result is usually available within 48 hours. A common indication for second-trimester or third-trimester placental biopsy is abnormal ultrasonic findings that put the pregnancy at an increased risk for a fetal chromosomal abnormality. The availability of rapid results is particularly important in late pregnancy when knowledge of the fetal karyotype is essential for obstetric management. Although the initial results of second-trimester or third-trimester placental biopsy are encouraging, the safety and accuracy of this procedure remain to be comprehensively assessed. In particular, the quality of the placental karyotype as well as the evaluation of diagnostic problems such as confined placental mosaicism still need to be addressed.

Percutaneous Umbilical Blood Sampling (Cordocentesis)

Percutaneous umbilical blood sampling is an outpatient procedure in which a fetal blood sample is obtained from the umbilical vein at the placental insertion site under ultrasonic guidance. The procedure is usually performed between 10 and 22 weeks gestation. A fetal blood sample is required for prenatal diagnosis of some genetic disorders and to assess other obstetric complications. It is also used to obtain a rapid fetal karyotype when an abnormal ultrasonic result suggests a chromosomal disorder or to assess further the fetal karyotype when mosaicism is detected by CVS or amniocentesis.

Ultrasonography

Ultrasonography by an experienced ultrasonographer is extremely useful as a diagnostic procedure to identify structural abnormalities of the fetus. It is the primary tool available to assess the fetus exposed to teratogenic agents. Structural defects that have been diagnosed with this technique include craniospinal abnormalities (anencephaly, hydrocephaly, spina bifida, holoprosencephaly, microcephaly), gastrointestinal anomalies (omphalocele, gastroschisis), excretory system anomalies (renal agenesis, renal dysplasia, urinary obstruction), skeletal dysplasias, and congenital heart defects.

Diabetic women are at an increased risk for delivering children with birth defects, such as congenital heart defects, skeletal defects, and neural tube defects. Echocardiograms of the fetus are now being used to delineate congenital heart defects in diabetic women and in women who have had a previously affected child or who themselves have a congenital heart defect. In addition, fetal cardiac arrhythmias can be studied by echocardiography.

Endovaginal ultrasonography is used primarily in the first trimester to establish fetal viability.

Recombinant DNA Technology

Over 4000 mendelian disorders are catalogued by McKusick. Only about 200 of these disorders can be identified by specific biochemical or enzymatic assays. Now using recombinant DNA technology, the gene structure can be studied at the molecular level even without knowing the underlying enzyme deficiency or abnormal gene product. In some cases, detection of a single nucleotide mutation in the nucleotide sequence can allow for the diagnosis of a single gene disorder, such as sickle cell anemia.

The first step in DNA analysis is the isolation of DNA from a particular cell type (villi, amniocytes, white blood cells, or skin fibroblasts). Restriction enzymes cut the DNA at specific sequences. The resulting DNA fragments are separated by size using agarose gel electrophoresis. The DNA is denatured and transferred to a nitrocellulose membrane called a Southern blot. The filterbound DNA fragments are hybridized to known radioactive DNA fragments or probes. Unhybridized DNA fragments are washed away, and the filter is autoradiographed. Depending on the specific banding pattern, a diagnosis of carrier status, noncarrier status or affected individual can be made.

Direct detection of genetic disorders can be accomplished when the specific mutation causes an identifiable nucleotide change, such as is seen with sickle cell anemia and some of the thalassemias. In other cases, such as Duchenne's muscular dystrophy, the disorder is caused by a deletion or absence of a number of nucleotides; restriction enzymes are available that recognize the specific site of the deletion. Most genetic disorders cannot be detected in this manner because the specific mutation or deletion is unknown.

In cases in which the disease mutation cannot be detected directly, family studies using indirect detection or linkage analysis can be used. Genes that are located close together on a chromosome are usually inherited together and are considered "linked." Linkage analysis uses normal variations, or polymorphisms, in the DNA makeup within a family to recognize a specific gene known to be very close to the disease-related gene under study. If the gene being studied is linked to known polymorphism, the transmission of the gene can be tracked within a family. Linkage analysis requires samples from the affected individual and from several close family members.

One of the problems associated with DNA analysis has been the large amount of tissue required to provide sufficient DNA. A new technique, polymerase chain reaction, has had a widespread impact on DNA analysis. Using this technique, very small amounts of DNA (e.g., a few cells obtained from CVS) can be amplified rapidly and used for direct and indirect molecular analysis.

TERATOLOGY

A teratogen is any agent or factor that can cause abnormalities of form or function (birth defects) in an exposed fetus. Such abnormalities include fetal wastage and intrauterine fetal growth retardation, malformations due to abnormal growth and morphogenesis, and abnormal central nervous system performance.

It was not until the teratogenic effects of rubella infection were demonstrated in 1941 that any notable consideration was given to environmental factors and their potential deleterious effects on human pregnancy. In the succeeding decades, the susceptibility of the fetus to many environmental factors has been appreciated.

Probably the best known teratogen is thalidomide, which was shown to cause phocomelia and other malformations in the offspring of mothers who had been given the drug during pregnancy. Thalidomide is unique in that it is the only example of a teratogen that when introduced to the pregnant population led to a dramatic epidemic of a specific malformation; withdrawal of the drug led to a virtual disappearance of the malformation. The thalidomide experience provided compelling evidence that, unless proved otherwise, chemical and physical agents must be seriously regarded as having a potential for adverse effects on the human fetus. In 1962, drug law amendments were enacted that led to regulations requiring that new drugs not be administered to pregnant women until preliminary studies indicated reasonable evidence of the drug's safety and effectiveness in animals and subsequently in men and nonpregnant women.

Although drugs are the most obvious source for teratogenic exposure, clinicians must also take measures to protect the pregnant patient from the potential hazards associated with today's technology and lifestyle. Chemical waste disposals, alcohol, tobacco, cosmetics, and occupational agents are substances that individuals are exposed to daily. Some of these agents are known teratogens, whereas the fetal effects of others are not known.

Exposure

Several studies indicate that pregnant women are being exposed to a large number of potential teratogens. Results of the Collaborative Perinatal Project indicate that during the first trimester alone, as many as 32 per cent of pregnant women are exposed to analgesics (mostly aspirin); 18 per cent to immunizing agents; 16 per cent to antimicrobial and antiparasitic agents; and 6 per cent to sedatives, tranquilizers, and antidepressants. Although some teratogenic exposures are unavoidable, the great majority of agents, including radiation and drugs, are readily avoidable.

Pathogenic Mechanisms

Teratogens may affect embryogenesis by the disturbance of one or more developmental processes. They may produce hypoplasia or hyperplasia of developing tissues, failure of cellular differentiation or interaction, or mechanical disruption of a cell. Often the end result of teratogenic action is an organ with too few cells. Subsequently, the organ system may fail to develop fully because of lack of a critical mass required for cellular differentiation.

Table 9–3. FACTORS THAT INFLUENCE THE EFFECT OF TERATOGENIC AGENTS
Nature and dose of agent Stage of embryonic development Fetal susceptibility Interaction with other environmental factors Maternal metabolism agent

Cell growth, differentiation, interaction, and migration are basic characteristics of embryologic development. Thus, environmental insults frequently affect more than one tissue or organ system. Cellular disturbances can occur as a result of many different teratogenic agents, and, conversely, the effect of a particular teratogen is influenced by a number of important factors (Table 9–3). In addition, congenital anomalies frequently caused by teratogenic agents also occur in fetuses not exposed to teratogens. Although teratogenicity is difficult to prove in humans, evidence of one or more of the observations listed in Table 9–4 provides support for a teratogenic insult.

Principles of Teratology

Fetal Susceptibility

The efficacy of a particular teratogen is, in part, dependent on the genetic makeup of both mother and fetus as well as on a num-

Table 9–4. INDICATORS OF POTENTIAL TERATOGENICITY IN HUMANS
Case-control studies demonstrate a relationship between exposure to agent and a particular anomaly The timing of exposure is consistent with embryologic development of malformed organs Incidence of an anomaly rises on introduction of a new drug Animal studies confirm relationship between a particular agent and a specific malformation

ber of factors related to the maternal-fetal environment. For instance, many congenital abnormalities, such as oral clefts, congenital heart disease, and neural tube defects, are inherited through multifactorial inheritance. These types of birth defects are thought to be due to a combination of several genetic and environmental insults. The recurrence risk for a similar abnormality in subsequent pregnancies is small but increased compared with the risk in the overall population. Thus, some fetuses are predisposed to certain malformations because of their genetic makeup; such fetuses would be particularly susceptible to teratogens that raise the risk for that malformation.

Fetal vulnerability may also be influenced by maternal variability in the ability to metabolize a teratogen, maternal variability in the rate of placental transfer, or differences in fetal metabolism.

Dose

Depending on the particular teratogen, there may be (1) no apparent effect at a low dose, (2) an organ-specific malformation at an intermediate dose, or (3) a spontaneous abortion at a high dose. Additionally, smaller doses administered over several days may produce a different effect from a single large dose.

Timing

Three stages of teratogenic susceptibility may be identified based on gestational age (Fig. 9–4). Prior to implantation (1 week in humans), there is no demonstrable teratogenic insult. The most vulnerable stage is between 3 and 8 weeks during the period of organogenesis. The timing determines which organ system or systems are affected. Unfortunately, most women do not realize they are pregnant until this critical period of development is well underway.

From about the fourth month of pregnancy to the end of gestation, embryonic development consists primarily of increasing organ size. With the exception of a limited number of tissues (brain and gonads), teratogenic exposure after the fourth month usually causes decreased growth without malformation.

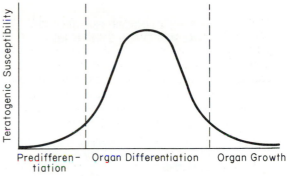

Figure 9–4. Schematic representation of embryonic periods of differential susceptibility to a teratogen. During the first weeks of embryogenesis, a teratogen can be lethal, but if the embryo survives, it will not necessarily be malformed. Following the period of maximum susceptibility, a teratogen can interfere with growth but will not directly affect organogenesis. Secondary effects (e.g., vascular occlusion) could still produce anomalies. (From Simpson LJ: Disorders of Sexual Differentiation. Etiology and Clinical Delineation. New York, Academic Press, 1976, p 46.)

Nature of Teratogenic Agents

Although few agents are known to cause serious malformations in a large proportion of exposed individuals, there are probably hundreds of potentially teratogenic agents, given the right set of circumstances (susceptible fetus, embryologically vulnerable period, large teratogenic dose). Furthermore, certain drugs combined with other drugs may be capable of producing malformations, although neither agent would be teratogenic when taken alone.

Teratogenic Agents

Teratogens may be categorized into three broad categories: (1) drugs and chemical agents, (2) infectious agents, and (3) radiation. The list that follows is far from exhaustive.

Drugs and Chemical Agents

Alcohol. Since ethanol is one of the most abused substances in the United States, it is perhaps surprising that the adverse effects of

Table 9–5. CLINICAL FEATURES OF FETAL ALCOHOL SYNDROME

CRANIOFACIAL
Eyes: Short palpebral fissures, ptosis, strabismus, epicanthic folds, myopia, microphthalmia
Ears: Poorly formed concha, posterior rotation
Nose: Short, hypoplastic philtrum
Mouth: Prominent lateral palatine ridges, micrognathia, cleft lip or palate, faulty enamel
Maxilla: Hypoplastic

CARDIAC
Murmurs, atrial septal defect, ventricular septal defect, tetralogy of Fallot

CENTRAL NERVOUS SYSTEM
Mild to moderate mental retardation, microcephaly, poor coordination, hypotonia

GROWTH
Prenatal onset growth deficiency

MUSCULAR
Hernias of diaphragm, umbilicus, or groin

SKELETAL
Pectus excavatum, abnormal palmar creases, nail hypoplasia, scoliosis

---

ethyl alcohol on fetal development were not fully realized until the 1970s. The frequency of the fetal alcohol syndrome runs as high as 0.2 per cent, and an additional 0.4 per cent of newborns show less severe features of the disorder.

The spectrum of anomalies caused by prenatal ingestion of ethanol is wide, and the frequency and severity appear to be dose-related. As little as one ounce of absolute alcohol twice per week appears to increase the risk of spontaneous abortion twofold to fourfold. One ounce of absolute alcohol daily (two drinks) may be enough to produce mild features of fetal alcohol syndrome, such as low birth weight.

The clinical features of FAS are summarized in Table 9–5. The most consistent findings in babies with this disorder include (1) prenatal growth deficiency for weight, height, and head circumference; (2) distinct craniofacial features; and (3) mild to moderate mental retardation. The average IQ among individuals with fetal alcohol syndrome is 65, but may range from 16 to 105. Hypotonia is a frequent finding, along with poor motor coordination.

It is of utmost importance that women of reproductive age be aware of the serious risks posed by prenatal alcohol consumption. It is not possible to state a safe level of ethanol intake. Until more detailed risk information becomes available, the safest advice is to avoid alcohol consumption during pregnancy.

Antianxiety Agents. This class of drugs is of special interest because it contains the now well-described teratogen thalidomide. Typical features of thalidomide exposure include phocomelia, ear anomalies, cardiac malformations, esophageal or duodenal atresia, and renal agenesis.

Antianxiety agents are currently used by a significant number of pregnant women. Data regarding their teratogenicity are conflicting, although exposure to meprobamate or chlordiazepoxide has been associated with a greater than fourfold increase in severe congenital anomalies. No specific pattern of anomalies is apparent.

Diazepam (Valium) crosses the placenta and accumulates in the fetal circulation. Pregnant women exposed to diazepam during the first trimester should be counseled as to the possible increased risk of oral clefts, although the incidence is probably well below 1 per cent.

Antineoplastic Agents. Aminopterin and methotrexate, both of which are folic acid antagonists, have been clearly established as teratogens. Exposure prior to 40 days' gestation is lethal to the embryo; later exposure during the first trimester produces fetal effects, including intrauterine growth retardation, craniofacial anomalies, abnormal positioning of extremities, mental retardation, early miscarriage, stillbirth, and neonatal death.

Alkylating agents have been associated with fetal anomalies, including severe intrauterine growth retardation, fetal death, cleft palate, microphthalmia, limb reduction anomalies, and poorly developed external genitalia. The first trimester is a particularly dangerous time for use of these drugs.

Antibiotics. The majority of studies on the teratogenicity of antibiotics have failed to reveal an increased risk to the fetus. A few, however, appear to pose potential harm. A history of antibiotic exposure should prompt physicians to obtain a detailed history of infectious disease and maternal fever during

Table 9–6. ETIOLOGIC FACTORS THAT MAY PLAY A ROLE IN ANTICONVULSANT TERATOGENICITY

Antiepileptic drugs
  Dose, serum levels, metabolism, teratogenicity, metabolic interactions
Genetic predisposition
  Maternal, paternal, and fetal metabolism
Maternal disease
  Teratogenicity, underlying disease, seizures

pregnancy because these factors, rather than the medication, may put the fetus at risk.

Although no consistent reports of fetal abnormalities have been associated with tetracycline exposure in the first trimester, fetal exposure beyond the fourth month of pregnancy has been shown to result in deciduous teeth that appear yellow, with hypoplasia of the enamel. There is also an increased susceptibility to caries.

About 10 to 15 per cent of fetuses exposed to streptomycin and closely related compounds, such as dihydrostreptomycin, will develop serious eighth cranial nerve damage with subsequent hearing loss.

Anticoagulants

Coumarin Derivatives. Use of coumarin during the first trimester is associated with an increased risk of spontaneous abortion, intrauterine growth retardation, central nervous system defects, stillbirth, and a characteristic syndrome of craniofacial features known as the fetal warfarin syndrome. Embryologically, the most vulnerable time appears to be between 6 and 9 weeks after conception. As many as 30 per cent of exposed fetuses suffer pregnancy loss or serious teratogenic consequences.

Heparin. Heparin has major advantages over coumarin anticoagulants during pregnancy because it does not cross the placenta. Therefore, it should be used routinely for anticoagulation during the first trimester and after 36 weeks' gestation.

Anticonvulsants. Approximately one of every 200 pregnant women is epileptic and faces an increased risk for significant fetal abnormalities. Table 9–6 lists the etiologic factors that may play a role in the congenital abnormalities associated with in utero exposure to anticonvulsants. The complexity in providing genetic counseling for pregnant epileptic women is underscored when one considers the interactive effects of these factors, the effect of combined anticonvulsant treatment, and the genetic aspects of the disease itself. The goals of counseling include providing the patient with the teratogenic risks of her medication, the risk of seizures during pregnancy, the effect of pregnancy on seizures, and the risk of her offspring developing epilepsy. From a medication standpoint, the benefits of seizure prevention need to be weighed against the teratogenicity of the drug.

Diphenylhydantoin (Dilantin). A specific syndrome, known as the fetal hydantoin syndrome, has been described, the clinical features of which include craniofacial abnormalities, limb reduction defects, prenatal onset growth deficiency, mental retardation, and cardiovascular anomalies. Overall, approximately 10 per cent of exposed fetuses demonstrate fetal hydantoin syndrome, whereas an additional 30 per cent may have isolated features of the syndrome. Furthermore, investigations suggest that hydantoins may have a prenatal carcinogenic effect in that several exposed infants with signs of fetal hydantoin syndrome have subsequently developed neuroblastomas.

Studies indicate that diphenylhydantoin is metabolized to form toxic oxidative metabolites. The epoxide metabolite, which is normally eliminated by epoxide hydrolase, is thought to be responsible for the increase in congenital abnormalities associated with diphenylhydantoin exposure prenatally. There is some evidence that epoxide hydrolase activity is genetically regulated by a single gene with at least two allelic forms, thus providing the potential for determining which infants are at increased risk for anticonvulsant-induced teratogenesis.

Oxazolidinedione Anticonvulsants. Trimethadione (Tridione) and paramethadione (Paradione), used to treat petit mal epilepsy, have been associated with a characteristic malformation syndrome in exposed fetuses. The clinical features include craniofacial abnormalities, prenatal onset growth deficiency, and an increased frequency of mental retardation and cardiovascular abnormalities. Additionally, exposure to these agents has been associated with an increased risk of fetal loss. Taken together, women using trimethadione or paramethadione face an 85 per cent risk for pregnancy loss or major congenital anomalies. Because of this serious teratogenic potential, and since petit mal epilepsy is rare during reproductive years, oxazolidinedione anticonvulsants are contraindicated during pregnancy.

Valproic Acid. Valproic acid (Depakene) was introduced in 1970 to treat petit mal seizures. Its use has now been broadened to treat other seizure disorders either alone or as an adjunct to other anticonvulsants. Valproic acid use during pregnancy is associated with a 1 to 2 per cent risk of open spina bifida and hypospadias. Other findings reported to be associated with valproic acid exposure include craniofacial and skeletal malformations. Since the introduction of valproic acid, animal studies have demonstrated a teratogenic effect in rabbits, rats, and mice causing vertebral or rib anomalies, exencephaly, and renal anomalies, depending on the species. Animal studies suggest that the teratogenic potential of valproic acid is related to the total dose and peak serum level, but this has not yet been confirmed in humans.

Women exposed to valproic acid during pregnancy should have genetic counseling and should be offered prenatal diagnosis including careful ultrasonography to check for skeletal or cranial abnormalities and an amniotic fluid AFP analysis to detect open neural tube defects.

Carbamazepine. Although the teratogenic effects of carbamazepine (Tegretol) are not yet well established, prenatal exposure has been associated with a malformation pattern that includes minor craniofacial defects, fingernail hypoplasia, and developmental delay. It is still unclear whether carbamazepine is associated with an increased risk for major malformations. Carbamazepine, like diphenylhydantoin, is thought to be metabolized through the arene oxide pathway, suggesting the possibility that toxic epoxide metabolites could be responsible for its teratogenic effect.

Phenobarbital. The true teratogenicity of phenobarbital is difficult to assess because other drugs are usually taken in combination with this agent, but the risk appears to be very low. A malformation pattern, such as is seen with diphenylhydantoin, is not associated with phenobarbital exposure. Other potential complications of phenobarbital include neonatal withdrawal symptoms and neonatal hemorrhage. Fetal addiction should not be a complication at the dosage levels required for seizure control.

Hormones

Progestins and Estrogen/Progestin Combinations. A large number of pregnant women are exposed to progestins or progestin/estrogen combinations for the management of threatened abortion or because they continue taking birth control pills unaware that they are pregnant. The main abnormality associated with the use of progestins during pregnancy is masculinization of the external genitalia in female fetuses. The magnitude of this risk, however, appears to be minimal.

The teratogenicity of estrogen and progestin combinations is more difficult to assess. Potential problems include congenital heart defects, nervous system defects, limb reduction malformations, and modified development of sexual organs. Except for the latter category, no firm evidence for a causal relationship exists.

Miscellaneous Agents

Diuretics. Although there is evidence of diuretic teratogenicity in rodents, teratogenicity has not been clearly demonstrated in humans.

Isotretinoin. Isotretinoin (Accutane) is prescribed for cystic acne or for acne that has not responded to other forms of treatment. Exposure during pregnancy is associated with isotretinoin embryopathy, which includes central nervous system, cardiovascular, and craniofacial defects (especially ear abnormalities). The risk of spontaneous abortion or congenital malformations is far greater than 50 per cent in patients who take isotretinoin throughout the first trimester. Thus, physicians have an important responsibility to discuss the risk with all female patients before beginning treatment.

Tobacco Smoking. Maternal tobacco smoking reduces the chance for a normal pregnancy outcome and is discussed further in Chapter 17.

Illicit Drugs. In the past few years, the problems associated with drug use during pregnancy have grown considerably. Cocaine is currently one of the most commonly used drugs during pregnancy, although polydrug abuse has become even more widespread, with many cocaine users additionally abusing marijuana, alcohol, and cigarettes. Most illicit drugs cross the placenta and lead to the potential for fetal problems including congenital abnormalities, fetal or neonatal growth retardation, and neurobehavioral abnormalities. Furthermore, fetal drug dependency develops with continued exposure. Symptoms of neonatal withdrawal include a high-pitched cry, sweating, tremulousness, and gastrointestinal upset. Illicit drug use during pregnancy is discussed in Chapter 17.

Infectious Agents

The exact frequency of significant infection during pregnancy is not known, but it is probably between 15 and 25 per cent. Viruses, bacteria, and parasites may have serious effects on the fetus, including fetal death, growth delay, congenital malformations, and mental deficiency. In more recent years, the AIDS epidemic has had a significant impact on pregnancy management. Approximately 50 per cent of infants born to HIV-1-seropositive mothers will also be HIV-1 positive. Intrauterine transmission has been demonstrated by identification of the virus in fetuses aborted in the second and third trimester. HIV-positive infants exhibit growth retardation, developmental delay, and dysmorphologic features. Women with a history of intravenous drug use, prostitution, or sexual intercourse with a bisexual or intravenous drug-using man should be considered high risk and should be encouraged to be tested for HIV-1 before becoming pregnant. A full discussion of infectious diseases occurring during pregnancy is provided in Chapter 16.

Radiation

Much attention has been directed to the potential adverse effects of radiation during pregnancy. Prenatal ultrasound and ionizing radiation exposure occur frequently as a result of therapeutic or diagnostic medical and dental procedures. The medical effects of ionizing radiation are dose-dependent and include teratogenesis, mutagenesis, and carci-

nogenesis. The most critical time period appears to be from about 2 to 6 weeks after conception. Exposures prior to 2 weeks either produce a lethal effect or produce no effect at all. Teratogenicity is still a possibility after five weeks, but the risk for deleterious consequences is relatively small.

Theoretically, any dose of ionizing radiation at a critical time could cause fetal damage. The incidence of serious effects, however, is significant only at doses greater than 50 cGy to the fetus. If a pregnant woman receives more than 10 cGy to the pelvis, available data indicate that abortion should be recommended; if exposure is between 5 to 10 cGy, termination of pregnancy should be considered, particularly if exposure occurs during the period of organogenesis. Teratogenic effects may include pregnancy loss, growth retardation, eye malformations, and central nervous system defects. Radiation doses of 5 to 15 cGy to the pelvis increase the risk of an anomaly by an additional 1 to 3 per cent over a background rate of 3 to 4 per cent. Radiation doses less than 5 cGy are not associated with fetal abnormalities, and patients should be reassured that their risk is not increased above that of the general population.

The mutagenic effect of radiation is also well known. It is thought that even doses around 5 cGy may produce mutations in an exposed fetus. It is estimated, however, that a dose of 50 cGy would be required to double the spontaneous mutation rate. Thus, the chance that prenatal radiation will produce a genetic disease in the exposed fetus is extremely small, especially since many of the induced mutations would be expressed only in the homozygous state.

Ionizing radiation has been shown to be related to the development of leukemia in exposed individuals. It is generally accepted that doses lower than 10 cGy increase the chance of leukemia from one in 3000 to one in 2000. Fortunately, under ordinary circumstances, only therapeutic levels of radiation present a significant risk to the fetus. Most diagnostic studies deliver substantially less than 5 cGy. For example, an upper and lower gastrointestinal series, an intravenous pyelogram, an extra-abdominal film, and a lower pelvic study would together deliver a total of less than 3 cGy to the fetus. Therefore, in most cases, women exposed to diagnostic radiation can be counseled that the risk is extremely small.

FUTURE DIRECTIONS

The field of prenatal diagnosis is expanding to provide earlier information about an increasing number of disorders caused by genetic or teratogenic factors. Advances in the understanding of an inherited predisposition to potential teratogens will allow for the identification of women who are specifically at risk for teratogen-induced malformations. The development of new medications will require continued evaluation of teratogenic effects. The increasing sensitivity of ultrasonography, however, along with information on genetic predisposition should allow the recognition of a larger number of affected fetuses during the second trimester. Molecular technology can now be applied to genetic screening to identify couples at risk for single gene disorders. Using this technology, diagnostic laboratory tests used in the first and second trimesters of pregnancy will soon be applied to the preimplantation embryo.

SUGGESTED READING

Botstein D, White RL, Skolnick M, Davis RW: Construction of a genetic linkage map in man using RFLPs. Am J Human Genet 32:314, 1980.

Brent RL: Radiation teratogenesis. Teratology 21:281,1980.

Buehler BA, Delimont D: Prenatal prediction of risk to the fetal hydantoin syndrome. N Engl J Med 332:1567, 1989.

Chasnoff IJ: Drug use in pregnancy: Parameters of risk. Pediatr Clin of North Am 35(6):1403, 1988.

Cronister AE, Hagerman RJ: Fragile X syndrome. J Pediatr Health Care 3:9, 1989.

Darras BT: Molecular genetics of Duchenne and Becker muscular dystrophy. J Pediatr 117(1):1, 1990.

Hall FG: Vitamin A: A newly recognized human teratogen: Harbinger of things to come? J Pediatr 105:583, 1984.

Hall JG, Pauli RM, Wilson KM: Maternal and fetal sequelae of anticoagulation during pregnancy. Am J Med 68:122, 1980.

Hanson FW, Zorn E, Tennant F, et al: Amniocentesis before 15 weeks' gestation: Outcome, risks and technical problems. Am J Obstet Gynecol 156:1524, 1987.

Hanson JL: Teratogenetic agents. In Emery AE, Rimoin DL (eds): Principles and Practice of Medical Genetics. Edinburgh, Churchill Livingstone, 1983, p 127.

Jones KL, Smith DW, Ulleland N, et al: Pattern of malformation in offspring of chronic alcoholic mothers. Lancet 1:1267, 1973.

Jones KL, et al: Pattern of malformations in the children of women treated with carbamazepine during pregnancy. N Engl J Med 320:1661, 1989.

Lindhout D: Teratogenicity of anticonvulsant drugs. In Moses AJ (ed): Pediatrics Update. New York, Elsevier, 1987.

Lindhout D, et al: Teratogenicity of antiepileptic drug combinations with special emphasis on epoxidation (of carbamazepine). Epilepsia 25:77, 1984.

Lustig L, Clarke S, Cunningham G, et al: California's experience with low MS-AFP results. Am J Med 31:211, 1988.

Lynch JR, Brown JM: The polymerase chain reaction: Current and future clinical applications. J Med Genetics 27:2, 1990.

McKusick V: Mendelian Inheritance in Man. 9th ed. Baltimore, The Johns Hopkins University Press, 1990.

Rommens JM, Riordon JR, Kerem BS, et al: Identification of the cystic fibrosis gene. Science 245:1059, 1989.

Wald NJ, Cuckle HS, et al: Maternal serum screening for Down's syndrome in early pregnancy. Br Med J 297(6653):883, 1988.

Weaver DD: Catalog of Prenatally Diagnosed Conditions. Baltimore, The Johns Hopkins University Press, 1989.

Wener CP: The role of cordocentesis in fetal diagnosis. Clin Obstet Gynecol 31(2):285, 1988.

Ten

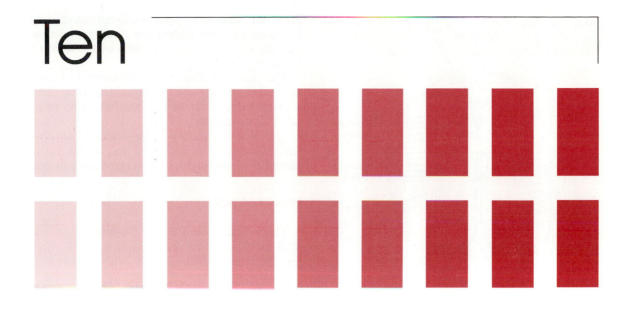

Anatomic Characteristics of the Fetal Head and Maternal Pelvis

CLIFFORD BOCHNER

Vaginal delivery necessitates the accommodation of the fetal head by the bony pelvis. Therefore, it is necessary to know the key landmarks and diameters of the fetal skull and to be able to identify the important sutures and fontanelles. The main consideration in assessing the maternal pelvis is to determine whether there is sufficient variation from a typical gynecoid pelvis to suggest the possibility of a difficult delivery.

FETAL HEAD

The head is the largest and least compressible part of the fetus. Thus, from an obstetric viewpoint, it is the most important part, whether the presentation is cephalic or breech.

The fetal skull consists of a base and a vault (cranium). The base of the skull has large, ossified, firmly united, and noncompressible bones. This serves to protect the vital structures contained within the brain stem.

The cranium consists of the occipital bone posteriorly, two parietal bones bilaterally, and two frontal and temporal bones anteriorly. The cranial bones at birth are thin, weakly ossified, easily compressible, and interconnected only by membranes. This allows them to overlap under pressure and to change shape to conform to the maternal pelvis, a process known as "molding."

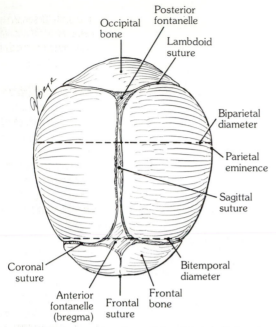

Figure 10-1. Superior view of the fetal skull showing the sutures, fontanelles, and transverse diameters.

Sutures

The membrane-occupied spaces between the cranial bones are known as sutures. The *sagittal suture* lies between the parietal bones and extends in an anteroposterior direction between the fontanelles, dividing the head into right and left sides (Fig. 10-1). The *lambdoid suture* extends from the posterior fontanelle laterally and serves to separate the occipital from the parietal bones. The *coronal suture* extends from the anterior fontanelle laterally and serves to separate the parietal and frontal bones. The frontal suture lies between the frontal bones and extends from the anterior fontanelle to the glabella (the prominence between the eyebrows).

Fontanelles

The membrane-filled spaces located at the point where the sutures intersect are known as fontanelles, the most important of which are the anterior and posterior. Clinically, they are even more useful in diagnosing the fetal head position than the sutures.

The posterior fontanelle closes at 6 to 8 weeks of life, whereas the anterior fontanelle does not become ossified until approximately 18 months. This allows the skull to accommodate the tremendous growth of the infant's brain after birth.

The anterior fontanelle (bregma) is found at the intersection of the sagittal, frontal, and coronal sutures. It is diamond-shaped, measures approximately 2 × 3 cm, and is much larger than the posterior fontanelle. The posterior fontanelle is Y-shaped and found at the junction of the sagittal and lambdoid sutures.

Landmarks

There are a number of landmarks on the fetal skull. Moving from front to back, they include (Fig. 10-2):

1. Nasion—the root of the nose.
2. Glabella—the elevated area between the orbital ridges.
3. Sinciput (brow)—the area between the anterior fontanelle and the glabella.
4. Anterior fontanelle (bregma).
5. Vertex—the area between the fontanelles and bounded laterally by the parietal eminences.
6. Posterior fontanelle (lambda).
7. Occiput—the area behind and inferior to the posterior fontanelle and lambdoid sutures.

Diameters

There are several important diameters of the fetal skull (see Figs. 10-1 and 10-2). The anteroposterior diameter presenting to the maternal pelvis depends on the degree of flexion or extension of the head and is important because the various diameters differ in length. The following measurements are considered average for a term fetus:

1. *Suboccipitobregmatic* (9.5 cm)—the presenting anteroposterior diameter when the head is well flexed, as in an occipitotransverse or occipitoanterior position. It extends from the undersurface of the occipital bone at the junction with the neck to the center of the anterior fontanelle.
2. *Occipitofrontal* (11 cm)—the presenting anteroposterior diameter when the head is deflexed, as in an occipitoposterior presentation; it extends from the external occipital protuberance to the glabella.

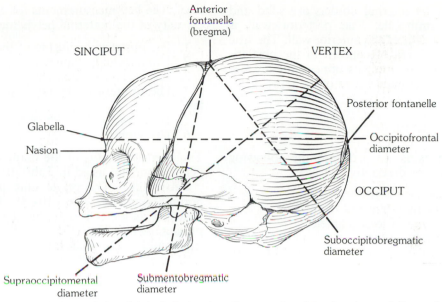

Figure 10-2. Lateral view of the fetal skull showing the prominent landmarks and the anteroposterior diameters.

3. *Supraoccipitomental* (13.5 cm)—the presenting anteroposterior diameter in a brow presentation and the longest anteroposterior diameter of the head; it extends from the vertex to the chin.

4. *Submentobregmatic* (9.5 cm)—the presenting anteroposterior diameter in face presentations; it extends from the junction of the neck and lower jaw to the center of the anterior fontanelle.

The transverse diameters of the fetal skull are:

1. *Biparietal* (9.5 cm)—the largest transverse diameter; it extends between the parietal bones.

2. *Bitemporal* (8 cm)—the shortest transverse diameter; it extends between the temporal bones.

The average circumference of the term fetal head, measured in the occipitofrontal plane, is 34.5 cm.

PELVIC ANATOMY

Bony Pelvis

The bony pelvis is made up of four bones: the sacrum, coccyx, and two innominates (composed of the ilium, ischium, and pubis). These are held together by the sacroiliac joints, the symphysis pubis, and the sacrococcygeal joint. The union of the pelvis and the vertebral column stabilizes the pelvis and allows weight to be transmitted to the lower extremities.

The sacrum consists of five fused vertebrae. The anterior superior edge of the first sacral vertebra is called the promontory, which protrudes slightly into the cavity of the pelvis. The anterior surface of the sacrum is usually concave. It articulates with the ilium at its upper segment, with the coccyx at its lower segment, and with the sacrospinous and sacrotuberous ligaments laterally.

The coccyx is composed of three to five rudimentary vertebrae. It articulates with the sacrum forming a joint, and occasionally there is fusion between the bones.

The pelvis is divided into the false pelvis above and the true pelvis below the linea terminalis. The false pelvis is bordered by the lumbar vertebrae posteriorly, an iliac fossa bilaterally, and the abdominal wall anteriorly. Its only obstetric function is to support the pregnant uterus.

The true pelvis is a bony canal and is formed by the sacrum and coccyx posteriorly and by the ischium and pubis laterally and anteriorly. Its internal borders are solid and relatively immobile. The posterior wall is twice the length of the anterior wall. The true pelvis is the area of concern to the obstetrician because at times its dimensions are not adequate to permit passage of the fetus.

Pelvic Planes

The pelvis is divided into the following four planes for descriptive purposes:

1. The pelvic inlet.
2. The plane of greatest diameter.
3. The plane of least diameter.
4. The pelvic outlet.

These planes are imaginary, flat surfaces extending across the pelvis at different levels. Except for the plane of greatest diameter, each plane is clinically significant.

The *plane of the inlet* is bordered by the pubic crest anteriorly, the iliopectineal line of the innominate bones laterally, and the promontory of the sacrum posteriorly.

The *plane of greatest diameter* is the largest part of the pelvic cavity. It is bordered by the midpoint of the pubis anteriorly, the upper part of the obturator foramina laterally, and the junction of the second and third sacral vertebrae posteriorly.

The *plane of least diameter* is the most important from a clinical standpoint, since most instances of arrest of descent occur at this level. It is bordered by the lower edge of the pubis anteriorly, the ischial spines and sacrospinous ligaments laterally, and the lower sacrum posteriorly.

The *plane of the pelvic outlet* is formed by two triangular planes with a common base at the level of the ischial tuberosities. The anterior triangle is bordered by the subpubic angle at the apex, the pubic rami on the sides, and the bituberous diameter at the base. The posterior triangle is bordered by the sacrococcygeal joint at its apex, the sacrotuberous ligaments on the sides, and the bituberous diameter at the base.

Pelvic Diameters

The diameters of the pelvic planes represent the amount of space available at each level. The key measurements for assessing the capacity of the maternal pelvis include:

1. The obstetric conjugate of the inlet.
2. The bispinous diameter.
3. The bituberous diameter.
4. The posterior sagittal diameter at all levels.
5. The curve and length of the sacrum.
6. The subpubic angle.

The average lengths of the diameters of each pelvic plane are listed in Table 10-1.

Pelvic Inlet. The pelvic inlet has five important diameters (Fig. 10-3). The anteroposterior diameter is described by one of two measurements. The *true conjugate* (anatomic conjugate) is the anatomic diameter and extends from the middle of the sacral promontory to the superior surface of the pubic symphysis. The *obstetric conjugate* represents the actual space available to the fetus and extends from the middle of the sacral promontory to the closest point on the convex posterior surface of the symphysis pubis.

The *transverse diameter* is the widest distance between the iliopectineal lines. Each *oblique diameter* extends from the sacroiliac joint to the opposite iliopectineal eminence.

The *posterior sagittal diameter* extends from the anteroposterior and transverse intersection to the middle of the sacral promontory.

Plane of Greatest Diameter. The plane of greatest diameter has two noteworthy diameters. The *anteroposterior diameter* extends from the midpoint of the posterior surface of the pubis to the junction of the second and third sacral vertebrae. The *transverse diameter* is the widest distance between the lateral borders of the plane.

Plane of Least Diameter (Midplane). The plane of least diameter has three important diameters. The *anteroposterior diameter* extends from the lower border of the pubis to the junction of the fourth and fifth sacral vertebrae. The *transverse (bispinous) diameter* extends between the ischial spines. The *posterior sagittal diameter* extends from the bispinous diameter to the junction of the fourth and fifth sacral vertebrae.

Pelvic Outlet. The pelvic outlet has four important diameters (Fig. 10-4). The *anatomic anteroposterior diameter* extends from the inferior margin of the pubis to the tip of

Table 10-1. AVERAGE LENGTH OF PELVIC PLANE DIAMETERS

PELVIC PLANE	DIAMETER	AVERAGE LENGTH (cm)
Inlet	True conjugate	11.5
	Obstetric conjugate	11
	Transverse	13.5
	Oblique	12.5
	Posterior sagittal	4.5
Greatest diameter	Anteroposterior	12.75
	Transverse	12.5
Midplane	Anteroposterior	12
	Bispinous	10.5
	Posterior sagittal	4.5–5
Outlet	Anatomic anteroposterior	9.5
	Obstetric anteroposterior	11.5
	Bituberous	11
	Posterior sagittal	7.5

the coccyx, whereas the *obstetric anteroposterior diameter* extends from the inferior margin of the pubis to the sacrococcygeal joint. The *transverse (bituberous) diameter* extends between the inner surfaces of the ischial tuberosities, and the *posterior sagittal diameter* extends from the middle of the transverse diameter to the sacrococcygeal joint.

PELVIC SHAPES

Based on the general bony architecture, the pelvis may be classified into four basic types (Fig. 10–5).

Gynecoid

This is the classic female type of pelvis and is found in approximately 50 per cent of women. It has the following characteristics:

1. Round at the inlet, with the widest transverse diameter only slightly greater than the anteroposterior diameter.
2. Side walls straight.
3. Ischial spines of average prominence.
4. Well-rounded sacrosciatic notch.
5. Well-curved sacrum.
6. Spacious subpubic arch, with an angle of approximately 90 degrees.

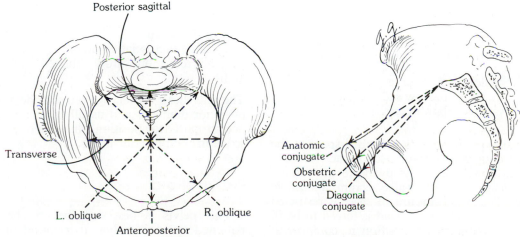

Figure 10–3. Pelvic inlet and its diameters.

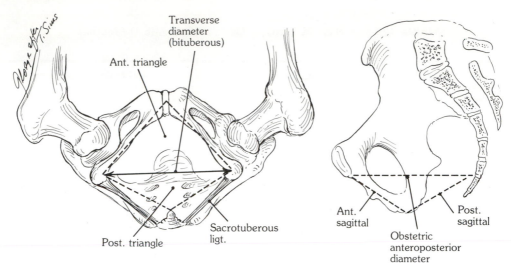

Figure 10–4. Pelvic outlet and its diameters.

These features create a cylindrical shape that is spacious throughout. The fetal head generally rotates into the occipitoanterior position in this type of pelvis.

Android

Although this is the typical male type of pelvis, it is found in approximately 30 per cent of women and has the following characteristics:

1. Triangular inlet with a flat posterior segment and the widest transverse diameter closer to the sacrum than in the gynecoid type.
2. Convergent side walls with prominent spines.
3. Shallow sacral curve.
4. Long and narrow sacrosciatic notch.
5. Narrow subpubic arch.

This type of pelvis has limited space at the inlet and progressively less space as one moves down the pelvis owing to the funneling effect of the side walls, sacrum, and pubic rami. Thus, the amount of space is restricted at all levels. The fetal head is forced to be in the occipitoposterior position to conform to the narrow anterior pelvis. Arrest of descent is common at the midpelvis.

Anthropoid

This type of pelvis resembles that of the anthropoid ape. It is found in approximately 20 per cent of women and has the following characteristics:

1. A much larger anteroposterior than transverse diameter, creating a long narrow oval at the inlet.
2. Side walls that do not converge.
3. Ischial spines that are not prominent, but are close, owing to the overall shape.
4. Variable, but usually posterior inclination of the sacrum.
5. Large sacrosciatic notch.
6. Narrow, outwardly shaped subpubic arch.

The fetal head can engage only in the anteroposterior diameter and usually does so in the occipitoposterior position, since there is more space in the posterior pelvis.

Platypelloid

This pelvis is best described as being a flattened gynecoid pelvis. It is found in only

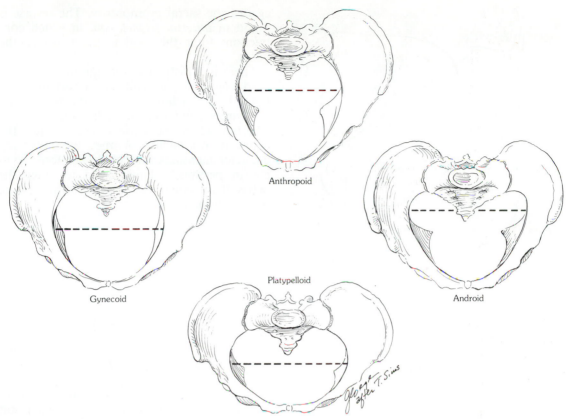

Figure 10–5. The four basic pelvic types. The dotted line indicates the transverse diameter of the inlet. Note that the widest diameter of the inlet is posteriorly situated in an android or anthropoid pelvis.

3 per cent of women, and it has the following characteristics:

1. A short anteroposterior and wide transverse diameter creating an oval-shaped inlet.
2. Straight or divergent side walls.
3. Posterior inclination of the sacrum.
4. A wide bispinous diameter.
5. A wide subpubic arch.

The overall shape is that of a gentle curve throughout. The fetal head has to engage in the transverse diameter.

ENGAGEMENT

Engagement occurs when the widest diameter of the fetal presenting part has passed through the pelvic inlet. In cephalic presentations, the widest diameter is the biparietal; in breech presentations, it is the intertrochanteric.

The *station* of the presenting part in the pelvic canal is defined as its level above or below the plane of the ischial spines. The level of the ischial spines is assigned as "zero" station and each centimeter above or below this level is given a minus or positive designation, respectively.

In the majority of women, the bony presenting part is at the level of the ischial spines when the head has become engaged. This is not true in women with a deep pelvis, in whom the presenting part may be up to 1 cm above the spines, even though engagement has taken place. When the presenting part is out of the pelvis (−3 station or higher) and is freely movable, it is considered to be *floating.* When it has passed through the plane of the inlet but is not yet engaged, it is considered to be *dipping.*

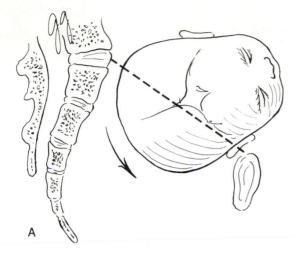

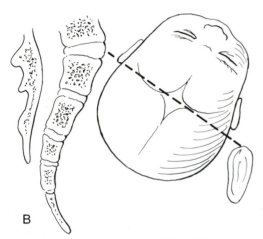

Figure 10–6. Anterior asynclitism (*A*) entering the pelvis, and synclitism in the pelvis (*B*).

The fetal head usually engages with its sagittal suture in the transverse diameter of the pelvis. The head position is considered to be *synclitic* when the biparietal diameter is parallel to the pelvic plane and the sagittal suture is midway between the anterior and posterior plane of the pelvis. When this relationship is not present, the head is considered to be *asynclitic* (Fig. 10–6).

When the posterior parietal bone is lower in the pelvis than the anterior parietal bone, the sagittal suture is closer to the pubis than the sacrum. This is called *posterior asynclitism.* Synclitism comes about as contractions force the head downward and into lateral flexion, and the posterior parietal bone pivots

against the sacral promontory. The reverse is found in *anterior asynclitism,* in which contractions force the head to pivot against the pubis.

There is a distinct advantage to having the head engage in asynclitism in certain situations. In a synclitic presentation, the biparietal diameter entering the pelvis measures 9.5 cm; but when the parietal bones enter the pelvis in an asynclitic manner, the presenting diameter measures 8.75 cm. Therefore, asynclitism permits a larger head to enter the pelvis than would be possible in a synclitic presentation.

PELVIMETRY

Clinical Pelvimetry

It is not possible to assess all of the pelvic dimensions by clinical mensuration. The diameters that can be clinically evaluated should be assessed at the time of the first prenatal visit to screen for obvious pelvic contractions.

Some obstetricians believe that it is better to wait until later in pregnancy when the soft tissues are more distensible and the examination is less uncomfortable and possibly more accurate. It should be remembered that the clinical examination is only an estimate, and there may be a considerable discrepancy from the measurements obtained via x-ray pelvimetry.

The clinical evaluation is started by assessing the pelvic inlet. The pelvic inlet can be evaluated clinically for its anteroposterior diameter, whereas the transverse diameter can be assessed only by x-ray film. The obstetric conjugate, previously described under pelvic anatomy, can be estimated from the diagonal conjugate, which is obtained on clinical examination.

The *diagonal conjugate* is approximated by measuring from the lower border of the pubis to the sacral promontory using the tip of the second finger and the point where the index finger meets the pubis (Fig. 10–7). The *obstetric conjugate* is then estimated by subtracting 1.5 to 2 cm, depending on the height and inclination of the pubis. Often the middle finger of the examining hand cannot reach the sacral promontory; thus, the obstet-

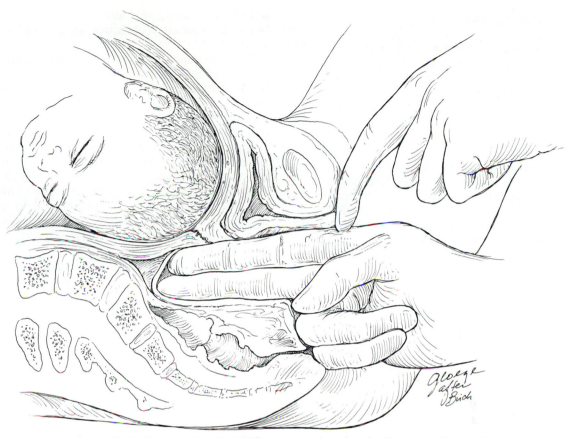

Figure 10–7. Clinical estimation of the diagonal conjugate diameter of the pelvis.

ric conjugate is considered adequate. If the diagonal conjugate is greater than or equal to 11.5 cm, the anteroposterior diameter of the inlet is considered to be adequate. The transverse diameter of the inlet cannot be evaluated clinically because of the inability to reach this area of the pelvis.

The anterior surface of the sacrum is then palpated to assess its curvature. The usual shape is concave. A flat or convex shape may indicate anteroposterior constriction throughout the pelvis.

The *midpelvis* cannot accurately be measured clinically in either the anteroposterior or transverse diameter. A reasonable estimate of the size of the midpelvis, however, can be obtained as follows. The pelvic side walls can be assessed to determine if they are convergent rather than having the usual, almost parallel, configuration. The ischial spines are palpated carefully to assess their prominence, and several passes are made between the spines to approximate the bispinous diameter. The length of the sacrospinous ligament is assessed by placing one finger on the ischial spine and one finger on the sacrum in the midline. The average length is three finger breadths. If the sacrosciatic notch located lateral to the ligament can accommodate two and a half fingers, the posterior midpelvis is most likely of adequate dimensions. A short ligament suggests a forward inclination of the sacrum and a narrowed sacrosciatic notch.

Finally, the pelvic outlet is assessed. This is done by first placing a fist between the ischial tuberosities. An 8-cm distance is considered to indicate an adequate transverse diameter. The infrapubic angle is assessed by placing a thumb next to each inferior pubic ramus and then estimating the angle where they meet. An angle of less than 90 degrees is associated with a contracted transverse diameter in the midplane and outlet.

X-Ray Pelvimetry

The purpose of x-ray pelvimetry is to aid in determining the need for a cesarean section. It can be used only to assess the bony landmarks, however, and, as such, should be considered one piece of information among many variables. Other factors determining the need for a cesarean section include the fetal head size, the force of contractions, the presentation and position of the fetus, and the degree of molding of the fetal head.

The advantage of x-ray over clinical pelvimetry is that it provides more accurate measurements and information about clinically unobtainable measurements.

Indications. Today x-ray pelvimetry is no longer considered necessary in the management of a cephalic presentation. If vaginal delivery is planned for a breech presentation, however, x-ray pelvimetry remains the standard of care. Other indications include:

1. Clinical evidence or obstetric history suggestive of pelvic abnormalities.
2. A history of pelvic trauma.

It should always be questioned whether the results obtained with x-ray pelvimetry will have sufficient influence on the patient's management to make the investigation worthwhile.

Dangers. There have been a number of epidemiologic studies purporting a greater risk of leukemia or other cancers in children exposed to x-rays in utero. Other studies have failed to confirm these findings, and at the present time there are arguments both for and against with no proven data for either side. In light of the present knowledge, it has been decided that if the circumstances dictate the procedure, the risk to the fetus is justifiable.

Method. There are a number of x-ray pelvimetry techniques. If the same reference points of measurement are used, the results from the various techniques should be the same.

The procedure requires two separate films. One is a lateral view, which is used for the anteroposterior measurements; the other is an inlet view, which is used for the transverse diameter. It is important that the landmarks of the pelvis be well visualized. Rotation, or tilting of the pelvis, results in distortion and should be avoided. Since there is distortion of the diameters owing to the distance from the x-ray plate, a correction must be made. This can be done by placing a centimeter grid at the same plane as the pelvis. Doses of radiation to the fetus from the pelvimetry range from 0.5 to 1 cGy.

Computed tomographic pelvimetry, although not extensively used at this time, results in less radiation exposure, more accuracy, and similar cost when compared with conventional x-ray pelvimetry. Ultrasonography has not proved useful in pelvic mensuration.

SUGGESTED READING

Adam PH, Alberge AY, Castellano S, et al: Pelvimetry by digital radiography. Clin Radiol 36:327, 1985.

Bithell J, Stewart A: Prenatal irradiation: A review of the British data from the Oxford survey. Br J Cancer 31:27, 1985.

Caldwell WE, Moloy HC: More recent conceptions of the pelvic architecture. Am J Obstet Gynecol 40:558, 1940.

Fine EA, Bracken M, Berkowitz RL: An evaluation of the usefulness of x-ray pelvimetry: Comparison of the Thoms and Ball methods with manual pelvimetry. Am J Obstet Gynecol 137:15, 1980.

Gimovsky ML, Willard K, Neglio M, et al: X-ray pelvimetry in a breech protocol: Comparison of digital radiology and conventional methods. Am J Obstet Gynecol 153:887, 1985.

Parsons MT, Spellacy WN: A prospective randomized study of x-ray pelvimetry in the primigravida. Obstet Gynecol 66:76, 1985.

Eleven

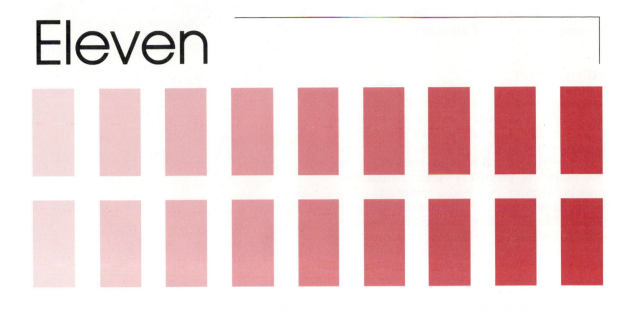

Normal Labor, Delivery, and the Puerperium

MICHAEL G. ROSS and CALVIN J. HOBEL

Labor is a physiologic process that permits a series of extensive changes in the mother to allow for the delivery of her fetus through the birth canal. It is defined as progressive cervical effacement, dilatation, or both, resulting from regular uterine contractions occurring at least every 5 minutes and lasting 30 to 60 seconds.

The role of the birth attendant is to anticipate and manage complications that may occur to either the mother or the fetus. When a decision is made to intervene, it must be considered carefully; each intervention carries not only potential benefits, but also potential risks. In the vast majority of cases, the best management may be "cautious observation."

PREPARATION FOR LABOR

Before actual labor begins, a number of physiologic preparatory events commonly occur.

Lightening

Two or more weeks before labor, the fetal head in most primigravid women settles into the brim of the pelvis. In multigravid women, this often does not occur until early in labor. Lightening may be noted by the mother as a flattening of the upper abdomen and an increased prominence of the lower abdomen.

Compression of the bladder often results in increased frequency of urination.

False Labor

During the last 4 to 8 weeks of pregnancy, the uterus undergoes irregular contractions that normally are painless. Such contractions appear unpredictably and sporadically and can be rhythmic and of mild intensity. In the last month of pregnancy, these contractions may occur more frequently, sometimes every 10 to 20 minutes, and with greater intensity. These "Braxton Hicks" contractions are considered false labor in that they are not associated with progressive cervical dilatation or effacement. They may serve, however, a physiologic role in preparing the uterus and cervix for true labor. When uterine contractions occur early in the third trimester of pregnancy, it is important to distinguish Braxton Hicks contractions from true preterm labor.

Cervical Effacement

Prior to the onset of parturition, the cervix is frequently noted to soften as a result of increased water content and collagen lysis. Simultaneous effacement, or thinning of the cervix, occurs as it is taken up into the lower uterine segment (Fig. 11–1). Consequently, patients often present in labor with a cervix that is already partially effaced. As a result of cervical effacement, the mucous plug within the cervical canal may be released. The onset of labor may thus be heralded by the passage of a small amount of blood-tinged mucus from the vagina ("bloody show").

STAGES OF LABOR

There are four stages of labor, each of which is considered separately. These stages in actuality are definitions of progress during labor, delivery, and the puerperium.

The first stage is from the onset of true labor to complete dilatation of the cervix. The second stage is from complete dilatation of the cervix to the birth of the baby. The third stage is from the birth of the baby to

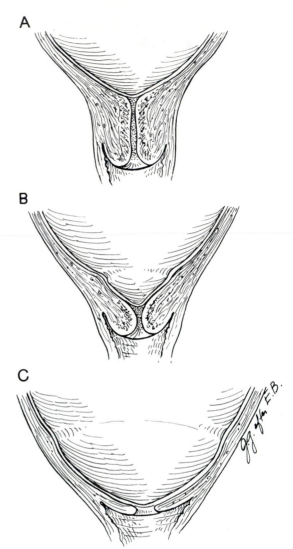

Figure 11–1. *A,* The absence of cervical effacement prior to labor. *B,* Cervix being progressively taken up into the lower segment of the uterus (approximately 50 per cent effaced). *C,* Cervix fully taken up; that is, cervix is completely effaced.

delivery of the placenta. The fourth stage is from delivery of the placenta to stabilization of the patient's condition, usually at about 6 hours postpartum.

First Stage of Labor

Phases

The first stage of labor consists of two phases: a latent phase during which cervical

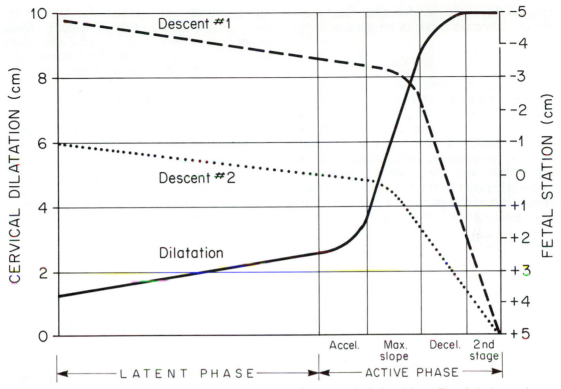

Figure 11-2. Cervical dilatation and descent of the fetal head during labor. The first descent curve represents a fetus with a floating presenting part at the onset of labor, whereas the second represents a fetus with the presenting part fixed in the pelvis prior to labor. (Modified from Friedman EA: Labor: Evaluation and Management, 2nd ed. East Norwalk, CT, Appleton-Century-Crofts, 1978, p 41.)

effacement and early dilatation occur and an active phase during which more rapid cervical dilatation occurs (Fig. 11-2). Although cervical softening and early effacement may occur before labor, during the first stage of labor the entire cervical length is retracted into the lower uterine segment as a result of myometrial contractile forces and pressure exerted by either the presenting part or fetal membranes.

Length

The length of the first stage may vary in relation to parity; primiparous patients generally experience a longer first stage than multiparous patients (Table 11-1). Because the latent phase may overlap considerably with the preparatory phase of labor, its duration is highly variable. It may also be influenced by other factors, such as sedation and stress. The duration of the latent phase has little bearing on the subsequent course of labor. The active

phase begins when the cervix is 3 to 4 cm dilated in the presence of regularly occurring uterine contractions. The minimal dilatation during the active phase of the first stage is nearly the same for primiparous and multiparous women: 1 and 1.2 cm per hour, respectively. Progress slower than this must be

Table 11-1. CHARACTERISTICS OF NORMAL LABOR

CHARACTERISTIC	PRIMIPARA	MULTIPARA
Duration of first stage	6-18 hr	2-10 hr
Rate of cervical dilatation during active phase	1 cm/hr	1.2 cm/hr
Duration of second stage	30 min to 3 hr	5-30 min
Duration of third stage	0-30 min	0-30 min

evaluated for uterine dysfunction, fetal malposition, or cephalopelvic disproportion.

Measurement of Progress

During the first stage, the progress of labor may be measured in terms of cervical effacement, cervical dilatation, and the descent of the fetal head. The clinical pattern of the uterine contractions alone is not an adequate indication of progress. After completion of cervical dilatation, the second stage commences. Thereafter, only the descent, flexion, and rotation of the presenting part are available to assess the progress of labor.

Clinical Management of the First Stage

Certain steps should be taken in the clinical management of the patient during the first stage of labor.

Maternal Position. The mother may ambulate during the first stage provided that intermittent monitoring ensures fetal well-being and the presenting part is engaged in patients with ruptured membranes. The mother may choose to sit or recline. If she is lying in bed, the lateral recumbent position should be encouraged to assure perfusion of the uteroplacental unit. The supine position should be discouraged.

Administration of Fluids. Because of decreased gastric emptying during labor, oral fluids are best avoided. Placement of a 16- to 18-gauge venous catheter is advisable during the active phase of labor. This intravenous route is used to hydrate the patient with crystalloids during labor, to administer oxytocin after the delivery of the placenta, and for the treatment of any unanticipated emergencies.

Preparing the Patient. Although once considered routine procedures for delivery, the use of enemas, pubic and vulvar shaves, and skin preparations may be individualized by physicians and patients. An enema should be considered in patients who are constipated and in those who have large amounts of stool palpable in the rectum during the pelvic examination.

Investigations. Every woman admitted in labor should have a hematocrit or hemoglo-bin measured and a blood clot held in the event that a crossmatch is needed. Blood group, rhesus type, and an antibody screen should be done if these are not known. Additionally, a voided urine specimen should be checked for protein and glucose.

Maternal Monitoring. Maternal pulse rate, blood pressure, respiratory rate, and temperature should be recorded every 1 to 2 hours in normal labor and more frequently if indicated. Fluid balance, particularly urine output and intravenous intake, should be monitored carefully.

Analgesia. Adequate analgesia, discussed in Chapter 12, is important during the first stage of labor.

Fetal Monitoring. Auscultation of the fetal heart rate should occur every 15 minutes, immediately following a contraction. The fetal heart rate can also be monitored continuously using either Doppler equipment (external monitoring) or a fetal scalp electrode (internal monitoring). Continuous fetal heart rate monitoring is not necessary in uncomplicated pregnancies.

Uterine Activity. Uterine contractions should be monitored every 30 minutes by palpation for their frequency, duration, and intensity. For high-risk pregnancies, uterine contractions should be monitored continuously along with the fetal heart rate. This can be achieved electronically using either an external tocodynamometer or an internal pressure catheter in the amniotic cavity. The latter is recommended when a patient's labor is being augmented with oxytocin (Pitocin).

Vaginal Examination. During the latent phase, particularly when the membranes are ruptured, vaginal examinations should be done sparingly to decrease the risk of an intrauterine infection. In the active phase, the cervix should be assessed approximately every 2 hours to determine the progress of labor. Cervical effacement and dilatation, the station and position of the presenting part, and the presence of molding or caput in vertex presentations should be recorded. Additional examinations may be performed if the patient reports the urge to push (to determine if full dilatation has occurred) or if a significant fetal heart rate deceleration occurs (to examine for a prolapsed umbilical cord).

Amniotomy. The artificial rupture of fetal membranes may provide information on the volume of amniotic fluid and the presence or absence of meconium. In addition, rupture of the membranes may cause an increase in uterine contractility. Amniotomy incurs risks of chorioamnionitis if labor is prolonged, however, and umbilical cord compression or cord prolapse if the presenting part is not engaged. It should not be routinely performed unless internal monitoring is indicated.

Second Stage of Labor

At the beginning of the second stage, the mother usually has a desire to bear down with each contraction. This abdominal pressure together with the uterine contractile force combines to expel the fetus. During the second stage of labor, fetal descent must be monitored carefully to evaluate the progress of labor. Descent is measured in terms of progress of the presenting part through the birth canal.

In cephalic presentations, the shape of the fetal head may be altered during labor, making the assessment of descent more difficult. Molding is the alteration of the relationship of the fetal cranial bones to each other as a result of the compressive forces exerted by the bony maternal pelvis. Some molding is necessary for delivery under normal circumstances. If cephalopelvic disproportion is present, the amount of molding will be more pronounced. Caput is a localized, edematous swelling of the scalp caused by pressure of the cervix on the presenting portion of the fetal head. The development of both molding and caput can create a false impression of fetal descent.

The second stage generally takes from 30 minutes to 3 hours in primigravidae and from 5 to 30 minutes in multigravidae. The median duration is 50 minutes in a primipara and slightly under 20 minutes in a multipara. These times may vary, depending on the type of analgesia.

Mechanism of Labor

Six movements of the baby enable it to adapt to the maternal pelvis: descent, flexion, internal rotation, extension, external rotation, and expulsion (Fig. 11–3). These movements are discussed here for both an occipitoanterior and occipitoposterior position at engagement. The mechanism of labor for other presentations is discussed in Chapter 20.

Descent. Descent is brought about by the force of the uterine contractions, maternal bearing-down efforts, and gravity if the patient is upright. A variable degree of fetal descent occurs before the onset of labor in primigravidae and during the first stage in both primigravidae and multigravidae. Descent continues progressively until the fetus is delivered; the other movements are superimposed on it.

Flexion. Partial flexion exists before labor as a result of the natural muscle tone of the fetus. During descent, resistance from the cervix, walls of the pelvis, and pelvic floor cause further flexion of the cervical spine with the baby's chin approaching its chest. In the occipitoanterior position, the effect of flexion is to change the presenting diameter from the occipitofrontal to the smaller suboccipitobregmatic (see Fig. 10–2). In the occipitoposterior position, complete flexion may not occur, resulting in a larger presenting diameter, which may contribute to a longer labor.

Internal Rotation. In the occipitoanterior positions, the fetal head, which enters the pelvis in a transverse or oblique diameter, rotates so that the occiput turns anteriorly toward the symphysis pubis. Internal rotation probably occurs as the fetal head meets the muscular sling of the pelvic floor. It is often not accomplished until the presenting part has reached the level of the ischial spines (zero station) and therefore is engaged. In the occipitoposterior positions, the fetal head may rotate posteriorly so the occiput turns toward the hollow of the sacrum. Alternatively, the fetal head may rotate more than 90 degrees, positioning the occiput under the pelvic symphysis and thus converting to an occipitoanterior position. Approximately 75 per cent of the fetuses commencing labor in the occipitoposterior position rotate to the occipitoanterior position during flexion and descent. In either case, the sagittal suture normally orients in the anteroposterior axis of the pelvis.

Extension. The flexed head in an occipitoanterior position continues to descend

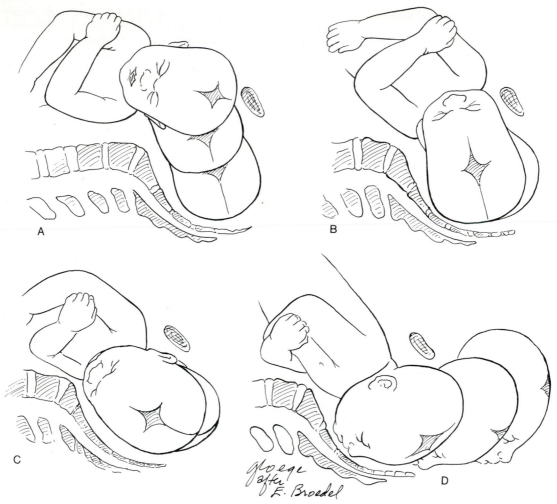

Figure 11–3. Mechanism of labor for a vertex presentation in the left occipitotransverse position. *A*, Flexion and descent; *B* and *C*, continued descent and commencement of internal rotation; *D*, completion of internal rotation to the occipitoanterior position, followed by delivery of the head by extension.

within the pelvis. Since the vaginal outlet is directed upward and forward, extension must occur before the head can pass through it. As the head continues its descent, there is bulging of the perineum followed by crowning. Crowning occurs when the largest diameter of the fetal head is encircled by the vulvar ring. At this time, the vertex has reached station 5. An incision in the perineum (episiotomy) may aid in reducing perineal resistance as well as in preventing tearing and stretching of perineal tissues. The head is born by rapid extension as the occiput, sinciput, nose, mouth, and chin pass over the perineum.

In the occipitoposterior position, the head is born by a combination of flexion and extension. At the time of crowning, the posterior bony pelvis and the muscular sling encourage further flexion. The forehead, sinciput, and occiput are born as the fetal chin approaches the chest. Subsequently, the occiput falls back as the head extends, and the nose, mouth, and chin are born.

External Rotation. In both the occipitoanterior and occipitoposterior positions, the delivered head now returns to its original position at the time of engagement to align itself with the fetal back and shoulders. Further head rotation may occur as the shoulders undergo an internal rotation to align themselves anteroposteriorly within the pelvis.

Expulsion. Following external rotation of the head, the anterior shoulder delivers under the symphysis pubis, followed by the posterior shoulder over the perineal body, then the body of the child.

Clinical Management of the Second Stage

As in the first stage, certain steps should be taken in the clinical management of the second stage of labor.

Maternal Position. With the exception of avoiding the supine position, the mother may assume any comfortable position for effective bearing down. If the birth is to occur in another room, primiparous patients should be moved at the beginning of crowning. Multiparous patients should be brought to the delivery room at the time of complete cervical dilatation.

Bearing Down. With each contraction, the mother should be encouraged to bear down with expulsive efforts. This is particularly important for patients with regional anesthesia because their reflex sensations may be impaired.

Fetal Monitoring. During the second stage, the fetal heart rate should be monitored either continuously or after each contraction. Fetal heart rate decelerations (head compression or cord compression) with recovery following the uterine contraction may occur during this stage.

Vaginal Examination. Progress should be recorded approximately every 30 minutes during the second stage. Particular attention should be paid to the descent and flexion of the presenting part, the extent of internal rotation, and the development of molding or caput.

Delivery of the Fetus. When delivery is imminent, the patient is usually placed in the lithotomy position, and the skin over the lower abdomen, vulva, anus, and upper thighs is cleansed with an antiseptic solution. Appropriate sterile leggings and drapes are applied. Uncomplicated deliveries, particularly in multiparous women, may be carried out in the supine position. The left lateral position may be used to deliver patients with hip or knee joint deformities that prevent adequate flexion or for patients with a superficial or deep venous thrombosis in one of the lower extremities.

As the perineum becomes flattened by the crowning head, an episiotomy may be performed, especially in the nulliparous patient, to prevent perineal lacerations and possible permanent relaxation of the pelvic outlet.

To facilitate delivery of the fetal head, a Ritgen's maneuver is performed (Fig. 11–4). The right hand, draped with a towel, exerts upward pressure through the distended perineal body, first to the supraorbital ridges and then to the chin. This upward pressure, which increases extension of the head and prevents it from slipping back between contractions, is counteracted by downward pressure on the occiput with the left hand. The downward pressure prevents rapid extension of the head and allows a controlled delivery.

Once the head is delivered, the airway is cleared of blood and amniotic fluid using a bulb suction. The oral cavity is cleared initially and then the nares. Suction of the nares is not performed if fetal distress or meconium stained liquor is present because it may result in gasping and aspiration of pharyngeal contents. A second towel is used to wipe secretions from the face and head.

After the airway has been cleared, an index finger is used to check whether the umbilical cord encircles the neck. If so, the cord can usually be slipped over the infant's head. If the cord is too tight, it can be cut between two clamps.

Following delivery of the head, the shoulders descend and rotate into the anteroposterior diameter of the pelvis and are delivered (Fig. 11–5). Delivery of the anterior shoulder is aided by gentle downward traction on the head. The brachial plexus may be injured if too much force is used. The posterior shoulder is delivered by elevating the head. Finally, the body is slowly extracted by traction on the shoulders.

After delivery, blood will be infused from the placenta into the newborn, provided that the baby is held below the introitus. It is therefore usual to wait 15 to 20 seconds before clamping and cutting the umbilical

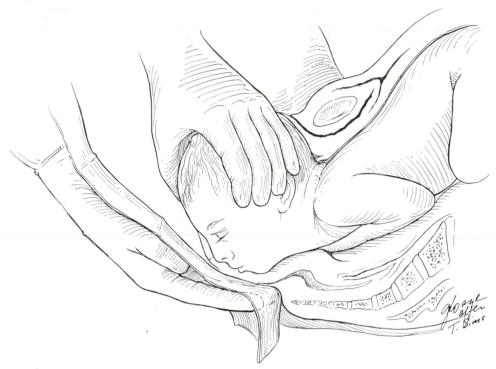

Figure 11–4. Ritgen's maneuver. The right hand is used to extend the head, while counterpressure is applied to the occiput by the left hand to allow a controlled delivery of the fetal head.

cord. The newborn is then placed under an infant warmer.

Third Stage of Labor

Immediately after the baby's delivery, the cervix and vagina should be thoroughly inspected for lacerations and surgical repair performed if necessary. The cervix, vagina, and perineum may be more readily examined before the separation of the placenta, since there should be no uterine bleeding to obscure visualization at this time.

Delivery of the Placenta

Separation of the placenta generally occurs within 5 to 10 minutes of the end of the second stage. Squeezing of the fundus to hasten placental separation is not recommended because it may increase the likeli-

hood of passage of fetal cells into the maternal circulation.

Signs of placental separation are as follows: (1) a fresh show of blood from the vagina, (2) the umbilical cord lengthens outside the vagina, (3) the fundus of the uterus rises up, and (4) the uterus becomes firm and globular. Only when these signs have appeared should the assistant attempt traction on the cord. With gentle traction and counterpressure between the symphysis and fundus, the placenta is delivered.

Following delivery of the placenta, attention should be paid to any uterine bleeding that may originate from the placental implantation site. Uterine contractions, which reduce this bleeding, may be hastened by uterine massage and the use of oxytocin. It is routine to add 20 units of oxytocin to the intravenous infusion after the baby has been delivered. The placenta should be examined to assure its complete removal. If the patient is at risk for postpartum hemorrhage (e.g., because of anemia, prolonged oxytocic augmentation of labor, multiple gestation, or

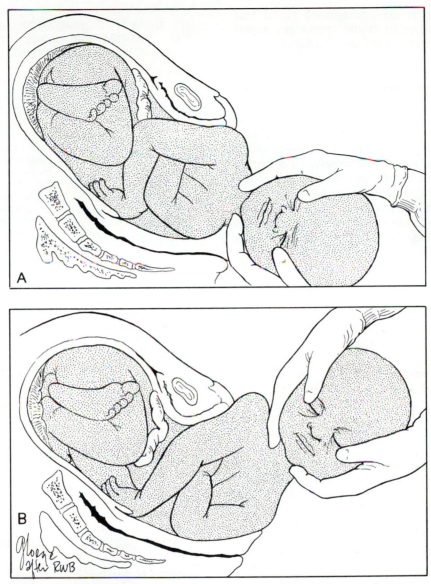

Figure 11-5. Delivery of the shoulders. *A,* Gentle downward traction on the head is applied to deliver the anterior shoulder, and *B,* gentle upward traction is used to deliver the posterior shoulder.

hydramnios), manual removal of the placenta, manual exploration of the uterus, or both may be necessary.

Perineal Lacerations

Perineal lacerations, with or without episiotomy, may be classified as follows:

First degree: A laceration involving the vaginal mucosa or perineal skin.

Second degree: A laceration extending into the submucosal tissues of the vagina or perineum with or without involvement of the muscles of the perineal body.

Third degree: A laceration involving the anal sphincter.

Fourth degree: A laceration involving the rectal mucosa.

The birth attendant should perform a digital rectal examination after delivery to be certain there is no undiagnosed rectal tear and that sutures from the episiotomy repair have not penetrated the rectal mucosa.

Fourth Stage of Labor

The hour immediately following delivery requires close observation of the patient. Blood pressure, pulse rate, and uterine blood loss must be monitored closely. It is during this time that postpartum hemorrhage commonly occurs, usually because of uterine relaxation, retained placental fragments, or undiagnosed lacerations. Occult bleeding (e.g., vaginal hematoma formation) may present with complaints of pelvic pain. There may be an increase in pulse rate, often out of proportion to any decrease in blood pressure.

INDUCTION AND AUGMENTATION OF LABOR

Induction of labor is the process whereby labor is initiated by artificial means; *augmentation* is the artificial stimulation of labor that has begun spontaneously.

The natural onset of labor at term involves complex interactions between the fetus and mother, which are discussed in Chapter 5. Oxytocin is identical to the natural pituitary peptide, and it is the only drug approved for induction and augmentation of labor. Pitocin and Syntocinon are the synthetic preparations. Currently, prostaglandin E_2 (PGE_2) is being investigated as a possible cervical ripening agent, but it has not yet been approved by the Food and Drug Administration.

Indications and Contraindications

The physician must be fully aware of both the indications and the contraindications for the use of oxytocin (Table 11–2). In general, induction of labor before term is indicated only when the continuation of pregnancy represents significant risk to the fetus or mother. In some situations, induction may be indicated at term, as in the case of premature rupture of the membranes. Induction at term

Table 11–2. INDICATIONS AND CONTRAINDICATIONS FOR INDUCTION AND AUGMENTATION OF LABOR

INDUCTION	AUGMENTATION
Indications	

Maternal
  Pre-eclampsia
  Diabetes mellitus
  Heart disease
	Abnormal labor (in the presence of inadequate uterine activity)
	  Prolonged latent phase
	  Prolonged active phase

Fetoplacental
  Prolonged pregnancy
  Intrauterine growth retardation
  Abnormal fetal testing
  Rh incompatibility
  Fetal abnormality
  Premature rupture of membranes
  Chorioamnionitis	

Contraindications	

Maternal
  Absolute
    Contracted pelvis
  Relative
    Prior uterine surgery
      Classic cesarean section
      Complete transection of uterus (myomectomy, reconstruction)
    Overdistended uterus
Fetoplacental
  Preterm fetus without lung maturity
  Acute fetal distress
  Abnormal presentation
	Same contraindications

for convenience is not appropriate unless the patient has a history of previous precipitous delivery (less than 3 hours) or lives an unusually long distance from the hospital.

In general, any condition that makes normal labor dangerous for the mother or fetus is a contraindication to induction or augmentation of labor. The most common contraindication is prior uterine surgery in which there has been complete transection of the uterine wall. However, a previous lower transverse uterine incision is no longer con-

Table 11-3. BISHOP SCORE TO ASSESS LIKELIHOOD OF SUCCESSFUL INDUCTION OF LABOR

PHYSICAL FINDINGS	RATING			
	0	1	2	3
Cervix				
Position	Posterior	Mid	Anterior	—
Consistency	Firm	Medium	Soft	—
Effacement (%)	0–30	40–50	60–70	≥80
Dilatation (cm)	0	1–2	3–4	≥5
Fetal head Station	−3	−2	−1	+1

for antibodies. A blood specimen should be held in the laboratory in case crossmatching becomes necessary (see under Complications). Continuous electronic monitoring of the fetal heart rate and uterine activity is required during induction. An internal uterine catheter for monitoring uterine pressure is suggested if intensity cannot be adequately assessed.

Oxytocin Infusion

There are several principles that should be followed when oxytocin is used to induce or augment labor.

1. Oxytocin must be given intravenously to allow the health care team to discontinue its use quickly if a complication such as uterine hypertonus or fetal distress develops. Since oxytocin has a half-life of 3 to 5 minutes, its physiologic effect will diminish within 15 to 30 minutes after discontinuation.

2. A dilute infusion must be used and piggybacked into the main intravenous line so that it can be stopped quickly if necessary, without interrupting the main intravenous route.

3. The drug is best infused with a calibrated infusion pump that can be easily adjusted to effect the required infusion rate accurately.

4. The induction of labor for a specific indication generally should not exceed 72 hours. In patients with a low Bishop Score, it is not unusual for an induction to progress slowly. If the cervix effaces and dilates, it is recommended that the membranes be ruptured on the third day. If adequate progress is not made within 12 hours of rupturing the membranes, a cesarean section should be performed.

5. If adequate labor is established, the infusion rate and the concentration can almost always be reduced, especially during the second stage of labor. This principle avoids the risks of hyperstimulation and fetal distress from excessive stimulation, which frequently occur once labor has been established.

The protocol for oxytocin induction or augmentation of labor is shown in Table 11-4.

sidered a contraindication to a trial of spontaneous labor. Thus, an induction of labor would not be contraindicated.

Induction of labor prior to term for maternal or fetal indications must not be undertaken without the assessment of fetal pulmonary maturity, provided that a delay will not jeopardize the mother or fetus. Fetal lung maturity can most often be accelerated within 24 to 48 hours by the use of glucocorticoids.

Technique for Induction and Augmentation

A hospital obstetric service must have guidelines for the proper use of oxytocin for induction and augmentation. In general, an assessment and plan of management must be outlined in the progress notes of the patient's medical record. Indications for induction of labor should be clearly stated. It is helpful to assess the likelihood of success by a careful pelvic examination to determine the *Bishop Score*, which evaluates the status of the cervix and the station of the fetal head (Table 11-3). A high score (9 to 13) is associated with a high likelihood of a vaginal delivery, whereas a low score (less than 5) is associated with a decreased likelihood of success (65 to 80 per cent). Prior to beginning induction, the patient must have her blood typed and screened

Table 11-4. METHOD OF OXYTOCIN INFUSION FOR INDUCTION/AUGMENTATION

Table 11-4. METHOD OF OXYTOCIN INFUSION FOR INDUCTION/AUGMENTATION

SOLUTION
10 units of oxytocin in 1000 ml of 5% dextrose or balanced salt solution (10 mU/ml)

ADMINISTRATION
Piggyback into main IV line
Administer solution by infusion pump
Initial rate is 0.5–1.0 mU/min
Increase every 15 min (every 20–30 min may be more appropriate for augmentation)
Maximum dose is 20 mU/min
Dosage progression as follows:
  0.5 mU/min
  1 mU/min
  2 mU/min
  5 mU/min
  7.5 mU/min
  10 mU/min
  15 mU/min
  20 mU/min

Amniotomy

Amniotomy alone is rarely used to induce labor. In general, induction with oxytocin facilitates the application of the presenting part to the lower uterine segment, thus reducing the likelihood for cord prolapse when the membranes are later ruptured. Amniotomy stimulates prostaglandin synthesis and secretion, which facilitates the induction of labor. Loss of amniotic fluid, however, significantly increases the likelihood of cord compression and possibly increases the likelihood of fetal distress.

Complications

There are three major complications from the use of oxytocin for the induction and augmentation of labor. First, an excessive infusion rate can cause *hyperstimulation* and thereby cause fetal distress. In rare situations, a tetanic contraction can occur and lead to *rupture of the uterus.* Second, since oxytocin has a similar structure to antidiuretic hormone, it has an intrinsic *antidiuretic effect* and will increase water reabsorption from the glomerular filtrate. Severe *water intoxication*

with convulsions and coma can rarely occur when oxytocin is infused continuously for more than 24 hours. Third, prolonged oxytocin infusions can result in *uterine muscle fatigue* (nonresponsiveness) and *postdelivery uterine atony* (hypotonus), which can increase the risk of postpartum hemorrhage.

PUERPERIUM

The puerperium consists of the period following delivery of the baby and placenta to approximately 6 weeks postpartum. During the puerperium, the reproductive organs and maternal physiology return toward the prepregnancy state.

Anatomic and Physiologic Changes

Involution of the Uterus. Through a process of tissue catabolism, the uterus rapidly decreases in weight from about 1000 gm at delivery to 50 gm at approximately 3 weeks postpartum. The cervix similarly loses its elasticity and regains its prepregnancy firmness. For the first few days after delivery, the uterine discharge (lochia) appears red *(lochia rubra)* owing to the presence of erythrocytes. After 3 to 4 days, the lochia becomes paler *(lochia serosa),* and, by the tenth day, it assumes a white or yellow-white color *(lochia alba).* Foul-smelling lochia suggests, but is not diagnostic of, endometritis.

Vagina. Although the vagina never returns to its prepregnancy state, the supportive tissues of the pelvic floor gradually regain their former tone.

Cardiovascular System. Immediately following delivery, there is a marked increase in peripheral vascular resistance due to the removal of the low-pressure uteroplacental circulation. The cardiac work and plasma volume gradually return to normal during the first 2 weeks of the puerperium. As a result of the loss of plasma volume and the diuresis of extracellular fluid, there is a marked weight loss in the first week. A significant granulocytic leukocytosis may be seen in the immediate postpartum period.

Psychosocial Changes. It is fairly common for women to exhibit a mild degree of depression a few days following delivery. The "postpartum blues" are probably due to both emotional and hormonal factors. With understanding and reassurance from both family and physician, this usually resolves without consequence.

Return of Menstruation and Ovulation. In women who do not nurse, menstrual flow will usually return by 6 to 8 weeks following delivery, although this is highly variable. Although ovulation may not occur for several months, particularly in nursing mothers, contraceptive counseling and use should be emphasized during the puerperium to avoid unwanted pregnancy (see Chapter 42).

BREAST FEEDING

There are many advantages to breast feeding. First, breast milk is the ideal food for the newborn, is inexpensive, and is usually in good supply. Second, nursing accelerates the involution of the uterus because suckling stimulates the release of oxytocin, thereby causing increased uterine contractions. Third, and probably most important, there are immunologic advantages for the baby from breast feeding. Various types of maternal antibodies are present in breast milk. The predominant immunoglobulin is secretory IgA, which provides protection in the infant's gut by preventing attachment of bacteria (e.g., *Escherichia coli*) to cells on the mucosal surface. This prevents the bacteria from penetrating the bowel wall. It is also thought that maternal lymphocytes pass through the infant's gut wall and initiate immunologic processes not yet well understood. Breast feeding thereby provides the newborn with passive immunity against certain infectious diseases until its own immune mechanisms become fully functional by 3 to 4 months.

Lactation

Various hormones, such as estrogen, progesterone, human chorionic gonadotropin, cortisol, insulin, prolactin, and placental lactogen play an important role in preparing the breasts for lactation. At delivery, two events are instrumental in initiating lactation. First, the drop in placental hormones (particularly estrogen) allows lactation to occur. (Prior to delivery, these hormones interfere with lactogenic action of prolactin.) Second, suckling stimulates the release of prolactin and oxytocin. The latter causes contraction of the myoepithelial cells in the alveoli and milk ducts. The suckling stimulus is thought important for milk production as well as the ejection of colostrum and milk.

On approximately the second day after delivery, colostrum is secreted. Its content is composed mostly of protein, fat, and minerals. It is the colostrum that contains secretory IgA. After about 3 to 6 days, the colostrum is replaced by mature milk. The content of milk varies considerably depending on the nutritional status of the mother and the gestational age at the time of delivery. In general, the major components of breast milk are proteins, lactose, water, and fat. The major proteins synthesized in the human breast, which are unique and not found in cows' milk, are casein, lactoalbumin, and beta-lactoglobulin. Essential amino acids are delivered from the mother's blood, and some of the nonessential amino acids can be synthesized in the breast. Lactose and fatty acids are synthesized in the breast.

Lactation Suppression

When the mother chooses not to breast feed, lactation suppression is indicated. The simplest, and probably safest, method to accomplish this is to use a tight-fitting bra to prevent breast distention. If breast distention does occur, pumping only makes the situation worse. Ice packs should be applied and the discomfort managed with analgesics. Drugs, such as estrogens in combination with testosterone, have been used to suppress lactation but must be given immediately after delivery to be effective, and there is concern that they may increase the risk of thromboembolism. Bromocriptine (Parlodel), a dopamine agonist, produces a fall in prolactin levels and inhibition of lactation. Therapy with bromocriptine should be started only after the patient's vital signs have stabilized

Table 11–5. EFFECTS OF MATERNAL DRUG INGESTION ON BREAST-FEEDING INFANTS

DRUG	REPORTED INFANT EFFECTS
Sedative-hypnotics	
Diazepam	Sedation
Meprobamate	Effects not known
Antipsychotics	
Chlorpromazine	No adverse effects reported
Haloperidol	No adverse effects reported
Non-narcotic analgesics	
Acetaminophen	No adverse effects reported
Salicylates	No known adverse effects; theoretical risk of platelet dysfunction
Naproxen	Effects not known
Anticonvulsants	
Phenobarbital	Sedation
Phenytoin	Sedation, decreased sucking
Narcotics	
Heroin	May cause addiction
Methadone	One infant death reported
Meperidine	No adverse effects reported
Antibiotics	
Penicillin	May modify bowel flora, cause allergy, or interfere with sepsis work-up
Ampicillin	Same as for penicillin
Erythromycin	Same as for penicillin
Nitrofurantoin	Theoretical risk of hemolytic anemia in infants with G6PD deficiency
Tetracycline	Same as for penicillin; theoretical risk of discoloration of teeth and inhibition of bone growth
Digoxin	No adverse effects reported
Thyroid drugs	
Thyroxine	May interfere with screening for hypothyroidism
Propylthiouracil	Nodular goiter
Antihypertensives	
Methyldopa	No adverse effects reported
Propranolol	No adverse effects reported
Theophylline	One case of infant irritability following maternal administration of a rapidly absorbed oral preparation

G6PD = Glucose-6-phosphate dehydrogenase.

and not sooner than 4 hours after delivery. The dosage is 2.5 mg twice daily for 14 days.

Complications of Breast Feeding

Cracked Nipples

If the nipples of the breast become fissured, nursing may become difficult. Since fissures are also a portal of entry for bacteria, they should be managed aggressively with a nipple shield and an appropriate cream, such as lanolin or Masse Breast Cream. Further breast feeding should be temporarily stopped. Milk can be expressed manually until the nipples heal, at which time breast feeding can be resumed.

Mastitis

This is an uncommon complication of breast feeding and usually develops 2 to 4 weeks after beginning breast feeding. The first symptoms are usually slight fever and chills. These are followed by redness of a segment of the breast, which becomes indurated and painful. The etiologic agent is usually *Staphylococcus aureus,* which originates from the infant's oral pharynx. Milk should be obtained from the breast for culture and sensitivity, and the mother should be started on antibiotics immediately. Since the majority of staphylococcal organisms are penicillinase-producing, a penicillinase-resistant antibiotic, such as cloxacillin, should be used. Breast feeding should be discontinued, and an appropriate antibiotic should be continued for 7 to 10 days. A breast pump can be used to maintain lactation until the infection has cleared, but the milk should be discarded. The infant, along with other family members, should be evaluated for staphylococcal infections that may be a source of reinfection if breast feeding is resumed.

Drug Passage to the Newborn

Since an infant may ingest up to 500 ml of breast milk per day, maternally administered drugs that pass into breast milk may have a significant effect on the infant. The amount of drug found in breast milk depends on the maternal dose, the rate of maternal clearance, the physicochemical properties of the drug, and the breast milk composition with respect to fat and protein. The gestational age of the infant may also be a determinant of the ultimate drug effect. Table 11–5 lists selected drugs with their reported newborn effects.

SUGGESTED READING

Bishop EN: Pelvic scoring for elective induction. Obstet Gynecol 24:266, 1964.

Briggs GG, Bodendorfer TW, Freeman RK, et al: Drugs in Pregnancy and Lactation. Baltimore, Williams & Wilkins, 1983.

Goldman AS, Smith CW: Host resistance factors in breast milk. J Pediatr 82:1082, 1973.

Herxheimer A (ed): Drugs which can be given to nursing mothers. Drug and Therapeutic Bulletin. London, Consumer's Association, 1983, p 5.

Hughey MJ, McElin TW, Bird CC: An evaluation of preinduction scoring systems. Obstet Gynecol 48:635, 1976.

McNeilly AS, Robinson ICA, Houston MJ, et al: Release of oxytocin and prolactin in response to suckling. Br Med J 286:257, 1983.

Pritchard JA, MacDonald PC, Gant NF (eds): Williams Obstetrics. 17th ed. East Norwalk, CT, Appleton-Century-Crofts, 1985.

Rovinsky JJ: Management of normal labor and delivery. In Sciarra JJ, Gerbie AB (eds): Gynecology and Obstetrics. Vol 2. Philadelphia, Harper & Row, 1984.

Tyson JE, Friesen HG, Anderson MS: Human lactational and ovarian response to endogenous prolactin release. Science 177:897, 1972.

Twelve

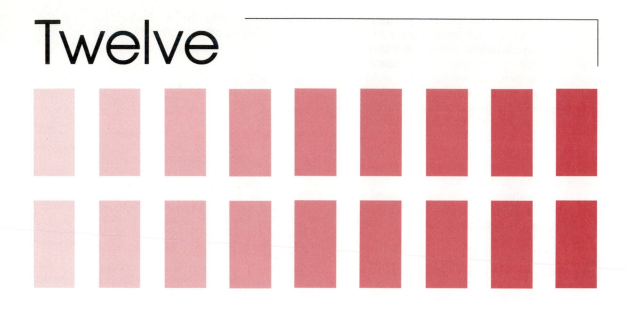

Obstetric Analgesia and Anesthesia

KENNETH A. CONKLIN

During labor and vaginal delivery, analgesia can be achieved with nonpharmacologic techniques, systemic medication, inhalation agents, or regional analgesia. For cesarean section, regional or general anesthesia may be used (Table 12–1). The obvious goal of obstetric anesthesia is to optimize maternal and neonatal outcome. Thus, the anesthesiologist must be aware of the maternal risks and benefits of the analgesic and anesthetic options that are available, the effects of analgesic techniques on the progress of labor, and the potential direct (due to placental drug transfer) and indirect (due to reduced uterine blood flow) adverse effects of the drugs and techniques on the fetus and neonate. Topics in this chapter that are relevant to these issues include placental drug transfer, the effects of obstetric analgesia and anesthesia on

uterine blood flow and uterine activity, and a description of the agents and techniques used for labor and vaginal delivery, cesarean section, and complicated obstetric situations.

PLACENTAL TRANSFER OF DRUGS

The direct effects of a maternally administered drug on the fetus and neonate depend on the amount of the drug that reaches the fetal circulation. The fetal to maternal ratio (FMR) of drug concentrations is used to assess placental drug transfer. This ratio is determined by measuring the drug level in samples of fetal and maternal blood obtained simultaneously (e.g., at the time of delivery). A high FMR suggests a high degree of placental transfer. Although all drugs cross the placenta to some extent, the degree of transfer is determined by maternal and fetal blood flow to the placenta as well as by factors that determine drug passage across the placental barrier itself.

Maternal Circulation of the Placenta

Maternal blood flow to the placenta is governed by the total uterine blood flow and the fraction that perfuses the intervillous space. Anything that reduces uterine blood flow, such as uterine contractions or maternal hypotension, reduces drug delivery to the placenta.

Drug Transfer Across the Placenta

Nearly all drugs cross the placenta by passive diffusion. The amount of transfer is pro-portional to the concentration gradient of the drug across the placenta and the diffusion constant of the drug. The latter is governed by the physicochemical properties of the drug, which include molecular weight, spatial configuration, lipid solubility, degree of ionization, and amount of drug binding to maternal plasma proteins. In general, if the molecular weight is under 1000, the size and spatial configuration do not affect placental transfer. As the amount of protein binding increases, transfer decreases, since only unbound drug crosses the placenta. A highly ionized drug also exhibits limited placental transfer. Drugs with high lipid solubility tend to cross the placenta readily.

Fetal Circulation of the Placenta

Fetal blood flow to the placenta via the umbilical arteries, returning to the fetus via the umbilical vein, has been estimated to be approximately 50 per cent of the combined ventricular output. An increase in fetal circulation of the placenta, as occurs with fetal asphyxia, may increase placental drug transfer. Fetal asphyxia, which is accompanied by a reduced pH of fetal blood, also results in the phenomenon of "ion trapping." In this situation, the lower pH causes a drug that is a weak base (e.g., a narcotic or local anesthetic) to become more highly ionized, thus trapping it in the fetal circulation. This may further enhance drug delivery to the fetus.

Evaluating Drug Effects in Newborns

The Apgar score, which is determined routinely for all newborn infants, assesses parameters that are essential to neonatal survival (see Chapter 13). A reduced Apgar score may occur in association with obstetric analgesia or anesthesia, for example, if reduced uterine blood flow results from hypotension with a spinal or epidural block, or if a high dose of narcotic or sedative-tranquilizer is administered during labor. Subtle effects of maternal medication or birth asphyxia, however, may be missed entirely by the Apgar score. Therefore, more sophisticated techniques have been developed for evaluating neurologic and behavioral parameters of the neonate that are controlled by higher central nervous system functions. These evaluations, which are primarily research tools, include the Brazelton Neonatal Behavioral Assessment Scale, the Early Neonatal Neurobehavioral Scale, and the Neurologic and Adaptive Capacity Score.

EFFECTS OF OBSTETRIC ANESTHESIA ON UTERINE ACTIVITY AND BLOOD FLOW

Analgesia and anesthesia must be administered to the parturient in a manner that neither reduces uterine activity, which may alter the progress of labor, nor reduces uterine blood flow, which may result in fetal distress or neonatal depression.

Effects on Uterine Activity and Labor

The uterus has alpha-1 and beta-2 adrenergic receptors. Alpha-1 adrenergic stimulants increase uterine tone. Conversely, agents with beta-2 adrenergic stimulating properties reduce uterine activity. Epinephrine, a beta-2 agonist, is released from the adrenal glands during the pain and stress of labor, and this may reduce uterine contractility and slow the progress of labor. Adrenal epinephrine secretion, however, may be affected by maternal analgesia or anesthesia.

Systemic Medication

Narcotics administered during the latent phase of the first stage of labor generally reduce uterine contractions. If given during the active phase, these agents increase or have no effect on uterine activity. Improvement of uterine contractility, when it occurs, is most likely attributable to a reduced maternal blood level of epinephrine. Tranquilizing agents have little effect on uterine activity when administered during the active phase of labor.

Inhalation Anesthetics

In circumstances such as therapy for a tetanic uterine contraction or for intrauterine manipulations, uterine relaxation is required. The most reliable technique for rapidly producing this effect is with general anesthesia using a high concentration of a halogenated anesthetic (halothane, isoflurane, or enflurane). These agents produce a dose-dependent decrease in uterine resting tone, uterine contractility, and uterine responsiveness to oxytocin. These actions, however, can also markedly increase uterine blood loss. Therefore, when these agents are needed for uterine relaxation, they are used for as short a period of time as possible.

Regional Analgesia and Anesthesia

The effect of well-conducted epidural analgesia on uterine activity depends, in part, on whether it is administered during the latent or the active phase of the first stage of labor. When given during the latent phase, epidural analgesia generally reduces uterine activity. Although it is uncertain as to the mechanism involved, interruption of oxytocin release in response to cervical dilatation (Ferguson's reflex) may cause uterine inhibition. During the active phase of the first stage of labor, epidural analgesia has either no significant effect or causes enhanced uterine activity. Beneficial effects are most likely due to reduced maternal epinephrine secretion from blockade of the sympathetic preganglionic innervation of the adrenal glands.

Improperly administered regional analgesia or anesthesia during labor or vaginal delivery may have adverse effects. Hypotension, for example, will reduce uterine activity and slow the progress of labor. Excessive anesthesia during the first stage of labor relaxes the pelvic musculature and may interfere with flexion and internal rotation of the fetal head, which can prolong the second stage. The second stage of labor may also be prolonged if the patient's abdominal muscles are relaxed by anesthesia. When this occurs, the parturient is unable to bear down efficiently. In some patients, this problem is compounded by the reduced desire to push when perineal analgesia is produced. In the parturient who is motivated to bear down and is properly instructed, however, the appropriate use of regional anesthesia without excessive motor blockade will not prolong the second stage of labor.

Effects on Uterine Blood Flow

Normal fetal respiratory gases depend on the maintenance of uterine blood flow. Since the uterine vascular bed does not possess autoregulatory mechanisms, uterine blood flow is solely dependent on uterine perfusion pressure (UPP) and uterine vascular resistance. A drop in uterine blood flow caused by a decrease in UPP or an increase in intrinsic (vascular tone) or extrinsic (intrauterine pressure) uterine vascular resistance may result in fetal hypoxia, hypercarbia, and acidosis.

UPP is the difference between uterine arterial pressure (UAP) and uterine venous pressure (UVP). UAP, which is proportional to maternal mean arterial pressure, is reduced by maternal hypotension. This may occur from blockade of the sympathetic nervous system during regional anesthesia if the parturient is not adequately hydrated or if deep general anesthesia with halothane (Fluothane), isoflurane (Forane), or enflurane (Ethrane) is administered. These effects may be enhanced by aortocaval compression, which results from compression of the great vessels by the gravid uterus when the parturient assumes the supine position. Compression of the inferior vena cava by the uterus elevates UVP, which reduces UPP, and decreases venous return to the heart, thereby causing a fall in cardiac output, maternal blood pressure, and UAP. Compression of the aorta above the origin of the uterine arteries further reduces UAP.

Intrinsic uterine vascular resistance may be increased if the concentration of local anesthetic in the uterine circulation is very high. This may occur with a paracervical block or if an unintentional intravascular injection is given when attempting epidural anesthesia. Vasopressor drugs that directly stimulate alpha-1 adrenergic receptors (for example, norepinephrine, epinephrine, and phenylephrine) also increase intrinsic vascular resistance. This effect is not seen with ephedrine (the vasopressor indicated for obstetric use), which possesses direct beta-1 adrenergic stimulating effects on the heart but only indirect alpha-1 adrenergic stimulating effects (release of norepinephrine from sympathetic nerve terminals). Intrinsic vascular resistance may also be increased by release of endogenous catecholamines when maternal sympathetic nervous system activity is high.

Extrinsic uterine vascular resistance is proportional to intrauterine pressure. It is elevated during uterine contractions and with an increase in resting uterine tone, as can occur following unintentional intravascular injection of a local anesthetic or with excessive intravenous infusion of oxytocin (tetanic uterine contraction).

PAIN PATHWAYS OF PARTURITION

Pain is the sensation of discomfort resulting from stimulation of specialized nerve endings. During labor and vaginal delivery, pain is caused by uterine contractions, dilatation of the cervix, and distention of the perineum. The visceral afferent nerve fibers that carry the sensory impulses from the uterus enter the spinal cord at the tenth, eleventh, and twelfth thoracic and first lumbar spinal segments (T10 to L1). Pain from the perineum travels via somatic afferent nerve fibers, primarily in the pudendal nerve, and reaches the spinal cord through the second, third, and fourth sacral segments (S2 to S4) (Fig. 12–1). These sensory fibers from the uterus and perineum make synaptic connections in the dorsal horn of the spinal cord with cells that provide axons that make up the spinothalamic tracts. During the early part of the first stage of labor, pain arises primarily from the uterus. During the latter part of the first stage and throughout the second stage of labor, pain impulses arise not only from the uterus but also from the perineum as the fetal presenting part passes through the pelvis.

SELECTION OF LOCAL ANESTHETICS FOR OBSTETRIC USE

The agents used clinically for regional anesthesia possess the general structure shown in Figure 12–2. The linkage between the

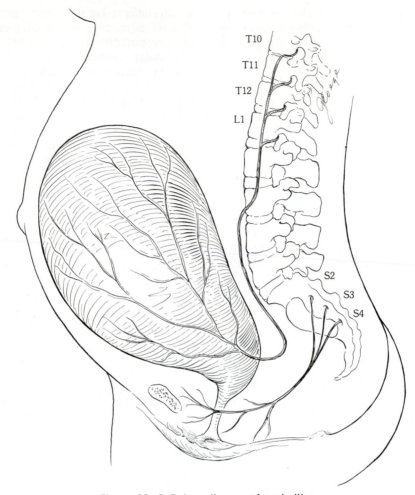

Figure 12-1. Pain pathways of parturition.

aromatic portion and the intermediate chain separates these agents into two groups with important distinctions. Although a rare occurrence, an ester-linked drug (e.g., chloroprocaine, procaine, or tetracaine) is more likely to be associated with allergic reactions than is an amide-linked agent (e.g., lidocaine or bupivacaine). The ester-linked local anesthetics are rapidly metabolized by plasma cholinesterase, which markedly reduces the potential for maternal systemic toxicity as well as limits fetal drug exposure and neonatal effects. The amide-linked local anesthetics are slowly degraded by the liver, thus allowing for a greater degree of placental transfer.

Placental transfer of the amide-linked local anesthetics, as reflected by FMR (Table 12-2), is most affected by their degree of ioniza-

tion and percentage of protein binding in maternal plasma. The low molecular weight (all under 350) and relatively high lipid solubility of these drugs do not significantly impair their passage across the placenta. The FMR of bupivacaine is 0.25, which is considerably lower than that of lidocaine (0.55). This is because the drug is more highly ionized and has a greater degree of protein binding. Despite the difference in placental transfer, however, use of either lidocaine or bupivacaine for well-conducted epidural blocks during labor or cesarean section does not affect Apgar scores or neurobehavioral performance. Therefore, since neonatal outcome is also unaffected by chloroprocaine because of rapid metabolism, the choice of local anesthetic for epidural analgesia or an-

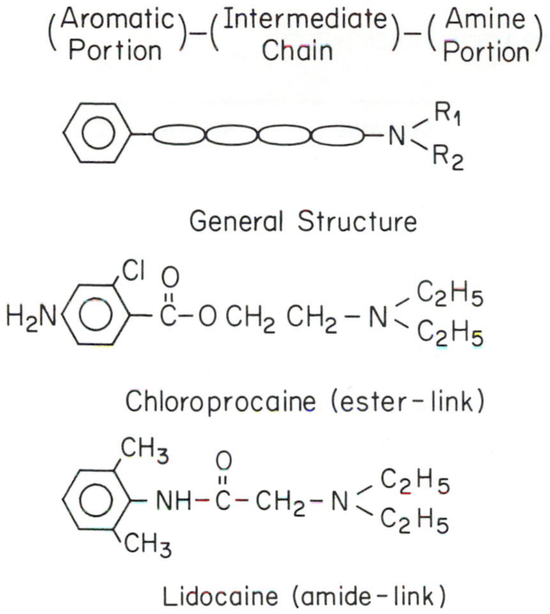

$$\left(\begin{array}{c}\text{Aromatic}\\\text{Portion}\end{array}\right) - \left(\begin{array}{c}\text{Intermediate}\\\text{Chain}\end{array}\right) - \left(\begin{array}{c}\text{Amine}\\\text{Portion}\end{array}\right)$$

General Structure

Chloroprocaine (ester-link)

Lidocaine (amide-link)

Figure 12–2. Structure of local anesthetics. The aromatic portion is primarily responsible for the lipophilic property (lipid solubility) of the local anesthetic, although this property is also affected by the -R groups. The intermediate chain serves to link the aromatic and amine portions of the molecule. The amine portion (generally a tertiary amine) confers on the local anesthetic the property of being a weak base and is responsible for the hydrophilic property (water solubility) of the drug.

esthesia is based on the onset and duration of action of the drugs (Table 12–2).

ANALGESIA AND ANESTHESIA FOR LABOR AND VAGINAL DELIVERY

Selection of the appropriate analgesic or anesthetic technique for labor and vaginal delivery depends on the desires of the parturient, the skills of available personnel, the stage of labor, and whether contraindications to a particular technique exist. Analgesia can be achieved by a drug at one of three different sites of action: the brain, the dorsal horn of the spinal cord, or the sensory nerve fiber. Agents such as narcotics, sedative-tranquilizers, and inhalation analgesics have an effect on the brain itself. Narcotics and alpha-2 agonists (e.g., clonidine and epinephrine), when injected into the epidural or subarach-

noid space, interfere with transmission of pain impulses by an action on receptors in the dorsal horn. Local anesthetics block conduction in sensory nerve fibers, thus preventing impulses arising from pain receptors in the periphery from reaching the central nervous system. In addition to its action in the dorsal horn, epinephrine also enhances the conduction block produced by local anesthetics by slowing their absorption from the epidural or subarachnoid space.

Systemic Medication

Systemic medication is more easily administered than spinal or epidural blocks but introduces potential adverse effects that are not seen with regional analgesia. Maternal awareness may be depressed, making the parturient less able to participate in the birth process. Systemic medications rapidly cross the placenta and may result in neonatal depression. Additionally, these agents do not provide the high degree of analgesia that can be easily achieved with a regional technique. Despite these limitations, systemic medication is still an appropriate means of providing analgesia, especially in situations when an anesthesiologist is unavailable, regional analgesia is contraindicated (e.g., in the presence of a coagulopathy or skin infection), or when the patient is fearful of regional anesthesia.

Narcotics

Meperidine (Demerol) is the most popular narcotic for the parturient during labor. It is generally administered in doses of 25 to 50 mg intravenously or 50 to 100 mg intramuscularly. After intravenous injection, the peak effect is seen in 7 to 8 minutes with a duration of action of 1.5 to 3 hours. The peak effect and duration of action after an intramuscular dose are 45 minutes and 3 to 4 hours, respectively. Fentanyl, two or three 25-μg doses 5 minutes apart, has a peak analgesic effect 5 to 6 minutes after (each) intravenous injection and a duration of action of 30 to 60 minutes. The narcotic agonist-antagonist butorphanol (Stadol) is also effective for providing analgesia during labor (1 mg intravenously or intramuscularly).

Table 12–2. PROPERTIES OF LOCAL ANESTHETICS

PROPERTY	CHLOROPROCAINE	TETRACAINE	LIDOCAINE	BUPIVACAINE
Trade name(s)	Nesacaine	Pontocaine	Xylocaine	Marcaine, Sensorcaine
pKa*	8.7	8.2	7.9	8.1
% Ionized (pH 7.4)	95	86	76	83
% Protein bound	—	76	64	95
FMR	—	—	0.55	0.25
Potency	0.7	4	1	4
Use	Epidural	Spinal	Epidural	Epidural
Onset	Rapid	Rapid	Intermediate	Slow
Duration	Short	Long	Intermediate	Long

* pKa: Dissociation constant for the drug.
FMR = Fetal to maternal ratio.

Morphine is rarely used because when it is administered in an equi-analgesic dose it is associated with a greater degree of neonatal respiratory depression than is meperidine.

Although narcotics provide both analgesia and sedation, they may be associated with maternal, fetal, or neonatal side effects (Table 12–3). Most side effects, however, can be reversed with naloxone (Narcan), a narcotic antagonist.

Sedative-Tranquilizers

These agents are generally given in combination with a narcotic. The phenothiazine promethazine (Phenergan), 25 mg intramuscularly or 12.5 mg intravenously, relieves anxiety, controls nausea and vomiting, and reduces narcotic requirements during labor. Hydroxyzine (Vistaril), 50 mg intramuscularly, has similar properties. These drugs are without significant maternal, fetal, or neonatal side effects when used in recommended doses. Diazepam (Valium) is rarely used in current obstetric practice because it is associated with significant neonatal side effects, including reduced Apgar scores, impaired neurobehavioral status, impaired thermogenesis (hypothermia when the infant is cold-stressed), and reduced feeding. Fetal tachycardia and reduced beat to beat variability are also seen when doses as small as 2.5 mg are given during labor.

Table 12–3. POTENTIAL SIDE EFFECTS OF NARCOTICS

Maternal
  Orthostatic hypotension
  Nausea and vomiting
  Delayed gastric emptying (increases aspiration risk)
  Slowing of labor (if given too early)
  Respiratory depression
Fetal
  Reduced beat to beat variability of fetal heart rate
Neonatal
  Respiratory depression
  Decreased Apgar score
  Altered neurobehavioral status

Inhalation Analgesia

This technique, which is infrequently used in the United States, involves the administration of subanesthetic concentrations of inhalation agents to provide analgesia during the first and second stages of labor. These drugs are administered with a mask or mouthpiece in a manner such that the parturient remains awake, cooperative, and in control of her airway so as to prevent pulmonary aspiration of gastric contents. Although not comparable with the degree of analgesia or safety of epidural anesthesia, the use of inhalation analgesia is associated with less risk of neonatal depression when compared with narcotics.

Nitrous oxide (N_2O) is the most commonly used inhalation agent. When administered during labor or vaginal delivery, the parturient intermittently breathes a 50 per cent concentration of N_2O in oxygen. Intermittent inhalation of methoxyflurane (Penthrane), 0.1 to 0.3 per cent in oxygen, or enflurane (0.5 per cent in oxygen) are alternative, but less popular, techniques.

Regional Analgesia and Anesthesia

Regional analgesic and anesthetic techniques for labor and delivery include peripheral (paracervical and pudendal) and central (lumbar epidural, caudal, and spinal) nerve blocks. Epidural anesthesia is the ideal anesthetic for the obstetric patient. It provides excellent analgesia during labor and anesthesia for vaginal delivery. Should it become necessary, an epidural block initiated during labor can be supplemented to provide anesthesia for cesarean section. A paracervical block, which is rarely used, provides analgesia during labor, but only for pain of uterine contractions and only during the early first stage of labor. A pudendal block provides perineal analgesia and is appropriate to administer for vaginal delivery as an alternative to an epidural or spinal block. A caudal anesthetic produces anesthesia that is comparable to spinal anesthesia for delivery but is infrequently used because a spinal block can be more quickly and easily administered.

Paracervical Block

This technique anesthetizes the sensory nerves of the uterus (T10 to L1) by the transvaginal injection of local anesthetic just lateral to the cervix on each side. Although the block is relatively easy to perform and does not produce maternal hypotension, it is associated with a high incidence of fetal distress as a result of vasoconstriction of the uterine vasculature, which follows the rapid absorption of the local anesthetic. Additionally, maternal toxicity from intravascular injection (e.g., a local anesthetic-induced seizure) or hematoma formation from uterine artery damage may occur.

Pudendal Block

A pudendal block (Fig. 12–3), which is administered shortly before delivery, anesthetizes the pudendal nerve (S2 to S4) as it travels just posterior to the junction of the ischial spine and sacrospinous ligament. After aspirating, so as to avoid intravascular injection, approximately 10 ml of 1 per cent lidocaine or 2 per cent chloroprocaine are injected on each side. The analgesia produced in the lower birth canal and perineum provides maternal comfort for low forceps delivery and episiotomy.

A pudendal block is easy to administer, is not associated with maternal hypotension, and is rarely associated with fetal distress. Disadvantages include incomplete analgesia at the time of delivery, since the pain of uterine contractions is unaffected, and incomplete perineal analgesia, especially if vaginal delivery is difficult or if there is extension of the episiotomy. This occurs because the perineum has sensory innervation from nerves other than the pudendal nerve. Analgesia may be improved by local anesthetic infiltration of the perineum in combination with the pudendal block. Complications include systemic toxic reactions, puncture of the rectum, hematoma formation, and sciatic nerve block if the needle is inserted too deeply.

Epidural Anesthesia

Continuous lumbar epidural analgesia should be initiated once labor is well established. Generally, this is when dilatation of the cervix is 4 to 5 cm in a multipara or 5 to 6 cm in a nullipara, uterine contractions are strong and regular, and the fetal head is engaged. When labor is being induced or augmented with oxytocin, however, the technique may be employed earlier. Anesthetic agents are usually injected through a 19- or 20-gauge indwelling catheter inserted into the epidural space at the L3–4 interspace through a special needle (e.g., Touhy).

During the early active phase of labor, relatively small doses of local anesthetic (e.g., 6 to 8 ml of 0.25 per cent bupivacaine every 1 to 1.5 hours) provide adequate segmental analgesia (T10 to L1) for pain arising from the uterus. During the latter part of the first

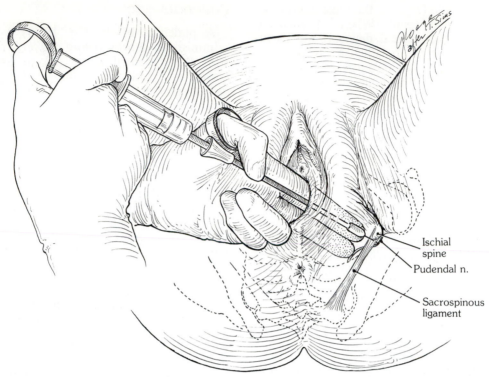

Figure 12-3. Technique for transvaginal pudendal block.

stage of labor and during the second stage of labor, the level of analgesia should be extended (T10 to S5) so that perineal discomfort is also relieved. This is accomplished by increasing the anesthetic dose (e.g., 8 to 12 ml of 0.25 per cent bupivacaine every 1 to 1.5 hours) and elevating the patient's head 20 to 30 degrees. Fentanyl (50 to 100 μg), administered with the dose of bupivacaine, prolongs analgesia to approximately 2.5 hours and produces an equivalent degree of analgesia with a reduced dose (30 to 40 per cent less) of local anesthetic. An alternative to repeated bolus injections throughout labor is the use of a continuous infusion, at the rate of approximately 10 ml per hour, of local anesthetic (0.125 per cent bupivacaine) or local anesthetic (0.0625 per cent bupivacaine) plus fentanyl (2 μg/ml) following institution of analgesia with an initial bolus injection. If perineal anesthesia (muscle relaxation) is needed to facilitate a difficult vaginal delivery (see later), this can be established by injection of 10 to 12 ml of 2 per cent lidocaine.

Certain precautions must be taken when administering an epidural anesthetic. After negative aspiration for blood and cerebrospinal fluid (CSF), an initial test dose of 3 ml is given and the patient is assessed for evidence of a spinal block (e.g., the rapid onset of sensory loss). Assuming that the initial test dose does not produce a spinal block, a second test dose of 5 ml is given to exclude the possibility of intravascular injection. If signs of intravascular injection, such as dizziness or tinnitus, do not occur, the remaining dose of local anesthetic is administered at the rate of 5 ml per minute. If the local anesthetic solution contains epinephrine (5 μg/ml), tachycardia occurring after a test dose also indicates an intravascular injection. A balanced salt solution must be administered intravenously concomitantly with an epidural anesthetic to prevent maternal hypotension.

Spinal (Subarachnoid) Anesthesia

A subarachnoid block is generally administered shortly before delivery by injecting a small amount of local anesthetic (e.g., 4 mg of tetracaine, 6 mg of bupivacaine, or 30 mg of lidocaine) through a spinal needle placed in the L3–4 interspace. To prevent the anesthetic level from ascending too high, the local anesthetic solution is made hyperbaric (with respect to CSF) by the addition of 10 per cent dextrose, and the injection is made with the parturient in the sitting position. The anesthetic level should extend to T10. As with an epidural block, an intravenous crystalloid solution (600 to 800 ml) must be given to prevent hypotension. Although some authors advocate the use of a "saddle block" (a spinal anesthetic of S1 to S5) for vaginal delivery, this procedure does not provide complete pain relief since the sensory nerves from the uterus are not anesthetized.

The main disadvantage of spinal anesthesia is the occurrence of a postspinal headache, a complication that is more likely in the pregnant than the nonpregnant patient. The cause of the headache is loss of CSF through the hole in the dura, which creates traction on the meninges. The incidence of this complication can be minimized by using either a small-gauge spinal needle (25- or 26-gauge) or a special spinal needle (Whitacre or Sprotte) that separates, but does not cut, the longitudinal fibers of the dura.

Caudal Anesthesia

This type of anesthesia is performed by injecting local anesthetic into the sacral epidural space. Entrance to this space is gained by placing an epidural needle through the sacrococcygeal membrane that covers the sacral hiatus. One advantage of a caudal block is that good perineal anesthesia can be achieved without placing the parturient in the sitting position. Disadvantages are the larger dose of local anesthetic needed to produce anesthesia (compared with a spinal or lumbar epidural block) and the technical difficulty that is commonly encountered when performing the procedure.

General Anesthesia

General anesthesia is not administered electively for vaginal delivery because the parturient, when unconscious, is at substantial risk of pulmonary aspiration of gastric contents. If an emergency arises in which rapid anesthesia is necessary, however, such as for shoulder dystocia, undiagnosed twins, or breech presentation, general anesthesia is indicated. A high concentration of halothane (2 per cent), isoflurane (3 per cent), or enflurane (4 per cent) is used if uterine relaxation is necessary.

ANESTHESIA FOR CESAREAN SECTION

Regional anesthesia is generally considered to be the technique of choice. It allows the parturient to be awake and the father to be present, reduces blood loss, is associated with less maternal risk of pulmonary aspiration of gastric contents or hypoxia from failed endotracheal intubation, and reduces neonatal drug effects. Although either a spinal or an epidural block is appropriate, the latter technique has several advantages. With epidural anesthesia, hypotension is less likely to occur because the sympathetic nervous system is blocked more slowly. Anesthesia is more controllable if an epidural catheter is placed since additional anesthetic doses can be given if necessary. Furthermore, a headache does not occur postoperatively since the dura is not punctured. A spinal anesthetic, however, is technically easier to administer and the anesthetic takes effect much more quickly. It is indicated when regional anesthesia is planned for cesarean section, but time does not permit placement of an epidural block. Compared with regional anesthesia, general anesthesia has the advantage of greater cardiovascular stability (i.e., less hypotension from sympathetic blockade). It is indicated when urgent cesarean section is required for maternal hemorrhage.

Regardless of the anesthetic technique selected, certain precautions should be taken to reduce maternal risk and to optimize fetal well-being and neonatal outcome. A clear, nonparticulate antacid (e.g., 30 ml of 0.3 molar sodium citrate) should be administered 10 to 15 minutes before anesthesia to reduce the maternal risk of pulmonary aspiration of acidic gastric contents. Monitors should include a maternal blood pressure cuff (automatic or manual), a chest stethoscope, an electrocardiograph, a pulse oximeter (for monitoring maternal arterial oxygen saturation), and, when general anesthesia is used, a capnograph (for monitoring maternal end-tidal carbon dioxide). Left uterine displacement should be used to prevent aortocaval compression. If regional anesthesia is selected, 1500 to 2000 ml of a balanced salt solution containing 0.5 to 1 per cent dextrose must be administered intravenously to prevent hypotension. Ephedrine should be available for treatment of hypotension, and supplemental oxygen should be given to the mother to increase placental oxygen transfer and reduce the chance of fetal distress if hypotension does occur.

If the anesthetic is administered appropriately, whether it be general or regional, Apgar scores will be unaffected regardless of the time from induction of anesthesia to delivery of the infant. Apgar scores after cesarean section, however, are depressed with prolonged uterine incision to delivery times (that is, greater than 90 seconds). Neurobehavioral status, which is unaffected by regional anesthesia, is temporarily impaired when general anesthesia is used. This is due to the thiopental or ketamine administered for induction of general anesthesia. The other drugs used for general anesthesia do not affect infant outcome, either because of the low concentration used (the inhalation anesthetics) or because of very limited placental transfer (as with muscle relaxants, which are fully ionized quaternary ammonium compounds).

Epidural Anesthesia

The local anesthetics used for cesarean section include lidocaine (1.5 or 2 per cent), chloroprocaine (3 per cent), and bupivacaine (0.5 per cent). A large dose (approximately 20 ml) of local anesthetic is used so as to achieve a level of anesthesia from T4 to S5. The quality of anesthesia can be enhanced by addition of epinephrine (100 μg), fentanyl (100 μg), or both agents.

Spinal Anesthesia

The block is generally performed with the patient in the lateral position. After identifying the subarachnoid space, 7 to 9 mg of tetracaine, 12 to 15 mg of bupivacaine, or 60 to 70 mg of lidocaine is slowly injected. The local anesthetic solution is made hyperbaric by the addition of dextrose (final concentration 5 to 7.5 per cent), and epinephrine (100 μg) may be added to prolong the duration and enhance the quality of anesthesia. The patient is then turned supine, and a wedge is placed under the right hip.

General Anesthesia

There are two primary concerns during induction of general anesthesia. The first is for maternal aspiration of acidic gastric contents, a risk that results from loss of protective laryngeal reflexes during induction. This risk is reduced by antacid administration and by application of pressure on the cricoid cartilage to occlude the esophagus until the airway is secured with a cuffed endotracheal tube. The second concern is for maternal and fetal oxygenation. When apneic, as during induction of anesthesia, the pregnant patient becomes hypoxic much more rapidly than a nonpregnant individual because of increased oxygen consumption and reduced functional residual capacity. Therefore, the patient should breathe 100 per cent oxygen for 3 to 4 minutes before induction of anesthesia.

Induction of general anesthesia is accomplished with intravenous injection of thiopental (Pentothal), 4 mg/kg. In certain circumstances, such as maternal hemorrhage, ketamine (Ketalar, 0.75 mg/kg) is used for induction of anesthesia because it causes less depression of the maternal cardiovascular system. Endotracheal intubation is facilitated by injection of succinylcholine (Anectine, 1.5 mg/kg), a depolarizing muscle relaxant, immediately following the thiopental or ketamine. Anesthesia is maintained until delivery of the fetus with 50 per cent N_2O in oxygen. A low concentration of halothane (0.5 per cent), isoflurane (0.75 per cent), or enflurane (1 per cent) is also administered to enhance the depth of anesthesia, thus reducing maternal blood levels of catecholamines and maintaining better uteroplacental perfusion. Following delivery of the infant, it is common practice to discontinue the halothane, isoflurane, or enflurane and deepen the anesthetic by administration of a narcotic. Muscle relaxation is maintained during the procedure with succinylcholine or a nondepolarizing muscle relaxant such as pancuronium, vecuronium, or atracurium.

POST-CESAREAN SECTION ANALGESIA

Periodic parenteral injection of narcotics for post-cesarean section analgesia has been replaced, in many institutions, by patient controlled analgesia. Patient controlled analgesia is administered by continuous intravenous infusion of a low concentration narcotic (e.g., morphine or meperidine) solution using a pump specifically designed for that purpose. If analgesia is insufficient, the patient is able to self-administer intermittent (e.g., every 10 to 15 minutes) small doses of narcotic from the patient controlled analgesia infusion pump. Compared with the use of periodic injections of narcotics, patient controlled analgesia provides superior analgesia with a lesser degree of respiratory depression.

Intraspinal (administration into the epidural or subarachnoid space) narcotics produce post-cesarean analgesia that is superior to that of patient controlled analgesia. A single dose of morphine, which is the most frequently used agent for this purpose, provides 18 to 24 hours of analgesia. Side effects include pruritus, nausea and vomiting, urinary retention, and (rarely) respiratory depression that occurs 10 to 18 hours after morphine is administered. Respiratory depression with intraspinal morphine is generally less than with patient-controlled analgesia. When intraspinal morphine is used, it is administered with the epidural (4.0 mg morphine) or spinal (0.2 mg morphine) anesthetic at the time of cesarean section.

ANESTHESIA FOR COMPLICATED OBSTETRICS

Pregnancy-Induced Hypertension (Pre-eclampsia)

Continuous lumbar epidural anesthesia is the technique of choice during labor and vaginal delivery. The epidural catheter is placed once active labor begins or earlier if labor is being induced or augmented with oxytocin. Epidural analgesia, which should be continuous throughout labor and vaginal delivery, provides optimal patient comfort, improves uterine blood flow, helps control blood pressure, and reduces the chance of seizures (low blood levels of local anesthetics depress the central nervous system).

When cesarean section is necessary, epidural anesthesia provides the greatest maternal and fetal safety. Spinal anesthesia is less desirable, since hypotension is more likely, although the risk of hypotension is less during regional anesthesia in a pre-eclamptic patient than in a normal parturient.

General anesthesia introduces several factors that increase maternal and fetal risk. Maternal blood pressure can increase significantly, causing a decrease in cardiac output and uterine blood flow, left ventricular failure with pulmonary edema, or intracranial hemorrhage. Therefore, use of a potent vasodilator (e.g., nitroglycerin or sodium nitroprusside) or an adrenergic blocker (e.g., labetalol) is necessary to prevent an exacerbation of maternal hypertension during induction and endotracheal intubation. Care must also be taken with administration of muscle relaxants, since magnesium, which is commonly used to treat pre-eclampsia, enhances their action. Because of the increased maternal risk during general anesthesia, invasive hemodynamic monitoring of blood pressure (intra-arterial catheter) and, possibly, cardiac filling pressures (pulmonary artery catheter) is indicated. Additionally, fluid administration should be somewhat restricted, with either regional or general anesthesia, to reduce the risk of pulmonary edema.

Heart Disease

The choice of analgesic or anesthetic technique for the parturient with heart disease depends, in general, on whether the hemodynamic changes brought about by a lumbar epidural block of the sympathetic nervous system will be tolerated. Patients with aortic stenosis or coarctation of the aorta have a fixed obstruction to ejection of left ventricular output that prevents increases in stroke volume. Thus, they may not be able to compensate for the reduction of venous return and systemic vascular resistance that occurs with epidural anesthesia, and hypotension may result. Patients with right to left shunts (tetralogy of Fallot, Eisenmenger's syndrome) may not tolerate epidural anesthesia because a fall in systemic vascular resistance will increase the shunt. Finally, patients with primary pulmonary hypertension do not tolerate decreases in preload. Therefore, for patients with these cardiac lesions, labor can be safely managed with systemic medication or intraspinal narcotics and a pudendal block for delivery. General anesthesia is preferred for cesarean section.

The clinical course of parturients with other cardiac lesions may actually be improved when epidural anesthesia is used. For example, patients with mitral stenosis, mitral regurgitation, aortic regurgitation, patent ductus arteriosus, and atrial or ventricular septal defects (with left to right shunts) may not tolerate the cardiovascular changes associated with pain and increased sympathetic activity during labor and delivery. Thus, lumbar epidural analgesia is the technique of choice. Generally, cesarean section for patients with these cardiac lesions is also best managed with epidural anesthesia.

Breech Presentation

Systemic medication during labor and pudendal block at the time of delivery may be used for breech presentations. Epidural anesthesia provides superior analgesia, however, without the side effects of systemic agents. At the time of delivery, the epidural block can provide perineal relaxation to facilitate delivery of the fetal head. Regardless of the technique employed, the anesthesiologist must be prepared to use general anesthesia to assist a difficult breech delivery.

Multiple Gestation

Use of continuous epidural anesthesia reduces infant mortality, shortens the interval between delivery of the first and second twin, facilitates forceps deliveries, and may allow for version and extraction when necessary. General anesthesia with halothane may be necessary to provide uterine relaxation should rapid delivery of the second twin become necessary.

SUGGESTED READING

Amiel-Tison C, Barrier G, Shnider SM, et al: A new neurologic and adaptive capacity scoring system for evaluating obstetric medications in full term newborns. Anesthesiology 56:340, 1982.

Apgar V: A proposal for a new method of evaluation of the newborn infant. Anesth Analg 32:260, 1953.

Caton D: Obstetric anesthesia and concepts of placental transport: A historical review of the nineteenth century. Anesthesiology 46:132, 1977.

Conklin KA: Effects of obstetric analgesia and anesthesia on uterine activity and uteroplacental blood flow. In Carsten M, Miller J (eds): Uterine Function: Molecular and Cellular Aspects. New York, Plenum Publishing, 1990, p 539.

Conklin KA, Murad SHN: Pharmacology of drugs in obstetric anesthesia. Semin Anesth 1:83, 1982.

Datta S, Alper MH: Anesthesia for cesarean section. Anesthesiology 53:142, 1980.

Norris MC: Preeclampsia. In Hood DD (ed): Problems in Anesthesia: Anesthesia in Obstetrics and Gynecology. Philadelphia, JB Lippincott, 1989, p 90.

Ralston DH, Shnider SM: The fetal and neonatal effects of regional anesthesia in obstetrics. Anesthesiology 43:34, 1978.

Scanlon JW, Brown WU, Weiss JB, et al: Neurobehavioral responses of newborn infants after maternal epidural anesthesia. Anesthesiology 40:121, 1974.

Thirteen

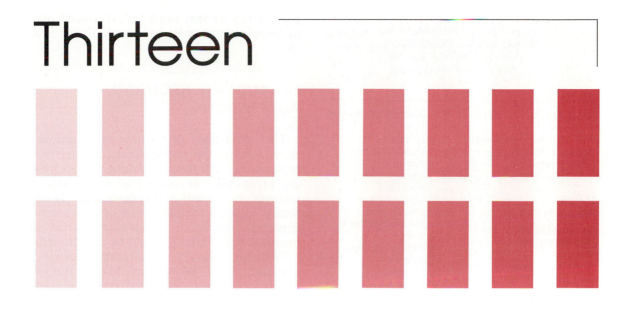

Resuscitation of the Newborn

CALVIN J. HOBEL

Improved surveillance using antenatal and intrapartum fetal heart rate monitoring, real time ultrasonography, amniocentesis, and fetal scalp blood sampling have allowed the clinician to recognize the fetus at risk who may need special care at birth. A problem-oriented assessment during prenatal visits allows identification of those patients who will need special assessment during labor.

PREPARATION FOR EXTRAUTERINE LIFE

Reaching maturity is the most important step for the fetus in utero. Prematurity is the leading cause of poor neonatal outcome because the fetus has not yet progressed through complete stages of anatomic development and biochemical maturation. Even

the fetus delivered at term undergoes changes prior to and with the onset of labor.

During pregnancy, fetal thyroxine (T_4) is converted to reverse triiodothyronine (rT_3), which is metabolically inactive. Several days before the onset of term labor, cortisol levels increase in the fetus and induce a change in thyroid hormone dynamics. Cortisol induces the enzyme system, allowing the conversion of T_4 to triiodothyronine (T_3), which is metabolically more active and necessary for neonatal thermogenesis. At birth, there is a surge of thyroid stimulating hormone (TSH), and at no time during life does this hormone reach such high levels as it does 30 minutes after birth. This is followed by a hyperthyroid neonatal state for several days, which is necessary for the newborn to maintain its body temperature.

A second change that occurs with the onset of labor is a change in fetal breathing activ-

Table 13−1. PRENATAL AND INTRAPARTUM CONDITIONS LIKELY TO PREDISPOSE TO ASPHYXIA NEONATORUM

ANTEPARTUM PROBLEMS	INTRAPARTUM PROBLEMS
Past Medical Problems	Preterm labor
Chronic hypertension	Premature rupture of
Diabetes mellitus	membranes
Renal disease	Fetal distress
Hyperthyroidism	Abnormal labor
Epilepsy	Prolonged labor
Pulmonary disease	Precipitous labor
	Abruptio placentae
Developing Problems	Amnionitis
Inaccurate gestational	Anesthetic problems
dates	Hypotension
Multiple pregnancy	Hypertension
Intrauterine growth retar-	Operative delivery
dation	
Fetal macrosomia	
Prolonged pregnancy	
Congenital anomalies	
Pregnancy-Induced	
Problems	
Hypertension	
Gestational diabetes	

ity. Fetal breathing, as observed by real time ultrasonography, is rarely observed once labor is established. This is thought to be associated with a decrease in pulmonary fluid dynamics that may be important for the onset of respiration after delivery and the retention of surfactant in the lungs.

Finally, labor is a stress to the fetus that stimulates the release of catecholamines. The latter may be responsible for the mobilization of glucose, lung fluid absorption, alterations in the perfusion of organ systems, and, possibly, the onset of respiration. Only at times of severe stress later in life do levels of catecholamines reach levels as high as those at birth.

ETIOLOGY OF NEONATAL CARDIORESPIRATORY DEPRESSION

At term, 0.5 per cent of infants will require vigorous resuscitation (positive pressure ventilation for more than 1 minute). At earlier stages of gestation, almost all infants require some type of supportive care.

Table 13−1 lists the antepartum and intra-partum factors that must be recognized during pregnancy in order to identify the fetus at risk.

FACILITATING NEONATAL ADAPTATION

The physician performing the delivery must delegate the responsibility for neonatal resuscitation. All nurses working in the delivery room must be trained in techniques of neonatal assessment and resuscitation. If risk factors increase the likelihood of delivering a depressed infant, a pediatrician trained in neonatal resuscitation should be summoned.

Following delivery of a normal newborn, attention should be directed toward the following important steps to assure optimal neonatal adaptation.

Clear the Airway

Descent through the birth canal causes compression of the chest wall, resulting in the discharge of fluid from the mouth and nose. When the head emerges from the vagina, the physician should use a towel or gauze pad to remove secretions from the face. In addition, a bulb suction may be used to aspirate secretions from the oral pharynx. The bulb suction should not be used to suction the nose because nasal stimulation may initiate a gasp and cause bradycardia. Also, nasal stimulation may cause aspiration of meconium, if present.

Dry the Newborn

An important part of neonatal adaptation is the initiation of thermogenesis. Excessive cooling from exposure of the wet skin is detrimental to all preterm infants and to depressed full-term infants. The physician should dry off the infant with a towel before cutting the cord. This also serves to stimulate the onset of respiration.

Clamp the Cord

The umbilical arteries usually close spontaneously within 45 to 60 seconds of birth, while the umbilical vein remains patent for 3 to 5 minutes or longer. Delayed cord clamping significantly increases the neonatal blood volume, which increases the likelihood of neonatal jaundice and tachypnea. The ideal time for clamping the cord is 20 to 30 seconds after birth.

Assure Onset of Respiration

The onset of respiration is usually within a few seconds of birth but may be delayed for up to 60 seconds. In the absence of clinical data to suggest a biochemical abnormality (hypoxia-acidosis), it is usually best to adopt an expectant policy of standing back and giving the infant a chance to breathe spontaneously.

Surfactant Replacement

For the premature infant, surfactant deficiency is the basic defect responsible for the development of the respiratory distress syndrome. After 10 years of clinical research, its usefulness has now been documented. Exogenous surfactant replacement varies from synthetic surfactant to modified or unmodified extracts of natural surfactant. These substances can be given by tracheal injection at birth to prevent the respiratory distress syndrome, or they can be given after the syndrome has developed to reduce its severity and prevent mortality.

APGAR SCORE

The Apgar score is an excellent tool for assessing the overall status of the newborn soon after birth (1 minute) and after a brief period of observation (5 minutes) (Table 13–2). A normal Apgar score is 7 or greater at 1 minute and 9 or 10 at 5 minutes.

RESUSCITATION OF THE ASPHYXIATED INFANT

The delivery of an asphyxiated infant should be predictable, based on a careful clinical assessment of those factors associated with biochemical abnormalities. During the past 10 years, increasing emphasis has been placed on transferring the mother with a high-risk pregnancy to a tertiary care regional center before labor, rather than transferring the sick neonate after delivery. The mother is considered to be a better and safer transport incubator.

Ideally, at the time of delivery, a segment of cord should be doubly clamped to allow blood gas determinations on cord arterial and venous blood. These serve as a baseline to assess the severity of the neonatal hypoxia and acidosis.

A stepwise sequence of procedures is necessary to enable a smooth transition to a normal metabolic state. This sequence is referred to as the ABCs of resuscitation and is summarized in Figure 13–1.

Establish an Airway

In any infant with a high likelihood of asphyxia, suctioning of the airway must be initiated after the delivery of the head. The asphyxiated neonate usually has meconium present in the upper airway, which must be cleared with an oral suction catheter before delivery of the shoulders. Immediately following the delivery of the infant, an endotracheal tube should be inserted to remove thick mucus or meconium from the trachea and upper airway.

Initiate Breathing

With an established airway, either bag-mask ventilation or ventilation via an endotracheal tube must be initiated to deliver oxygen to the lungs. Usually, the heart rate increases rapidly after the apnea is corrected, and intermittent bag-mask ventilation with supplemental oxygen can be given until spontaneous respiration commences.

Assure Cardiac Performance

If cardiac performance is poor (heart rate less than 50 beats per minute after 1 minute), external cardiac massage must be initiated. The best technique for cardiac massage in the newborn is to compress the middle third of

Table 13-2. THE APGAR SCORE FOR DETERMINING THE CONDITION OF A NEWBORN INFANT

SIGN	0	1	2
Heart rate	Absent	Below 100	Over 100
Respiratory effort	Absent	Slow, weak cry	Good, strong cry
Muscle tone	Limp	Some flexion of extremities	Active motion
Reflex irritability (response to stimulation of sole of foot)	None	Grimace	Strong cry
Color	Pale, blue	Body: pink Extremities: blue	Completely pink

the sternum with two fingers at a rate of 100 times per minute. The middle finger and either the index or ring finger should be used (Fig. 13-2). The sternum should be depressed approximately 2 cm. Placement of the other hand beneath the infant's back can facilitate compression of the heart between the sternum and spine. Cardiac arrest is rare. If cardiac massage and artificial ventilation are not successful in re-establishing cardiac function, an intracardiac injection of a dilute solution of epinephrine may be given through the chest wall.

Correct Biochemical Abnormalities

Acidosis. In the case of a very sick newborn, an umbilical arterial catheter is placed and blood gases obtained to monitor the severity of the acidosis and the effectiveness of the resuscitation. Severe acidosis can be corrected by the infusion of sodium bicarbonate.

Anemia. On rare occasions, the newborn may have abnormal perfusion secondary to blood loss (for example, from vasa previa or abruptio placentae), which can be corrected only by immediate transfusion with blood from the mother, a blood bank, or a walk-in donor. A solution of plasmanate can be used to maintain an adequate vascular volume temporarily.

Narcotic Depression. Respiratory depression secondary to medication is unusual in today's practice of natural childbirth and the increased use of conduction anesthesia. If

respiratory depression from excessive use of narcotics is suspected, naloxone (Narcan) is effective. It is just as effective and more easily administered intramuscularly as intravenously. There is a very high toxic ratio of neonatal naloxone, so dosage is less critical than for most drugs. Table 13-3 lists the drugs commonly used in resuscitation and their dosages.

Hypoglycemia. Hypoglycemia can also contribute to unsuccessful resuscitation, especially in infants with intrauterine growth retardation or those with diabetic mothers. Glucose administration should be considered after the other issues have been addressed. The use of high concentrations of glucose (for example, 25 to 50 per cent) is contraindicated in asphyxiated newborns because in the absence of oxygen, the glucose is converted to lactic acid, which may increase the likelihood of brain damage.

Evaluate Other Factors

Following a systematic resuscitation effort, it is necessary to search for other contributing factors if cardiorespiratory depression persists. Hypothermia is one of the most critical aggravating factors, and temperature control must be continuously supported. A pneumothorax is not uncommon following a difficult resuscitation (especially with intubation). It must be recognized promptly and decompressed with a chest tube. A diaphragmatic hernia can result in the displacement of stomach, bowel, or both into the thoracic cavity, thus limiting the expansion of the left

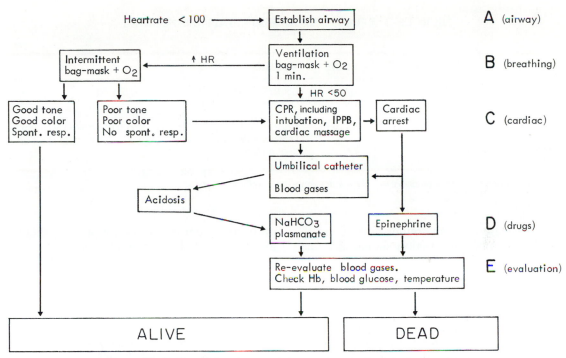

Figure 13-1. The ABCs of resuscitation for the asphyxiated neonate.

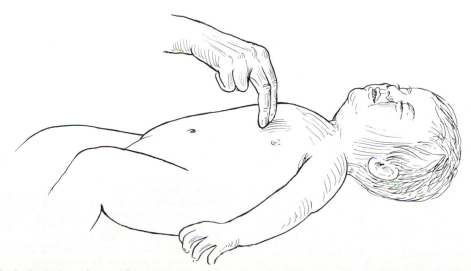

Figure 13-2. Technique for cardiac massage in the neonate. Note that the middle third of the sternum is depressed with two fingers of the physician's right hand. The infant's back may be supported with the left hand if necessary.

Table 13-3. DRUGS USED TO RESUSCITATE THE NEONATE

DRUG	DOSE	ROUTE	VOLUME
Sodium bicarbonate	1–3 mEq/kg	UA	Dilute 1:1 with sterile water to 0.5 mEq/ml
		UV	Dosage 2–6 ml/kg
Epinephrine	0.1 mg/kg	IV	0.1 ml/kg of a 1:10,000 solution
Naloxone	0.1 mg/kg	IM or IV	Neonatal dosage: 0.5 ml/kg of a 0.02 mg/ml solution
			Maternal dosage: 0.025 ml/kg of a 0.4 mg/ml solution
Plasmanate		IV	4–5 ml/kg

UA = umbilical artery; UV = umbilical vein; IV = intravenous; IM = intramuscular

lung. Decreased breath sounds and failure to improve pulmonary function should alert the team to this possible diagnosis.

NEONATAL RESPIRATORY FAILURE

Neonates in imminent danger of death from a narrow range of conditions causing hypoxemia and respiratory distress not responsive to conventional forms of therapy are now candidates for extracorporeal membrane oxygenation. Infants with a congenital diaphragmatic hernia, severe meconium aspiration, or other forms of persistent pulmonary hypertension have been saved using this procedure performed in selected regional centers. Data concerning long-term outcome of infants treated with extracorporeal membrane oxygenation are limited. Concerns exist about the consequences of carotid artery and/or jugular vein ligation, prolonged anticoagulation, and long-term circulatory bypass.

LONG-TERM OUTCOME

Data have indicated that low birth weight (less than 2500 gm), whether caused by prematurity or intrauterine growth retardation, is an independent risk factor for cerebral palsy. By contrast, for infants weighing more than 2500 gm, Apgar scores less than or equal to 3 at 5 minutes are not associated with an increased risk of cerebral palsy, provided that there is no associated obstetric complication. If both a low Apgar score and an obstetric complication are present, there is an increased risk of cerebral palsy.

SUGGESTED READING

Apgar V, James LS: Further observations on the newborn scoring system. J Dis Child 104:419, 1962.

Chernick V, Manfreda J, DeBooy V, et al: Clinical trial of naloxone in birth asphyxia. J Pediatr 113:519, 1988.

Committee on Drugs: Naloxone dosage and route of administration for infants and children: Addendum to emergency drug doses for infants and children. Pediatrics 86:484, 1990.

Committee on Fetus and Newborn: Recommendations on extracorporeal membrane oxygenation. Pediatrics 85:618, 1990.

Cordero J, Hon EG: Neonatal bradycardia following nasopharyngeal stimulation. J Pediatr 78:441, 1971.

Fujiwara T, Konishi M, Chida S, et al: Surfactant replacement therapy with a single postventilatory dose of a reconstituted bovine surfactant in preterm neonates with respiratory distress syndrome: Final analysis of a multicenter, double blind, randomized trial and comparison with similar trials. Pediatrics 86:753, 1990.

Gregory GA, Gooding CA, Phibbs RA, et al: Meconium aspiration in infants—a prospective study. J Pediatr 85:848, 1974.

Hobel CJ: Management of the high risk fetus and neonate. In Bolognese RJ, Schwarz RH, Schneider J (eds): Perinatal Medicine. 2nd ed. Baltimore, Williams & Wilkins, 1982, p 3.

Hobel CJ, Hyvarinen MA, Okada DM, et al: Prenatal and intrapartum high-risk screening. Am J Obstet Gynecol 117:1, 1973.

Hobel CJ, Oh W, Hyvarinen MA, et al: Early versus late treatment of neonatal acidosis in low birth weight infants: Relation to respiratory distress syndrome. Pediatrics 81:1178, 1972.

MacDonald HM, Mulligan JC, Allen AC, et al: Neonatal asphyxia. I. Relationship of obstetric and neonatal complications to neonatal mortality in

38,405 consecutive deliveries. J Pediatr 96:898, 1980.

Milner AD, Vyas H: Lung expansion at birth. J Pediatr 101:879, 1982.

Modanlou H, Yeh SY, Hon EH, et al: Fetal and neonatal biochemistry and Apgar scores. Am J Obstet Gynecol 117:942, 1973.

Nelson KB, Ellenberg JH: Obstetrical complications as risk factors for cerebral palsy or seizure disorders. JAMA 251:1843, 1984.

O'Rouke PP, Crone RK, Vacanti JP, et al: Extra-corporeal membrane oxygenation and conventional medical therapy in neonates with persistent pulmonary hypertension of the newborn. A prospective randomized study. Pediatrics 84:959, 1989.

Rudolph AM: The changes in the circulation after birth. Circulation 41:343, 1970.

Soll RF, Hoekstra RE, Fangman JJ: Multicenter trial of single dose modified bovine surfactant extract (Survanta) for prevention of respiratory distress syndrome. Pediatrics 85:1092, 1990.

Todres ID, Rogers MC: Methods of external cardiac massage in the newborn infant. J Pediatr 86:781, 1975.

Fourteen

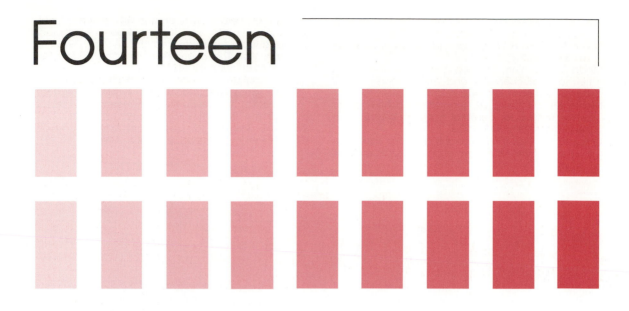

Antepartum Hemorrhage

JEAN M. RICCI

Vaginal bleeding in the third trimester complicates 4 per cent of all pregnancies. It is considered an obstetric emergency because hemorrhage remains the most frequent cause of maternal death in the United States. It is critical for the well-being of both the mother and fetus that the patient who presents with third-trimester bleeding be managed expediently. The differential diagnosis of third-trimester bleeding is outlined in Table 14–1.

INITIAL EVALUATION

Principles of Management

The initial evaluation of a patient with an antepartum hemorrhage should include a history, physical examination, and special investigative studies designed to establish the cause of the bleeding. If a patient is bleeding profusely, a team approach to the assessment and management should be instituted to maintain hemodynamic stability. This team should include an obstetrician, an anesthesiologist, and nurses who are knowledgeable about the management of the critically ill patient. At least one large-bore intravenous line should be placed. A central venous pressure line or preferably a Swan-Ganz catheter is helpful in the management of hypovolemic shock.

History

Any history of trauma or sexual intercourse prior to the onset of bleeding should be determined, and the duration and amount of bleeding should be established. The patient should be asked about any abdominal pain, uterine contractions, or both. The obstetric history should be reviewed for prior cesarean section(s), preterm labor, or placenta previa. Medical history should be checked for known

Table 14–1. CAUSES OF ANTEPARTUM BLEEDING
Placenta previa
Abruptio placentae
Uterine rupture
Fetal vessel rupture
Cervical lesions/lacerations
Vaginal lesions/lacerations
Congenital bleeding disorder
Unknown

bleeding disorders or liver disease. Social history should be reviewed for tobacco or cocaine abuse. The prenatal course should be reviewed with particular reference to any prior ultrasonic examinations and any criteria to establish gestational age (e.g., last menstrual period, ultrasonic findings, time of first fetal heart tones, onset of fetal movements, fundal height measurements).

Physical Examination

The vital signs and amount of bleeding should be checked immediately as should the patient's mental status. Whether the skin is moist or dry, pale or mottled should be noted, as should the presence of petechial hemorrhages or bleeding from any site other than the vagina, such as the nose or rectum. The abdominal examination must include fundal height measurement and assessment of uterine tenderness. A pelvic examination should *not* be performed until placenta previa has been excluded by ultrasonography. Once excluded, a sterile speculum examination can be safely done to rule out genital tears or lesions (e.g., cervical cancer) that may be responsible for the bleeding. If none are identified, a digital examination may be performed to determine if cervical dilatation is present.

Investigations

Laboratory Tests. A complete blood count should be obtained and compared with previous evaluations to help assess the amount of blood loss. An assessment of the patient's coagulation profile should be done by obtaining a platelet count, serum fibrinogen, prothrombin time, and partial thromboplastin time. It is often helpful to do a "wall clot" test, whereby a red topped tube of blood is drawn, taped to the wall, and timed for clot formation. If no clot develops within 6 minutes, coagulopathy is most likely present. The patient should be typed and cross-matched for at least 4 units of blood.

Ultrasonography. The most accurate means of determining the cause of third-trimester bleeding is with ultrasonography. The ultrasonic evaluation should include not only the location and character of the placenta, but also an assessment of gestational age, an estimate of fetal weight, determination of the fetal presentation, and a screening for fetal anomalies.

Monitoring. Uterine activity and the fetal heart rate should be monitored to rule out labor and establish fetal well-being.

PLACENTA PREVIA

The incidence of placenta previa is 0.5 per cent. Bleeding from a placenta previa accounts for approximately 20 per cent of all cases of antepartum hemorrhage. Seventy per cent of patients with placenta previa present with painless vaginal bleeding in the third trimester, 20 per cent have contractions associated with bleeding, and 10 per cent have the diagnosis of previa made incidentally by ultrasonography or at term.

Predisposing Factors

Factors that have been associated with a higher incidence of placenta previa include (1) multiparity, (2) increasing maternal age, (3) prior placenta previa, and (4) multiple gestation. Patients with a placenta previa have a 4 to 8 per cent risk of having a previa in a subsequent pregnancy.

Classification

Placenta previa is classified according to the relationship of the placenta to the internal cervical os (Fig. 14–1). *Complete placenta previa* implies that the placenta totally

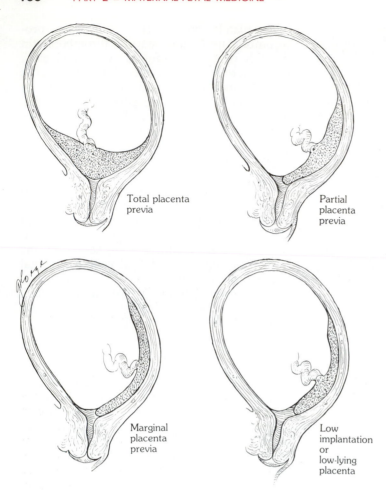

Figure 14–1. Types of placenta previa.

Total placenta previa

Partial placenta previa

Marginal placenta previa

Low implantation or low-lying placenta

covers the cervical os. A complete previa may be central, anterior, or posterior, depending on where the center of the placenta is located relative to the os. *Partial placenta previa* implies that the placenta partially covers the internal cervical os. A *marginal placenta previa* is one in which the edge of the placenta extends to the margin of the internal cervical os. The term *low-lying placenta* implies that the placenta is implanted in the lower uterine segment, but does not extend to the cervical os, and is therefore not a previa.

Diagnosis

The classic presentation of placenta previa is painless vaginal bleeding in a previously normal pregnancy. In general, those with a complete previa bleed earlier and heavier than do those with a partial or marginal previa. Bleeding occurs owing to the disruption of the placental attachment resulting from the development and thinning of the lower uterine segment in the third trimester. The mean gestational age at onset of bleeding is 30 weeks, with one third presenting before 30 weeks.

Placenta previa is almost exclusively diagnosed today by ultrasonography (Fig. 14–2). Between 4 and 6 per cent of patients have some degree of previa on ultrasonic examination before 20 weeks, gestation. With the development of the lower uterine segment, there is a relative upward placental migration, with 90 per cent of these resolving by the third trimester. Complete previas are the least likely to resolve, however, with only 10

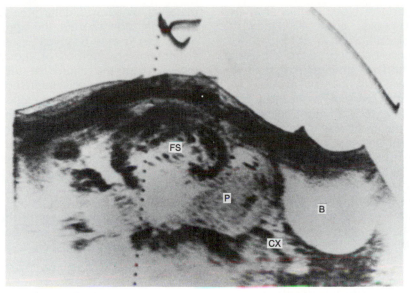

Figure 14–2. Ultrasonic examination of a patient with a complete placenta previa. Placenta (P), cervix (C), and bladder (B) are indicated.

per cent resolving by the third trimester. When placenta previa is diagnosed in the second trimester, a repeat sonogram is indicated at 30 to 32 weeks for follow-up evaluation.

Transabdominal ultrasonography has an accuracy for previa detection of 95 per cent. If the placenta is implanted posteriorly and the fetal vertex is low, the lower margin of the placenta may be obscured and the diagnosis of previa missed. A false-positive diagnosis of previa by a transabdominal scan is also possible, particularly with an anterior placenta. Transvaginal ultrasonography has been introduced, and this can accurately diagnose placenta previa in virtually 100 per cent of cases. Theoretically, transvaginal ultrasonography could precipitate bleeding, so it should be done in a hospital setting with informed consent.

Clinically, the diagnosis of placenta previa can be made by palpating the placenta through the cervical os during a procedure called a *double set-up examination.* Although the double set-up was used frequently in the past, the introduction of high-resolution ultrasonography has left little indication for it today. The double set-up procedure dictates that the patient be in the operating room prepared for cesarean delivery with a complete operating team in attendance. The pa-

tient is placed in the lithotomy position, and the examiner inserts a speculum to inspect the cervix. If no local source of bleeding is identified, the speculum is removed and the fornices gently palpated to determine if there is placental tissue between the cervix and the presenting part. The presence of the placenta is indicated by a cushion-like sensation. A finger is then inserted carefully into the cervical canal and gently advanced toward the internal os. If placental tissue is palpated, the procedure is terminated and a cesarean section performed.

The only indication for a double set-up in modern obstetrics is when ultrasonography is inconclusive and the patient is in labor with non–life-threatening vaginal bleeding. Typically this applies to the patient in whom a low-lying placenta or a marginal previa is suspected, rather than a partial or complete previa. The procedure otherwise should be considered an anachronism, which in the presence of active hemorrhage or clear evidence of previa on ultrasonography could place the patient at greater risk of morbidity.

Management

As with any third-trimester bleeding, the patient should initially be stabilized, fetal monitoring instituted, blood studies sent, and blood products made available. Once the diagnosis of placenta previa is established, management decisions depend on the gestational age of the fetus and the extent of the vaginal bleeding.

With a preterm pregnancy, the goal is to attempt to obtain fetal maturation without compromising the mother's health. If bleeding is excessive, delivery must be accomplished by cesarean section regardless of gestational age. When the bleeding is not profuse, however, the patient is managed expectantly in hospital on bed rest. Her hematocrit should be followed, and blood should always be available. Autologous blood donation is indicated if the patient is a candidate, or blood may be donated by a family member. With expectant management, 70 per cent of patients will have recurrent vaginal bleeding prior to completion of 36 weeks' gestation and will require delivery. If the patient reaches 36 weeks, fetal lung maturity should be determined at that time by amniocentesis and the patient delivered by cesarean section if the lungs are mature. Elective delivery is preferable, as spontaneous labor places the mother at greater risk for hemorrhage and the fetus at risk for hypovolemia and anemia.

Twenty per cent of patients with placenta previa will present with vaginal bleeding and uterine contractions. Concomitant placental abruption must always be considered in this differential diagnosis. If abruption is comfortably ruled out, however, tocolysis may be attempted, with magnesium sulfate being the drug of choice. Tocolysis with β-agonists (i.e., ritodrine, terbutaline) is contraindicated.

If a patient presents in labor with vaginal bleeding at term, delivery should proceed by cesarean section if placenta previa is documented by ultrasonography. If the ultrasonic diagnosis is uncertain, a double set-up examination can be done as previously described. In rare circumstances, a patient with a marginal placenta previa can deliver vaginally, provided that the fetal head tamponades the site of bleeding during labor.

Patients who are Rh-negative and bleed from a placenta previa are at increased risk of fetomaternal transfusion and immunization. Therefore, RhoGAM is indicated in such cases. A Kleihauer-Betke test on the maternal blood will determine the extent of the transfusion so that the appropriate dose of RhoGAM may be given.

The delivery method of choice is cesarean section, with the choice of uterine incision dependent on the placental location. A low transverse incision is selected if the lower uterine segment is well developed. In many cases, however, the lower uterine segment is poorly developed and a vertical incision is required. All efforts should be made to avoid the placenta during delivery, because this can be associated with massive maternal hemorrhage and fetal blood loss. Blood loss can also be significant after delivery of the placenta as a result of lower uterine segment atony. It is not uncommon to sustain a blood loss of 1500 ml or more at cesarean section for placenta previa.

Low-Lying Placenta

A patient with a low-lying placenta may present in the same way as a patient with placenta previa. That is, she may experience painless antepartum vaginal bleeding, experience bleeding at term in labor, or remain asymptomatic. By definition, placental tissue is implanted in the lower uterine segment but does not cover the os. As the lower uterine segment develops and thins in the third trimester, the placental attachment is disrupted, and bleeding may occur from the implantation site. The management of antepartum or intrapartum bleeding is the same as that previously outlined. A vaginal delivery is usually accomplished, although it should be done in a well-controlled setting. It may be difficult to distinguish a low-lying placenta from a marginal previa, and a double set-up examination may be done if the diagnosis is uncertain.

Maternal-Fetal Risks

The maternal mortality from placenta previa has dropped precipitously over the past 50 years from 30 per cent to less than 1 per cent. This has primarily been due to the liberal use of cesarean section and careful expectant management.

The risk of antepartum or intrapartum

hemorrhage, or both, is a constant threat to the patient with placenta previa. Bleeding may be due to an associated accreta, uterine atony, or the placenta previa itself. Placenta accreta implies an abnormal attachment of the placenta to the uterine myometrium caused by defective decidual formation (absent Nitabuchs layer). This abnormal attachment may be superficial *(accreta),* or the placental villi may invade partially through the myometrium *(increta)* or extend to the uterine serosa *(percreta).* Two thirds of patients with this complication require hysterectomy. Patients with a history of uterine surgery are at greatest risk of developing an accreta. In fact, those with a prior cesarean section carry a 25 per cent risk. Disseminated intravascular coagulopathy (DIC) may result if a massive hemorrhage or an associated abruption occurs.

Preterm delivery poses the greatest risk to the fetus. Fortunately, as a result primarily of advances in obstetric and neonatal care, the perinatal mortality rate (PMR) has declined over the past decade. The PMR is, however, significantly higher than in the general population and is presently quoted as 40 to 80 deaths per 1000 births. Twenty per cent of pregnancies will be complicated by intrauterine growth retardation, and there is a twofold higher incidence of congenital abnormalities. The incidence of malpresentation is 30 per cent. In addition, there is a higher incidence of preterm premature rupture of the membranes in pregnancies complicated by placenta previa. Vasa previa is rare but can be associated with placenta previa, carrying a perinatal mortality rate of 75 per cent.

ABRUPTIO PLACENTAE

Abruptio placentae, or premature separation of the normally implanted placenta, complicates 0.5 to 1.5 per cent of all pregnancies (1 in 120 births). Abruption severe enough to result in fetal death occurs in 1 per 500 deliveries.

Predisposing Factors

Factors associated with an increased incidence of abruption include (1) hypertension, (2) trauma, (3) polyhydramnios with rapid decompression on membrane rupture, (4) cocaine use, (5) tobacco use, (6) preterm premature rupture of the membranes, and (7) a short umbilical cord. The most common of these risk factors is maternal hypertension, whether chronic or as a result of pre-eclampsia. The recurrence risk of abruption is high, being 10% after one abruption and 25% after two.

Pathophysiology

Placental separation is initiated by hemorrhage into the decidua basalis with formation of a decidual hematoma. The resulting separation of the decidua from the basal plate predisposes to further separation and bleeding as well as compression and destruction of placental tissue. The inciting cause of placental separation is unknown. It has been postulated that it may be due to an inherent weakness or anomaly in the spiral arterioles. Blood may either dissect upward toward the fundus, resulting in a *concealed hemorrhage,* or extend downward toward the cervix, resulting in an external or *revealed hemorrhage.* Hemoglobin may penetrate the chorion and amnion and discolor the amniotic fluid. Blood may also infiltrate the myometrium, causing a blue discoloration of the uterus, the so-called *Couvelaire uterus.*

Diagnosis

Clinically, the diagnosis of a placental abruption is entertained if a patient presents with vaginal bleeding in association with uterine tenderness, hyperactivity, and increased tone. The signs and symptoms of placental abruption are, however, variable. The most common finding is vaginal bleeding, seen in 80 per cent of cases. Usually the blood is dark red, commonly described as port-wine colored. It is important to recognize that in 20 per cent of cases bleeding will be concealed, and so there will be no external evidence of hemorrhage. A concealed hemorrhage is a greater hazard, since the extent of placental separation may not be appreciated and management may be delayed. An increasing fundal height, determined by periodic measurements, may give an indication of continued concealed bleeding. Abdominal pain and uterine tenderness are seen in 66 per cent, fetal distress in 60 per cent, uterine hyperactivity and increased uterine tone in 34 per cent, and fetal demise in 15 per cent of cases.

The diagnosis of placental abruption is primarily a clinical one. Ultrasonography will detect only 2 per cent of abruptions. Because placental abruption may coexist with a placenta previa, the reason for doing an initial ultrasonic examination is to exclude the latter diagnosis. Identification of a retroplacental clot with underlying placental destruction at delivery will confirm the diagnosis, but this is not always found if the abruption is a recent one.

Maternal-Fetal Risks

Abruption places the fetus at significant risk of hypoxia and ultimately death. The perinatal mortality rate due to placental abruption is presently 35 per cent, and the condition accounts for 15 per cent of third-trimester stillbirths. Fifteen per cent of live-born infants have significant neurologic impairment.

Placental abruption is the most common cause of DIC in pregnancy. It results from release of thromboplastin from the disrupted placenta and the subplacental decidua into the maternal circulation, causing a consumptive coagulopathy. Clinically significant DIC complicates 20 per cent of cases and is most commonly seen when the abruption is massive or fetal death has occurred. Hypovolemic shock and acute renal failure due to massive hemorrhage may be seen with a severe abruption if hypovolemia is left uncorrected. Acute tubular necrosis due to impaired renal perfusion may result.

Management

Management of the patient with an abruption includes careful maternal hemodynamic monitoring, fetal monitoring, serial evaluation of the hematocrit and coagulation profile, and delivery. Intensive monitoring of both the mother and the fetus are essential because rapid deterioration of either can occur. Blood products for replacement should always be available, and a large-bore intravenous line must be secured. A Foley catheter should be placed to assess urine output accurately. A Swan-Ganz catheter may be indicated to manage the patient's hemodynamic status. Fluid resuscitation should be with Ringer's lactate solution, and blood (whole or packed red blood cells) should be given liberally if indicated.

Typically, patients with an abruption labor and deliver rapidly, owing to uterine irritability. Vaginal delivery is preferred as long as there is no fetal distress or other contraindication for it. Cesarean delivery should be reserved for obstetric indications only. Once the decision is made to proceed with delivery, labor needs to be aggressively managed to remove the inciting cause of the hemorrhage and DIC, namely, the separated placenta. The membranes should be ruptured as soon as possible, and oxytocin should be used for augmentation or induction of labor.

Because the patient with placental abruption is at risk for developing DIC, blood (whole or packed red blood cells), fresh frozen plasma, cryoprecipitate, and platelets should be given as indicated. After delivery, DIC will correct spontaneously, although it may take several days before the coagulation profile returns to normal.

Rarely is placental abruption managed conservatively owing to the great risks associated with it. Very mild forms of abruption in the premature fetus can be managed expectantly in carefully selected cases. In the majority of cases, however, delivery is indicated.

UTERINE RUPTURE

Uterine rupture implies complete separation of the uterine musculature through all of its layers, with all or a part of the fetus being extruded from the uterine cavity. The overall incidence is 0.5 per cent.

Predisposing Factors

Uterine rupture may be spontaneous, traumatic, or associated with a prior uterine scar, and it may occur during or before labor or at the time of delivery. A prior uterine scar is associated with 40 per cent of cases. Most commonly, the scar is from a prior cesarean section, although any uterine procedure that extends through the myometrium into the endometrial cavity (e.g., myomectomy, cornual resection, metroplasty) places the patient at risk for uterine rupture. With a prior lower segment transverse incision, the risk for rupture is 0.5 per cent, whereas the risk with a vertical (classic) scar is 5 per cent. Sixty per cent of uterine ruptures occur in previously unscarred uteri. Factors associated with an increased risk of rupture of the unscarred uterus include (1) the injudicious use of oxytocin, (2) grand multiparity, (3) marked uterine distention, (4) abnormal fetal lie, (5) cephalopelvic disproportion, (6) external version/extraction, (7) shoulder dystocia, (8) midforceps delivery, (9) uteroplacental pathology, and (10) trauma.

Diagnosis

The signs and symptoms of uterine rupture are highly variable. Classically, rupture is characterized by the sudden onset of intense abdominal pain. Impending rupture may be heralded by hyperventilation, restlessness, agitation, and tachycardia. After the rupture has occurred, the patient may be free of pain momentarily and then complain of diffuse pain thereafter. The patient may or may not have vaginal bleeding, and if it occurs it can vary from spotting to severe hemorrhage. The presenting part may be found to retract on pelvic examination, and fetal parts may be more easily palpable abdominally. Abnormal contouring of the abdomen may also be seen. Fetal distress develops commonly, and the mother may become hypotensive and develop hypovolemic shock.

Management

A high index of suspicion is required. Immediate laparotomy is essential. In most cases, total abdominal hysterectomy is the treatment of choice, although debridement of the rupture site and primary closure may be considered in women of low parity who desire more children.

Maternal-Fetal Risk

Delay in management places both mother and child at significant risk. The major risk to the mother is hemorrhage and shock. Although the associated maternal mortality rate is now less than 1 per cent, if the mother is left untreated she will die. For the fetus, rapid intervention will minimize morbidity and mortality. The associated fetal mortality rate today is still 32 per cent.

FETAL BLEEDING

Rupture of a fetal vessel complicates 0.1 per cent to 0.8 per cent of pregnancies. This often results when the cord insertion is *velamentous,* implying that the vessels of the cord insert between the amnion and chorion away from the placenta. The incidence of velamentous cord insertion varies from 1 per cent in singleton pregnancies to 10 per cent in twins and 50 per cent in triplets. If the unprotected vessels pass over the cervical os, this is termed a *vasa previa.* The incidence of vasa previa is 1 per 5000 pregnancies. Velamentously inserted vessels need not pass over the os to rupture, although the risk of rupture is greatest with a vasa previa.

The patient with a ruptured fetal vessel will present with vaginal bleeding in association with progressive changes in the fetal heart tracing from tachycardia to bradycardia to a sinusoidal pattern, indicating increasing fetal anemia. An Apt test, which differentiates fetal from adult hemoglobin, may help in making the diagnosis. This test is done by mixing a sample of vaginal blood with an equal amount of water and examining the supernatant after centrifugation. If the supernatant is pink, hemoglobin is present. One part of 0.25 per cent sodium hydroxide is then added to 5 parts of the supernatant. If fetal hemoglobin is present, the pink color will deepen and persist for more than 2 minutes. A change to a yellow color indicates the presence of hemoglobin A.

Rupture of a fetal vessel necessitates immediate abdominal delivery. Vasa previa alone carries a perinatal mortality rate of 50 per cent, which increases to 75 per cent if the membranes rupture.

BLEEDING OF UNKNOWN ETIOLOGY

In many cases of antepartum hemorrhage, no definite cause is ever found. The bleeding is usually minimal in amount. This diagnosis can be made only after exclusion of all other causes.

SUGGESTED READING

Abdella TN, Sibai BM, Hayes JM, Anderson GD: Perinatal outcome in abruptio placentae. Obstet Gynecol 63:365, 1984.

Cotton DB, Reed JA, Paul RH, et al: The conservative aggressive management of placenta previa. Am J Obstet Gynecol 137:687, 1980.

Farine D, Fox HE, Timor-Tritsch I: Vaginal ultrasound for ruling out placenta previa. Br J Obstet Gynaecol 96:117, 1989.

Lavery JP: Placenta previa. Clin Obstet Gynecol 33:414, 1990.

Lockwood CJ: Placenta previa and related disorders. Contemp Obstet Gynecol 34:47, 1990.

Lowe TW, Cunningham FG: Placental abruption. Clin Obstet Gynecol 33:406, 1990.

O'Sullivan MJ, Ricci JM: Uterine rupture: Management alternatives. Contemp Obstet Gynecol 32:83, 1988.

Phelan JP: Uterine rupture. Clin Obstet Gynecol 33:432, 1990.

Silver R, Depp R, Sabbagha RE, et al: Placenta previa: Aggressive expectant management. Am J Obstet Gynecol 150:15, 1984.

Thomas RL: How to manage third-trimester bleeding. The Female Patient 15:17, 1990.

Fifteen

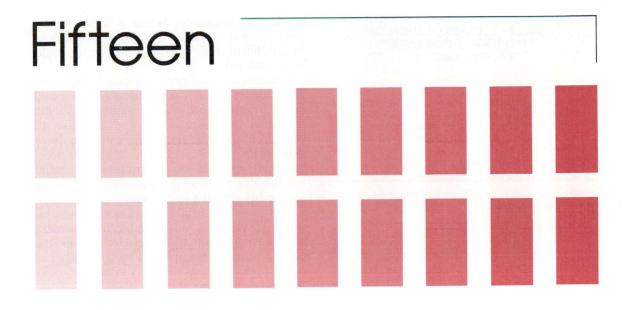

Hypertensive Disorders of Pregnancy

CHARLES R. BRINKMAN III

The hypertensive disorders of pregnancy are major contributors to maternal and perinatal morbidity and mortality. Complications from hypertensive disorders of pregnancy are consistently listed among the three most common causes of maternal death in virtually all developed countries. The reported incidence depends on the criteria for diagnosis, and there is a distinct lack of uniformity. In Great Britain, with primarily a white population, some form of hypertension occurs in 25 per cent of pregnancies. In the United States, the incidence reported by the Task Force on Toxemia of the Collaborative Perinatal Project was 28 per cent for whites and 36 per cent for blacks.

CLASSIFICATION AND DEFINITIONS

The classification of hypertensive disorders recommended by the American College of Obstetricians and Gynecologists is outlined in Table 15–1. The general term *toxemia* should not be used, since it represents the entire spectrum of hypertensive disorders of pregnancy and, on occasion, may also include patients with proteinuria only.

The clinical criteria for the diagnosis of hypertension in pregnancy merit some discussion. There is uniform agreement that an absolute blood pressure of 140/90 mm Hg is

Table 15-1. CLASSIFICATION OF HYPERTENSIVE DISORDERS OF PREGNANCY*

1. Pre-eclampsia–eclampsia (hypertension peculiar to pregnancy)
2. Chronic hypertension (of whatever cause)
3. Chronic hypertension with superimposed pre-eclampsia
4. Late or transient hypertension

* Recommended by the American College of Obstetricians and Gynecologists.

abnormal because the normal resting arterial pressure is lower in pregnant than in non-pregnant subjects. An increase of 30 mm Hg in the systolic pressure or 15 mm Hg in the diastolic pressure also represents a pathologic change. The problem with this latter criterion is the lack of a standardized baseline from which the increase should be calculated if the patient is first seen after the fifth or sixth month of pregnancy.

Because of the many potential errors associated with the clinical determination of blood pressure, the diagnosis of hypertension should be reserved for those having an abnormal reading, taken with the patient at rest on two occasions at least 6 hours apart. The NIH Consensus Report on Hypertension in Pregnancy recommends that blood pressure be taken in the sitting position and that the fifth Korotkoff's sound (disappearance) be used for determining diastolic pressure. It is probably advisable that both the fourth (muffling) and fifth sounds be recorded because there is some controversy as to which sound more closely represents true intra-arterial diastolic pressure.

Pre-eclampsia

This acute syndrome is peculiar to pregnancy and is referred to as pregnancy-induced hypertension or acute hypertensive disease of pregnancy. Pre-eclampsia is primarily, although not exclusively, confined to the young woman in her first pregnancy. It most commonly occurs during the last tri-

mester of pregnancy. When it arises in the early second trimester (14 to 20 weeks), a hydatidiform mole or choriocarcinoma should be considered.

The diagnosis of pre-eclampsia is made by the presence of pathologic edema (hands and face), hypertension, and proteinuria. Edema per se is not essential for the diagnosis of pre-eclampsia; hydrostatic edema of the lower extremities occurs frequently in normal pregnancy. Hypertension is absolutely essential for the diagnosis of pre-eclampsia. There is agreement that the combination of hypertension and proteinuria is diagnostic. When either hypertension or proteinuria is present alone, it is difficult to be certain whether the patient has pre-eclampsia in its early stage of development or a hypertensive disorder unrelated to pregnancy.

Pre-eclampsia is divided into mild and severe forms, depending on the height of the blood pressure and the degree of proteinuria (Table 15-2).

In addition to the blood pressure and proteinuria criteria for severe pre-eclampsia listed in Table 15-2, any of the following conditions arising in a mild pre-eclamptic patient would place her in the severe category:

1. Oliguria (less than 400 ml/24 hr).
2. Altered consciousness, headache, scotomata, or blurred vision.
3. Pulmonary edema or cyanosis.
4. Epigastric or right upper quadrant pain.
5. Significantly altered liver function.
6. Significant thrombocytopenia.

Eclampsia

Eclampsia is defined as the addition of grand mal seizures to either the mild or severe pre-eclamptic syndrome. Patients with severe pre-eclampsia are at greater risk to develop seizures, but 25 per cent of eclamptic patients have only mild pre-eclampsia. In general, 25 per cent of eclamptic patients develop the syndrome before labor, 50 per cent during labor, and 25 per cent after delivery.

Table 15–2. CRITERIA FOR DETERMINING SEVERITY OF PREGNANCY-INDUCED HYPERTENSION

CONDITION	BLOOD PRESSURE	PROTEINURIA	EDEMA
Pre-eclampsia			
Mild	140/90 to 160/110 or Systolic: ≥30 mm Hg increase Diastolic: ≥15 mm Hg increase	<5 gm/24 hr 1 to 2 plus	Hands and/or face
Severe	>160/110	>5 gm/24 hr 3 to 4 plus	Hands and/or face
Eclampsia	Any of the above with seizures		

Chronic Hypertension

The diagnosis of chronic hypertension is made in those patients in whom hypertension is known to antedate pregnancy or in whom hypertension is first noted before the twentieth gestational week. These patients may have any of the diseases that cause hypertension, including essential hypertension, acute and chronic glomerulonephritis, chronic pyelonephritis, and collagen vascular diseases, particularly systemic lupus erythematosus. It is not uncommon for the physiologic stress of pregnancy to bring to clinical attention for the first time a previously unapparent or subclinical vascular or renal disease. In these situations, it may be very difficult to determine whether one is dealing with a pregnancy-induced (pre-eclampsia) or aggravated (chronic hypertension) condition.

Chronic Hypertension with Superimposed Pre-eclampsia

Pre-eclampsia may become superimposed on chronic hypertensive disease. In most instances, there is an underlying hypertensive disorder of renal or other origin, and the process is aggravated by pregnancy. If the diagnosis of superimposed pre-eclampsia is to be used, it should be reserved for those chronic hypertensive patients who either have a marked increase in pre-existing proteinuria during the pregnancy or demonstrate significant proteinuria for the first time in the latter half of pregnancy. The perinatal risk is greatly increased in these patients.

Late or Transient Hypertension

Also called gestational hypertension, this confusing hypertensive syndrome occurs in the second half of pregnancy, during labor, or within 48 hours of delivery, without significant proteinuria (less than 300 mg/L). It is extremely difficult to differentiate this condition from pre-eclampsia. The diagnosis should be made only in retrospect, when the pregnancy has been completed without the development of proteinuria. Even then, renal disease should be ruled out first.

HELLP Syndrome

This is an uncommon, although highly morbid, variant of pre-eclampsia associated with hemolysis, elevated liver enzymes, and low platelet count. In contrast to pure pre-eclampsia, the typical HELLP syndrome patient is more likely to be multiparous, greater than 25 years of age, and at less than 36 weeks' gestation. Hypertension may be absent in 20 per cent of the patients, whereas 30 per cent will have mild pre-eclampsia and 50 per cent severe pre-eclampsia.

PRE-ECLAMPSIA – ECLAMPSIA

Etiology

Pre-eclampsia–eclampsia is justly called a disease of theories. Despite extensive interest and investigation, no definite cause has been identified. As the term *toxemia* indicates, the search for a toxin has been long, arduous, and fruitless. An infectious etiology has also been sought unsuccessfully.

Because of the prompt resolution of the disease following delivery, most attention has been focused on the placenta and its membranes and the fetus. A hormonal etiology has been postulated, but no hormone or combination of hormones has been experimentally proved to produce pre-eclampsia.

Currently three hypotheses are in the forefront of investigation. The first hypothesis relates pre-eclampsia to an immunologic factor or deficiency. Suggestions have been made for both excessive compatibility and excessive incompatibility between mother and fetus. The second hypothesis relates the syndrome to prostaglandins and proposes an imbalance between the vasodilators PGE_2 and prostacyclin and the vasoconstrictor PGF series and thromboxanes.

In normal pregnancy, prostacyclin (PGI_2) synthesis increases fourfold to fivefold, whereas thromboxane A_2 production remains relatively unchanged or increases slightly. PGI_2 is associated with decreased vascular resistance and decreased platelet aggregation. In hypertensive pregnancies, PGI_2 production does not increase to the same degree as in normal pregnancy and thromboxane A_2 is reported to be unchanged. The result will be a relatively reduced PGI_2 to thromboxane A_2 ratio compared with normotensive pregnancy, resulting in increased peripheral vascular resistance and increased platelet activation.

The third hypothesis, which relates the disease to uteroplacental ischemia, suggests the following:

1. Pre-eclampsia begins with uteroplacental ischemia, which is thought to be related to various factors. One is an increased intramural resistance in the myometrial vessels, which could be related to a heightened myometrial tension produced by a large fetus in a primipara, twins, or hydramnios. Alternatively, ischemia could be due to underlying vascular changes such as occur in chronic hypertensive disease or failure of the normal physiologic changes in the spiral and radial arteries of the uterus, as described under Pathology and Pathogenesis.

2. The uteroplacental ischemia leads to the production of a vasoconstrictor substance, which, on entering the circulation, produces renal vasoconstriction; this latter condition leads to the increased production of renin-angiotensin and aldosterone.

3. The renin-angiotensin produces a generalized vasoconstriction and aggravates further the uteroplacental ischemia.

4. Aldosterone leads to water and electrolyte retention and generalized edema, including edema of the intima of the arterioles. These changes produce arteriolar stiffness, which increases sensitivity to angiotensin. Further vasoconstriction leads to capillary hypoxia and increased permeability of the glomerular membrane, leading to proteinuria and further edema. Vasoconstriction and hypoxia in certain areas of the brain would produce convulsions and coma.

In favor of the hypothesis relating the disease to uteroplacental ischemia is the more frequent occurrence of pre-eclampsia in primiparae with large babies and in patients with multiple pregnancy, polyhydramnios, or hydatidiform mole. In all of these conditions, there is increased distention of the uterine walls, which probably increases vascular resistance. Opposing the hypothesis, however, are the following findings:

1. No vasoconstrictor substance has been isolated from the blood of patients with pre-eclampsia, even when the blood is collected from the uterine veins.

2. Blood levels of renin-angiotensin and aldosterone are not significantly different in patients with pre-eclampsia from those in patients with a normal pregnancy.

The search for the cause or causes of pre-eclampsia is hampered by the lack of an animal model. All efforts to reproduce the human disease in animals have been unsuccessful.

Pathophysiology

Although the etiology of the pregnancy-induced hypertensive syndrome is unknown, it is well accepted that the underlying pathophysiologic abnormality is a generalized arteriolar constriction or vasospasm. A rise in blood pressure can be elicited by an increase in either cardiac output or systemic vascular resistance. Cardiac output in pregnant patients with pre-eclampsia and eclampsia is not significantly different from that of normal pregnant subjects in the last trimester of pregnancy. On the other hand, the systemic vascular resistance has been shown to be significantly elevated.

Renal blood flow and glomerular filtration rate (GFR) in patients with pre-eclampsia and eclampsia are significantly lower than in those patients with a normal pregnancy of a comparable gestational period. The decrease in renal blood flow has been shown to be related to constriction of the afferent arteriolar system. This afferent vasoconstriction may eventually lead to damage to the glomerular membranes, thereby increasing their permeability to proteins. The renal vasoconstriction and the decrease in GFR could also account for the oliguria.

The few studies that have been done on cerebral hemodynamics have shown that the cerebral vascular resistance is always high in patients with pre-eclampsia and eclampsia. In hypertensive patients without convulsions, cerebral blood flow may remain within normal limits as a result of autoregulatory phenomena. In convulsive cases, however, cerebral blood flow and oxygen consumption are below those of normal pregnant subjects. Likewise, the few studies that have been done in human subjects on uteroplacental circulation have shown a decreased blood flow and increased vascular resistance in pre-eclamptic patients.

Pathology and Pathogenesis

There are three major pathologic lesions primarily associated with pre-eclampsia and eclampsia: (1) hemorrhage and necrosis in many organs, presumably secondary to arteriolar constriction; (2) glomerular capillary endotheliosis; and (3) lack of decidualization of the myometrial segments of the spiral arteries. Arteriolar vasospasm of relatively short duration (1 hour) may cause hypoxia and necrosis of sensitive parenchymal cells. Vasospasm of longer duration (3 hours) may cause infarction in vital organs, such as the liver, placenta, and brain. In the liver, periportal necrosis and hemorrhage may occur, with a subcapsular hematoma—a rare complication. In the brain, focal areas of hemorrhage and necrosis may occur. In the retina, the clinical window to the arterial vasculature, vasospasm may be visualized on ophthalmoscopic examination. Retinal hemorrhage is considered to be an extremely ominous sign, since it may signal similar phenomena in other vital organs.

The typical renal lesion of pre-eclampsia–eclampsia is "glomerular capillary endotheliosis," which is best seen by electron microscopy. This disorder is manifested by marked swelling of the glomerular capillary endothelium, with deposits of fibrinoid material in and beneath the endothelial cells. On light microscopy, the glomerular diameter is increased, with protrusion of the glomerular tufts into the neck of the proximal tubules and variable degrees of endothelial and mesangial cell swelling.

The uteroplacental pathology in pre-eclampsia–eclampsia is characterized by a lack of "decidualization" of the myometrial segments of the spiral arteries. Under normal circumstances, the invasion of trophoblast results in the replacement of the muscular and elastic layers of the spiral arteries by fibrinoid and fibrous tissue, resulting in large tortuous channels that extend through the myometrium. In pre-eclampsia, this change is limited to the decidual segments of the vessels and may result in a 60 per cent reduction in the diameter of the myometrial segment of a spiral artery. The extent of placental infarction is increased in almost all hypertensive pregnancies.

Clinical and Laboratory Manifestations

Many of the clinical manifestations of pre-eclampsia and eclampsia can be explained on the basis of vasospasm.

Angiotensin Sensitivity

One of the earliest signs of developing pre-eclampsia is a change in the effective pressor dose of infused angiotensin II. In normal pregnancy, there is an increase in the amount of angiotensin necessary to increase the diastolic pressure 20 mm Hg, whereas those patients destined to develop pre-eclampsia have an effective pressor dose similar to the nonpregnant state.

Weight Gain and Edema

Abnormal weight gain and edema occur early and reflect an expansion of the extravascular fluid compartment. This expansion is related to the increased capillary permeability produced by the arteriolar vasoconstriction. The increased capillary permeability allows fluid to diffuse from the intravascular space with resultant expansion of the extracellular space.

Excessive weight gain and edema, especially if confined to the lower extremities, do not establish a diagnosis of pre-eclampsia. Edema that includes the face and hands is of more concern but is still not diagnostic.

Elevation of Blood Pressure

The next sign usually detected is an elevation of blood pressure, particularly the diastolic pressure (greater than 90 mm Hg), which more closely mirrors changes in peripheral vascular resistance. In the antepartum period, the blood pressure changes may occur days to weeks after the onset of pathologic fluid retention.

Proteinuria

Proteinuria completes the classic clinical triad of pre-eclampsia. In the antepartum period, this sign may occur days or weeks after the onset of hypertension. If the disease first manifests during labor or in the immediate postpartum period, this progression of events is compressed into hours and sometimes minutes. The proteinuria of pre-eclampsia–eclampsia can be explained on the basis of afferent arteriolar constriction with increased glomerular permeability to proteins.

Renal Function

It is usually only during the stage of renal involvement, clinically denoted by proteinuria, that detectable changes in renal function appear. The earliest change may be an increase in serum uric acid concentration. Creatinine clearance may decrease, and serum creatinine and blood urea nitrogen may increase; the hematocrit may also increase, reflecting the relative hypovolemia. Renal involvement may progress to significant oliguria and frank renal failure.

Liver and Placental Function

In the liver, vasospasm may produce focal hemorrhages and infarctions. Therefore, elevated serum enzyme levels are usually present. Thrombocytopenia and disseminated intravascular coagulation may occur, reflecting an increased platelet destruction. Spasm in the uteroplacental vascular bed results in placental infarcts, which may become extensive and lead to a retroplacental hemorrhage. The indirect evidence for a reduced uteroplacental blood flow is the increased incidence of placental infarctions and intrauterine fetal growth retardation.

Central Nervous System Effects

Visual disturbances, such as blurred vision, spots, and scotomata, represent degrees of retinal vasospasm. Increased reflex irritability and hyperreflexia are extremely worrisome signs of central nervous system (CNS) involvement and may denote imminent seizures related to cerebral vasospasm and hypoxia.

Diagnosis and Evaluation

In the prenatal history and physical examination, particular attention should be directed to any previous history of hypertension, proteinuria, or both in either the pregnant or nonpregnant state. Review of medical records from previous hypertension or proteinuria evaluations or from previous hypertensive pregnancies is frequently helpful in establishing a working diagnosis and in

**Table 15–3. INITIAL EVALUATION OF A PATIENT
WITH CHRONIC HYPERTENSION**

BLOOD	URINE	OTHER
Electrolytes	Sediment	Electrocardiogram
Blood urea nitrogen (BUN)	Culture	Obstetric ultrasonography
Creatinine	24-hr protein	
Antinuclear antibody (ANA)	24-hr creatinine	

guiding further evaluation and management. During the initial physical examination, particular attention should be given to the funduscopic examination to record baseline findings. Blood pressure taken in both arms may point toward the rare aortic coarctation.

For the purposes of clinical diagnosis and further evaluation, patients may be divided into two working groups: chronic hypertension and pre-eclampsia. The chronic hypertension group includes most multiparae, those with a previous history of hypertension, and those developing hypertension prior to 20 weeks. Pre-eclampsia is predominantly limited to those women in their first pregnancy who develop the syndrome after 20 weeks.

Table 15–3 outlines the baseline studies recommended for those patients falling into the chronic hypertension group. Table 15–4 outlines the baseline tests to be performed once the diagnosis of pre-eclampsia is suspected. Although some of these tests will result in a low yield, the establishment of normality or abnormality as early in the course as practical may be very helpful as the pregnancy progresses.

Management of Pre-eclampsia

The management of pre-eclampsia should begin at the first sign of abnormality, well before the diagnosis is confirmed. When excessive weight gain or fluid retention is documented in the absence of other pathognomonic changes, a brief dietary history should be obtained, looking for indiscretions and excesses. Appropriate counseling should follow. The patient should be advised of the concerns and be requested to practice bed rest, preferably in the left lateral position. For the following 48 hours, activity out of bed should be limited to eating meals (not preparing them) and using the bathroom. A no-added-salt diet may be prescribed. More severe sodium restriction is contraindicated for all but those in frank renal failure. Follow-up is requested 48 hours later to confirm continued normal blood pressure and to determine the efficacy of treatment for the weight gain and fluid retention. Successful treatment dictates no further intervention other than perhaps the continuation of the no-added-salt diet. If there has been no weight loss, continued reduction of activity with periods of bed rest and more frequent prenatal visits are indicated.

The treatment of hypertension depends to a great extent on the duration of the pregnancy and the height of the blood pressure. At the lowest end of the hypertensive spectrum, 140/90, and in the absence of protein-

**Table 15–4. INITIAL EVALUATION
OF A PATIENT WITH
PRE-ECLAMPSIA**

BLOOD	URINE
Electrolytes	Sediment
Blood urea nitrogen (BUN)	24-hr protein
Creatinine	24-hr creatinine
Uric acid	
Platelet count	
Liver function studies	

uria, outpatient management is possible. Mild salt reduction (no added salt) and bed rest in the left lateral position are again advised. The patient and her family should be counseled regarding warning symptoms of deterioration. Follow-up should occur no later than 48 hours. Many patients in this category respond to bed rest with a normalization of their blood pressure. These women merely require more frequent follow-up than usual.

For the nonresponders, the next step should be a trial of bed rest and a no-added-salt diet in the more controlled environment of the hospital. If blood pressure normalizes, observation should be continued for an additional 24 to 48 hours and the patient discharged on a continued regimen of bed rest and diet with frequent follow-up. Nonresponders who are greater than 36 gestational weeks should be considered for induction of labor. Those less than 37 weeks should continue bed rest and diet in the hospital for several days while undergoing the work-up detailed in Table 15–4. Patients with continued mild hypertension (not greater than 150/100) without proteinuria and with normal laboratory values may be considered for discharge and close follow-up.

The advent of proteinuria in the hypertensive primigravida confirms the diagnosis of pre-eclampsia and requires prompt hospitalization and evaluation (see Table 15–4). For those meeting the criteria for mild pre-eclampsia (see Table 15–2) who are less than 37 gestational weeks, a period of bed rest, no-added-salt diet, and observation, during which appropriate laboratory tests are carried out, is indicated. For those greater than 36 weeks, induction of labor is the treatment of choice, since delivery is the ultimate treatment for this disease.

Patients meeting the criteria for severe pre-eclampsia should have a period of evaluation and stabilization before a final management decision. Those with persistent blood pressure greater than or equal to 160/110 are candidates for antihypertensive therapy (Table 15–5). Prompt response to therapy may allow temporization in those pregnancies of less than 37 weeks. Patients greater than 36 weeks should be delivered, along with those who fail to stabilize and improve, regardless of gesta-

tional age. Intrapartum fetal monitoring is mandatory for all patients (see Chapter 21).

Antihypertensive Therapy

Antihypertensive therapy has two main objectives in both pregnancy-induced and pregnancy-aggravated hypertension: (1) to reduce the maternal morbidity and mortality associated with cerebral vascular accidents and (2) to reduce the perinatal morbidity and mortality associated with intrauterine growth retardation, placental infarcts, and placental abruption. In the absence of underlying abnormalities in the maternal cerebral vasculature, arterial pressures below 160/100 probably do not need therapy for maternal indications. Acute elevations in maternal blood pressure above that level should be promptly brought under control with an intravenous agent, such as hydralazine, or, in a very critical or refractory situation, nitroprusside.

Caution must always be exercised not to lower the arterial pressure too far or too rapidly, for either may result in a decreased uteroplacental blood flow and fetal distress. Although the fetus may certainly derive some benefit from the antihypertensive therapy instituted for maternal indications, it is within the diastolic range of 90 to 100 mm Hg that therapy has been instituted primarily for fetal indications. Controversy continues to exist as to whether effective antihypertensive therapy improves perinatal outcome, although the weight of evidence is increasing in favor of such treatment.

In the near-term and laboring patient, short-term control can best be achieved with intravenous hydralazine. In the patient in whom long-term control is the objective, one of the oral agents is the treatment of choice. Extensive experience on the efficacy and safety of methyldopa (Aldomet) has been published from randomized trials, and it is probably the most commonly prescribed antihypertensive for the ambulatory patient. There is increasing evidence that selective β blockers such as atenolol (Ternormin) and metoprolol (Lopressor) are equally safe and efficacious, although small-for-dates infants, fetal and neonatal bradycardia, and hypoglycemia have been reported. The alpha-1/non-

Table 15–5. ANTIHYPERTENSIVE THERAPY DURING PREGNANCY

AGENT	ROUTE	ACTION	PEAK RESPONSE	SIDE EFFECTS	COMMENT
Hydralazine (Apresoline)	IV or PO	Direct vasodilator	20–30 min 1–2 hr	Headache, palpitations, lupus-like syndrome	Increases cardiac output and probably uterine and renal blood flow. Drug of choice for short-term control
Nifedipine (Adalat, Procardia)	PO	Calcium ion influx inhibitor	30 min	Edema, dizziness	Exaggerated response in patients on magnesium
Methyldopa (Aldomet)	PO	False neurotransmitter	3–5 days	Postural hypotension, drowsiness, fluid retention	Frequently used for long-term control of mild hypertension
Diazoxide (Hyperstat)	IV	Direct vasodilator	2–4 min	Hypotension, hyperglycemia	Hard to control; may cause rapid decrease in blood pressure
Prazosin (Minipress)	PO	Alpha-1 blocker (postsynaptic)	1–3 hr	Hypotension (especially first dose), drowsiness	Limited obstetric experience reported
Atenolol (Tenormin)	PO	Selective beta-1 blocker	1–2 wk	Lassitude, breathlessness	Limited experience
Labetalol (Trondate)	PO	Nonselective beta-1 and alpha-1 blocker	2 hr	Tremulousness, headache	Increasing experience and efficacy reported. May be drug of choice in future
Nitroprusside (Nipride)	IV	Direct vasodilator	1–2 min	Hypotension, cyanide toxicity in fetus	Useful only for short-term control in hypertensive crisis

selective β blocker labetalol (Trondate) appears to be as effective as methyldopa and is used extensively in Europe and Great Britain. Calcium-channel blockers such as nifedipine have been suggested as second-line drugs, but caution must be exercised in anyone also receiving magnesium. Converting-enzyme inhibitors should be avoided because fetal death has been reported in several animal species.

Anticonvulsant Therapy

Because of the risk of seizures and their attendant morbidity and even mortality, a great deal of attention must be given to the level of CNS irritability. Peripheral reflexes, particularly of the patella and ankle, are most frequently used as determinants of increased instability. Sustained clonus is a clinically significant finding.

Seizure prophylaxis should be instituted in all pre-eclamptics during labor and delivery and continued for 12 to 24 hours following delivery. All severe pre-eclamptics should have seizure prophylaxis instituted on admission and continued during the period of evaluation and observation. Magnesium sulfate is the agent of choice because of its efficacy and associated low neonatal morbidity. Both intramuscular and intravenous routes are effective.

Table 15–6 outlines the protocols for magnesium administration, and Table 15–7 reviews the relationship of serum concentrations to clinical response. The magnesium ion is excreted exclusively through the kidneys, so caution must be exercised in those

Table 15-6. MAGNESIUM SULFATE THERAPY

TYPE OF TREATMENT	IM	IV
Prophylactic		
Loading	5 gm each buttock	4 gm over 10 min
Maintenance	5 gm/4 hr	1-2 gm/hr
Therapeutic (for seizure treatment)	—	1 gm/min until seizure controlled; 4-6 gm maximum

IM = Intramuscular; IV = intravenous.

patients with compromised renal function. As already indicated, caution must also be exercised in patients receiving a calcium-channel blocker.

Management of Fluid Balance

The management of fluid balance is of major importance in all hypertensive patients receiving intravenous therapy. Accurately recorded intake and output data must be kept to calculate requirements. These patients are vasoconstricted and may have some relative degree of reduced intravascular volume, both of which may reduce urinary output. In addition, they may be receiving several different therapeutic infusions, such as magnesium sulfate and oxytocin, which have a direct or indirect effect on urinary output.

The most common errors that occur in the management of these patients are volume overload and water intoxication. The conservative approach is to replace documented output plus insensible loss with an appropriate electrolyte-containing fluid. Because of the multifaceted pathophysiology of this disease, central hemodynamic monitoring may aid in the management of the more severe cases. Pulmonary artery and pulmonary capillary wedge pressures are more helpful in guiding fluid therapy than is central venous pressure, which on occasion may be misleading.

Prophylaxis

Although the etiology of pre-eclampsia is not known, there is some evidence that inadequate intake of protein and calcium have been associated with an increased incidence. Much attention has focused on attempts to correct the abnormal PGI_2 to thromboxane A_2 ratio. Low-dose aspirin (60 to 80 mg) is known to inhibit thromboxane A_2 synthesis and is currently undergoing rigorous evaluation. Low-dose aspirin is also known to reduce platelet aggregation, which would potentially have a positive effect on the presumed pathologic mechanisms of this disease. At this time the jury is still out on the risk/benefit of low-dose aspirin as a means to prophylaxis and treatment of pre-eclampsia.

Management of HELLP Syndrome

Delivery is the definitive treatment for those pregnancies beyond 34 weeks or with evidence of fetal lung maturity, or in those patients with deteriorating maternal or fetal condition. Initial maternal evaluation should include those studies listed in Table 15-8. In addition, a significant percentage of these patients will have a disseminated intravascular coagulation syndrome. Management is directed toward stabilization of the fluid bal-

Table 15-7. CLINICAL CORRELATES OF SERUM MAGNESIUM SULFATE LEVELS

SERUM CONCENTRATION (mg/dl)	(mEq/L*)	OBSERVED RESPONSE
1.2-1.8	1.5-2.1	Normal
3-8	2.5-6.7	Therapeutic range
6-8	5-6.6	CNS depression
8-10	6.6-8.3	Absent reflexes
12-17	10-14.2	Respiratory depression
13-17	10.8-14.2	Coma
19-20	15.8-16.6	Cardiac arrest

* 1 mEq/L = 1.2 mg/dl.

Table 15–8. LABORATORY EVALUATION FOR HELLP SYNDROME

Hemolysis
  Peripheral smear
  Bilirubin
  LDH

Liver enzymes
  SGOT
  LDH

Platelets
  Platelet count

LDH = lactate dehydrogenase; SGOT = serum glutamic-oxaloacetic transaminase.

ance and coagulopathy. The syndrome slowly corrects following delivery.

Management of Eclampsia

If the patient develops convulsive seizures at home, she is usually brought to the hospital in a comatose condition. The management of these patients should be carried out by a team of physicians and well-trained nurses in an isolated labor room, with minimal noise and not too much light. As with any epileptic condition, the initial requirement is to clear the airway and give oxygen by face mask to relieve airway obstruction and hypoxia. Blood pressure should be recorded every 10 minutes with the patient in the lateral position. An intravenous line should be placed for drawing blood and administering drugs and fluids. Intravenous fluids should be limited to sufficient 5 per cent dextrose in water to replace urine output, plus about 700 ml per day to replace insensible losses. An indwelling catheter should be placed in the bladder, urine sent to the laboratory for urinalysis, and all urine output recorded.

Pharmacologic management necessitates an antihypertensive drug (hydralazine) to lower blood pressure and relieve vasoconstriction. The aim is to decrease the diastolic pressure by 25 to 30 per cent from the hypertensive values. Magnesium sulfate is given intravenously to decrease hyperreflexia and prevent further convulsions (Table 15–6). Agents such as diazepam (Valium) may also be used.

If the patient is prenatal, no attempt should be made to deliver her either vaginally or by cesarean section until the acute phase of convulsive eclampsia and coma has passed. Induction of labor or cesarean section during the acute phase may aggravate the oliguria and other manifestations of the disease. When the urine output increases and the coma and convulsions are controlled, delivery should be expedited, preferably by the vaginal route. If this is not feasible, cesarean section is indicated.

Management of Chronic Hypertension

The management of pregnancy-aggravated or chronic hypertension is in many ways more clear-cut. Despite the fact that the blood pressure of these patients may be "normal" in the first and second trimesters, existing antihypertensive medication should be stopped only for unusually low pressures or other strong indications. Those women who are not taking antihypertensive agents should be started once the diastolic pressure is consistently greater than 90 mm Hg. The foundations of conservative management include reduced physical activity and bed rest.

Because these women have a high incidence of intrauterine fetal growth retardation, both early and serial ultrasonic examinations are indicated. The early ultrasonogram (16 to 20 weeks) is primarily for confirmation of pregnancy dates, whereas serial ultrasonic examinations (every 3 weeks from 24 to 28 weeks) are of great assistance in detecting growth retardation. Significant growth retardation may be an indication for early delivery.

Because of the concern for chronic uteroplacental insufficiency in this group of patients, the various tests for fetal well-being are indicated (see Chapter 7). Depending on the clinical circumstances, fetal monitoring may start as early as 28 weeks and, in all hypertensive patients, should be commenced by 36 weeks.

A significant increase in hypertension or the addition of proteinuria to a previously nonproteinuric chronic hypertensive patient is of great concern. Many would regard these as signs of superimposed pre-eclampsia. The incidence of superimposed pre-eclampsia varies from 15 to 25 per cent. These patients should undergo further laboratory evaluation, as outlined in Table 15–4. Management should follow that outlined for severe pre-eclampsia.

In general, the timing of delivery in the chronic hypertensive group is more difficult. For those without fetal growth retardation in whom the blood pressure is well controlled and proteinuria is not present, a full-term gestation may be allowed, provided that there is normal fetal well-being. Any progression beyond the fortieth week should be very carefully considered. The presence of growth retardation or blood pressure deterioration or the advent of proteinuria may dictate earlier delivery. If delivery is desirable but not imperative prior to 37 weeks, confirmation of fetal lung maturity should be initially obtained. There is no contraindication to vaginal delivery in the hypertensive patient; therefore, the route of delivery should be decided on obstetric criteria.

Sequelae and Outcome

There are essentially no long-term maternal sequelae to an episode of uncomplicated pre-eclampsia or eclampsia in the primigravid patient. Such patients are at no greater risk of subsequently developing hypertensive cardiovascular disease than any other individual. Interestingly, their female offspring do have an increased risk of pre-eclampsia in their own pregnancies. Similarly, pregnancy does not seem to affect the subsequent course of a patient with chronic hypertension. Some of the more serious complications of both pregnancy-induced and pregnancy-aggravated hypertension, such as cerebrovascular accidents and renal failure, may have long-term maternal sequelae.

Fetal and neonatal sequelae are more difficult to determine, since some of the prenatal morbidity and mortality of these hypertensive syndromes are related to intrauterine growth retardation and acute and chronic fetal distress. All of these may have long-term CNS effects. Overall, the mortality rate in women with hypertensive disease of pregnancy is about 10 per cent, but this figure varies according to economic level and the quality of care received. Maternal mortality is virtually nonexistent in women with pre-eclampsia, but the mortality rate is in the vicinity of 10 per cent in women with eclampsia and HELLP.

SUGGESTED READING

Assali NS (ed): Pathophysiology of gestation. In Maternal Disorders. Vol 1. New York, Academic Press, 1972.

Brosens IA, Robertson WB, Dixon HG: The role of the spiral arteries in the pathogenesis of pre-eclampsia. Obstet Gynecol Annu 1:117, 1972.

Chamberlain G, Philipp E, Howlett B, et al: British Births, 1970. In Obstetric Case. Vol 2. London, Heinemann, 1978.

Chesley LC: Hypertensive Disorders in Pregnancy. New York, Appleton-Century-Crofts, 1978, p 57.

Gant NF, Chand S, Worley RJ, et al: A clinical test useful for predicting the development of acute hypertension in pregnancy. Am J Obstet Gynecol 120:1, 1974.

Gant NF, Daley GL, Chand S, et al: A study of angiotensin II pressor response throughout primigravid pregnancy. J Clin Invest 52:2682, 1973.

Michelson EL, Fuschman WH: Labetalol: An alpha- and beta-adrenoceptor blocking drug. Ann Intern Med 99:553, 1983.

Report on Confidential Enquiries into Maternal Deaths in England and Wales, 1973–1975. Report on Health and Social Subjects. Department of Health and Social Security, 1975.

Rubin PC, Butters L, Clark DM, et al: Placebo-controlled trial of atenolol in treatment of pregnancy-associated hypertension. Lancet 1(8322): 431, 1983.

Schiff E, Peleg E, Goldenberg M: The use of aspirin to prevent pregnancy-induced hypertension and lower the ratio of thromboxane A2 to prostacyclin in relatively high risk pregnancies. N Engl J Med 321:351, 1989.

Sheehan HL, Lynch JB: Pathology of Toxemia of Pregnancy. Baltimore, Williams & Wilkins, 1973.

Sibai, BM: The HELLP syndrome (hemolysis, elevated liver enzymes and low platelets). Much ado about nothing? Am J Obstet Gynecol 162:311, 1990.

Symonds EM: Etiology of pre-eclampsia: A review. J Royal Soc Med 73:871, 1980.

Vollman RF: Study design, population and data characteristics. In Friedman MA (ed): Progress in Clinical and Biological Research. Blood Pressure, Edema and Proteinuria in Pregnancy. Vol 7. New York, Alan R. Liss Inc, 1976.

Sixteen

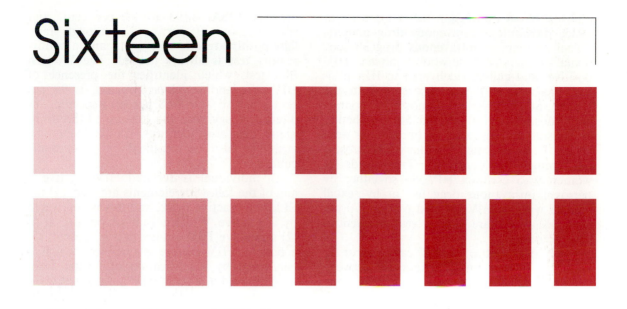

AIDS and Infectious Diseases in Pregnancy

JEAN M. RICCI

Infections in pregnancy are a recognized cause of maternal and neonatal morbidity. Many cases are preventable, and in this chapter the more common infectious disease entities which may be seen in pregnancy are discussed.

VIRAL INFECTIONS

Acquired Immunodeficiency Syndrome

Incidence. Infection with the human immunodeficiency virus (HIV) results in the development of the acquired immunodeficiency syndrome (AIDS), which has been a recognized disease in the United States since 1981. There are no precise data on the exact number of individuals infected with HIV at the present time, but its spread definitely has reached epidemic proportions. It is estimated that between 5 and 10 million people are now infected with HIV in the world, with 1.5 million of these individuals living in the United States. Estimates for 1991 showed that 74,000 people will have developed AIDS in the United States, including 7200 cases in women of childbearing age and 1000 cases in the children of these infected women.

Epidemiology. HIV has been isolated from blood, semen, vaginal secretions, urine, saliva, tears, cerebrospinal fluid, amniotic fluid, and breast milk. There are three primary modes of HIV transmission: (1) intimate contact with infected bodily secretions, (2) exposure to infected blood and blood products, and (3) maternal-infant spread. Therefore, individuals who are at high risk for contracting HIV include homosexuals, hemophiliacs, blood transfusion recipients prior to 1985, prostitutes, intravenous drug abusers, sexual partners of intravenous drug abusers, sexual partners of those who are already HIV positive, and children delivered to HIV-positive mothers. HIV was first spread in the United States through homosexual contact and transmission of infected blood, whether as a result of transfusion or intravenous drug abuse. However, transmission via heterosexual contact is increasing. Two thirds of women who contract HIV do so either by personal intravenous drug use or by sexual contact with an HIV infected partner, 70 per cent of whom are themselves intravenous drug abusers.

Eight per cent of AIDS cases occur in women, 80 per cent of whom are between the ages of 13 and 39. AIDS can strike any ethnic or social group. The prevalence of HIV carriage in pregnant women in inner city hospitals is 8 per 1000, whereas in the suburban sector the prevalence is 0.9 per 1000.

The Virus. HIV is an RNA retrovirus. Virus-infected cells are the major source of transmission of HIV (for example, in tears or saliva). Free virus rarely is a source of infection except if the concentration of free virus is very high. HIV replicates in certain cell types, in particular cells of the hematopoietic system (T-helper lymphocytes*) and the central nervous system. As with all retroviruses, HIV contains a reverse transcriptase in its core. HIV has specific surface proteins gp120 and gp41 and core proteins p18 and p24. The HIV infects a cell by first making contact with the gp120 protein. It then enters the cell, releases its core RNA, and using its own reverse transcriptase, makes a DNA copy of itself and inserts this DNA into the host genome. This viral gene then either enters into a latent state or begins making viral RNA and proteins with production of an infectious virus.

Laboratory Diagnosis. Serology is the most common method of diagnosis. Indirect serologic methods that detect HIV antibody include the enzyme-linked immunosorbent assay (ELISA), Western Blot, and immunofluorescence assay (IFA) tests. The sensitivity

of the ELISA is 93 to 99 per cent, and specificity is 99 per cent. Although rare, false-positive results may occur and a confirmatory test is always needed. The Western Blot test, which identifies the presence of HIV core and envelope antigens, is 99 per cent sensitive and 99.8 per cent specific. Indirect serology with the capture ELISA technique can also identify HIV antigen. The virus can also be identified by direct tissue culture.

An individual is declared HIV positive if any of the following elements are true: (1) the ELISA is reactive twice, and this is confirmed by a positive Western Blot or positive IFA; (2) a positive HIV antigen test is present; (3) a positive HIV culture is obtained, which is confirmed by identification of reverse transcriptase and a specific HIV antigen test.

Disease Course. Infection with HIV results in a chronic progressive disease. Seroconversion typically occurs 3 to 14 weeks after exposure but rarely may take 6 months or more. In 90 per cent of cases, seroconversion is associated with a mononucleosis-like syndrome or aseptic meningitis. Once the virus has been acquired, the patient enters an asymptomatic period but should be assumed to be infected for life. Because HIV has a predilection for helper (T_4) cells, there is a gradual destruction in the patient's cell-mediated immunity, rendering the host susceptible to opportunistic infections. Eventual reversal of the T_4/T_8 ratio to less than 1 is seen on laboratory analysis. Typically, the patient develops asymptomatic lymphadenopathy, followed by the onset of constitutional symptoms (anorexia, fever, weight loss, diarrhea, nausea and vomiting). Eventually, opportunistic infections, secondary cancers (Kaposi's sarcoma, non-Hodgkin's lymphoma) or neurologic diseases (dementia, neuropathy) develop. Opportunistic infections that may be seen include: *Pneumocystis carinii* pneumonia (PCP), tuberculosis, cryptococcal meningitis, cytomegalovirus (CMV) retinitis, atypical mycobacterial disease, cerebral toxoplasmosis, severe herpes and cryptospiridiosis.

The average interval from initial infection to the onset of AIDS is 7.5 years in adult male homosexuals. This information is presently unknown in women. The disease progresses more rapidly in infants, with most living only a few years.

---

* T, Thymus-dependent lymphocyte; T_4, helper cells; and T_8, suppressor cells.

Table 16–1. RISK FACTORS FOR HIV TRANSMISSION

Multiple sexual partners
Intravenous drug abuse
Sexual partner of an intravenous drug abuser
Sexual partner of HIV-infected person
Prostitution
Transfusion prior to 1985
History of sexually transmitted diseases (especially ulcerative)
Birth in, or sexual partner of those born in Africa, or the Caribbean

Screening for HIV Infection. Patients who are at risk for HIV transmission (Table 16–1) should be offered screening. Given the risk of perinatal transmission, screening for HIV should be offered to all pregnant women. Testing requires that the patient give informed consent, with adequate counseling before and after testing. When counseling a newly identified HIV positive pregnant woman, it is necessary to discuss the risk of perinatal transmission, the potential for disease progression during the pregnancy, and the effect of HIV on pregnancy. Counseling on disease prevention, including a discussion of safe sexual practices and avoidance of breast feeding, is imperative. In addition, the option of pregnancy termination as well as future family planning must also be discussed.

Effect of Pregnancy on HIV Infection. It remains controversial as to whether pregnancy is associated with a decrease in cell-mediated immunity. Concern has been raised that this possible natural depression superimposed on the T_4 suppression seen in HIV-infected patients may adversely affect the pregnant HIV-infected patient. At this point in time, pregnancy has not been shown to result in an acceleration of disease in HIV-infected women, but long-term studies are needed to clarify this.

Effect of HIV Infection on Pregnancy. There is no confirmed evidence that maternal AIDS can result in a fetal embryopathy. In addition, not all infants delivered to HIV-infected mothers contract the disease. Present estimates of vertical transmission from the mother to her fetus range from 25 to 35 per cent. It has been postulated that women with more severe disease, evidenced by T_4 counts less than $300/\mu l$, may be more likely to transmit their infection to the fetus. Transplacental transmission accounts for 80 per cent of AIDS-related infections in infants. Because the HIV virus has been isolated from breast milk, transmission is probable with breast feeding. The risk of maternal-fetal transmission from amniocentesis, chorionic villus sampling, and umbilical blood sampling is unknown. Therefore, if these procedures are indicated, the patient must first be counseled regarding the potential for fetal transmission. There is no evidence that the mode of delivery affects transmission rates.

It is extremely difficult to determine which infant will be infected in the newborn period. This is because newborns delivered to HIV-infected mothers will test positive for the HIV IgG antibody, which is acquired via transplacental passage, for up to 18 months. Of those infants who eventually show signs of disease, half develop AIDS in the first year of life and 85 per cent develop AIDS by age 3. The median age of onset of AIDS in children is 8 months of age. Children have an extremely poor prognosis, with an average survival time from time of diagnosis of 3 years.

Studies are under way to determine whether or not HIV has any effect on pregnancy outcome. It is believed that women with blood T_4 counts of less than $300/\mu l$ are at increased risk for developing infectious complications in their pregnancies. These infections include opportunistic infections, postpartum infections, antepartum urinary tract infections, and sexually transmitted diseases. Studies to date have not shown an increased risk of growth retardation, preterm labor, or premature rupture of the membranes.

Care of the Pregnant HIV Patient. At the present time, there is no cure for HIV-related disease. The main focus of management is directed toward early detection of infection and prevention of further transmission. Baseline evaluation of the HIV-positive pregnant patient should include a detailed history of risk factors for transmission and a careful medical history, including questioning about weight change, headaches, diarrhea, nausea, vomiting, anorexia, fever, night sweats, cough, shortness of breath, and sore throat.

The patient should also be questioned about exposure to tuberculosis, varicella, or herpes simplex, contact with cats, and recent travel, because all of these factors may expose the immunocompromised patient to opportunistic infection. On physical examination, particular attention should be given to the oral cavity (thrush, leukoplakia), eyegrounds (CMV retinitis), lungs, lymph nodes, liver, spleen, vagina (candida), and perirectal area (herpes). In addition, a complete neurologic examination is essential. Initial laboratory tests should include a complete blood count (CBC) along with differential leucocyte count, platelet count, liver function tests, T_4 cell count, T_4/T_8 ratio, PPD, syphilis serology, and serum titers for hepatitis B surface antigen, toxoplasmosis, rubella, and CMV. T_4 cell counts should be repeated each trimester. Cervical cultures should be obtained for chlamydia, yeast, and gonorrhea. Prenatal visits need not be any more frequent unless specifically indicated. Fetal surveillance testing should be reserved for obstetric indications.

Prophylaxis against PCP with Bactrim is indicated in pregnancy if T_4 counts fall below $200/\mu l$. Azidothymidine (AZT) is under investigation for use in asymptomatic HIV-infected pregnant women to determine its impact on disease progression and transmission. At this time, its use is limited to study protocols, women with low T_4 counts ($<500/\mu l$), or those who are severely ill. It is unknown whether or not AZT has a teratogenic effect, although there is no evidence to suggest this.

Human Parvovirus B19 Infection

Clinical Manifestations. Human parvovirus B19 is a single-stranded DNA virus that is cytotoxic for erythroid progenitor cells. Clinical infection is most common in school children, with only 20 per cent of clinical infections occurring in adults. The severity of clinical infection also decreases with increasing age, with high rates of asymptomatic infection in older patients. The virus is spread via a respiratory route primarily but may also be spread by infected blood products or transplacentally. The adult who is symptomatic usually experiences a vague flu-like syndrome with symmetric polyarthralgias

and arthritis. Infection with parvovirus B19 infection is, however, a cause of aplastic crisis in patients with sickle cell disease, hereditary spherocytosis, or any immunodeficiency syndrome.

Diagnosis. The serologic response to parvovirus includes an elevation of IgM by 2 weeks, and this persists for approximately 60 days. IgG is present 3 weeks after exposure and may persist for years.

Impact on Pregnancy. Less than one third of maternal infections are associated with fetal infection. However, 10 per cent of in utero infections are associated with adverse outcomes, specifically spontaneous abortion, stillbirth, and nonimmune hydrops fetalis. Fetal risk is greatest if maternal infection occurs between 10 and 20 weeks of gestation. There is no known antiviral therapy for treatment nor evidence that giving gamma globulin after exposure is preventative. Intrauterine blood transfusion may prove to be helpful for the fetus with severe hydrops, which results from hemolysis and marrow aplasia. Management of the exposed or symptomatic gravida includes testing for IgM and IgG. If tests are positive for IgM, a maternal serum alpha-fetoprotein sample should be obtained and ultrasonic examinations should be performed serially to identify hydrops. The presence of both hydrops and an elevated maternal serum alpha-fetoprotein level correlates with a very poor fetal outcome. If hydrops is present, umbilical blood sampling and intrauterine transfusion may be considered.

Rubeola (Measles)

Clinical Manifestations. Measles is an exanthematous infection caused by a paramyxovirus, which is spread by direct or indirect contact with respiratory secretions, particularly aerolized ones. It is communicable from 4 days before to 7 days after the onset of the rash. Time from exposure to onset of clinical disease is 10 days.

Diagnosis. Diagnosis is primarily by clinical presentation. However, a measles-specific IgM antibody will appear 5 to 10 days after the onset of the rash.

Impact on Pregnancy. Fortunately most women have acquired immunity to measles by reproductive age. There is no difference in the disease course in pregnancy. For the exposed woman without a prior history of measles, immunoglobulin, given within 6 days of exposure, may prevent the infection. Measles vaccine is contraindicated in pregnancy because it is a live attenuated virus. Maternal infection has been associated with a higher risk of spontaneous abortion, preterm labor, and low birth weight. The fetus can become infected by transplacentally transmitted virus, but there is no increased risk of congenital anomalies. When maternal infection occurs near delivery, the fetus may appear infected at birth or develop an exanthem within the first 10 to 12 days of life. Neonatal infection due to congenital measles may be mild or rapidly fatal, with a case-fatality ratio of 56 per cent in preterm infants and 20 per cent in the term fetus. This is in contrast to postnatally acquired measles in which the disease course is usually mild.

Rubella (German Measles)

Clinical Manifestations. Rubella results from infection with a single-stranded RNA togavirus transmitted via the respiratory route, with highest attack rates occurring between March and May. It is highly contagious, with 75 per cent of those infected becoming clinically ill. The incubation period is 14 to 21 days.

Diagnosis. The diagnosis of rubella is best made by serologic testing. The IgM response is a rapid one that begins at the onset of the rash, and then declines and disappears by 4 to 8 weeks. IgG response also begins at the onset of the rash and remains elevated for life. The diagnosis can be made by the presence of a fourfold rise in the hemagglutination-inhibiting antibody (HAI) titer in paired sera obtained 2 weeks apart or by the presence of IgM. Rubella can also be diagnosed by culture and isolation of the virus during the acute phase of infection, although this technique is slow. The presence of IgM in cord blood or IgG in an infant after 6 months of age supports the diagnosis of perinatal rubella infection.

Impact on Pregnancy. Between 10 and 15 per cent of adult women are susceptible to rubella. The disease course is unaltered by pregnancy, and the mother may or may not

Table 16-2. CONGENITAL RUBELLA SYNDROME
Symmetric IUGR
Congenital deafness (detected after age 1 year)
Cardiac malformations
Patent ductus arteriosus
Pulmonary artery hypoplasia
Eye lesions
Cataracts
Retinopathy
Micropthalmia
Hepatosplenomegaly
Central nervous system involvement
Microcephaly
Panencephalitis
Brain calcifications
Psychomotor retardation
Hepatitis
Thrombocytopenic purpura

exhibit the full clinical disease. The severity of the mother's illness does not impact on the risk of fetal infection. Rather, it is the trimester in which infection occurs that has the greatest impact on fetal risk. Fetal infection may result in either a normal baby, spontaneous abortion, or the congenital rubella syndrome (CRS). Specifically, infection in the first trimester carries a 25 per cent risk of CRS (50 per cent risk in the first 4 weeks), whereas the risk of CRS drops to less than 1 per cent if infection occurs in the second or third trimesters. Components of CRS are outlined in Table 16-2.

Routine rubella susceptibility testing should be performed in all pregnant women with a single IgG level. Those who are nonimmune should be vaccinated in the immediate postpartum period. Follow-up antibody titers should then be obtained, because up to 20 per cent will fail to develop an antibody response at the time of the first test. Postpartum vaccination is not a contraindication to breast feeding. There is no specific treatment for rubella, and routine prophylaxis with gamma globulin after exposure is not recommended because it has not been shown to change the risk of fetal involvement.

Cytomegalovirus

Clinical Manifestations. CMV is a DNA virus and a member of the herpes virus family and, therefore, has the ability to establish latency. The virus is transmitted in a number of ways, including blood transfusion, organ transplant, sexual contact, breast milk, urine, saliva, transplacentally, or at delivery by direct contact. Between 30 and 60 per cent of school-aged children are seropositive for CMV, as are 57 per cent of all pregnant women, which suggests that a prior infection occurred. Infection may be expressed as a mononucleosis-like illness, although subclinical infection is more common. Viral excretion may continue for months, and the virus may establish latency in lymphocytes, salivary glands, renal tubules, and the endometrium. Reactivation may occur years after primary infection, and reinfection with a different strain of the virus is also possible.

Diagnosis. The virus may be isolated on urine culture or by culture of other body secretions or tissues. Serologic testing is possible, with an elevation in IgM that peaks 3 to 6 months after infection and resolves by 1 to 2 years. IgG elevates rapidly and persists for life. Problems with serologic testing include (1) the prolonged elevation in levels of IgM, making delineation of timing of infection difficult and (2) a 20 per cent false-negative rate in IgM testing. In addition, the presence of IgG does not rule out the presence of persistent disease.

Impact on Pregnancy. CMV is the most common congenital viral infection in the United States, affecting 0.5 to 2.5 per cent of all liveborn infants per year. Placental infection may occur without fetal infection, and fetal infection can occur when the mother does not exhibit symptoms. The risk of transmission is constant across trimesters, with a 40 to 50 per cent maternal-infant transmission rate. Ten to twenty per cent of infected infants are symptomatic at birth, exhibiting nonimmune hydrops, symmetric intrauterine growth retardation (IUGR), chorioretinitis, microcephaly, cerebral calcifications, hepatosplenomegaly, and hydrocephaly. Eighty to ninety per cent are asymptomatic at birth but later exhibit mental retardation, visual impairment, progressive hearing loss and delayed psychomotor development. How severely an infant will be affected is unrelated to when in pregnancy maternal infection occurred. Recurrent CMV infection is associated with a much lower fetal risk, with a 0.15 to 1 per cent maternal-fetal transmission rate. Only three cases of severely affected infants have ever been reported.

There is no treatment available for CMV infection. Preventive measures include good hygiene in high-risk settings such as the neonatal intensive care unit, day care centers, and dialysis units. Maternal transfusion with CMV positive blood should be avoided. Aids to making the diagnosis of fetal infection in a suspected case include ultrasonography (to identify symmetric IUGR, nonimmune hydrops or ascites, or central nervous system [CNS] abnormalities), and amniotic fluid CMV culture. Percutaneous umbilical cord blood sampling may also be performed to obtain fetal blood for culture and IgM testing.

Varicella-Zoster

Clinical Manifestations. Acute varicella infection, or chickenpox, is caused by the varicella-zoster virus, which is a DNA herpes virus transmitted by direct contact or via the respiratory route. The attack rate in susceptible individuals is over 90 per cent. The incubation period is 10 to 21 days. Infection is believed to be more severe in adults, and potential complications include encephalitis and pneumonia. Because it is a herpes virus, the varicella virus has the ability to establish latency and does so in nerve ganglia. Reactivation of the virus results in herpes zoster (shingles).

Diagnosis. The diagnosis of chickenpox is usually determined by the patient's clinical presentation, although the virus may be cultured from vesicles during the first 4 days of the rash. On serologic testing, varicella-zoster IgM will rise in 2 weeks on ELISA or complement fixation. Paired sera for IgG obtained 2 weeks apart may also detect infection. Fluorescent antibody membrane antigen (FAMA) is the most useful test to determine whether or not a woman is immune.

Impact on Pregnancy. Between 5 and 10 per cent of adult women are susceptible to the varicella virus. Acute varicella infection complicates 1 in 7500 pregnancies. Potential maternal complications include preterm labor, encephalitis, and varicella pneumonia. Varicella pneumonia complicates 16 per cent of cases and carries a mortality rate of 40 per cent. Maternal management should be symptomatic, but a chest x-ray study should be obtained to rule out pneumonia. If pneumonia is confirmed or suspected, the patient requires immediate admission and institution of antiviral therapy, because rapid respiratory decompensation is not uncommon.

Congenital varicella syndrome, which occurs in up to 10 per cent of first-trimester infections, has been identified. The risk of this syndrome is 2 per cent overall up to 30 weeks, with no cases having occurred after 30 weeks' gestation. Diagnosis of the syndrome is based on IgM-positive cord blood and clinical findings in the newborn, which include limb hypoplasia, cutaneous scars, chorioretinitis, cataracts, cortical atrophy, microcephaly, and symmetric IUGR. There are no reliable methods of prenatal diagnosis.

If maternal infection occurs within 3 weeks before delivery, the fetus has a 24 per cent risk of developing infection after delivery. If maternal infection occurs 5 to 21 days before delivery and the infant develops infection, it is typically mild and self-limited. However, if maternal infection occurs between 4 days before delivery and 2 days after delivery, the infant is at great risk of developing a fulminant infection with a 30 per cent mortality rate. Varicella-Zoster immune globulin (VZIG) is given to these infants within 72 hours of birth, and they are placed in contact isolation. The placenta and fetal membranes should be considered potentially infectious.

For the exposed gravida who has no knowledge of a prior infection, a varicella IgG titer should be sent immediately. If results are delayed or if the patient proves to be nonimmune, VZIG should be administered within 96 hours of exposure, although it is unclear whether or not this therapy will indeed modify the disease course and risk to the fetus. Administration of VZIG is also recommended after exposure to zoster. Varicella vaccine is composed of a live attenuated virus and, therefore, is contraindicated in pregnancy.

Herpes zoster does not occur more frequently in pregnancy. If it does occur it poses no risk to the fetus. If zoster develops close to delivery, varicella may be transmitted through contact with a lesion, so this problem should be avoided.

Hepatitis B

The hepatitis B virus is a DNA virus that is transmitted via blood, saliva, vaginal secretions, semen, breast milk, and across the placenta. The population at greatest risk for contracting the virus includes intravenous drug abusers, homosexuals, individuals of Asian descent, and health care workers. Infection with the virus is either asymptomatic or expressed as acute hepatitis. Ten per cent of individuals then go on to develop chronic active or persistent hepatitis.

Impact on Pregnancy. The course of acute hepatitis is unaltered in pregnancy. Fetal infection may occur and is most likely if maternal infection occurs in the third trimester. Chronic active hepatitis is associated with an increased risk of prematurity, low birth weight, and neonatal death. Maternal prognosis is very poor if the disease is complicated by cirrhosis, varices, or liver failure.

The incidence of hepatitis B surface antigen (HBsAG) positivity in pregnancy in the United States is 0.2 per cent, or 1 in 300 deliveries. Women who are asymptomatic HBsAG carriers are at no higher risk for antepartum complications than are the general population. However, newborns delivered to mothers positive for HBsAG have a 10 per cent risk of developing acute infection at birth. This is in contrast to those delivered to mothers positive for both HBsAG and hepatitis Be antigen (HBeAG), in which the infant's risk increases to 70 to 90 per cent. Infection in the infant may be fulminant and lethal. If the infant survives, it has an 85 to 90 per cent chance of becoming a chronic hepatitis carrier and a 25 per cent chance of developing liver cirrhosis, hepatocellular carcinoma, or both. Therefore, it is recommended that all pregnant women be screened for HBsAG carriage during their pregnancy. Those women in high-risk groups (Table 16–3) should be rescreened in the third trimester if the initial screen is negative. If a pregnant woman is found, on screening, to be HBsAG positive, liver function tests and a complete

Table 16-3. HIGH-RISK GROUPS FOR HBsAG CARRIAGE

Birth in Haiti or Africa
Asian, Pacific Island, or Eskimo descent (immigrant or born in the United States)
Work or treatment in hemodialysis unit
Work or residence in institutions for mentally handicapped
History of repeated transfusion
Occupational exposure to blood
Repetitive episodes of sexually transmitted diseases
Intravenous drug abuse
Prostitution
Household contact with hepatitis carrier
Household contact with hemodialysis patient

hepatitis panel should be performed. Household members and sexual contacts should be tested and offered vaccination if they are susceptible. Transmission to the infant is believed to occur by direct contact during delivery. The newborn is given hepatitis immune globulin and hepatitis vaccine soon after delivery.

Herpes Simplex

Clinical Manifestations. The herpes simplex virus (HSV) is a member of the DNA herpes virus family and is transmitted by intimate mucocutaneous contact. Because the virus has the ability to establish latency in sensory ganglia, it is an incurable sexually transmitted disease and is highly contagious. The clinical manifestations of herpes genitalis and its diagnosis are discussed in Chapter 35.

Impact on Pregnancy

Primary Genital Herpes. Patients who acquire primary herpes in pregnancy have an increased risk of obstetric and neonatal complications. Maternal infection has been associated with an increased risk of spontaneous abortion, IUGR, and preterm labor. Fifty per cent of infants born vaginally to mothers with a primary infection at delivery have HSV infection.

Recurrent Genital Herpes. Complications from a recurrence in pregnancy are rare. However, 4 per cent of infants born to mothers with recurrent infection at the time of delivery have HSV infection.

Neonatal Herpes. The incidence of neonatal herpes is 0.01 to 0.04 per cent of all deliveries, with infection acquired by the infant via passage through an infected birth canal or via an ascending infection in 90 per cent of cases. Transplacental infection has also been documented as a route of transmission, as has close contact with an infected individual after delivery. Premature infants are at the greatest risk for contracting infection and account for over two thirds of reported cases. Symptoms typically present on day 2 to 3 of life, with rapid progression of disease thereafter. Sixty per cent of infected infants die in the neonatal period, and 50 per cent of survivors have significant sequelae, including microcephaly, mental retardation, seizures, and microphthalmos.

Management in Pregnancy. Because of lack of correlation with cervical shedding at the time of delivery, antepartum surveillance cultures are of little clinical use and are not recommended. Women with a prior history of herpes should be allowed to deliver vaginally if no genital lesions are present at the time of labor. Patients with active lesions, either recurrent or primary, at the time of labor should be delivered by cesarean section. Those with active lesions at sites distant from the genital area may be delivered vaginally if the lesions are covered. Once delivered, isolation of the mother from her infant is not necessary as long as direct contact with lesions is avoided. Mothers may breast feed as long as there are no lesions on the breasts.

BACTERIAL INFECTIONS

Urinary Tract Infections

Urinary tract infections occur more frequently in pregnancy and the puerperium and are the most common medical complications of pregnancy. This increased incidence appears to be a result of both hormonal (progesterone) and mechanical factors that increase urinary stasis. A decrease in ureteral tone and motility, and dilatation of the ureters and renal pelvis are seen as early as the second month of pregnancy. Also, the enlarging uterus compresses the bladder, which may result in distortion of the ureteral orifices.

Urinary tract infections in pregnancy may be either asymptomatic or symptomatic (cystitis, pyelonephritis). By definition, *asymptomatic bacteriuria* is the presence of 100,000 organisms per milliliter or greater in a clean urine specimen from an asymptomatic patient. The incidence of asymptomatic bacteriuria in pregnancy is the same as in the nonpregnant sexually active population, ranging from 2 to 10 per cent. Highest rates are found in inner city populations, and in patients with sickle cell disease or trait. *Escherichia coli* is the organism most frequently isolated (60 per cent). Other organisms encountered are *Proteus mirabilis,* enterococci, *Klebsiella* pneumoniae, and Group B streptococci. If the condition is left untreated, roughly 20 per cent of pregnant women will develop either acute cystitis or pyelonephritis later in pregnancy. Treatment consists of a 7- to 10-day course of either an ampicillin or a first-generation cephalosporin. Nitrofurantoin has also safely been used in pregnancy. After treatment it is wise to follow with monthly urine cultures because up to 25 per cent of patients will have a recurrence later in their pregnancy. *Acute cystitis* complicates 1 to 2 per cent of pregnancies and is characterized by dysuria, frequency, urgency, and hematuria. Systemic signs and symptoms such as flank pain or fever are absent. Urinalysis reveals bacteriuria, pyuria, and often, hematuria. As in patients with asymptomatic bacteriuria, treatment is instituted on an outpatient basis while awaiting the results of sensitivity tests. Monthly surveillance cultures are indicated. *Acute pyelonephritis* occurs in approximately 2 per cent of pregnancies, most frequently in the third trimester. It is characterized by flank pain, fever, rigors, and the urinary complaints of cystitis. A rare associated complication is septic shock and adult respiratory distress syndrome. Often, nausea and vomiting may be present and the patient may be markedly dehydrated. Physical examination reveals fever and costovertebral angle tenderness. As a result of sepsis, premature uterine contractions are frequent. Urinalysis reveals the same findings as found with acute cystitis; blood cultures are positive in 10 per cent. Organisms responsible are the same as those causing asymptomatic bacteriuria and cystitis.

The presence of pyelonephritis mandates hospitalization and intravenous antibiotic therapy. Usually, ampicillin or cefazolin are initiated, with cefazolin gaining a great deal of popularity in areas where resistance to ampicillin is prominent. Most patients (>80 per cent) become asymptomatic and afebrile within 48 hours of initiation of antibiotics and may be discharged at this point and told to continue oral antibiotics for a 10-day course. Serial urine cultures are indicated because 10 to 25 per cent of patients will have a recurrence later in their pregnancy. Those with recurrent pyelonephritis should have antibiotic suppression and an intravenous pyelogram performed 6 weeks postpartum to rule out urinary tract abnormalities.

Group B Streptococcus

Epidemiology. Group B streptococci (GBS) are considered part of the normal flora of humans. The gastrointestinal tract is the major resevoir, although the organism has been isolated from the vagina, cervix, throat, skin, urethra, and urine of healthy individuals. GBS may be transmitted to the genital tract by fecal contamination or sexual transmission from a colonized partner. Vaginal carriage rates vary from 5 to 35 per cent, but are the same in pregnancy as in sexually active nonpregnant women. Carriage rates do not appear to be affected by age, race, socioeconomic status, or parity. The majority (two thirds) of pregnant women who carry GBS do so intermittently or transiently, and only one third of all pregnant GBS carriers have the organism chronically.

Diagnosis. Group B streptococci grow readily on routine bacteriologic media and are easy to isolate from clinical specimens. A number of rapid assays for the detection of GBS have been developed over recent years. These include assays based on ELISA and latex agglutination. Though these assays are specific when compared with culture, their sensitivity is low (60 to 70 per cent).

Impact on Pregnancy. GBS may be transferred from a colonized mother to her infant via vertical transmission at delivery. Transmission rates of 35 to 70 per cent have been reported, with the highest transmission rates occurring in women with heavy vaginal colonization. Other risk factors for increased rates of transmission are preterm labor or delivery, preterm rupture of the membranes, low birth weight, prolonged labor, and intrapartum fever.

GBS sepsis is the most common cause of neonatal sepsis in the United States with 2 to 3 cases per 1000 live births per year reported. Neonatal infection with GBS is of two clinically distinct types, early-onset and late-onset disease. *Late-onset GBS infection* has been linked to a nosocomial source in the nursery, occurs after the first week of life (mean onset 4 weeks), and usually is exhibited as meningitis (80 per cent) or another type of focal infection. *Early-onset GBS infection* is characterized by its rapid onset and fulminant course, with presentation typically within the first 48 hours of life. Pathogenesis of this form of GBS sepsis is best explained by direct maternal-infant transmission at delivery. The infant presents with respiratory distress and pneumonia, and 30 per cent develop meningitis. Septicemia, shock, and death may result even when antibiotics are begun expediently. The overall infant mortality rate from early-onset disease is 50 per cent. Colonized preterm infants have an 8 to 10 per cent risk of developing sepsis and account for over 90 per cent of deaths reported. The risk of a colonized full-term infant developing sepsis is 1 to 2 per cent.

GBS is the second most common cause of bacteriuria in pregnancy and is a major cause of puerperal infection. Infection with GBS accounts for 20 per cent of cases of endomyometritis and is unique in its acute onset within the first 48 hours postpartum and typical fulminant course. The organism is sensitive to penicillin, but ampicillin is usually used because many of these infections are polymicrobial. Erythromycin is effective for the penicillin-allergic patient.

Many protocols have been developed in an attempt to eradicate maternal-infant transmission of GBS. Mass antepartum screening to identify GBS carriers and antepartum antibiotic therapy has proved ineffective because of the nature of GBS carriage. It has been shown, however, that treating carriers in labor prevents transmission to the infant. Therefore, most management protocols are now focused on intrapartum therapy. For an intrapartum approach to be most effective, a good predictor of GBS colonization at the time of labor is needed. Culture is believed to be the gold standard for GBS detection but requires 24 to 48 hours for completion. Some centers have chosen to culture patients deemed high risk for GBS carriage at 26 to 28 weeks (e.g., those with a prior history of preterm labor, premature rupture of the membranes, or neonatal sepsis) and to base intrapartum treatment on the findings of those cultures.

Listeriosis

Clinical Manifestations. Fortunately, listeriosis is a rare infection, with 2 to 3 cases per million population reported per year. It is caused by infection with *Listeria monocytogenes,* a gram-positive rod, which can usually be traced to unpasteurized milk or milk products. High carriage rates are also found in pigs and chickens. In addition, the organism may be a normal part of fecal flora in humans. The most prevalent sources of transmission are infected animal fecal matter and soil.

Impact on Pregnancy. Listeriosis in pregnancy is usually a mild, self-limited illness. However, maternal infection may result in chorioamnionitis or preterm labor. A characteristic murky brown color to the amniotic fluid is present. Fetal infection occurs primarily by transplacental passage, although listeria can also be transmitted intrapartum via passage through a colonized genital tract or by ascending infection. Neonatal infection may also result from cross contamination in the nursery. Fetal infection may result in spontaneous abortion, intrauterine fetal demise, or respiratory infection and sepsis at delivery, with significant associated morbidity and mortality. Neonatal infection is exhibited as pneumonitis, meningitis, conjunctivitis, or a skin rash.

Diagnosis. The only reliable method of diagnosis is culture with selective media of any suspected infected fluid or tissue. Therefore, a high index of suspicion for listeriosis must be held in order to request such a specific test. Histopathologic examination of infected tissue reveals miliary granulomas and focal necrosis. The placenta classically contains multiple small gray necrotic foci, which are abscesses and are pathognomonic for listeriosis.

Management. The pregnant patient who ingests contaminated food and is symptomatic should have cultures for *Listeria* performed from the vagina, rectum, stool, CSF, urine, and blood. A combination of ampicillin and gentamicin is the recommended therapy for listeriosis in pregnancy. Erythromycin may be substituted for ampicillin if a penicillin-allergy is present. *Listeria* is not sensitive to cephalosporins. For the pregnant patient who has ingested contaminated food but is asymptomatic, vaginal, rectal, and stool cultures should be performed. If these cultures are positive, the patient should be treated with ampicillin for a 7- to 10-day course to eradicate carriage.

Gonorrhea

Impact on Pregnancy. The incidence of asymptomatic cervical gonorrhea in inner-city populations is 1 to 2 per cent. The incidence of disseminated gonococcal infection in pregnancy is higher than in the nonpregnant population. Pelvic inflammatory disease in the first trimester has been reported, although it is an extremely rare occurrence. An association with preterm labor and preterm rupture of the membranes has been made, although it is controversial. Chorioamnionitis and postpartum endometritis may result from ascending infection or by hematogenous spread in the presence of disseminated gonorrhea. Fetal infection in utero is associated with spontaneous abortion and stillbirth. Gonorrhea is transmitted to the fetus at delivery in 25 to 50% of cases if the mother is left untreated; neonatal gonococcal ophthalmia, arthritis, sepsis or abscesses at scalp electrode sites may result.

The treatment for gonorrhea carriage is a single dose (250 mg) of intramuscular ceftriaxone. Spectinomycin may be used in the penicillin-allergic patient. Because coexistent chlamydial carriage is very common, a course of erythromycin therapy also should be given. Tetracycline, the usual treatment for chlamydia, is contraindicated because of the potential for adverse effects on fetal teeth and long bones. All sexual contacts should be empirically treated for both infections. All newborns empirically receive erythromycin eye therapy at delivery. Disseminated gonorrhea requires hospital admission and prolonged intravenous penicillin. Chorioamnionitis may be treated with ampicillin, ampicillin/sulbactam, or ceftriaxone.

Chlamydia

Impact on Pregnancy. Chlamydial cervical carriage has been associated with a higher incidence of premature labor, premature rupture of the membranes, and late postpartum endometritis. The neonate may acquire the organism at delivery and develop conjunctivitis, pneumonitis, and otitis media. Screening of women in the first trimester who are at high risk for carriage is recommended. High-risk groups include adolescents, single mothers, nonwhite women of lower socioeconomic status, patients with multiple sexual partners, and those with other sexually transmitted diseases. High-risk groups may have a carriage rate as high as 30 per cent.

Diagnosis. Culture on cyclohexamide-treated McCoy cells is the most sensitive means of diagnosis, but this technique is costly, slow, and limited in availability. Rapid antigen detection tests such as Chlamydiozyme or Microtrak have gained popularity as they are reliable, inexpensive, and rapid.

Treatment. Erythromycin is the therapy of choice in pregnancy. Sexual contacts should be traced and treated empirically. Infants receive eye therapy with erythromycin empirically at delivery. Erythromycin is also the drug of choice for the neonate if pneumonia or otitis media develops.

Tuberculosis

Although the incidence of active tuberculosis (TB) in the United States is very low (0.6 to 1 per cent), approximately 10 per cent of all women of childbearing age test positive on purified protein derivative (PPD) testing. A positive PPD test indicates that the patient has had a tuberculosis infection at one time. It does not indicate active disease.

Tuberculin skin testing is not a routine component of prenatal screening but is performed in high-risk populations. High-risk groups include lower socioeconomic minority women and women who live in areas where large numbers of immigrants from Southeast Asia, Central America, or South America reside.

Pregnancy does not alter the course of active tuberculosis, nor does it place the known PPD-positive woman at greater risk of disease reactivation. Tuberculosis can, however, be passed to the fetus by a hematogenous route across the placenta or as a result of the fetus swallowing infected amniotic fluid. The risk of pregnancy wastage is increased, and congenital tuberculosis may be evident at birth. An affected infant exhibits low birth weight, failure to thrive, fever, respiratory distress, adenopathy, and hepatosplenomegaly and is at high risk of dying if not treated rapidly. Treatment of the mother with active disease during her pregnancy removes such fetal risks.

The pregnant patient who tests positive for tuberculosis should have a chest x-ray study performed with abdominal shielding to rule out active disease. If the chest x-ray study is suspicious for active disease, three sets of sputum cultures should be obtained. If the cultures are positive, therapy should be instituted without delay. If the chest x-ray study is normal, no further treatment is required, but the patient should be followed with annual chest x-ray studies. Prophylactic treatment with single-agent therapy is recommended for patients who are recent PPD converters, those who live with someone with active TB, and those who are immunosuppressed and PPD positive, for example, AIDS sufferers and diabetics.

Several drugs are available for therapy, but all have potential maternal and fetal risks. Untreated TB is believed, however, to be of greater risk to both the mother and infant. Isoniazid (INH) is considered the safest for use in pregnancy. Fetal risks include potential CNS toxicity but treating the mother with vitamin B_6 supplements eliminates this risk. The main risk to the mother is hepatitis, so monthly liver function tests should be performed. *Rifampin* has been linked to limb reduction defects in the fetus and hepatitis in the mother. *Ethambutol* is safer than rifampin but not as effective and has been associated with a reversible maternal optic neuritis in 6 per cent. *Streptomycin* is to be avoided in pregnancy because of the risk of nephrotoxicity and permanent cranial nerve VIII damage in the fetus. For women with active disease, current recommendations are for 9 months of therapy with INH and rifampin. After delivery, newborns should be isolated from their mothers with active disease until the mothers are culture negative. INH prophylaxis of the infant is recommended because 50 per cent of infants develop active TB by 1 year of age if they are not given prophylaxis. Once the mother is culture negative, she may breast feed because only small concentrations of the drugs pass into the milk.

SPIROCHETE INFECTIONS

Syphilis

The clinical manifestations of syphilis during pregnancy are the same as those in the nonpregnant state and are outlined in Chapter 35. All pregnant women should be screened for syphilis at the first prenatal visit with either a Venereal Disease Research Laboratories (VDRL) test or a rapid plasma reagin (RPR) test. These tests carry a false-positive rate between 0.5 and 14 per cent because they are nonspecific for treponemas. Common causes of false-positive results are drug addiction, autoimmune disease, recent viral infection or immunization, or pregnancy itself. False-positive titers are usually 1:4. Specific treponemal tests, such as the fluorescent treponemal antibody absorption test (FTA-ABS) are performed to confirm the diagnosis.

Impact on Pregnancy. Maternal infection can result in transplacental transmission to the fetus at any gestational age. Mothers with primary and secondary syphilis are more likely to transmit the infection, with more severe manifestations occurring in the fetus. Transmission rates for primary and secondary disease are between 50 and 80 per cent. There is a wide range of fetal responses to infection and latent congenital infection.

Components of early congenital syphilitic infection include nonimmune hydrops, hepatosplenomegaly, profound anemia and thrombocytopenia, skin lesions, rash, osteitis and periostitis, pneumonia, and hepatitis. The perinatal mortality rate from congenital syphilis is roughly 50 per cent.

Late congenital syphilis (diagnosis after 2 years of age) is a multisystem disease characterized by dental abnormalities (Hutchinson's teeth, mulberry molars); saber shins; destruction of the nasal septum, resulting in a saddle-nose; interstitial keratitis; eighth nerve deafness; and failure to thrive.

Treatment. Treatment of the condition in pregnancy is the same as that in the nonpregnant state. Penicillin G is the therapy of choice. Patients with primary, secondary, or latent syphilis of less than 12 months duration are treated with a single dose of benzathine penicillin, 2.4 million units, intramuscularly. Those with syphilis of undetermined length or with latent infection for longer than 1 year receive this therapy weekly for 3 weeks. For patients with penicillin allergy, erythromycin therapy has been used but has been associated with an 11 per cent failure rate. Therefore, desensitization and use of penicillin is recommended. Ceftriaxone may be an alternative in the future, but it is presently under investigation. Patients with neurosyphilis require admission and prolonged intravenous penicillin therapy.

Women treated for syphilis during their pregnancy require careful follow-up with monthly VDRL or RPR titers to ensure that the treatment is successful. Patients with syphilis remain positive on FTA-ABS testing for the remainder of their lives. Patients' sexual contacts should be referred for treatment. Neonates are evaluated and treated as indicated.

Lyme Disease

The spirochete *Borrelia burgdorferi* is responsible for Lyme disease, which is characterized by a multisystem inflammatory illness in which neurologic, rheumatic, and cardiac problems are present. The deer tick is the carrier of *Borrelia,* with the most common mode of transmission to humans being through a cat or dog intermediary that has been infected with the tick. Human infection results from a tick bite or contact through infected cat or dog urine. Lyme disease is seasonal, occurring primarily between May and August, with the peak occurring in July. Ninety per cent of cases have occurred in Connecticut, New York, New Jersey, Rhode Island, Massachusetts, Maryland, Wisconsin, Minnesota, and California. An increase in IgM and cryoglobulins containing IgM occurs with a profound immune complex response, thus explaining the cardiac, neurologic and arthritic manifestations.

Impact on Pregnancy. When infection occurs in pregnancy, a higher incidence of preterm labor, spontaneous abortion, low birth weight, and stillbirth has been reported. Transplacental transfer to the fetus is known to occur but the consequences of it are controversial. Preliminary reports suggest that there is no increased risk of birth defects. The neonate can, however, manifest signs of infection at birth with relapsing fevers.

Diagnosis. Diagnosis is by clinical presentation alone. Antibody tests are being developed but are not yet sensitive enough to be used for diagnostic testing.

Treatment. With early treatment, the prognosis is good. Treatment outside of pregnancy is tetracycline. In pregnancy, penicillin or erythromycin is used. After delivery, the placenta should be examined for spirochetes. To prevent the disease, pregnant women should be advised to avoid tick exposure in endemic areas in the summer months and direct contact with an exposed animal's urine.

PARASITIC INFECTIONS

Toxoplasmosis

Toxoplasmosis is a systemic disease caused by the protozoan *Toxoplasma gondii.* Between 15 and 40 per cent of women of reproductive age have antibodies (IgG) to toxoplasmosis and, therefore, are immune to future infection. Occasionally, toxoplasmosis presents as a mononucleosis-like syndrome, but most infections are subclinical. The organism is acquired by ingesting undercooked meat, unpasteurized goat's milk, or by exposure to feces from an infected cat.

Impact on Pregnancy. The incidence of primary infection in pregnancy is 1 in 1000. Routine screening for toxoplasmosis is not recommended in pregnancy. The risk of transmission to the fetus is 15 per cent in the first trimester, 25 per cent in the second trimester, and 65 per cent in the third trimester. However, the severity of fetal infection is greatest with first trimester infection. The classic triad of hydrocephalus, intracranial calcifications, and chorioretinitis is rarely seen. Approximately 75 per cent of infected infants are asymptomatic at birth. Between 25 and 50 per cent exhibit sequelae of toxoplasmosis including chorioretinitis, hydrocephaly, microcephaly, micropthalmia, hepatosplenomegaly, adenopathy, convulsions, or mental delay. The presence of IgM in cord blood confirms the diagnosis. In addition, placental culture reveals the organism in over 90 per cent of cases of congenital infection.

Diagnosis. Because it is very often a subclinical infection, toxoplasmosis is rarely diagnosed. It should be considered in the differential diagnosis of anyone with a mononucleosis-like syndrome. Diagnosis by serologic testing for both IgG and IgM is by a positive finding of IgM or a fourfold rise in IgG titer in paired sequential samples obtained 2 to 3 weeks apart. IgM titers may, however, remain elevated for 4 months.

Treatment. Toxoplasmosis is a self-limiting infection. Therapy with pyrimethamine and sulfadiazine plus folinic acid is available, although these drugs carry potential fetal risks and their use in pregnancy is controversial.

To prevent infection, pregnant women should be advised to avoid contact with cat litter or feces, to wear gloves while gardening, and to avoid ingestion of raw meat or unpasteurized goat's milk.

SUGGESTED READING

ACOG Technical Bulletin. Perinatal Viral and Parasitic Infections. No 114, 1988.

ACOG Technical Bulletin. Perinatal Herpes Simplex Virus Infections. No 122, 1988.

Brown Z: Is neonatal herpes a preventable disease? A review of the risks and mechanisms of neonatal transmission. Am J Gyn Health 4:17, 1990.

Centers for Disease Control: 1989 Sexually transmitted diseases treatment guidelines. MMWR 38:1, 1989.

Centers for Disease Control: Increase in rubella and congenital rubella syndrome—United States, 1988–1990. MMWR 40:1, 1991.

Centers for Disease Control: Protection against viral hepatitis. MMWR 39:1, 1990.

Edly SJ: Lyme disease during pregnancy. N Engl J Med 87:557, 1990.

Greenspoon JS, Wilcox JG, Kirschbaum TH: Group B streptococcus: The effectiveness of screening and chemoprophylaxis. Obstet Gynecol Surv 46:499, 1991.

McNeeley SG, Ryan GM, Baselski V: Treatment of chlamydial infections of the cervix during pregnancy. Sex Transm Dis 16:60, 1989.

Medchill MT, Gillum M: Diagnosis and management of tuberculosis during pregnancy. Obstet Gynecol Surv 44:81, 1989.

Minkoff HL: Care of pregnant women infected with human immunodeficiency virus. JAMA 19:2714, 1987.

Nanda D, Minkoff HL: HIV in pregnancy—transmission and immune effects. Clin Obstet Gynecol 32:456, 1989.

Paryani SG, Arvin AM: Intrauterine infection with varicella-zoster virus after maternal varicella. N Engl J Med 314:1542, 1986.

Ricci JM, Fojaco RM, O'Sullivan MJ: Congenital syphilis: The University of Miami/Jackson Memorial Medical Center experience, 1986–1988. Obstet Gynecol 74:687, 1989.

Sever JO, Ellenberg JH, Ley AC, et al: Toxoplasmosis: Maternal and pediatric findings in 23,000 pregnancies. Pediatrics 82:181, 1988.

Shmoys S, Kaplan C: Parvovirus and pregnancy. Clin Obstet Gynecol 33:268, 1989.

Seventeen

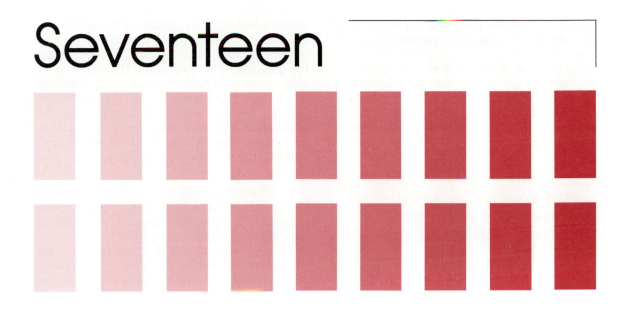

Licit and Illicit Drug Use in Pregnancy

CAROL L. ARCHIE

The National Institute of Drug Abuse reports 70 to 90 per cent of Americans between the ages of 15 to 40 years have used mood-altering chemicals, approximately half of whom are women with reproductive potential. Among women in this group, approximately 60 per cent (34 million) are current drinkers, 32 per cent (18 million) are smokers, and 11 per cent (6 million) use marijuana. Screening a single urine sample for alcohol, cannabinoids, cocaine, and opiates in women presenting for prenatal care reveals positive urine toxicology results in about 15 per cent of cases. This applies to both private and public clinic patients.

Substance use by an expectant mother can affect reproduction from fertility through pregnancy and lactation. In addition, this behavior can affect the developing fetus and neonate. Ideally, a woman's primary care physician should take advantage of routine gynecologic examinations, prepregnancy, and other office visits to provide information and counseling about substance use effects. These are valuable opportunities for informing women of the risks involved, especially since most congenital structural anomalies are induced in the 58 days following conception, which is often prior to recognition of pregnancy by the woman. Unfortunately, most women who use social and illicit substances will not have that optimal interaction before pregnancy. Hence it is important for those providing prenatal care to be familiar with possible adverse effects of commonly used and abused drugs. In most cases, continued substance use beyond the period of embryogenesis carries risks for both mother and

189

fetus. These are the risks that the obstetrician most frequently has the opportunity to reduce.

The purpose of this chapter is to outline an approach to the identification and effective treatment or referral of cases of substance abuse in pregnancy. Additionally, specific maternal and fetal effects of commonly abused social and illegal substances are reviewed.

PATIENT EDUCATION ABOUT SUBSTANCE USE AND ABUSE IN OBSTETRICS AND GYNECOLOGY

Opportunities for substance use screening and patient education are presented by any patient encounter and include routine gynecologic, prenatal, and postnatal visits as well as encounters during obstetric emergencies. The focus of patient education will vary with the nature of the encounter. During routine gynecologic visits, emphasis may be placed on the effects of various substances on fertility. The woman should also be informed of potential fetal effects and obstetric problems should she become pregnant and continue substance use. When counseling a woman during routine prenatal visits, fetal and obstetric effects associated with initial or continued use should be discussed. At this time, the benefits to the mother and the fetus of treatment or abstinence should be emphasized. The risks of passive smoking should also be reviewed. The postnatal visit invites discussion of the effects of substance use on lactation. The effects of substances transmitted to the baby through breast milk should be explained as should the effects of passive smoking on the infant and child. Substance abuse may interfere with a woman's contraceptive plans, either through chemical interaction or by affecting the woman's ability to comply with the regimen. These issues should be frankly discussed.

SCREENING FOR SUBSTANCE USE: THE ROLE OF THE CLINICAL INTERVIEW

The substance use interview should take place within the context of a comprehensive medical history. The quality of the substance use history obtained, like that of the general medical history, is frequently dependent on the quality of the relationship the physician is able to establish with the patient. In addition to reassuring the patient that all information will be treated with strict confidence, the following five specific steps have been shown to enhance the establishment of an optimal working relationship with patients.

1. Establish a partnership with the patient: "We will work together throughout your pregnancy in order for you and your baby to have the best outcome possible."
2. Assure the patient that you intend to be supportive: "I will be available to work with you and answer any questions you might have."
3. Demonstrate respect for the patient: "I know it has been difficult, but it sounds as if you have been coping with the morning sickness and managing to get adequate nutrition."
4. Demonstrate empathy by identifying emotions expressed by the patient and expressing them in words: "You seem sad."
5. It can be important to legitimate the patient's concerns: "It is understandable that you might be concerned because of your last experience with childbirth."

Specific substance use screening is often best addressed while discussing other patient-controlled health issues such as nutrition and exercise. It is important to specifically address the use of prescription drugs. The dosage and indication as well as the frequency and duration of usage should be carefully noted. Similarly, any nonprescription medication use must be carefully evaluated. The intake of caffeine, tobacco, and alcohol as well as the use of illicit drugs must be recorded.

ADDRESSING POTENTIAL SUBSTANCE ABUSE PROBLEMS

One commonly used screening test that can be easily integrated into the clinical interview is the CAGE questionnaire. For any alcohol or drug use mentioned in the initial interview, ask the following CAGE questions:

CAGE Questions:

1. Have you ever felt the need to *cut down* on your drinking or drug use?
Yes—Why? When? What did you do? What happened?
2. Have you ever been *annoyed* by criticism of your drinking or drug use?
Yes—Who criticized you? What happened? How often did this happen?
3. Have you ever felt *guilty* about your drinking or drug use?
Yes—Under what circumstances? Did you try to change?
4. Have you ever had a morning *eye-opener*? (Used drugs first thing in the morning to get started.)
Yes—How often? What were the feelings you had that made you think you needed it? Did the drug relieve these feelings?

One positive response indicates problem use and possible dependence. The follow-up questions provide important information for making a diagnosis of dependence or addiction and offer clues to the level of intervention that will be required. In pregnancy, any substance use that is potentially harmful to the fetus is problematic and requires intervention. In addition to establishing the level of current use, it is important to assess the amount of alcohol and drug use at the time of conception.

PRESENTING THE DIAGNOSIS

When problematic substance use is discovered, the manner in which the diagnosis is presented to the patient becomes a factor in determining the level of cooperation with intervention that is likely to be obtained. It is crucial that a nonjudgmental approach be taken. Begin by providing valid, factual information about substance use and its effects. Explain carefully the implications and consequences of future use, especially fetal effects and effects on the reproductive system. Describe the benefits of stopping or decreasing substance use, or, in some cases, substituting medication (e.g., methadone) for substances of abuse. Allow the patient to describe her understanding of the problem, and check the patient's understanding of information provided. Finally, correct any misunderstandings.

MANAGEMENT STRATEGIES

All obstetric patients can be categorized into one of three groups by the substance use interview. The majority will be found to have no substance problems. Some will be found to be currently using or abusing substances harmful to mother or fetus or both. Others will be found to have a previous substance abuse problem but to be currently in recovery. Each individual should be managed appropriately based on the outcome of the interview.

For those with no substance abuse problem, management should be directed toward prevention. As always, the physician should provide factual information about the effects of substance use, including prescription drugs, over-the-counter drugs, tobacco, and caffeine. The physician should reinforce positive attitudes expressed by the patient regarding avoidance of damaging substances.

The management of those with a current substance use or abuse problem is more difficult. Once the diagnosis has been made and appropriately presented to the patient (see earlier), the urgency of treatment, especially in pregnancy, must be stressed. Where appropriate, referrals should be made. Whether the referral is for drug/alcohol treatment or support group only, the patient must understand that the primary physician will continue to manage her medical and obstetric care while supporting her drug treatment.

When referral is not indicated or possible, the obstetrician should approach management by beginning with clear, definite treatment recommendations. At times, it may be necessary to make reasonable compromises in the treatment plan to secure the patient's acceptance. For example, if a woman consumes three drinks every night and smokes one pack of cigarettes each day, it may be necessary to accept a decrease in smoking while the woman attempts to achieve abstinence from alcohol. The specifics of the treatment plan should be reviewed with the patient, and the patient's verbal or written agreement should be obtained.

Pregnancy can be stressful for a woman in the best of circumstances, and for recovering substance users this may be particularly true. This group of women requires close follow-up and monitoring. The physician should stress the importance of strict self-monitoring and of continuing in treatment or self-help group activities. She should understand the risks to herself and the fetus and neonate of a full relapse.

EFFECTS OF RECREATIONAL AND ILLICIT DRUG USE ON PREGNANCY

In most cases, the limitations of the data concerning substance use in pregnancy do not allow full assessment of either maternal or fetal risks. In many cases, the available information is confounded by complications that may arise from the lifestyle of the addicted woman. Malnutrition, frequently seen with the use of various substances including alcohol, opioids, and amphetamines, is associated with anemia and fetal growth retardation. Sexually transmitted and other infectious diseases occur more frequently in pregnancies of substance abusers and cause complications. For example, intravenous drug use is associated with endocarditis, phlebitis, hepatitis and acquired immunodeficiency syndrome (AIDS), all of which cause problems in pregnancy. Another important confounder in analyzing information on drug use in pregnancy is the fact that substance abusers rarely take a single drug. This makes it difficult to discern which drug is causing a given effect or whether the drugs are acting synergistically to cause a given finding.

SPECIFIC DRUGS FREQUENTLY COMPLICATING PREGNANCY

Tobacco

The chemically complex nature of tobacco smoke, which contains potentially harmful components such as nicotine, carbon monoxide, hydrogen cyanide, and potential carcinogens such as diazolemzopyrene, makes specific identification of factors responsible for deleterious effects elusive. Nonetheless, several specific perinatal problems have been identified as complications of this addiction. These include an increased frequency of spontaneous abortion, low birth weight, and prematurity. These complications appear to be dose-related effects. Maternal smoking has also been associated with placental abruption, premature rupture of the membranes, intra-uterine fetal death, increased neonatal mortality, and sudden infant death syndrome. Long-term follow-up studies of children of smokers have described impaired growth, impaired intellectual development, and behavioral disorders. The frequency of major structural congenital anomalies has not been shown to be increased among neonates of mothers who smoked during pregnancy.

Alcohol

An estimated 70 per cent of Americans use alcohol socially. Typical periconceptual alcohol consumption (the period of maximum vulnerability to the anatomic defects of this recognized teratogen) is nearly as heavy as that in the nonpregnant state. During pregnancy, alcohol use varies considerably. Alcohol abuse has been defined as four or more drinks per day and has been found to occur in approximately 2 per cent of pregnant women. As many as one in 300 infants born in the United States have some degree of stigmata of fetal alcohol exposure. *Fetal alcohol syndrome* is the most commonly identifiable cause of mental retardation in live-born infants.

The anatomic abnormalities detectable in the neonate are related in a dose-response fashion to prenatal alcohol exposure. Moreover, as would be expected embryologically, the critical period for precipitating these abnormalities is in the early first trimester. The consumption of more than three cans of beer, or three glasses of wine or mixed drinks per day, and repetitive binge drinking, greatly increase the risk of alcohol teratogenicity. A precise intake threshold has not been established, and lower doses may still be related to an increased incidence of cranial, facial, or other abnormalities. Because of the uncertainty of how little alcohol is required to cause fetal disruption and because many women may become aware of pregnancy after possible effects of their drinking habit have occurred, women contemplating pregnancy should consider avoidance of all alcohol in order to eliminate the possibility of alcohol-related birth defects. Those women who conceive while maintaining their normal drinking patterns are advised to stop alcohol as soon as they become aware of pregnancy.

Fetal Alcohol Effects

There is a continuum of effects of alcohol on the fetus. The most severe complications of alcohol are abortion and stillbirth. Of lesser severity are the *fetal alcohol syndrome* and alcohol-related birth defects, including abnormal growth and neurobehavioral development.

The complex of newborn findings characterizing the diagnosis of fetal alcohol syndrome was defined by the Research Society on Alcoholism in 1980. The diagnosis requires the presence of characteristic manifestations in each of three areas: (1) prenatal and postnatal growth retardation, (2) central nervous system involvement, and (3) characteristic facial morphology.

Growth retardation of the fetus or neonate is defined as weight below the tenth percentile. Central nervous system abnormalities include tremulousness, poor suckling, abnormal muscle tone, hyperactivity, attention defects, or mental retardation. At least two characteristics facial anomalies are required for the diagnosis. The range of possible dismorphology includes microcephaly (head circumference less than the third percentile), thin upper lip vermilion, short upturned nose, flattened nasal bridge, and general underdevelopment of the midfacial area.

Alcohol-related birth defects are congenital anomalies attributable to alcohol but not meeting the criteria for fetal alcohol syndrome. Possible congenital anomalies include congenital heart defects and brain abnormalities. Other major congenital anomalies such as spinal bifida, limb defects, and genitourinary defects are seen much less frequently.

Marijuana

Among women of reproductive age, marijuana is the most commonly used illicit substance and, after alcohol and tobacco, the most commonly used recreational drug in pregnancy. Epidemiologic studies show women who use marijuana outside of and during early pregnancy are often young and tend to use other substances. The minority of women who continue to use marijuana throughout pregnancy tend to be less well educated, of lower social class, and much more likely to use other substances.

Studies on the use of marijuana in pregnancy have generated inconclusive data. None of the studies distinguishes between exposure in early versus late pregnancy, dosage is vaguely defined, and potency of tetrahydrocannabinol (THC), the active ingredient in marijuana, varies greatly, if reported at all. Because women who use marijuana during pregnancy are more likely to use other substances as well, the effect of polydrug use and other factors that correlate with marijuana use during pregnancy need to be addressed when analyzing data on the impact of THC on the fetus and infant. This has not been consistently done.

Some studies of marijuana use in pregnancy have reported intrauterine growth retardation, neurobehavioral effects, and increased prematurity. The results have not, however, been consistently replicated across studies. Most available data do not show an increased risk of major congenital anomalies among infants prenatally exposed to marijuana. Long-term effects of marijuana use in pregnancy have not been identified, but few studies have been reported.

Cocaine

Cocaine is derived from the leaves of the *Erythroxylon coca* plant, which is native to South America. In addition to its local anesthetic properties, cocaine is a potent central nervous system stimulant through its sympathomimetic action. It blocks dopamine and norepinephrine uptake at nerve terminals. These actions are manifested physiologically as tachycardia, hypertension, and muscle twitching immediately after intake. The intense sense of euphoria experienced with intake and the decreasing cost of this drug over the past decade have contributed to its becoming one of the most widely abused recreational drugs. Cocaine use crosses all ethnic, geographic, and socioeconomic lines. The prevalence in obstetric populations varies. Approximately 10 per cent of an average obstetric population may be using the drug.

Cocaine may result in numerous maternal medical complications, including but not limited to acute myocardial infarction, arrhythmias, hyperthermia, hypertensive crisis, stroke, seizures, and sudden death. Cocaine use in pregnancy has been implicated in a wide spectrum of adverse pregnancy sequelae. Pregnancy complications include abruption, spontaneous abortion, intrauterine growth retardation, low birth weight, and prematurity.

Embryo-fetal and neonatal adverse outcomes have also been found attributable to cocaine exposure prenatally. Many congenital anomalies such as segmental intestinal atresia, limb reduction defects, and disruptive brain anomalies have been thought to result from vascular disruption caused by cocaine exposure. Congenital heart defects, prune belly syndrome, and urinary tract anomalies have also been reported in higher than expected numbers of cocaine-exposed neonates.

Postnatal problems have also been associated with cocaine use in pregnancy. An increased risk of sudden infant death syndrome has been reported. Early neurobehavioral studies have suggested depression of interactive behavior and poor organizational responses to environmental stimuli. Studies are under way to evaluate this population for possible long-term sequelae.

Narcotics

Heroin and methadone are the two narcotics most frequently encountered in pregnancy. Heroin is a widely abused illegal narcotic that is used intravenously and often irregularly. Methadone is taken orally and usually under medical supervision. The use of narcotics in pregnancy has not been associated with an increased incidence of congenital anomalies in prenatally exposed infants, but other morbidity is common. The ecology of the heroin addict includes dirty needles and other high-risk behaviors, including lack of prenatal care, that complicate pregnancy. These behaviors result in a high incidence of skin and subcutaneous tissue infections, phlebitis, endocarditis, urinary tract infections,

and sexually transmitted diseases (including HIV transmission) in heroin-addicted women. An increased incidence of inflammation or infection of the placenta, chorion, and amnion has also been reported. Adverse pregnancy effects include an increased incidence of premature labor and delivery, intrauterine growth retardation, low birth weight, fetal distress, and meconium passage as well as neonatal infections.

The pharmacologic effects of narcotic use in pregnancy are marked by the development of physical dependence in both mother and fetus when the drugs are used regularly. In these patients, failure to take the drug or use of a narcotic antagonist will precipitate the narcotic abstinence syndrome: agitation, lacrimation, rhinorrhea, yawning, mydriasis, and perspiration. Prolonged narcotic withdrawal may produce abdominal and uterine cramps, diarrhea, and myalgias. Although extremely uncomfortable, narcotic withdrawal is rarely injurious to the mother. Maternal withdrawal is, however, potentially fatal to the fetus. During the first trimester, abortion may occur during severe withdrawal. Later in pregnancy, maternal withdrawal is accompanied by fetal withdrawal, which results in hyperactivity, hypoxia, meconium passage, and possibly intrauterine fetal death. Because of the risks to the fetus, narcotic withdrawal is not encouraged during pregnancy and narcotic antagonists are used with caution.

Some patients use heroin irregularly, and because the content of heroin available in the community is highly variable, physical dependence may not develop. It is among these less tolerant users that serious narcotic overdosage is most likely to occur. The overdosed patient presents with respiratory depression or arrest with pinpoint pupils and may be comatose. Naloxone, a narcotic antagonist without respiratory depressive activity, should be given intravenously in a dose of 2 mg/kg. The same dose may be given intramuscularly, subcutaneously, or via an endotracheal tube.

Pregnant heroin addicts are best managed in methadone maintenance programs. Methadone is a long-acting, synthetic opiate that blocks heroin-induced euphoria and blunts heroin craving. Detection and treatment of infections, improved nutrition, provision of prenatal care, and psychosocial support all contribute to an improved outcome for the pregnancy. Medication without prenatal care and psychosocial support is less effective.

Neonatal withdrawal syndrome in children of heroin addicted mothers tends to occur within the first 12 to 24 hours after birth. It is characterized by high-pitched crying, frantic fist sucking or searching for food, and tremulousness, and it can be associated with seizures, disrupted sleep-wake cycles, and muscle hypertonia. Withdrawal in children of methadone-maintained mothers tends to be less severe (although this depends in part on the mother's dosage and use of other drugs) and occurs 2 to 4 weeks after birth. Subacute withdrawal of methadone-exposed infants may last for months.

Postnatally, growth patterns in small for gestational age children of narcotic addicts (heroin or methadone) tend to normalize. Long-term effects of narcotics have been difficult to identify because of numerous environmental confounders. Pregnant women who are found to have a narcotic use habit should be cared for and delivered in a high-risk obstetric and neonatal center with a methadone maintenance program. In this way, the special needs of both mother and neonate can be identified and optimally managed.

Amphetamines

These drugs are central nervous system stimulants that can be obtained by prescription or illegally acquired as street drugs. Amphetamines are traditionally ingested orally or administered intravenously. An inhalable form of methamphetamines known as "crystal" has begun to gain popularity as a recreational drug. Amphetamines may be used in cycles following binges of sedative and alcohol abuse. They have also been used to "cut" or mix with other street drugs. Therefore, use of multiple substances must be screened for in any amphetamine abuser.

Tolerance develops with regular use of amphetamines. Patients actively abusing amphetamines are hyperactive and paranoid, have insomnia and hallucinations, and, because of lack of appetite, are usually badly malnourished. Patients who use amphetamines intravenously are subject to all the complications of intravenous drug use. Amphetamine use may increase the risk of serious arrhythmias during obstetric anesthesia. Withdrawal is characterized by the abstinence syndrome of lethargy and profound depression, which should be closely monitored.

Most case-control and large cohort studies have shown no increase in major or minor congenital anomalies among infants exposed to amphetamines prenatally. The major fetal effect that has been documented is symmetrical fetal growth retardation.

Hallucinogens

Lysergic acid diethylamide (LSD, "acid") and phencyclidine (PCP, "angel dust") are the most commonly used agents in this class of drugs. The major maternal risks associated with their use are psychiatric and environmental: Patients high on these drugs often place themselves in physically dangerous situations. Reports describing infants with congenital anomalies born to mothers who used LSD or PCP during pregnancy have shown no consistent pattern of anomalies. There is little evidence, based on available data, that these drugs are human teratogens. Studies of exposed neonates have suggested an association with decreased birth weight and head circumference, but well-controlled studies of use of other drugs and other environmental risk factors for these findings have not been done. Neonatal withdrawal, characterized by tremors, jitteriness, and irritability, has been described in some prenatally exposed children. Developmental delays are suggested by ongoing studies that seek to determine long term effects.

SUMMARY

The use of substances that are potentially harmful to both mother and fetus is widespread in pregnancy and involves both legal and illegal drugs. Efforts should be made to educate all pregnant and potentially pregnant women about the risks of substance use as well as to identify all patients who have a substance abuse problem. Women who are identified as users of potentially harmful drugs require intensified maternal and fetal surveillance as well as psychosocial support. Referral to a high-risk obstetric center is sometimes necessary and usually advisable.

SUGGESTED READING

Abel EL: Smoking during pregnancy: A review of effects on growth and development of offspring. Hum Biol 52:593, 1980.

Abel EL, Solol RJ: Incidence of fetal alcohol syndrome and economic impact of FAS-related anomalies. Drug Alcohol Depend 19:51, 1987.

AMA Council on Scientific Affairs: Fetal effects of maternal alcohol use. JAMA 249:2517, 1983.

American College of Obstetricians and Gynecologists: Cocaine abuse: Implications for pregnancy. ACOG Committee Opinion, Number 81, March 1990.

Aselton P, Jick H, Milunsky A, et al: First-trimester drug use and congenital disorders. Obstet Gynecol 65:451, 1985.

Bingol N, Fuchs M, Diaz V, et al: Teratogenicity of cocaine in humans. J Pediatr 110:93, 1987.

Chasnoff IJ, Burns KA, Burns WJ: Cocaine use in pregnancy: Perinatal morbidity and mortality. Neurotoxicol Teratol 9:291, 1987.

Chasnoff IJ, Burns KA, Burns WJ, Schnoll SH: Prenatal drug exposure: Effects on neonatal and infant growth development. Neurobehav Toxicol Teratol 8:357, 1986.

Chasnoff IJ, Landress HJ, Barrett ME: The prevalence of illicit drug or alcohol use during pregnancy and discrepancies in mandatory reporting in Pinellas County, Florida. N Engl J Med 322:1202, 1990.

Ewing JA: Detecting alcoholism: The CAGE questionnaire. JAMA 252:1905, 1984.

Fried PA, Buckingham M, Von Kulmiz P: Marijuana use during pregnancy and perinatal risk factors. Am J Obstet Gynecol 146:992, 1983.

Little BB, Snell LM, Gilstrap LC: Methamphetamine abuse during pregnancy: Outcome and infant effects. Obstet Gynecol 72:541, 1988.

Little BB, Snell LM, Klein VR, et al: Maternal and fetal effects of heroin addiction during pregnancy. J Reprod Med 35:159, 1990.

Voight LF, Hollenbach KA, Brohn MA, et al: The relationship of abruptio placentae with maternal smoking and small for gestational age infants. Obstet Gynecol 75:771, 1990.

Eighteen

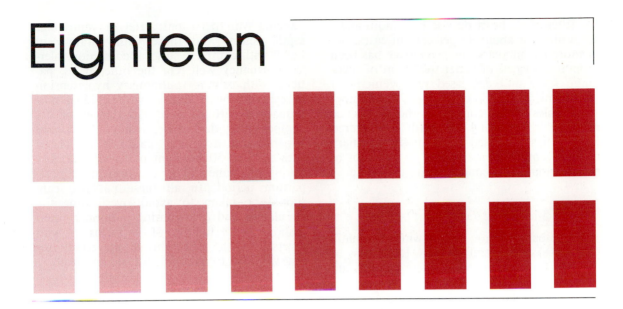

Medical Complications of Pregnancy

BAHIJ NUWAYHID AND SAMIR KHALIFÉ

Physiologic adaptation to pregnancy involves the cardiovascular, pulmonary, endocrine, hematologic, neurologic, renal, and gastrointestinal systems. In a normal, healthy pregnant woman, the adaptive responses are appropriate and well tolerated. When there is underlying pathology, the responses of the different organ systems are less well tolerated, and organ failure may occur. Physiologic changes in pregnancy are discussed in Chapter 6 and briefly summarized in this chapter.

CARDIOVASCULAR SYSTEM

Physiologic Changes During Pregnancy

During human pregnancy, cardiac output increases by almost 40 per cent. Most of this increase is due to an increase in stroke volume, since heart rate increases by only about 10 beats per minute during the third trimester. Cardiac output peaks at around 18 to 24 weeks and then stabilizes. Because of the increase in cardiac output, grade 2 systolic flow murmurs may be frequently heard at the left sternal border, with no radiation. Additionally, a third heart sound might be heard, with wide splitting of S1. Diastolic murmurs should be considered pathologic and investigated. Because of the increased venous return, cardiac fullness, and hypertrophy, the heart is displaced superiorly, laterally, and anteriorly, and the point of maximum impulse is shifted superiorly and laterally. Electrocardiographic changes include a left axis deviation and a flattened T wave.

Heart Disease

Heart disease in pregnancy can be divided into two categories: rheumatic and congenital. Rheumatic heart disease has traditionally accounted for about 90 per cent of cases, but in more recent years this percentage has been dropping because of better treatment of rheumatic fever and decreased pathogenicity of the organism. On the other hand, the number of females with congenital heart disease reaching childbearing age with unimpaired fertility has increased. In a modern tertiary referral center, approximately 35 per cent of patients may have congenital heart disease.

Rheumatic Heart Disease

The most common lesion with rheumatic heart disease is mitral stenosis. Regardless of the specific valvular lesion, these patients are at higher risk of developing heart failure, pulmonary edema, subacute bacterial endocarditis, and thromboembolic disease. They also have a high rate of fetal wastage.

Pure mitral stenosis is found in about 90 per cent of rheumatic heart disease patients. During pregnancy, the cardiac output increases, and the mechanical obstruction worsens. Asymptomatic patients may develop symptoms of cardiac decompensation or pulmonary edema.

Atrial fibrillation is more common in patients with severe mitral stenosis, and its onset during pregnancy is ominous. Nearly all women who develop atrial fibrillation during pregnancy experience congestive heart failure. On the other hand, if atrial fibrillation predates pregnancy, only half of the women will develop pulmonary congestion and heart failure.

Patients with mitral insufficiency or aortic stenosis are in less danger of having cardiac decompensation in the third trimester of pregnancy. The myocardium of these young women is able to increase its workload without decompensation.

Congenital Heart Disease

This entity includes patients with atrial or ventricular septal defects, primary pulmonary hypertension (Eisenmenger's syndrome), and cyanotic heart disease. If the anatomic defect has been corrected during childhood with no residual damage, the patient will go through pregnancy with no apparent complications.

Patients with persistent atrial or ventricular septal defects and those with tetralogy of Fallot with complete surgical correction tolerate pregnancy well. On the other hand, patients with primary pulmonary hypertension or cyanotic heart disease with residual pulmonary hypertension are in danger of decompensating during pregnancy. Pulmonary hypertension from any cause is associated with a 25 to 50 per cent maternal mortality during pregnancy or in the immediate postpartum period. In all these patients, care should be taken to avoid overloading the circulation and precipitating pulmonary congestion, heart failure, or hypotension with reversal of the left-right shunt, conditions that will lead to hypoxia and sudden death.

Cardiac Arrhythmias

Paroxysmal atrial tachycardia is the most common cardiac arrhythmia. Usually it is benign and not associated with underlying heart disease. It is generally provoked by strenuous exercise. Atrial fibrillation and atrial flutter are more serious and usually associated with underlying cardiac disease.

Peripartum and Postpartum Cardiomyopathy

This entity is very rare, but is exclusively associated with pregnancy. These patients have no underlying cardiac disease, and symptoms of cardiac decompensation appear during the last weeks of pregnancy or 2 to 20 weeks postpartum. Pregnant individuals at risk to develop cardiomyopathy are those with a history of pre-eclampsia or hypertension and those with poor nutrition. No etiologic factor has been found, although Coxsackie B virus and fetal antimyocardial antibodies have been incriminated.

Management of Cardiac Disease During Pregnancy

The New York Heart Association's functional classification of heart disease is of value in assessing the risk of pregnancy for a patient with cardiac disease and in determining the optimal management during preg-

Table 18–1. NEW YORK HEART ASSOCIATION'S FUNCTIONAL CLASSIFICATION OF HEART DISEASE

Class I	No signs or symptoms of cardiac decompensation
Class II	No symptoms at rest, but minor limitation of physical activity
Class III	No symptoms at rest, but marked limitation of physical activity
Class IV	Symptoms present at rest, discomfort increased with any kind of physical activity

nancy, labor, and delivery (Table 18–1). In general, the maternal and fetal risks for patients with class I and II disease are small, whereas they are greatly increased with class III and IV disease. This does not imply that less attention should be given to the former group. Pulmonary edema leading to maternal death has been reported in patients with class I and II cardiac disease.

Prenatal Management

As a general principle, all pregnant cardiac patients should be managed with the help of a cardiologist. Frequent prenatal visits are indicated, and frequent hospital admissions may be needed, especially for patients with class III and IV cardiac disease. It is important to keep in mind a number of guidelines during the prenatal period.

Avoidance of Excessive Weight Gain and Edema. Cardiac patients should be placed on a low-sodium diet (2 gm per day) to prevent excessive expansion of blood volume. They should be encouraged to rest in the lateral decubitus position for at least 1 hour every morning, afternoon, and evening to promote diuresis, especially during the latter part of gestation. Adequate sleep should be encouraged.

Avoidance of Strenuous Activity. All cardiac patients should avoid strenuous activity. Individuals with heart disease are unable to increase their cardiac output to the same extent as healthy individuals to meet the increased metabolic demands associated with exercise. Consequently, they tend to extract more oxygen from the arterial blood, resulting in a larger arteriovenous oxygen difference. With strenuous exercise or tissue hypoxia or both, blood is shifted from the uteroplacental circulation to other organs.

Avoidance of Anemia. With anemia, the oxygen carrying capacity of the blood decreases. This is compensated for by an increase in cardiac output, brought about mainly by an increase in heart rate. An increase in heart rate, especially with mitral stenosis, leads to a decrease in left ventricular filling time, so pulmonary congestion and edema may result. Another factor that might lead to cardiac decompensation is the inability of the right ventricle to pump all of the venous return.

Early Detection of a Problem. During every prenatal visit, the patient should be carefully examined to exclude infection, cardiac decompensation, pulmonary congestion, and cardiac arrhythmias.

Aside from the increased metabolic demands and cardiac output associated with a febrile illness, bacteremia may lead to the development of bacterial endocarditis.

With heart failure, the pulse increases to a rate greater than 100 beats per minute; the neck veins become congested; and the liver and spleen become enlarged and tender. Excessive weight gain is usual, and generalized edema might be present. Digitalization and diuretics are required if heart failure develops.

With pulmonary congestion, a history of dyspnea and orthopnea might be elicited, and pulmonary rales and crepitations are usually present. Vital capacity, which can be measured in a clinic setting, is decreased.

The apical heart rate should be auscultated because the peripheral pulse may not be sensitive to changes in cardiac rhythm. The onset of dysrhythmias, a change in the character of a murmur, or a change in heart sounds necessitates further cardiac work-up and specific treatment.

Although cardiac decompensation may occur at any phase of pregnancy, it is most likely to occur during the period of peak increase in cardiac output (18 to 24 weeks), during labor, during delivery, or during the immediate postpartum period. A pregnant patient with sufficient cardiac reserve to tolerate the peak increase in cardiac output without cardiac decompensation has a good chance of continuing the pregnancy without complications.

Management of Labor

During labor, cardiac output increases by about 40 to 50 per cent when compared with prelabor levels and by about 80 to 100 per cent when compared with prepregnancy levels. Although part of the increase in cardiac output during labor is due to catecholamine release brought about by pain and apprehension, most of the increase is due to abdominal and uterine muscle contraction. To minimize the increase in cardiac output, assurance, sedation, and epidural anesthesia are encouraged early in labor. Prophylactic antibiotics (penicillin and gentamicin) against subacute bacterial endocarditis are started once labor is established and continued for 48 hours postpartum. To reduce the risk of supine hypotension and increase the oxygen carrying capacity of the blood, patients should be nursed on the side and given oxygen by mask.

In patients with severe cardiac disease (class III and IV, pulmonary hypertension), monitoring of the cardiovascular status is essential during labor and delivery. Arterial and Swan-Ganz catheters should be inserted to monitor arterial pressure and cardiac output, together with right atrial, main pulmonary artery, and pulmonary wedge pressures. The cardiac rhythm should be monitored continuously. Fluid intake and urine output, arterial blood gases, hemoglobin concentration, and electrolytes are also monitored. Labor monitoring may be accomplished by external or internal means, depending on the obstetric needs, although the former is preferred. It is desirable to limit the number of pelvic examinations and to avoid the use of the intrauterine catheter in order to reduce the incidence of intrauterine infection.

Management of Delivery and the Immediate Postpartum Period

Cardiac patients should be delivered vaginally unless there are obstetric indications for cesarean section. It is important to shorten the second stage of labor by performing an outlet forceps delivery or by the use of a vacuum extractor. The patient should be instructed to avoid pushing during uterine contractions because the associated increase in intra-abdominal pressure increases venous return and cardiac output and might lead to cardiac decompensation.

The immediate postpartum period presents special risks to the cardiac patient. After delivery of the placenta, the uterus contracts and about 500 ml of blood are added to the effective blood volume. To minimize the risk of overloading the circulation, the lower extremities are kept at the level of the body by lowering the stirrups, the uterus is not massaged to expedite placental separation, and pitocin is not given after delivery of the placenta. A small postpartum hemorrhage is frequently desirable, and if cardiac decompensation occurs, phlebotomy, rotating tourniquets, or both should be considered.

Thromboembolic Disorders

These disorders include superficial thrombophlebitis, deep venous thrombosis, and pulmonary embolism. The overall incidence of these disorders during pregnancy is about 1.4 per cent. About 80 per cent occur during the postpartum period.

Superficial Thrombophlebitis

The incidence of superficial thrombophlebitis during pregnancy is one in 600 during the antepartum period and one in 95 in the immediate postpartum period. It is more common in patients with varicose veins, obesity, and limited physical activity. In most patients, superficial thrombophlebitis is limited to the calf area, and symptoms include swelling and tenderness of the involved extremity. On physical examination, there is erythema, tenderness, warmth, and a palpable cord over the course of the involved superficial veins.

Superficial thrombophlebitis is not life-threatening and does not lead to pulmonary embolization. If not treated promptly and adequately, however, the inflammatory process might extend to the deep veins. Pain medications, local application of heat (thermal blanket), and elevation of the lower extremities to promote improved venous flow are often sufficient treatment. There is no need for anticoagulants or anti-inflammatory agents. After 5 to 7 days of bed rest and when symptoms disappear, the patient may be ambulated gradually. Postrecovery residual effects frequently persist in the form of valvular incompetence. Patients should be instructed to avoid standing for prolonged periods of time and to wear support hose to help avoid a repeat infection, which is prone to occur during pregnancy and the immediate postpartum period.

Deep Venous Thrombosis

The incidence of deep venous thrombosis is one in 2000 antepartum and one in 700 postpartum. The risk of pulmonary embolization is high, and immediate treatment is indicated. Vascular injury, infection, and tissue trauma, coupled with the hypercoagulability and venous stasis of pregnancy, are the triggering factors for deep venous thrombosis.

Clinical Features. The clinical diagnosis of deep venous thrombosis is difficult. Pain in the calf areas in association with dorsiflexion of the foot (positive Homans' sign) is a clinical sign of deep venous thrombosis in the calf veins. Acute swelling and pain in the thigh area, plus tenderness in the femoral triangle, are suggestive of iliofemoral thrombosis.

Investigations. Noninvasive techniques such as Doppler ultrasonography and plethysmography are helpful and may be used as screening techniques, but a negative result does not exclude the diagnosis, especially in women in whom the clinical picture is highly suggestive of deep venous thrombosis. Iodine-125 labeled fibrinogen and technetium-99 scans are sensitive to calf and iliac thrombosis, respectively. They are infrequently used, however, because of unavailability or radiation hazard. The best single test for the diagnosis of deep venous thrombosis is a well-performed venogram. Although some iliac lesions are missed and there is a 2 per cent incidence of phlebitis induced by the dye, the greatest concern is about radiation exposure, which is about 1 cGy.

Treatment. When a clinical diagnosis of deep venous thrombosis is made, anticoagulant therapy should be started and further diagnostic work-up delayed several hours until adequate heparin levels have been reached. If the work-up fails to identify any ileofemoral or calf thrombosis, heparin may be discontinued.

Many obstetricians and patients are not willing to accept the risks and limitations of a venogram and maintain anticoagulant therapy on the basis of clinical findings. Such an empiric approach is not without risks. In addition, these patients will forever carry such a diagnosis, necessitating special precautions during any subsequent pregnancy or surgical procedure.

Treatment of active deep venous thrombosis during pregnancy is initiated with intravenous heparin therapy. An initial dose of 10,000 units followed by a continuous infusion of intravenous heparin at a rate of about 1000 units per hour is maintained for 5 to 7 days or until symptoms disappear. For the first 1 to 2 days, the heparin dose should be increased or decreased to keep the prothrombin time (PT) at 2 to 2.5 times the normal control values. Since anticoagulant therapy must be continued for the duration of pregnancy and up to 6 weeks postpartum, either subcutaneous full-dose heparin or warfarin (Coumadin) by mouth might be given. If warfarin is chosen, a partial thromboplastin time (PTT) should be obtained weekly. PTT values should be maintained in the range of 2 to 2.5 times control.

Heparin is a high-molecular-weight substance that does not cross the placental barrier and is not secreted in the breast milk, so there are no untoward effects for the fetus and neonate. For this reason, most physicians prefer to maintain their patients on heparin given subcutaneously for the duration of pregnancy. Heparin therapy may be continued until the onset of labor, stopped during active labor and delivery, and resumed 6 to 12 hours postpartum. If prothrombin time remains prolonged during labor, 5 gm of protamine sulfate are enough to reverse the action of heparin. There is no evidence to suggest an increased incidence of postpartum uterine bleeding or bleeding from the episiotomy site when patients are restarted on anticoagulant therapy. Complications of long-term therapy include (1) hemorrhage, (2) heparin-associated thrombocytopenia, and (3) heparin-induced osteoporosis.

Warfarin has a low molecular weight and crosses the placental barrier. If given during the period of fetal organogenesis, its teratogenic potential should be kept in mind. If given late in the pregnancy, fetal ecchymoses and intracranial bleeding may occur with the onset of uterine contractions. Warfarin may, therefore, be given during the second trimester and up until 36 weeks of gestation. Thereafter, heparin is reinstituted and continued until the onset of labor. During the postpartum period, warfarin may be resumed.

Pulmonary Embolism

The incidence of pulmonary embolism during pregnancy is about one in 2500. The maternal mortality is less than 1 per cent if treated early and greater than 80 per cent if left untreated. In about 70 per cent of cases, deep venous thrombosis is the instigating factor.

Clinical Features. Clinical and laboratory findings parallel the degree of insult to tissues but may be deceptively nonspecific. Suggestive symptoms include pleuritic chest pain, shortness of breath, air hunger, palpitations, hemoptysis, and syncopal episodes. Suggestive signs include tachypnea, tachycardia, low-grade fever, a pleural friction rub, chest splinting, pulmonary rales, an accentuated pulmonic valve second heart sound, and even signs of right heart failure. In most obstetric patients, the signs and symptoms of a pulmonary embolus are subtle.

Investigations. An electrocardiogram might show sinus tachycardia with or without premature heart beats or right ventricular axis deviation. Cardiac enzymes are not helpful. On chest film, atelectasis, pleural effusion, obliteration of arterial shadows, and elevation of the diaphragm might be present. Arterial blood gases taken on room air show an oxygen tension below 80 mm Hg. If there is any doubt about the diagnosis, a ventilation-perfusion scan should be done. A technetium-99 ventilation-perfusion scan has a high level of sensitivity for detecting pulmonary embolism, provided that there is no heart failure, obstructive or constrictive lung disease, or pulmonary infiltrate. It can be performed with minimal risk to the fetus. Pulmonary angiography is rarely required, but its main value is to diagnose a large embolus in patients on whom embolectomy is planned.

Treatment of acute episodes and follow-up during pregnancy, labor, delivery, and the postpartum period are the same as for deep venous thrombosis.

Prophylactic Anticoagulant Therapy. In pregnant patients with a history of a pulmonary embolus or deep venous thrombosis during a previous pregnancy, prophylactic anticoagulants are given during pregnancy and the immediate postpartum period. Most patients are given full-dose anticoagulation, but some studies have suggested that minidose heparin (10,000 to 15,000 units per day) might be given. For patients with a history of deep venous thrombosis or pulmonary embolism not related to pregnancy, prophylactic minidose heparin might also be given, although there are no firm data to support such an approach.

PULMONARY DISORDERS

Obstructive Lung Disease

Bronchial Asthma

The incidence of bronchial asthma in pregnancy is approximately 1 per cent, and about 15 per cent of these individuals develop one or more severe attacks during pregnancy. Although the effect of pregnancy on bronchial asthma is variable, severe asthma is associated with a high abortion rate and an increased incidence of intrauterine fetal death and fetal growth retardation, most probably secondary to intrauterine hypoxia. Pulmonary function studies done during an acute episode show (1) increased airway resistance; (2) increased residual volume, functional residual capacity, and total lung capacity; (3) decreased inspiratory and expiratory reserve volume; (4) decreased vital capacity; and (5) decreased 1-second forced expiratory volume (FEV_1), peak expiratory flow rate, and maximum midexpiratory flow rate.

Obstetric Management. Pregnant asthmatics should be followed closely during pregnancy to assure adequate maternal and fetal assessment. In most asthmatics, no drug treatment is needed. Adequate bed rest; the avoidance of dehydration; early and aggressive treatment of respiratory infections; and the avoidance of hyperventilation, excessive physical activity, and allergins are sufficient to prevent an exacerbation of symptoms. Additionally, minimal studies are needed to assess respiratory status. Cough medications containing iodine should be used with care because of the risk of causing a congenital goiter in the fetus.

In moderately affected asthmatics, baseline pulmonary function studies and a chest film (with abdominal shielding) are essential to assess cardiopulmonary status. Follow-up studies are repeated as clinically indicated, although vital capacity may be assessed in the clinic at every visit. Most of these patients will respond well to β-adrenergic receptor stimulant inhalers, such as salbutamol (Ventolin) and isoproterenol (Isuprel), used two to three times per day. If symptoms persist or the inhalers are needed more than three to four times per day, selective beta-2 receptor stimulants, such as terbutaline (2.5 mg every 4 to 6 hours), may be added to the aforementioned regimen.

Patients with more complicated cases should be managed in consultation with pulmonary internists and respiratory therapists. If glucocorticoids are needed, every effort should be made to taper the dose gradually and then stop it. If continuous steroids are deemed necessary, 5 to 10 mg of prednisone every other day is usually sufficient.

For severe attacks, hospitalization is usually necessary. High dose steroids plus inhaler therapy (Ventolin) are the preferred methods of treatment. Many respirologists stay away from the use of intravenous aminophylline for the treatment of acute asthmatic attacks. Once the acute episode is over, β-sympathomimetic preparations are substituted and steroids tapered gradually.

Because most of the medications the mother receives during pregnancy cross the uteroplacental barrier, the potential of added risk to the fetus must be emphasized to parents. Although β-stimulants seem to be safe for the fetus, glucocorticoids are associated with fetal intrauterine growth retardation and rarely cleft palate.

Antepartum monitoring of the fetus to assess growth and development is essential. Early and serial pelvic ultrasonography, together with nonstress or oxytocin challenge tests as indicated, is usually employed.

The timing of delivery is dependent on the status of both the mother and the fetus. If pregnancy is progressing well, there is no need for early intervention, and it is advisable to await the spontaneous onset of labor. If the maternal condition is deteriorating or there is fetal growth retardation, early delivery is recommended.

Management of Labor and Delivery. If the patient has been taking oral steroids during pregnancy, the intravenous administration of glucocorticoids is recommended during labor, delivery, and the postpartum period. A selective epidural block during labor benefits the patient in that it reduces pain, anxiety, hyperventilation, and respiratory work, all of which are known to aggravate the disease or precipitate an attack. Vaginal delivery should be anticipated, but if cesarean section is indicated for obstetric reasons, general anesthesia is desirable, in spite of the fact that endotracheal intubation represents the most common stimulus precipitating asthma during general anesthesia. Spinal or epidural anesthesia for cesarean section poses potential hazards to the asthmatic patient. The supine position will limit respiration, while the high thoracic level of the block might impair coughing and the sensation of breathing and lead to increased patient anxiety. Additionally, the high sympathetic nerve blockade may lead to parasympathetic dominance and bronchoconstriction. Nausea, vomiting, and coughing may then develop with peritoneal traction during surgical manipulation.

Other Forms of Obstructive Lung Disease

The most severe form of obstructive lung disease observed during pregnancy is in patients with cystic fibrosis. The abnormal mucus results in airway plugging, inflammation, bronchiectasis, and recurrent pulmonary infections. Approximately half of these patients develop serious and progressive pulmonary decompensation during and after pregnancy. Although fetal outcome depends on the severity of the maternal disease, available data suggest excellent fetal survival rates. Chronic bronchitis and emphysema are not common in women of childbearing age.

Restrictive Lung Disease

Tuberculosis

The incidence of tuberculosis in the indigent population varies from 0.6 to 4.8 per

Table 18–2. CLASSIFICATION OF DIABETES MELLITUS (NONPREGNANT)

Diabetes mellitus
  Type I—Ketosis-prone
  Type II—Ketosis-resistant
  Diabetes associated with certain conditions or syndromes
Impaired glucose tolerance
Gestational diabetes

cent. About 10 to 12 per cent of these cases are active. Tuberculosis during pregnancy is discussed in Chapter 16.

ENDOCRINE DISORDERS

Only the most common endocrine disorders are discussed in this section. Emphasis is on diabetes mellitus and thyroid disease.

Diabetes Mellitus

Incidence and Classification

The incidence of diabetes mellitus in pregnancy is less than 0.5 per cent. In addition to the uniform classification of diabetes during the nonpregnant state (Table 18–2), White's classification of diabetes during pregnancy is used and is of more prognostic value (Table 18–3).

Complications

Fetal and maternal complications associated with diabetes mellitus during pregnancy are listed in Table 18–4.

Diagnosis

Screening for diabetes mellitus is discussed in Chapter 8. If the fasting and 1-hour or 2-hour screening plasma glucose levels are abnormal, a glucose tolerance test may not be required. For borderline screening tests, a 3-hour glucose tolerance test should be performed, preceded by a special diet containing about 300 gm of carbohydrate for 3 days (Table 18–5). If any two values are abnormal, excluding the fasting blood glucose, the patient is classified as having gestational diabetes class A_1. If the fasting blood glucose is also abnormal, the patient is classified as class A_2.

The best time to screen for gestational diabetes is between 24 and 28 weeks gestation because peripheral insulin resistance and insulin response to a glucose load start to increase at that time.

Management—Diabetic Team

Management of the gestational diabetic requires patient teaching and counseling, medical-nursing assessments and interventions, strategies to achieve maternal euglycemia, and avoidance of fetal-neonatal compromise. A diabetic team works together to achieve these objectives. This team includes the pa-

Table 18–3. WHITE'S CLASSIFICATION OF DIABETES IN PREGNANCY

CLASS	DESCRIPTION	THERAPY
A_1	Gestational diabetes. Glucose intolerance developing during pregnancy; fasting blood glucose is normal	Diet alone
A_2	Gestational diabetes with fasting plasma glucose greater than 105 mg/dl; or 2-hr postprandial plasma glucose greater than 120 mg/dl	Diet and insulin
B	Overt diabetes developing after age 20 and duration less than 10 yr	Diet and insulin
C	Overt diabetes developing before age 20 or duration greater than 10 yr	Diet and insulin
D	Overt diabetes developing between the ages of 10 and 19, or duration 10–19 yr, and/or background retinopathy.	Diet and insulin
F	Overt diabetes at any age or duration with nephropathy	Diet and insulin
R	Overt diabetes at any age or duration with proliferative retinopathy	Diet and insulin
H	Overt diabetes at any age or duration with arteriosclerotic heart disease	Diet and insulin

Table 18-4. MATERNAL AND FETAL COMPLICATIONS OF DIABETES MELLITUS

ENTITY	MONITORING
Maternal Complications	
Obstetric complications	
Polyhydramnios	Close prenatal surveillance; ultrasonography
Pre-eclampsia	
Diabetic emergencies	Blood glucose monitoring; insulin and dietary adjustment;
Hypoglycemia	check for infection, including urine culture every 6 wk
Ketoacidosis	
Diabetic coma	
Vascular and end organ involvement or deterioration	
Cardiac	ECG, first visit and as needed
Renal	Renal function studies, first visit and as needed
Ophthalmic	Funduscopic evaluation, first visit and as needed
Peripheral vascular	Check for ulcers, foot sores; noninvasive Doppler studies as needed
Neurologic	
Peripheral neuropathy	Neurologic and gastrointestinal consultations as needed
Gastrointestinal disturbance	
Fetal Complications	
Macrosomia with traumatic delivery	Repeat pelvic ultrasonography prior to delivery
Delayed organ maturity (pulmonary, hepatic, neurologic, pituitary-thyroid axis)	Amniocentesis for lung profile
Congenital anomalies	
Cardiovascular	Prior to 22 wk gestation, maternal serum alpha-fetoprotein; Hgb A1C monthly; pelvic ultrasonography and fetal echocardiogram; amniocentesis and genetic counseling, if necessary
Neural tube defects	
Caudal regression syndrome	
Intrauterine growth retardation	
Intrauterine fetal death	Repeat ultrasonography every 4 wk; NST and OCT; biophysical profile weekly or biweekly
Abnormal FHR patterns	
Small-for-dates babies	

FHR, fetal heart rate; NST, nonstress test; OCT, oxytocin challenge test.

tient, obstetrician, clinical nurse specialist, dietitian, psychosocial worker, and neonatologist.

Patient. The most significant change in diabetic management during pregnancy has been the inclusion of the patient as an active participant in formulating management strategies. In addition to teaching the patient survival skills, such as the identification and management of hypoglycemic and hyperglycemic episodes, she is taught the techniques for home glucose monitoring, insulin administration, and dietary adjustments.

Obstetrician. The obstetrician, as the head of the diabetic team, coordinates its activities and presents a unified concept of medical care strategies to the patient. The physician plays a very important role in the prevention

and early identification of prognostically poor indices, such as hypertension, infection, poor control of blood glucose, polyhydramnios, and fetal macrosomia.

Clinical Nurse Specialist. The clinical nurse specialist is involved in teaching the patient basic concepts about the pathophysiology of diabetes during pregnancy; assessing patient compliance and well-being; and teaching the patient methods of insulin administration, home glucose monitoring, and survival skills.

Psychosocial Worker. The psychosocial worker helps the patient to deal emotionally with her diabetes and explores the avenues to help her avoid stress.

Dietitian. The dietitian evaluates the patient's knowledge about the American Dia-

Table 18–5. THREE-HOUR GLUCOSE TOLERANCE TEST*

TEST	NORMAL PLASMA GLUCOSE (mg/dl)
fasting	105
1 hr	190
2 hr	165
3 hr	145

* 100 gm of oral glucose given after an overnight fast.

betic Association's (ADA) diet and food exchange lists and provides dietary information as necessary.

Achieving Euglycemia

In more recent years, the importance of stricter metabolic control before and during pregnancy in decreasing perinatal morbidity and mortality has been appreciated and emphasized. It has been suggested that better control of blood glucose levels reduces the incidence of congenital anomalies, although other data are less supportive of this association. To achieve euglycemia, diet, insulin, and exercise must be regulated.

Diet. An ADA diet with at least 1800 calories should be prescribed. Caloric requirements are calculated on the basis of 30 to 35 calories per kilogram of ideal body weight, plus 300 calories for anticipated weight gain during pregnancy. For an obese patient, additional calories are needed to prevent starvation ketonemia, whereas for underweight and adolescent patients, additional calories are needed for an appropriate weight gain during pregnancy. In general, 50 to 60 per cent of the caloric requirements are given as carbohydrates, 18 to 22 per cent as protein, and the remainder (about 25 per cent) as fat. Less than 10 per cent of the fat is saturated, up to 10 per cent polyunsaturated fatty acids, and the remainder is nonsaturated. Inclusion of a high-fiber content in the diet is also recommended.

A comprehensive meal plan must be devised for the patient. It is particularly impor-

tant in the pregnant diabetic to have a bedtime snack.

Insulin. Oral hypoglycemic agents are not recommended during pregnancy because they cross the placental barrier and may induce fetal and neonatal hypoglycemia. Short-acting, intermediate-acting, or long-acting insulins may be used in a combination of dosage schedules to effect maternal euglycemia. The peak action of short-acting (regular) insulin is about 4 hours, intermediate-acting insulin about 12 hours, and long-acting insulin 14 to 20 hours. For tight diabetic control during pregnancy, long-acting insulins are rarely used, but a combination of short-acting and intermediate-acting insulins are given as a split morning and evening dose. A method for calculating insulin dosage is shown in Table 18–6. Beef and pork combinations or pork insulin alone may be used. These are now available as purified insulin products (less than 50 particles/million of impurities). Synthetic human insulin has been introduced; its promise lies in reducing the antibody production, which increases insulin resistance.

Blood glucose levels drawn at specified hours to coincide with the peak action of insulin are used to assess the adequacy of insulin therapy. For a split (morning and evening), mixed (short and intermediate) dose of insulin, blood glucose levels are drawn before breakfast and at lunch, dinner, and evening snack, respectively. Postprandial values may also be helpful. The fasting and predinner blood glucose levels reflect the adequacy of evening and morning intermediate insulin dosage, respectively. Similarly, the

Table 18–6. METHOD FOR CALCULATION OF STARTING DOSE OF INSULIN

Insulin units
= body weight (kg) × 0.6 (First trimester)
0.7 (Second trimester)
0.8 (Third trimester)

Dosage schedule: Give ⅔ in AM and ⅓ in PM.
AM   ⅔ NPH, ⅓ regular
PM   ½ NPH, ½ regular

prelunch and presnack levels reflect the adequacy of morning and evening short-acting insulin dosages. In some individuals, 2:00 AM blood glucose levels might be indicated to adjust the insulin dosage adequately and avoid nocturnal hypoglycemia. A mean daily serum glucose level of less than 100 mg/dl is encouraged, with fasting levels 60 to 90 mg/dl, premeal blood glucose levels between 60 and 105 mg/dl, postprandial levels less than 120 mg/dl, and levels greater than 60 mg/dl between 2 and 6 AM.

Adjusting the insulin dosage to achieve euglycemia is facilitated by careful home glucose monitoring using a glucose refractometer. It is important to keep the following principles in mind:

1. Initial adjustment should be directed toward achieving a fasting plasma glucose level of 70 to 90 mg/dl.

2. Only one change in insulin dosage should be attempted at any given time, and changes in insulin dosage should not exceed 2 to 3 units/day. Additionally, at least 24 hours should be allowed after a dosage change to evaluate blood glucose response adequately.

3. Prior to changing the insulin schedule, careful attention should be given to compliance with diet, change in physical activity, or other temporary mitigating factors, such as stress or infection, that alter insulin requirements.

4. Patients who fail to maintain adequate glucose control in spite of multiple insulin injections might be candidates for insulin infusion pump therapy.

Exercise. Diabetic patients should be encouraged to exercise about half an hour after meals. Use of a stationary bike or mild to moderate aerobic exercises are adequate. A hospitalized, sedentary patient who achieves euglycemia during her hospital stay may encounter frequent episodes of hypoglycemia once she is discharged and returns to her usual daily activities.

Antepartum Obstetric Management

Aside from achieving euglycemia, adequate surveillance should be maintained during pregnancy to avoid maternal complications and to assure fetal growth and development. A detailed ultrasound study, fetal echocardiogram, and maternal serum alpha-fetoprotein level should be obtained at 16 to 20 weeks to alert the obstetrician to the presence of congenital malformations in the fetus. Maternal renal, cardiac, and ophthalmic function are closely monitored. The glycosylated hemoglobin levels (Hgb A1C) are monitored monthly. The percentage of Hgb A1C has been shown to correlate with long-term (up to 4 weeks) blood glucose levels. Elevated levels of Hgb A1C suggest that diabetic control is not adequate. Regular electronic, biochemical, and ultrasonographic fetal monitoring should be performed, as shown in Figure 8–1 (Chapter 8). For diabetic classes A, B, and C, fetal macrosomia should be sought, whereas for classes D, E, and F, fetal growth retardation is more commonly found.

Timing of Delivery

Advances in the management of the diabetic patient, such as tight metabolic control, availability of the fetal lung profile, and fetal biophysical profile determinations, have obviated the need for early delivery. If the maternal state is stable, blood glucose is in the euglycemic range, and fetal studies indicate continued growth of a healthy baby, delivery may be delayed until fetal lung maturity is achieved. Early intervention is indicated if these conditions are not met. For macrosomic babies, increased birth trauma to both mother and fetus should be kept in mind, and judicious use of cesarean section is preferable to protracted induction.

Intrapartum Management

Adequate intrapartum management of a diabetic patient requires maternal euglycemia during labor, which may be achieved by giving a continuous infusion of regular insulin in 5 or 10 per cent dextrose at a rate of 0.5 to 2 units of insulin per hour. Plasma glucose levels are measured every 2 hours and insulin dosage adjusted accordingly to maintain a plasma glucose level of between 80 and 100 mg/dl. In calculating the 24-hour insulin requirements, the ratio of insulin requirements to total caloric intake per day may be used as a rough estimate. This ratio multiplied by caloric intake during labor (600 calories) yields an estimate of anticipated total insulin requirements for the day. Provided that plasma glucose is monitored frequently and insulin administered when plasma glucose exceeds 100 mg/dl, not all insulin-dependent patients will require exogenous insulin during labor.

Fetal monitoring is recommended for all diabetic patients, especially for those who are insulin-dependent.

Standard obstetric criteria should guide the individual as to the mode of delivery. Regardless of mode of delivery, a neonatologist should be available in the labor area for immediate neonatal evaluation.

Postpartum Period

After delivery of the fetus and placenta, insulin requirements drop sharply because the placenta, which is the source of many insulin antagonists, has been removed. Most insulin-dependent diabetic patients do not require exogenous insulin for the first 48 to 72 hours after delivery. Plasma glucose levels should be obtained every 6 hours and regular insulin given when plasma glucose levels exceed 150 mg/dl. Prior to hospital discharge, patients may be restarted on two thirds of their prepregnancy insulin dosage and gradual adjustments made as necessary. Gestational diabetics (class A_1 and A_2) frequently do not need insulin therapy postpartum; an oral glucose tolerance test, however, should be repeated at 6 weeks postpartum.

Patients should be counseled about changes in diet. Except for gestational class A diabetics, the ADA diet with the same distribution of carbohydrates, proteins, and fat should be maintained. If the mother is breast feeding, 700 calories per day should be added to the maintenance diet.

Contraceptive counseling is an important aspect of total patient care, especially in the diabetic patient (see Chapter 42). Tubal ligation is recommended for patients who are desirous of permanent sterilization or for those with advanced vascular involvement.

Thyroid Diseases

Normal Thyroid Physiology During Pregnancy

With the increase in glomerular filtration rate that occurs during pregnancy, the renal excretion of iodine increases, and plasma inorganic iodine levels are nearly halved. Whether goiter ensues depends on the ability of the thyroid gland to compensate, which in turn depends on the concentration of plasma inorganic iodine and dietary iodine intake. Goiters due to iodine deficiency are not likely if plasma inorganic iodine levels are greater than 0.08 μg/dl. Only in patients who have plasma inorganic iodine levels that are borderline before pregnancy is there an increased incidence of goiter during pregnancy. Inorganic iodine supplementation up to a total of 250 μg per day is sufficient to prevent goiter formation during pregnancy.

Thyroid Function Tests. The free thyroxine concentration is the only direct method of estimating thyroid function that compensates for changes in thyroxine-binding globulin (TBG) capacity. Although serum levels of bound triiodothyronine (T_3) and thyroxine (T_4) are increased during pregnancy (as discussed in Chapter 6), free thyroxine levels remain within the normal range. The uptake of triiodothyronine by resin (T_3 resin uptake), which is an indirect measure of T_4-binding capacity, tends to be in the hypothyroid range during pregnancy, an indication that more binding sites are available. Since serum T_4 increases and the T_3 resin uptake decreases, the free T_4 index remains the same during pregnancy. Determination of free T_4 levels is time-consuming, difficult, and expensive, and the free thyroxine index may be used as an indirect approximation of the free thyroxine concentration during pregnancy. Values of thyroid function tests during pregnancy are shown in Table 18–7.

Fetal Thyroid Function. Prior to 10 weeks gestation, no organic iodine is present in the fetal thyroid. By 11 to 12 weeks, the fetal thyroid is able to produce iodothyronines and

Table 18-7. THYROID FUNCTION TESTS IN NONPREGNANT WOMEN AND IN MATERNAL AND CORD BLOOD AT TERM

TEST	NONPREGNANT	PREGNANT	CORD
Serum thyroxine (μg/dl)	5–12	10–16	6–13
Free thyroxine (ng/dl)	1.0–2.3	2.5–3.5	1.5–3.0
Serum triiodothyronine (ng/dl)	110–230	150–250	40–60
Reverse triiodothyronine (ng/dl)	—	35–65	80–360
Resin T_3 uptake (per cent)	20–30	10	10–15
TBG (μg/dl)	12–28	40–50	10–16
Serum TSH (μU/ml)	1.9–5.4	0–6	0–20

Note: Absolute values for these tests may vary according to the method used, but the ratio between maternal and cord values should remain constant.
Modified from Burrow GN, Ferris T (eds): Medical Complications During Pregnancy. Philadelphia, WB Saunders, 1972, p 194.

T_4, and by 12 to 14 weeks it is able to concentrate iodine. Fetal thyroid-stimulating hormone (TSH), T_4, and free thyroxine levels suggest that a mature, autonomous, thyroid-pituitary axis exists as early as 12 weeks of gestation.

In the amniotic fluid, T_4 and reverse T_3 concentrations reach a peak at 25 to 30 weeks and then decrease, whereas T_3 concentrations continue to increase throughout pregnancy. Whether amniotic fluid levels of thyroid hormone activity reflect the fetal compartment is unknown, although levels of T_3 in the amniotic fluid have been used for the prenatal diagnosis of fetal thyroid abnormalities.

Placental Transfer of Thyroid Hormone. There is minimal transfer of T_4 and T_3 across the placenta. Thyroid hormone analogs, with smaller molecular weights, decreased protein binding, and increased fat solubility, cross the placental barrier much more easily and could potentially be used to affect the fetal status without producing maternal thyrotoxicosis.

Maternal Hyperthyroidism

The incidence of maternal thyrotoxicosis is about 1 per 500 pregnancies. Although the incidence of fetal wastage is not increased, there is an increased incidence of prematurity, intrauterine growth retardation, and neonatal morbidity and mortality.

Graves' disease or toxic diffuse goiter is the most common cause of hyperthyroidism associated with pregnancy. Other causes of hyperthyroidism in pregnancy include hydatidiform mole and toxic nodular goiter. Patients with Graves' disease tend to have a remission during pregnancy and an exacerbation during the postpartum period. There is evidence to suggest that the increased immunologic tolerance during pregnancy may lead to a decrease in thyroid antibodies and amelioration of symptoms.

Clinical Features. The clinical diagnosis of hyperthyroidism in pregnancy is difficult because many of the signs and symptoms of the hyperdynamic circulation associated with hyperthyroidism are present in a normal euthyroid pregnant individual. A resting pulse rate greater than 100 beats per minute that fails to slow with a Valsalva maneuver, eye changes, loss of weight, failure to gain weight in spite of normal or increased food intake, and heat intolerance are all helpful in making the clinical diagnosis.

Investigations. A total serum T_4 level of greater than 15 μg/dl or a greatly elevated free thyroxine index are diagnostic. The free T_4 index is not an actual measure of free T_4 concentration; therefore, free T_4 levels are helpful in confirming the diagnosis.

Therapy. Since radioactive iodine treatment is contraindicated during pregnancy, either medical treatment or partial surgical ablation of the thyroid gland is employed.

The mainstay of antithyroid therapy is thioamides, which block the synthesis but not the release of thyroid hormone. It usually takes about 1 week for amelioration of symptoms and 4 to 6 weeks for full control. Propylthiouracil (PTU) and methimazole (Tapazole) have been used interchangeably, although PTU has the added advantage of blocking conversion of T_4 to T_3.

Once a diagnosis of hyperthyroidism has been made, the patient should be started on 100 to 150 mg of PTU every 8 hours. After the symptoms have subsided and serum levels of T_4 have returned toward normal, the dose of PTU should be lowered gradually to about 100 mg/day and maintained for the duration of pregnancy. Postpartum, the dose might be increased to about 300 mg/day to avoid an exacerbation of symptoms.

Since PTU crosses the placenta without difficulty, a major concern during maternal treatment is the development of fetal goiter and hypothyroidism. Clinical follow-up of these patients suggests that only 1 to 5 per cent of children exposed to PTU develop goiter. The neonatal goiter associated with PTU therapy is not large and obstructive, and there is no conclusive evidence that PTU treatment can lead to cretinism. Children exposed to thioamides in utero attain full physical and intellectual development and have normal thyroid function studies. PTU excretion in breast milk does not exceed 0.025 per cent of the administered daily maternal dose, and no changes occur in the thyroid function tests of breast-fed neonates.

There has been interest in the use of β-receptor blockers in conjunction with PTU. Propranolol in a dose of 40 mg every 6 hours may be used. There are scattered reports, however, implicating propranolol as an etiologic agent in intrauterine growth retardation, fetal demise, impaired fetal responses to hypoxic stress, and postnatal hypoglycemia and bradycardia. Therefore, the drug should be used only in acute situations to control acute symptoms until PTU achieves its effect.

Surgical management of the hyperthyroid pregnant patient is recommended only if medical treatment fails. Today few patients undergo subtotal thyroidectomy during pregnancy. It is advisable to delay surgery until the second trimester, since the rate of spontaneous abortion is highest during the first trimester. For rapid control of thyrotoxicosis prior to surgery, the addition of propranolol, 40 mg every 6 hours, and potassium iodide, 100 mg per day for 5 to 7 days, usually results in a marked improvement within a week.

Thyroid Storm

The major risk for a pregnant patient with thyrotoxicosis is the development of a thyroid storm. Precipitating factors include infection, labor, cesarean section, or noncompliance with medication. The maternal mortality exceeds 25 per cent in spite of good medical management. The signs and symptoms associated with a thyroid storm include hyperthermia, marked tachycardia, perspiration, and severe dehydration. Specific treatment is directed at (1) blocking β-adrenergic activity with propranolol, 20 to 80 mg every 6 hours; (2) blocking secretion of thyroid hormone with sodium iodide, 1 gm intravenously; (3) blocking synthesis of thyroid hormone and conversion of T_4 to T_3 with 1200 to 1800 mg PTU given in divided doses; (4) further blocking the deamination of T_4 to T_3 with 8 mg dexamethasone per day; (5) replacing fluid losses with at least 5 L of fluid; and (6) rapidly lowering the temperature with hypothermic techniques.

Neonatal Thyrotoxicosis

About 1 per cent of pregnant women with a history of Graves' disease give birth to children with thyrotoxicosis. Although it is transient and lasts less than 2 to 3 months, it is not a benign condition, since it is associated with a neonatal mortality rate of about 16 per cent.

Neonatal thyrotoxicosis is most likely related to placental transfer of thyroid-stimulating immunoglobulins (TSIG) of the 7S (IgG) variety, previously referred to as long-acting thyroid stimulator (LATS). The presence of TSIG in maternal and cord blood and the decline in neonatal serum concentrations of TSIG as neonatal thyrotoxicosis improves gives credence to this hypothesis. It has been found that TSIG protector is more commonly found in the serum of mothers whose infants develop thyrotoxicosis, and levels of TSIG-P exceeding 20 units/ml are almost always associated with neonatal thyrotoxicosis.

Hypothyroidism

Hypothyroidism is relatively uncommon during pregnancy, and fetal and neonatal outcome is normally good.

Maternal Hypothyroidism. The most important laboratory finding to confirm the diagnosis of hypothyroidism is an elevated TSH level. Other findings include low levels of serum T_3 and T_4 and a decreased T_3 resin uptake.

Once a diagnosis of hypothyroidism has been made in a pregnant woman, thyroid replacement should be started immediately. L-thyroxine in a dose of 0.15 mg daily is usually sufficient to ameliorate the symptoms. Later adjustments in the dosage schedule depend on the increase in serum T_3 and T_4 and the decrease in serum TSH levels.

Not infrequently, pregnant women are encountered who are receiving maintenance doses of T_4 for obscure reasons. Although some physicians have recommended discontinuation of thyroid treatment for 5 to 6 weeks to allow for a re-evaluation of thyroid function, most have opted for continuation of treatment during pregnancy and re-evaluation during the postpartum period.

Neonatal Hypothyroidism. Thyroid hormone deficiency during the fetal and early neonatal periods leads to generalized developmental retardation. The severity of symptoms depends on the time of onset and the severity of the deprivation. If the disease is diagnosed and treated during the early neonatal period, the damage may be greatly minimized.

The incidence of congenital hypothyroidism (cretinism) is about one in 4000 births. The etiologic factors include thyroid dysgenesis, inborn errors of thyroid function, and drug-induced endemic hypothyroidism. The most common cause of neonatal goiter is maternal ingestion of iodides present in cough syrup. The goiters associated with maternal iodine ingestion are large and obstructive, unlike those associated with maternal PTU treatment.

The clinical diagnosis of neonatal hypothyroidism is very difficult. Hypothyroidism should be suspected in a large neonate with respiratory and feeding difficulties, an umbilical hernia, and rough dry skin. Screening of all neonates before discharge with serum T_4 and serum TSH levels should identify almost all affected infants.

HEMATOLOGIC DISORDERS

Anemia

Physiologic Anemia in Pregnancy

During pregnancy, the blood volume increases by 40 to 50 per cent. The red cell mass increases by 25 per cent, so there is a relative increase in plasma volume, compared with red cell mass. The hematocrit and hemoglobin concentrations decrease. The term *physiologic anemia of pregnancy* is applied to this drop in hematocrit. The serum iron levels decrease slightly but remain within the normal range, while the total iron binding capacity increases by about 15 per cent. Hemoglobin levels less than 10 gm/dl indicate the presence of anemia. Only hemoglobin levels less than 6 gm/dl are associated with an increased incidence of stillborn and premature infants.

Iron-Deficiency Anemia

Primary iron deficiency is responsible for about 80 per cent of nonphysiologic anemias during pregnancy. Approximately 1000 mg of additional iron is required during pregnancy for the expanded maternal red cell mass, for fetal hemoglobin, and for iron lost through bleeding at the time of delivery. Therefore, at least 4 mg of elemental iron are needed per day. This amount exceeds the 1.3 to 2.6 mg per day that is absorbed from a normal diet, even in an iron-deficient person. As a result, iron supplementation during pregnancy is necessary. A 325-mg ferrous sulfate tablet taken daily (60 mg of elemental iron) is usually sufficient for prophylactic purposes, although more is needed with iron-deficiency anemia.

Laboratory findings depend on the severity and chronicity of anemia. Initially, the iron stores are depleted, followed by a decrease in the serum iron and an increase in the total iron-binding capacity. Finally, morphologic changes in the red cells occur. Serum ferritin levels less than 10 ng/ml, serum iron levels less than 60 μg/dl, and transferrin saturation rates (total iron binding capacity/serum iron) less than 16 per cent are suggestive of iron-deficiency anemia. A peripheral smear may show microcytosis, hypochromia, and a reticulocyte count that is low for the degree of anemia. If the diagnosis of iron-deficiency anemia is equivocal or the patient is not responding to iron supplementation, bone marrow aspiration is recommended. The absence of stainable iron on a bone marrow aspirate is diagnostic for iron deficiency.

The thalassemia trait must be differentiated from iron deficiency anemia, since both entities exhibit microcytic, hypochromic red blood cells. With the thalassemia trait, the serum iron, total iron-binding capacity, and stainable iron on bone marrow aspirate are within normal limits. The hemoglobin A_2 level is elevated.

Up to 1 gm of oral ferrous sulfate per day (180 mg of elemental iron) is usually sufficient to reverse the anemia. Occasionally, when more rapid iron supplementation is required in a severely anemic patient at or close to term, intramuscular or intravenous administration of iron has been suggested. This latter approach is not recommended, since side effects are numerous.

Folic Acid Deficiency Anemia

The incidence of folic acid deficiency anemia varies from 0.5 to 25 per cent, depending on the region of the United States, the population, and the diet. Where leafy green vegetables are available all year around, the incidence of folate deficiency is low, whereas the reverse is true in cold, mountainous, and isolated areas. Non-nutritional factors also contribute to folate deficiency, including (1) chronic hemolytic anemias with increased red blood cell turnover; (2) medications, such as phenytoin (Dilantin) and methotrexate; (3) malabsorption entities, such as sprue; and (4) increased demand, as in a twin gestation. Rarely, folic acid deficiency presents as a single entity, but more commonly it is found in association with iron-deficiency anemia.

In about 50 per cent of patients, anemia develops in the latter part of pregnancy or during the postpartum period, since it takes about 18 weeks of a folate-deficient diet to produce anemia. Initially, the serum folate level decreases, followed by hypersegmentation of neutrophils. Much later, the red blood cell folate levels fall, urinary formiminoglutamic acid (FIGLU) excretion increases after a histidine load, and megaloblastic anemia develops. A bone marrow aspirate showing megaloblasts is diagnostic, although it is rarely used.

For prophylactic and treatment purposes, 0.7 to 1 mg of folic acid may be given daily, either alone or with ferrous sulfate. Patients with chronic hemolytic anemia or those on antifolate medications might require 2 mg of folic acid per day.

Combined Iron and Folate Deficiency

In this group of patients, the diagnosis of either entity is difficult, since laboratory findings are equivocal and changes in red blood cell morphology are inconsistent. A complete hematologic response does not occur until both iron and folic acid are given. If the anemia is severe and there is a partial response to treatment, a bone marrow aspirate is indicated.

Hemoglobinopathies

Careful medical, family, and obstetric histories are usually helpful in uncovering hemoglobinopathies. The presence of severe anemia or failure to respond to iron and folic acid supplementation, however, should alert the physician to look for these disorders. Hemoglobin electrophoresis differentiates normal adult hemoglobin A from sickle hemoglobin S, fetal hemoglobin F, and hemoglobin C.

Sickle-Cell Disease

This entity includes sickle-cell anemia, which has a homozygous S-S pattern, sickle-cell trait (S-A), sickle-cell β-thalassemia (S-B-Thal), and sickle-cell hemoglobin C disease (S-C). The maternal mortality-morbidity and the fetal complication rate reflect the percentage of S hemoglobin and the degree of anemia in the pregnant patient. Patients with S-A and S-B-Thal tolerate pregnancy well with lower rates of maternal-fetal complications, since the hemoglobin A level is higher than the hemoglobin S level. The incidence of sickle-cell anemia (S-S) in blacks is about one in 2000, whereas the incidence of sickle-cell trait is about one in 11.

Maternal mortality in patients with sickle-cell disease is about 2 per cent. Morbidity rates still average about 80 per cent and involve sickle-cell crises, pyelonephritis, severe anemia, neurologic manifestations, and sickle-cell lung syndrome. Fetal wastage is highest during a sickle-cell crisis, and even if the fetus survives, the incidence of intrauterine growth retardation is increased. Pregnancy has an adverse effect on sickle-cell disease.

Antepartum Management. Pregnant patients with sickle-cell disease should seek early prenatal care, be seen frequently, and be informed of the maternal-fetal risks associated with their pregnancy. Recommended initial studies include (1) early ultrasonography to assess fetal viability and exclude gross congenital anomalies; (2) hemoglobin electrophoresis to assess the percentage of hemoglobin S; (3) a complete blood and reticulocyte count with red blood cell indices to assess the degree of anemia; (4) serum iron, total iron-binding capacity, and serum folate to assess iron and folic acid stores; (5) renal function studies, including microscopic urine analysis and culture; and (6) pulmonary function studies in patients with frequent episodes of respiratory infection.

Supplemental iron should not be given to patients with a history of repeated blood transfusions or those with a diagnosis of hemochromatosis. Supplements of folic acid (1 to 2 mg/day) are recommended.

Several studies have suggested that prophylactic simple or exchange transfusions might be of value in preventing sickle-cell crises, fetal growth retardation, perinatal mortality, premature labor, and maternal infection. The theoretic benefits are (1) an increase in the oxygen-carrying capacity of the blood; (2) a reduction in the percentage of sickled hemoglobin; and (3) suppression of production of cells with S-S hemoglobin. The National Institutes of Health Consensus Report, however, does not support the use of prophylactic

transfusions. At most institutions, sickle-cell patients are transfused (1) when hemoglobin levels fall below 9 gm/dl in spite of iron and folic acid supplementation and the patient becomes symptomatic; (2) when the patient is having a sickle-cell crisis and not responding to supportive measures; (3) late in the third trimester or prior to labor and delivery to raise the hemoglobin above 10 gm/dl; and (4) postpartum in the presence of severe infection.

Maternal surveillance studies are repeated at least every 4 to 6 weeks. Episodes of sickle-cell crisis and urinary or pulmonary infections are treated aggressively. During the third trimester, fetal surveillance studies (pelvic ultrasonography and stress and nonstress testing) are indicated to assess fetal growth and development.

Intrapartum Care. Labor and delivery pose additional maternal and fetal risks for an individual with sickle-cell disease. The risk of development of a sickle-cell crisis is increased if oxygen and fluid demands are not met. Similarly, the growth-retarded fetus might not tolerate the stress of labor as a result of uteroplacental insufficiency. To safeguard against these complications, the following measures are indicated:

1. Oxygen supplementation to the mother.
2. Administration of intravenous fluids.
3. Reassurance and early sedation to prevent excessive anxiety.
4. Adequate fetal monitoring.
5. Avoidance of a prolonged and traumatic labor and delivery.
6. Administration of prophylactic antibiotics if an operative delivery is necessary.

Disorders of Blood Coagulation and Platelets

The presence of ecchymoses and hematomas is usually associated with a deficient coagulation mechanism, whereas petechial lesions are associated with platelet disorders. A drug history is important, since certain drugs might affect coagulation factors, platelets, and blood vessels. Simple tests, such as a PT and PTT, are appropriate for the initial diagnosis of coagulation disorders, whereas a platelet count is sufficient for differentiation of thrombocytopenic and nonthrombocytopenic purpura.

Inherited Disorders of Plasma Coagulation Factors

The most common inherited plasma coagulation disorders are hemophilia A (factor VIII deficiency), hemophilia B (factor IX deficiency), and von Willebrand's disease. Hemophilias A and B are X-linked recessive disorders, and the typical female carrier is not clinically affected.

Von Willebrand's disease accounts for about 10 per cent of the inherited coagulation disorders and can lead to a hemorrhagic diathesis in the pregnant patient. The laboratory diagnosis of von Willebrand's disease is based on (1) factor VIII, procoagulant (VIII:C), and related antigen (VIII R:Ag) deficiency; (2) prolonged bleeding time; (3) positive tourniquet test; and (4) delayed response to infused plasma with production of new factor VIII in vivo. Treatment for von Willebrand's disease is with fresh frozen plasma or cryoprecipitate.

Thrombocytopenia

With thrombocytopenia, the bleeding time becomes prolonged, clot retraction becomes decreased, and the tourniquet test becomes positive. Although a peripheral smear is sufficient for determining the platelet count, a bone marrow aspirate is needed to quantitate the megakaryocytes. Idiopathic thrombocytopenic purpura and thrombotic thrombocytopenic purpura are discussed in Chapter 7.

Disseminated Intravascular Coagulopathy

The factors usually responsible for disseminated intravascular coagulopathy (DIC) in pregnancy are varied and may be grouped into several categories: (1) abruptio placentae, (2) severe pre-eclampsia or eclampsia, (3) intrauterine fetal demise, (4) sepsis, (5) transfusion reaction, and (6) amniotic fluid embolism.

Impaired clot retraction; decreased serum fibrinogen; decreased platelet count; and an increase in fibrin split products, PT, and PTT are diagnostic of DIC.

Treatment is directed at resolving the underlying etiologic factor. In most obstetric situations, emptying the uterus is sufficient to reverse the process. Occasionally, fresh frozen plasma, cryoprecipitate, and whole blood and platelet transfusions are needed to establish hemostasis, especially if delivery is not imminent or a cesarean section is planned. Continuous heparin infusion may be useful in reversing DIC occurring in association with an intrauterine fetal death, but heparin is contraindicated in an actively bleeding patient.

NEUROLOGIC DISORDERS

Seizures

There are no specific neurologic disorders related to pregnancy; therefore, only seizure disorders are discussed in this section.

Seizure frequency during pregnancy may increase, decrease, or remain the same. It is difficult to relate the worsening of seizure control during pregnancy to the lower plasma levels of anticonvulsant drugs, since seizure control improves in more than 50 per cent of patients. Rarely, grand mal seizure may occur for the first time during pregnancy or in the puerperium and must be distinguished from eclampsia.

Treatment

If patients have had no seizure activity for a few years, medication may be discontinued before conception. If they are pregnant and well controlled, no change in therapy should be attempted unless the drugs are teratogenic.

The two most commonly used drugs for seizure treatment are diphenylhydantoin (Dilantin) and phenobarbital. Phenobarbital has less teratogenic effects, so is the drug of first choice in early pregnancy. Phenobarbital at a dose of 100 to 250 mg per day may be given in divided doses. The serum levels are monitored, and the dose is increased gradually until a therapeutic level (10 to 40 μg/ml) is reached. Dilantin may be given at 300 to 500 mg per day in single or divided doses to achieve serum levels of 10 to 20 $\mu g/ml$ (1 to 2 $\mu g/ml$ free level), whereas primidone can be given at 750 to 1500 mg per day in three divided doses to give 5 to 15 $\mu g/ml$ serum levels. Other anticonvulsant drugs, such as clonazepam (Clonopin) and carbamazepine (Tegretol), should be used with care. Valproic acid (Depakene) and trimethadione pose special risks to the mother and fetus and should be avoided.

Maternal megaloblastic anemia and fetal congenital malformations due to folic acid deficiency occur as a rare complication of anticonvulsant therapy. Most of the reported cases have followed the administration of Dilantin. The use of folic acid supplementation is recommended, but careful attention should be paid to plasma levels of Dilantin since folic acid supplements are known to reduce plasma levels of Dilantin. Dilantin is also reported to interfere with intestinal calcium absorption leading to maternal and fetal hypocalcemia. In patients taking phenobarbital, primidone, or Dilantin, vitamin D supplements (10 mg per day) are recommended starting at about 34 weeks. Antacids and antihistamines should be avoided in patients receiving Dilantin, since they also lower plasma levels of Dilantin and may precipitate a seizure attack.

For the treatment of status epilepticus, immediate hospitalization is required. Patency of the airway should be ascertained. After blood is drawn for plasma levels of anticonvulsants, 10 mg of intravenous diazepam (Valium) should be given slowly, followed by 200 to 500 mg of diphenylhydantoin. If seizure patterns continue, 500 mg of amobarbital sodium may be added. If the above measures fail, general anesthesia may be employed. Therapeutic levels of diphenylhydantoin must be maintained during the rest of the pregnancy and postpartum period.

All patients who receive anticonvulsant therapy should have detailed ultrasonography and fetal echocardiography at about 18 weeks to look for fetal congenital anomalies.

The management of labor and delivery follows obstetric indications. During labor and in the immediate postpartum period, anticonvulsant drugs may be given intravenously. Cord blood should be sent for the measurement of PT because of the possibility of a coagulopathy in the neonate. Postpartum, the dose of the anticonvulsant drug may be lowered, provided that a therapeutic level is maintained. Although anticonvulsants are excreted in breast milk in small amounts, breast feeding is not contraindicated.

Complications

Pregnant patients with epilepsy have a twofold increase in such maternal complications as pre-eclampsia, vaginal bleeding, hyperemesis, prolonged labor, and premature labor.

In the fetus, there is a high incidence of intrauterine fetal demise, coagulopathy, and congenital anomalies. In the neonate, higher rates of coagulopathy, drug withdrawal symptoms, and neonatal morbidity and mortality are reported. (Teratogenic effects of anticonvulsants are discussed in Chapter 9). Anticonvulsants alone may not be responsible for the twofold to threefold increase in the rate of congenital anomalies. Other risk factors include the occurrence of frequent convulsions during pregnancy, the increased incidence of maternal complications during pregnancy, and the socioeconomic status of the pregnant epileptic.

RENAL DISORDERS

Acute Renal Failure

Acute renal failure during pregnancy or in the postpartum period may be due to deterioration of renal function secondary to a pre-existing renal disease or to a pregnancy-related disorder. The underlying causative factors may be prerenal, renal, or postrenal. With prerenal causes, a history of blood or fluid loss is usually elicited from the patient or implied from reviewing the medical history. Renal causes are usually suspected in a patient with a history of pre-existing renal disease or with a hypercoagulable state, such as thrombotic thrombocytopenic purpura or hemolytic uremic syndrome. With prolonged hypotension, acute cortical necrosis or acute tubular necrosis may occur. Postrenal causes are less common but should be suspected in situations in which urologic obstructive lesions are present or in which there is a history of kidney stones.

Laboratory Studies

Laboratory tests are directed at assessing renal function, cardiovascular status, and patency of the urologic tract.

Renal Studies. These include urine output, blood urea nitrogen (BUN) to creatinine ratio, fractional excretion of sodium, and urine osmolality.

Oliguria is defined as urine output of less than 25 ml/hr, whereas anuria is the cessation of urine output. With acute renal failure, the urine output may not decrease, although oliguria or anuria are usually present. Not infrequently, a decrease in urine output alerts the physician to an impending crisis.

During pregnancy, the serum values of BUN and creatinine decrease, but the BUN to creatinine ratio remains about 20:1. A ratio greater than 20:1 suggests tubular hypoperfusion (prerenal failure).

The fractional excretion of sodium (FENa) is calculated as follows:

$$\text{FENa} = \frac{\text{Urine sodium/plasma sodium}}{\text{Urine creatinine/plasma creatinine}} \times 100$$

An FENa less than 1 per cent is suggestive of hypovolemia and tubular hypoperfusion. Alternatively, a value greater than 3 per cent is highly indicative of tubular damage.

Urine osmolality greater than 500 mOsm/L or a urine to plasma osmolality ratio greater than 1.5:1 is highly suggestive of renal hypoperfusion. Urine specific gravity is of limited value, especially when there is protein or hemolyzed blood in the urine.

Cardiovascular Studies. Acute blood and fluid losses are usually associated with orthostatic hypotension, tachycardia, decreased skin turgor, and reduced sweating. In a pregnant hypertensive or pre-eclamptic patient who is in labor, many of these signs are overlooked. A Swan-Ganz catheter introduced through the external jugular vein into the pulmonary artery allows monitoring of right and left ventricular filling pressures, cardiac output, and pulmonary capillary wedge pressure. Systemic vascular resistance may also be calculated. This can help to distinguish between congestive heart failure, cardiac tamponade, and volume depletion, any of which can lead to acute renal failure.

Urologic Tract Studies. A Foley catheter and renal sonogram are usually sufficient to diagnose obstructive lesions. Rarely, a one-shot intravenous pyelogram is needed.

Treatment

Prerenal Causes. Restoration of intravascular volume, cardiac output, and arterial pressure to normal values is sufficient to reverse oliguria. Careful attention should be given to electrolyte imbalance when large amounts of crystalloids are infused.

Renal Causes. Acute tubular necrosis, acute cortical necrosis, or both may be present. Because acute cortical necrosis is generally irreversible, treatment is directed toward preventing further damage. A trial of diuretic therapy to increase urinary output appears to decrease the duration and severity of acute tubular necrosis and increase survival rates. Intravenous administration of 25 gm of mannitol and 40 mg of furosemide (Lasix) is given initially and then repeated every 4 to 6 hours for 48 hours in the presence of adequate urinary response. If the diuretic therapy fails to increase the urine output, an oliguric fluid regimen is initiated. Fluid intake should be limited to replacement of urine output and insensible water loss, and renal function studies should be monitored on a daily basis. For the first few days after the renal ischemic episode, renal function may worsen; within 7 to 10 days, however, most patients with acute tubular necrosis show marked improvement. If renal function deteriorates rapidly or fails to recover, hemodialysis is recommended.

In some patients in whom acute renal failure is accompanied by oliguria, a diuretic phase coincides with the recovery period. The urine output might exceed 10 L per day, and if fluid and electrolyte losses are not replaced promptly, death ensues.

About 50 per cent of obstetric patients who develop acute renal failure during pregnancy or the postpartum period will recover enough renal function during the first year to survive without dialysis.

Postrenal Causes. In many instances, simple measures, such as turning the patient to the side to displace the gravid uterus from the ureters or inserting a Foley catheter into the bladder to overcome urethral obstruction, will resolve the problem. In situations in which a ureteral or renal pelvic obstruction is present (e.g., stones) surgical intervention is indicated to relieve the obstruction.

Chronic Renal Failure

The outcome of pregnancies complicated by chronic renal disease is less favorable. Good pregnancy outcome may be expected in nonhypertensive pregnant patients who have serum creatinine levels below 1.5 mg/dl prior to conception. When the serum creatinine levels exceed 3 mg/dl, continuation of pregnancy until fetal viability is rare. Hypertensive individuals with chronic renal disease do not fair as well as normotensive patients with the same degree of renal impairment.

Pregnancy has no effect on the natural course of the renal disease in patients who have mild impairment of renal function and are normotensive. The deterioration in renal function, superimposition of hypertension, and substantial increase in proteinuria seen during pregnancy subside after delivery. Patients with nephrotic syndrome do well during pregnancy in spite of the massive urinary protein losses. In most of these individuals, proteinuria partially abates postpartum.

Pregnancy Following Renal Transplantation

Pregnancy after renal transplantation should not be considered before a thorough assessment of maternal, fetal, and neonatal risk factors. Fetal complications include steroid-induced adrenal and hepatic insufficiency, prematurity, and intrauterine growth retardation. Decrease in thymus size, lymphopenia, and lethargy have been reported. In addition, the infant may inherit the primary disease of the mother or other family members. The mother and neonate are at increased risk of infection because of immunosuppressive therapy.

Table 18–8. CRITERIA FOR SELECTING SUITABLE RENAL TRANSPLANTATION PATIENTS FOR PREGNANCY

Two years post-transplant with good health
Anatomic status compatible with good obstetric outcome
No proteinuria
No significant hypertension
No evidence of active allograft rejection
No evidence of pelvicalyceal distention on recent IVP
Serum creatinine less than 2 mg/dl
Prednisone dosage 15 mg/day or less and azathioprine dosage 2 mg/kg/day or less

Adapted from Davison JM, Lindheimer MD: Pregnancy in renal transplant recipients. J Reprod Med 27:613, 1982.

The criteria shown in Table 18–8 may be used to identify renal transplantation patients who are good candidates for pregnancy.

GASTROINTESTINAL DISORDERS

Nausea and Vomiting During Pregnancy

About 60 to 80 per cent of pregnant women complain of nausea and vomiting during the first 8 to 12 weeks of gestation. The symptoms are usually mild and disappear during the early part of the second trimester. In a small number of patients, the severity of the symptoms necessitates hospital admission.

The underlying causes of nausea and vomiting during pregnancy are not well delineated. Several hypotheses are proposed:

1. Psychic events. Patients under emotional stress are more likely to experience nausea and vomiting.

2. Neuroendocrine alterations. The appearance of nausea and vomiting is thought to parallel the increase in serum chorionic gonadotropin. Several studies, however, have shown no correlation between the frequency and severity of nausea and vomiting and serum chorionic gonadotropin levels.

3. Adrenal and pituitary dysfunction. Patients with Addison's disease or adrenocor-

tical insufficiency following adrenalectomy complain of nausea and vomiting. Administration of adrenocorticotropic hormone (ACTH) to patients with hyperemesis gravidarum often produces a therapeutic response. Both glands function normally, however, in the hyperemetic patient.

4. Hyperthyroxinemia. Hyperthyroxinemia is present in about 70 per cent of patients with hyperemesis.

5. Sex steroid imbalance. Progesterone deficiency and estrogen excess have been implicated, although no data substantiate either claim.

6. Drugs. Drugs and chemicals may evoke nausea and vomiting through their alteration of the chemoreceptors in the base of the fourth ventricle. Prostaglandins, chemotherapeutic and noxious agents, and cardiac glycosides are thought to work through such a mechanism.

Hyperemesis Gravidarum

This term is reserved for the intractable nausea and vomiting that occurs in a few gravidas; the overall incidence is about 1 per cent. Cultural, racial, and personality factors are known to influence the prevalence of this disorder. It is more commonly found in the white population, and less frequently seen in blacks, Eskimos, and some African tribes. It is also seen in oppressive cultural environments and in individuals stereotyped as having an immature personality. The disorder appears more frequently with first pregnancies but tends to recur with subsequent pregnancies. Pregnancy outcome is usually good, with no added risk to mother, fetus, or neonate.

Clinical diagnosis is based on history and physical findings. A history of intractable vomiting and inability to retain food and fluid intake is usually elicited. Physical findings of weight loss, dry and coated tongue, and decreased skin turgor are very suggestive. The initial laboratory work-up includes urine tests for ketonuria and blood tests for electrolytes and acetone. Electrolyte disturbances may include hypokalemia, hyponatremia, and hypochloremic alkalosis.

Additional laboratory work-up should include hematologic, renal, and hepatic studies. Although the condition is self-limiting, occasionally severe complications result from metabolic deterioration with hepatic or renal involvement. Other diseases that may have similar clinical manifestations should be excluded, such as gastroenteritis, cholecystitis, pancreatitis, hepatitis, peptic ulcer, and pyelonephritis.

Treatment

Nonhospital management includes psychological support, assurance, dietary alterations, and avoidance of spicy foods and other foods that induce emesis. Patients are encouraged to take small, frequent meals and to eat solid foods. Antiemetic drugs such as prochlorperazine (Compazine), promethazine hydrochloride (Phenergan), dimenhydrinate (Gravol or Dramamine), doxylamine succinate (Diclectin), and pyridoxine are frequently used in pregnancy. Their use should be limited to patients who are well informed about the potential fetal risks and in whom conservative approaches fail.

If electrolyte disturbances are present or outpatient management fails, patients are admitted to the hospital for further work-up and treatment. Intravenous hydration, correction of electrolyte and acid-base imbalance, and psychological counseling are instituted. Frequently, stressful life events are identified, and intervention may facilitate improvement. Gastroscopy may sometimes be indicated to rule out gastric pathology. In refractory patients in whom there is persistent weight loss and starvation ketosis, enteral and parenteral hyperalimentation may be necessary.

Reflux Esophagitis

During pregnancy, physiologic alterations occur that increase the potential for esophageal reflux. Early in pregnancy, the lower esophageal sphincter tone remains unchanged, but the responses to pharmacologic and humoral manipulations are reduced. During late pregnancy, with the increase in serum progesterone levels, the sphincter tone decreases. Additionally, during pregnancy, the intragastric pressure increases and the intraesophageal pressure decreases. Gastric pH and gastric acid output remain unchanged.

Reflux esophagitis or heartburn is a common complaint during pregnancy. It occurs in about 70 per cent of gravidas and gets worse during the latter part of gestation.

Symptoms and Diagnosis

The main symptoms include substernal discomfort aggravated by meals and the recumbent position and occasional hematemesis. An unusual symptom peculiar to reflux esophagitis is water brash, which is best described as the sudden filling of the mouth with clean, watery material that has a salty taste and produces a nauseous sensation.

The diagnosis of reflux esophagitis is usually based on symptoms and response to treatment. In severe cases, in those with atypical clinical manifestations, and in those that are unresponsive to treatment, endoscopy is indicated.

Treatment

Treatment is usually symptomatic. Patients are instructed to refrain from eating large and late meals, to avoid the recumbent position, especially after meals, and to use an extra pillow to elevate the head when sleeping. Patients with more severe symptoms also require liquid antacids, which should be taken 1 to 3 hours after meals and at bedtime.

Peptic Ulcer

Pregnancy conveys relative protection against the development of peptic ulceration and may ameliorate an already present ulcer. Gastric acid secretion is probably not altered during pregnancy, although some studies suggest modest suppression.

Diagnosis

The diagnosis of ulcer disease is mainly based on symptomatic improvement in response to conservative treatment. Endoscopy is reserved for those patients who do not respond to antacid treatment, have more severe gastrointestinal symptoms, or manifest significant gastrointestinal hemorrhage. Radiographic studies, such as a barium swallow or upper gastrointestinal series, have no advantage over endoscopy and are unnecessary, especially during pregnancy.

Treatment

Treatment involves avoiding caffeine, alcohol, tobacco, and spicy foods, all of which stimulate acid secretion. Liquid antacids with a low sodium content are recommended and should be continued for at least 6 weeks. These include Maalox TC Suspension, Mylanta II liquid, and Gelusil II liquid. Cimetidine (Tagamet) should be reserved for complicated, recurrent, and refractory cases. Cimetidine, an H_2 histamine receptor antagonist, inhibits gastric acid secretion but has no effect on gastric volume, gastric emptying, or lower esophageal sphincter tone. The drug has been associated with cardiac arrhythmias, cardiac arrest, and an increased risk of gastric carcinoma. It crosses the placenta and reaches the fetus in substantial quantities.

Acid Aspiration Syndrome (Mendelson's Syndrome)

The pregnant patient in labor is at an increased risk of having acid aspiration because of (1) delayed gastric emptying, which is made worse when associated with increased anxiety or the use of sedatives, narcotics, and anticholinergic agents; (2) increased gastric acidity; and (3) increased intra-abdominal and intragastric pressure, making regurgitation more likely. Damage to the pulmonary tissue is greatest when the pH of the aspirated fluid is less than 2.5 or the volume of the aspirate is greater than 25 ml.

Preventive efforts are directed at decreasing the acidity of the gastric contents or decreasing the acid secretion by the stomach. Toward this end, women in labor should be advised not to eat before coming to the hospital. Liquid magnesium and aluminum antacids given every 3 to 4 hours during labor decrease the gastric acidity but increase the volume of the gastric acid-antacid emulsion. If the patient is to undergo any surgical procedure that requires general anesthetic, intubation should be performed.

The signs and symptoms of acid aspiration syndrome vary depending on the volume, acidity, and consistency of the aspirate. Solid aspirates may obstruct the tracheobronchial tree and lead to cyanosis, atelectasis, and mediastinal shift. Liquid aspirates tend to produce segmental rather than lobar signs, affect the right lung more than the left, and produce a burn-like injury to the lung parenchyma. Increased airways resistance, decreased lung compliance, and pulmonary edema may develop.

Gastrointestinal Bypass and Pregnancy

A pregnant patient with a jejunoileal bypass poses special problems. The overall capacity for nutrient and mineral absorption is drastically reduced because of anatomic diversion and decreased transit time. The overall absorption of fat is reduced 30 to 80 per cent, with profound effects on water and electrolyte absorption. Serum triglycerides, cholesterol, calcium, magnesium, and fat-soluble vitamins (A, D, E, and K) are usually low. Hepatic dysfunction may occur as a result of deposition of fat in the liver parenchyma. Dietary counseling is aimed at emphasizing the need for the pregnant patient to ingest enough calories and nutrients to avoid weight loss and mineral and vitamin deficiency. If this conservative approach fails, total parenteral nutrition is recommended.

The outcome of pregnancy in patients with a jejunoileal bypass is usually good, provided that specific metabolic and nutritional deficiencies are corrected. Currently, jejunoileal bypass surgery is rarely done. It has been replaced by gastric stapling procedures, which are tolerated well during pregnancy.

Chronic Inflammatory Bowel Disease

The two entities described under this disorder are Crohn's disease (regional enteritis) and ulcerative colitis. In about 25 per cent of patients with inflammatory bowel disease, differentiation between these two disorders is difficult.

Patients with inflammatory bowel disease do well during pregnancy, provided that there are no acute exacerbations. It seems unlikely that the natural history of the disease changes during pregnancy. Patients with regional enteritis are thought to have higher rates of abortion and fetal loss than normal individuals or patients with ulcerative colitis. This difference might be related to the fact that patients with regional enteritis are usually thin and debilitated.

Treatment

Treatment of an acute exacerbation of inflammatory bowel disease is the same for pregnant and nonpregnant patients, although some of the more experimental drugs should not be used during pregnancy. If diarrhea is the main complaint, dietary restriction of lactose, fruits, and vegetables is necessary. If a lactose-free diet is used, calcium supplementation is needed. Constipating agents, such as Pepto-Bismol and psyllium hydrophilic mucilloid (Metamucil), may be used daily and are quite effective. The use of diphenoxylate/atropine (Lomotil) or loperamide (Imodium) should be restricted to patients in whom conservative management fails. For those patients with mild to moderate symptoms, sulfasalazine may be beneficial. Although its action is not well understood, current views suggest that it inhibits prostaglandin synthesis. The usual daily dose is 2 to 12 gm, although lower dosage is recommended during pregnancy. Initial studies suggested that sulfasalazine might induce neonatal kernicterus, so its use during the third trimester of pregnancy and during breast feeding was not recommended. More recent studies suggest it is safe during both pregnancy and the postpartum period.

Steroid treatment is indicated when there is excessive weight loss, anorexia, partial intestinal obliteration, or persistent rectal bleeding. Prednisone, 20 to 40 mg daily, may be given and the dose tapered gradually when symptoms resolve. Other more experimental drugs, such as azathioprine and 6-mercaptopurine, should be avoided during pregnancy.

Patients with severe disease require hospitalization. Treatment strategies should be directed at relieving psychological stress, hydration, correction of iron-deficiency anemia by iron supplements or transfusions, increasing caloric intake (including utilization of the parenteral route), and enhancement of drug treatment.

HEPATIC DISORDERS

Liver disorders that are peculiar to pregnancy are discussed.

Intrahepatic Cholestasis of Pregnancy

Although the pathogenesis of this syndrome is not known, some distinctive features are present: (1) cholestasis and pruritus without other major liver dysfunction, (2) a tendency to recur with each pregnancy, (3) an association with oral contraceptives, and (4) a benign course in that there are no maternal hepatic sequelae. The disease may be inherited as an autosomal dominant disorder.

The main symptom in a patient with cholestasis of pregnancy is itching, which may occur early in pregnancy. Jaundice may be observed late in pregnancy, although it is rare. Laboratory tests are variable and of little help except for serum bile acid level, which is elevated.

Abdominal ultrasonography should be performed to exclude gallbladder obstruction, and liver enzymes should be assessed to exclude hepatitis.

Treatment

Treatment is partially effective in relieving the itching. Cholestyramine, which binds the bile acids in the gut, has been used with mixed results. The recommended dose is 12 gm per day (range 8 to 16 gm) taken in divided doses with meals. Since this resin binds fat-soluble vitamins (A, D, E, and K), oral daily supplements of vitamin K should be given. Phenobarbital to induce liver enzymes has been used in the treatment of this syndrome with a minor degree of success. Termination of pregnancy is the only effective cure. Itching disappears within hours or days of delivery.

Complications

Although this entity is benign in nature and leaves no maternal sequelae, the outcome of pregnancy is not as favorable. The incidence of prematurity and stillbirth is increased. At term, and especially during labor, prothrombin time should be checked. If prolonged, vitamin K should be given parenterally to decrease the risk of postpartum hemorrhage.

Acute Fatty Liver Atrophy

This is a very serious complication that is peculiar to pregnancy. It most commonly occurs in the third trimester of pregnancy or the early postpartum period. Although the etiology is unknown, many physicians tend to regard it as a form of severe hepatic toxemia. Presentation is variable, with abdominal pain, nausea and vomiting, jaundice, and increased irritability. Invariably these patients go into hepatic coma. Laboratory findings include an increase in PT and PTT, hyperbilirubinemia, hyperammonemia, and a moderate elevation of the transaminases. Hematemesis and spontaneous bleeding become manifest as the patient develops DIC.

Prognosis was once very poor, with about 80 per cent of patients dying while in a coma. With early recognition and immediate delivery, however, up to 72 per cent of these patients survive. Treatment is mainly directed at supportive measures such as intravenous fluids with 10 per cent glucose to prevent dehydration and severe hypoglycemia. For the coagulopathy of hepatic failure, vitamin K supplementation is not effective, and fresh frozen plasma or cryoprecipitate should be given. Survivors of liver failure have no hepatic sequelae. Even subsequent pregnancies in these patients have progressed well with no increased maternal or fetal risks.

SUGGESTED READING

Burrow GN, Ferris T (eds): Medical Complications in Pregnancy. Philadelphia, WB Saunders, 1982.

Creasy B, Resnik R: Maternal and Fetal Medicine. Philadelphia, WB Saunders, 1984.

Davison JM, Lindheimer M: Pregnancy in renal transplant recipients. J Reprod Med 27:613, 1982.

Gabbe S (guest editor): Obstetric ultrasound up-date. In Clinical Obstetrics and Gynecology. Vol. 31, no. 1, 1988.

Gabbe SG, Niebyl JR, Simpson JL (eds): Obstetrics, Normal and Problem Pregnancies, New York, Churchill Livingstone, 1986.

Garite TJ: Antepartum fetal surveillance. Clin Obstet and Gynecol 30(4):885, 1987.

Gilstrop LC III: Heart disease during pregnancy. Clin Obstet Gynecol 33(1), 1989.

Malkosian GD Jr, Moller KL, Aoro LA, et al: Miscellaneous medical complications. In Iffy L, Kaminelzky H (eds): Principles and Practice of Obstetrics and Perinatology. New York, Wiley, 1981.

Metcalfe J, AcAnultz JH, Ueland K (eds): Burwell and Metcalfe's Heart Disease and Pregnancy. Boston, Little, Brown, 1986.

Nuwayhid B, Brinkkman CR III, Lieb S (eds): Management of the Diabetic Pregnancy. New York, Elsevier, 1987.

Nineteen

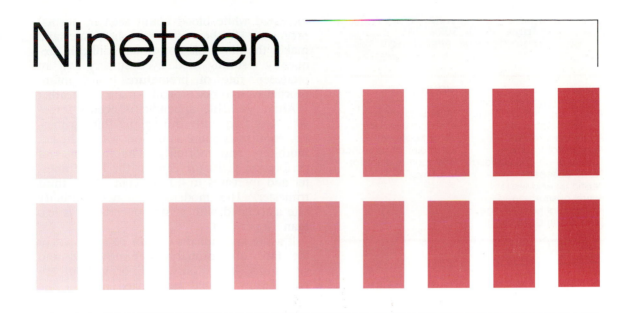

Surgical Conditions in Pregnancy

J. GEORGE MOORE

Pregnancy substantially enhances the problems associated with surgery. Physiologic changes and the altered immunologic responses of pregnancy change the diagnostic parameters of surgical diseases. Reluctance to operate during pregnancy may add to critical delays and increase the morbidity for both the fetus and the mother.

Common surgical conditions complicating pregnancy include acute appendicitis, acute cholecystitis, acute pancreatitis, and ovarian neoplasms (Table 19–1). Cancer of the breast, cervix, bowel, and skin are occasionally diagnosed during pregnancy and may require relatively urgent surgery.

The general approach to acute surgical conditions during pregnancy (e.g., acute appendicitis) is to manage the problem regardless of the pregnancy. Because of the possible teratogenic risk of anesthesia and the possi-

bility of inducing an abortion in the first trimester, surgery for some semi-urgent conditions (e.g., an ovarian neoplasm) is better delayed until the more stable second trimester. If the uterus is to be removed (e.g., stage Ib cervical cancer), surgery may be delayed in the interests of fetal maturity (see Chapter 55).

Generally, a surgical procedure in itself undertaken during pregnancy has very little effect on the pregnancy. The most common untoward outcome is related to peritonitis, which may result in premature delivery. Tocolytics and antibiotics may play an important adjuvant role.

ACUTE SURGICAL CONDITIONS

Acute nonobstetric surgical emergencies occur in all three trimesters of pregnancy.

223

Table 19-1. SURGICAL CONDITIONS IN PREGNANCY

ACUTE	NONEMERGENT
Acute appendicitis	Adnexal tumors
Acute cholecystitis	Cervical cancer
Acute pancreatitis	Breast cancer
Abdominal trauma	Gastrointestinal cancer
Torsion of uterine adnexae	Melanoma, osteosarcoma
Pelvic abscess	
Peptic ulcer disease	
Bowel obstruction	
Intracranial hemorrhage	
Thromboembolic disease	

The overall incidence is one per 500 pregnancies.

ACUTE APPENDICITIS

The incidence of acute appendicitis in pregnancy is one per 1500 gestations. The usual symptoms of acute appendicitis, such as epigastric pain, nausea, vomiting, and lower abdominal pain, are not uncommon during normal pregnancy. Hence, the diagnosis is often difficult, and the differential diagnosis may be especially confusing (Table 19–2). The enlarging uterus displaces the appendix superiorly and laterally as pregnancy progresses so the point of maximal tenderness also rises and may be masked by the overlying uterus and broad ligament (Fig. 19–1). Tenderness and guarding are elicited more laterally than expected. The somewhat

Table 19-2. DIFFERENTIAL DIAGNOSIS OF ACUTE APPENDICITIS IN PREGNANCY

Ruptured corpus luteum
Pyelonephritis
Ectopic pregnancy
Acute mesenteric lymphadenitis
Regional enteritis (Crohn's disease)
Salpingo-ovarian abscess
Acute mesenteric thrombosis

increased white blood count seen in normal pregnancy further confuses the issue and makes the diagnosis notoriously difficult, frequently resulting in delayed surgery and an increased rate of premature labor, infant morbidity, and occasionally, maternal death.

Although acute appendicitis occurs somewhat less frequently during the third trimester, rupture is more common with a higher morbidity and mortality. The incidence of perforation is 10 per cent in the first trimester and increases to 40 per cent in the third trimester. The modern perinatal mortality rate associated with acute appendicitis is less than 10 per cent.

If acute appendicitis cannot be ruled out in the face of reasonably definite signs and symptoms, laparotomy with or without appendectomy should be carried out. In the first trimester with a fairly certain diagnosis, a McBurney or a transverse or Rocky-Davis incision is employed. If the diagnosis is equivocal, a right paramedian incision should be made to allow a more extensive exploration. If acute appendicitis is encountered late in pregnancy, appendectomy should be carried out without a concurrent cesarean section. Appropriate antibiotics along with the judicious use of tocolytics should be employed postoperatively. If labor does occur with a recent laparotomy incision, it can be managed quite well with epidural anesthesia and shortening of the second stage of labor with a low forceps delivery.

Abdominal pain and tenderness with nausea or vomiting in pregnancy should be carefully evaluated, and laparotomy should not be delayed if acute appendicitis cannot be ruled out.

ACUTE CHOLECYSTITIS AND CHOLELITHIASIS

An increase in serum cholesterol and lipids in pregnancy, along with biliary stasis, leads to a higher incidence of cholelithiasis, biliary obstruction, and cholecystitis. The high levels of estrogens in pregnancy increase the saturation of cholesterol in the bile. Virtually all of the gallstones associated with pregnancy are composed of crystallized cholesterol. The incidence of hospitalization for cholecystitis in pregnancy is 1 to 2 per cent; one in 2000

Figure 19–1. The changing position of the right colon and appendix as pregnancy progresses.

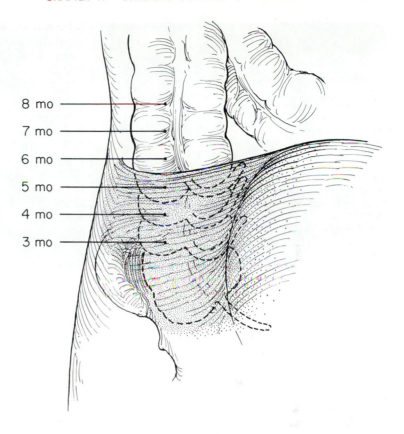

8 mo

7 mo

6 mo

5 mo

4 mo

3 mo

pregnant women require cholecystectomy. In more recent years, ultrasonography has revealed a fairly high incidence of cholelithiasis in pregnancy (4 per cent), and the incidence of cholecystectomy in pregnancy has appreciably increased.

Nausea and vomiting, along with right upper quadrant tenderness and guarding, generally suggest biliary tract disease. In the third trimester, the large uterus may make it difficult to evaluate any tenderness and guarding. An increasing white blood cell count with slightly elevated alkaline phosphatase and bilirubin levels or jaundice along with the presence of stones or increased thickness of the gallbladder wall on ultrasonography (Fig. 19–2) serve to authenticate the diagnosis. Parenteral fluids, gastric decompression, and dietary management should be the primary approach to management. Fifty per cent of patients with cholelithiasis are asymptomatic, and the severity of biliary colic varies considerably.

The nausea and vomiting, leukocytosis, and somewhat increased alkaline phosphatase

of normal pregnancy serve to make the diagnosis more difficult. Pernicious nausea and vomiting of pregnancy and viral hepatitis must be considered in the differential diagnosis. Markedly elevated serum glutamic-oxaloacetic transaminase and serum glutamate pyruvate transaminase levels (above 200), especially without leukocytosis, should suggest viral hepatitis and mitigate against the diagnosis of acute cholecystitis. Generally, cholecystitis can be managed medically in pregnancy, but if symptoms and signs persist with progressive peritonitis, cholecystectomy is indicated.

ACUTE PANCREATITIS

Generally, pancreatitis is associated with cholecystitis, cholelithiasis, or acute alcoholism, but occasionally it is idiopathic (Table 19–3). Acute pancreatitis is seen less often in pregnancy, probably because the age-related contributing factors of alcoholism and cholelithiasis are more common later in life, but

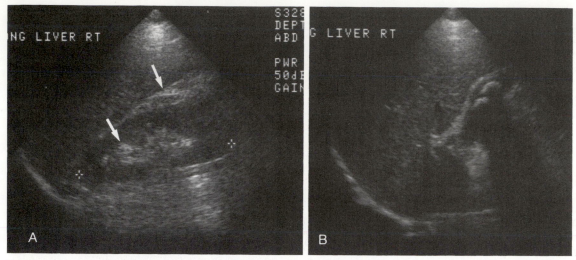

Figure 19–2. Ultrasound photo showing cholelithiasis and cholecystitis in the third trimester of pregnancy. Arrows show gallstones and the thickened gallbladder wall.

mortality from pancreatitis is significantly higher when it does occur in pregnancy. As noted in Table 19–4, some drugs not uncommonly prescribed in pregnancy are associated with acute pancreatitis.

The prime symptom is severe, noncolicky epigastric pain radiating to the high back, relieved somewhat by leaning forward. Nausea and vomiting generally are present but initially may not be prominent. Upper abdominal guarding may be difficult to assess in late pregnancy because of muscular tightness occasioned by the enlarging uterus. An elevated serum amylase level (>200 U/dl, or urinary amylase excretion exceeding 300

units/hour) generally confirms the diagnosis, although cholecystitis, peptic ulcer, and diabetic ketoacidosis may also be associated with less marked elevations of serum amylase.

Generally, the disease is self-limiting and responds within 1 to 10 days to bed rest, parenteral fluids, pain relief, and nasogastric suction. Any complications must be managed as they arise. In the occasional patient, the disease may become severe and protracted, with extensive pancreatic edema and autodigestion, massive ascites, fever, and paralytic ileus. In such cases, the mortality is high and may require peritoneal lavage, operative drainage, partial pancreatic resection, or some combination of these procedures.

Table 19–3. RISK FACTORS ASSOCIATED WITH ACUTE PANCREATITIS

Alcohol abuse
Cholecystitis and cholelithiasis
Abdominal trauma
Infectious disease: mumps, hepatitis
Elevated lipids
Drugs: steroids, isoniazid, diuretics
Familial: pancreatitis
Rare: Ischemic vascular disease, systemic lupus erythematosis

Table 19–4. DRUGS ASSOCIATED WITH ACUTE PANCREATITIS

Thiazide diuretics
Furosemide
Acetaminophen
Isoniazid
Rifampin
Tetracycline
Propoxyphene
Clonidine

PEPTIC ULCER

Peptic ulcer is uncommon in pregnant women. It generally occurs in men and older women, but when it does occur in younger women, the symptoms tend to lessen during pregnancy. Several factors such as the decreased gastric motility and the relative achlorhydria of pregnancy may account for this effect. Another ameliorating factor may be the increase in histaminase secreted by the placenta.

The symptoms of peptic ulcer, as in the nonpregnant patient, are epigastric pain, nausea and vomiting, and occasionally hematemesis. Persistent bleeding may result in anemia and melena. Diagnosis does not vary appreciably from that in nonpregnant patients, although diagnostic irradiation must be minimized with more reliance on endoscopic procedures. When marked abdominal guarding and generalized board-like rigidity are noted, perforation should be strongly suspected. An upright abdominal x-ray film should be obtained to detect free air under the diaphragm.

Treatment consists mainly of antacids (e.g., Gelusil, Maalox, Mylanta), taking care to avoid preparations that deplete calcium or provide excessive sodium. After the first trimester, anticholinergic drugs or even histamine antagonists (e.g., cimetidine) may be used in refractory cases, although the latter does not have Food and Drug Administration (FDA) approval for use in pregnancy.

If perforation or substantial bleeding occurs, corrective surgery must not be delayed. Massive hemorrhage can lead to hypotension, which is a threat to the fetus. If endoscopic or embolic procedures do not control the bleeding or if perforation occurs, an emergency laparotomy is indicated.

BOWEL OBSTRUCTION

Bowel obstruction in pregnancy is most often associated with postoperative adhesions, although volvulus and intussusception are rare causes. It generally occurs in late pregnancy associated with traction on adhesions as the uterus enlarges. The nausea and vomiting often seen in early pregnancy may confuse the issue, but the more colicky character of the pain along with abdominal tenderness, distention and abnormal peristalsis are very helpful in making the diagnosis. An upright x-ray film of the abdomen showing characteristic dilated loops of bowel and air-fluid levels serves to confirm the obstruction.

Management does not differ from that in the nonpregnant patient. Nasogastric suction should be instituted and fluid and electrolyte balance carefully monitored. If the obstruction does not resolve after 48 to 96 hours, an exploratory laparotomy should be carried out through an appropriate incision (usually a right or left paramedian incision). The appropriate surgical procedure should be carried out without disturbing the uterus. If uterine contractions occur postoperatively, tocolytics should be employed.

ADNEXAL TORSION

Torsion of the uterine adnexae tends to occur more commonly in pregnancy, possibly because their supporting ligaments elongate as the gestation progresses. Ovarian tumors (e.g., cystic teratomas, corpus luteum cysts) may become ischemic if their vascular pedicles undergo torsion. Such ischemic events are usually heralded by the sudden onset of severe abdominal pain, which may radiate to the flank and down the anterior thigh.

During the first and early second trimesters, a mass is usually felt on pelvic examination or is visualized by ultrasonography. Later in the pregnancy it may be impossible to palpate a mass clinically. There may be a low-grade fever, leukocytosis, and serum creatine phosphokinase levels may be elevated depending on the extent of the infarction. The most likely differential diagnoses include ectopic pregnancy and hemorrhagic corpus luteum, both of which seldom occur beyond 10 to 12 gestational weeks.

Although the pain may diminish somewhat after 24 hours, removal of the infarcted organ is indicated. If the excised ovary contains the corpus luteum, progesterone supplementation is generally necessary prior to 6 to 8 weeks gestation.

PELVIC ABSCESS

Tubo-ovarian infections are rare in pregnancy, probably because thick cervical mucus and the gestational sac block the ascent of lower genital tract infections. Occasionally, tubo-ovarian abscesses do occur, and if the process extends with progressive peritonitis, drainage is in order. The abscess is best drained extraperitoneally through a McBurney or flank incision, or if necessary the tubo-ovarian abscess may be excised transperitoneally as a salpingo-oophorectomy. In such circumstances, the prognosis for continuation of the pregnancy is poor.

ABDOMINAL TRAUMA

By far the most common abdominal trauma in pregnancy occurs in automobile accidents. Abruptio placentae, uterine contusions, and fetal skull fractures may result. Abruptio placentae is treated expectantly unless fetal monitoring indicates distress, in which case immediate abdominal delivery is in order if the fetus is at a reasonably safe gestational age (28 weeks or greater). Abdominal exploration may be necessary to stop bleeding and repair uterine lacerations. Lap-shoulder harness seat belts rather than lap belts are advisable for pregnant women after 12 weeks gestation.

Gunshot wounds of the abdomen are treated as in nonpregnant patients, with measures taken to stop bleeding and repair visceral or uterine injuries. As long as the pregnancy is intact, the uterus should not be disturbed. Careful monitoring of fetal well-being should be maintained before and after the operation.

INTRACRANIAL HEMORRHAGE

Intracranial hemorrhage is most commonly associated with hypertensive episodes during pregnancy and is generally managed by medical measures directed toward reducing the blood pressure and alleviating intracranial pressure, rather than by surgical intervention. Rupture of a congenital intracranial aneurysm, however, may present an acute surgical emergency during pregnancy. Symptoms and signs are those of a subarachnoid hemorrhage, with severe headache, nuchal rigidity, papilledema, bradycardia, and coma. The diagnosis is made by computed tomographic scan. Efforts should be made initially to reduce intracranial pressure (diuretics, burr holes, or both), and at an appropriate interval, craniotomy and surgical occlusion of the aneurysm must be carried out. Every effort must be made to maintain cardiovascular integrity of the mother and oxygenation of the fetus.

Following a subarachnoid hemorrhage or repair of an intracranial aneurysm, vaginal delivery is usually recommended, although some authorities would opt for cesarean section. If vaginal delivery is planned, every effort should be made to keep pushing to a minimum by using epidural anesthesia and low forceps delivery.

PULMONARY EMBOLUS

Deep venous thrombosis and pulmonary embolism in pregnancy are generally treated medically with heparin, as discussed in Chapter 18. Occasionally pregnant patients develop repeat pulmonary emboli while on full heparin anticoagulation. On such occasions, percutaneous placement of a filter or umbrella into the vena cava is indicated. Occasionally, it may be necessary to perform a laparotomy with vena caval and ovarian vein ligation. In most instances, both mother and fetus tolerate the procedure well.

NONEMERGENT SURGICAL CONDITIONS IN PREGNANCY

Ovarian Tumors

Adnexal masses are not at all uncommon in pregnancy and can best be identified by pelvic examination early in the pregnancy. Most of these ovarian masses are functional cysts (e.g., corpus luteal cysts) and regress as the gonadotropin levels fall during the second trimester. All adnexal masses should be evaluated by ultrasonography. Solid ovarian tumors larger than 5 cm or cystic tumors larger than 10 cm deserve exploration without undue delay. Cystic tumors 6 cm or less should be followed into the second trimester and removed if they persist. The incidence of ovarian carcinoma in pregnancy is one in 5000.

Breast Cancer

Breast cancer in pregnancy is managed much the same as in the nonpregnant patient. Survival rates, stage for stage, are essentially the same as in the nonpregnant patient. If estrogen receptors are present, therapeutic abortion should be considered.

Bowel Cancer

Bowel cancer, usually colorectal cancer, is fairly uncommon in pregnancy. Diagnosis is suggested by hematochezia and a positive stool guaiac test and is confirmed by biopsy at colonoscopy. Management by surgical resection does not differ from that in the nonpregnant patient.

Cervical Cancer

The diagnosis of cervical cancer in pregnancy is often delayed because the bleeding is attributed to some pregnancy-related cause (e.g., threatened abortion). All patients should have a Papanicolaou smear at the first antenatal visit, and all patients with vaginal bleeding during pregnancy should have a speculum examination to allow visualization of the cervix. The management of this condition is discussed in Chapter 54.

Melanoma

Melanoma growth may be enhanced during pregnancy because of the increased melanocytic stimulating hormone present. In addition, some melanomas have been shown to contain estrogen receptors. Treatment is generally by wide local excision, although some would recommend regional lymph node resection. In the first trimester, therapeutic abortion is generally recommended if the tumor contains estrogen receptors. Maternal melanomas have been observed to spread to the placenta and the fetus.

Osteogenic Sarcoma

Osteogenic sarcoma occasionally is diagnosed in pregnancy and is treated as in the nonpregnant state with surgery and perhaps therapeutic abortion. If chemotherapy is required in the first trimester, therapeutic abortion is indicated.

SUGGESTED READING

American College of Obstetrics and Gynecology: Trauma During Pregnancy. ACOG Technical Bulletin 161. Washington, DC, November, 1991.

Block P, Kelly TR: Management of gallstone pancreatitis during pregnancy and the postpartum period. Surg Gynecol Obstet 168:426, 1989.

Cope Z: The Early Diagnosis of the Acute Abdomen. London, Oxford University Press, 1940.

Hess LW, Peaseman A, O'Brien WF: Adnexal mass occurring with an intrauterine pregnancy: A report of 54 cases requiring laparotomy for definitive management. Am J Obstet Gynecol 158:1029, 1988.

McKay AJ, O'Neill J, Imrie CW: Pancreatitis, pregnancy and gallstones. Br J Obstet Gynaecol 87:47, 1980.

Nakhegivany KB, Clark LE: Acute appendicitis in women of childbearing age. Arch Surg 121:1053, 1986.

Stauffer RA, Adams A, Wygal J, Labery JP: Gall bladder disease in pregnancy. Am J Obstet Gynecol 144:661, 1982.

Thornton JG, Wells M: Ovarian cysts in pregnancy: Does ultrasound make traditional management inappropriate. Obstet Gynecol 69:717, 1987.

Whitworth CM, Whitworth PW, Sanfillipo J, et al: Value of diagnostic laparoscopy in young women with possible appendicitis. Surg Gynecol Obstet 167:187, 1988.

Twenty

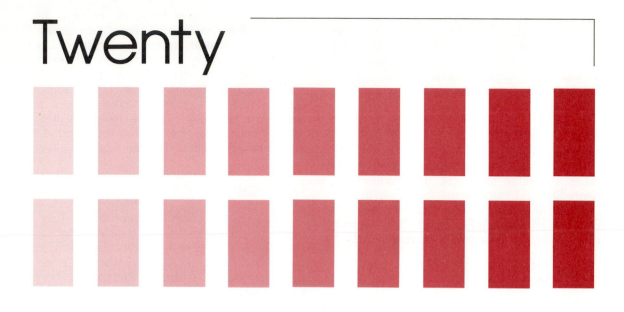

Fetal Malpresentations

JAMES R. SHIELDS AND ARNOLD L. MEDEARIS

Malpresentation occurs when the fetus presents in any manner other than vertex. This includes breech, face, brow, shoulder, and compound presentations. Both fetal and maternal factors contribute to the occurrence of malpresentation. The most common type of malpresentation is breech.

BREECH PRESENTATION

Breech presentation occurs when the fetal buttocks or lower extremities present into the maternal pelvis. The incidence of breech presentation is 3 per cent of all deliveries. Prior to 28 weeks, approximately 25 per cent of fetuses are breech in presentation. As the fetus grows and occupies more of the uterus, it tends to assume a vertex presentation to accommodate best to the confines and shape of the uterus. By 34 weeks gestation, most fetuses will have assumed the vertex presentation.

Etiology

The major predisposing factor toward breech presentation is prematurity. Approximately 20 to 30 per cent of all singleton breeches are of low birth weight (less than 2500 gm). The incidence of congenital anomalies with breech presentations is in excess of 6 per cent, which is two to three times that of vertex presentations. Fetal anomalies may restrict the ability of the fetus to assume a vertex presentation. Common congenital anomalies associated with breech presentation include anencephaly and hydrocephalus, in both of which the form, function, or movement of the fetus may be affected. Other etiologic factors include uterine anomalies,

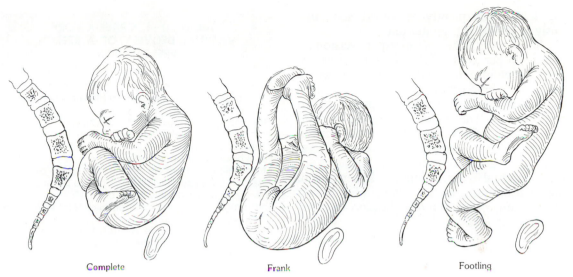

Complete   Frank   Footling

Figure 20–1. Types of breech presentation.

multiple gestation, placenta previa, hydramnios, contracted maternal pelvis, and pelvic tumors that obstruct the birth canal.

Classification

There are three types of breech presentation: frank, complete, and incomplete (Fig. 20–1). Frank breech occurs when both fetal thighs are flexed and both lower extremities are extended at the knees. Complete breech is represented when both fetal thighs are flexed and one or both knees are flexed. An incomplete (or footling) breech occurs when one or both fetal thighs are extended and one or both knees or feet lie below the buttocks. With term gestations, 65 per cent of breech presentations are frank, 25 per cent are complete, and 10 per cent are incomplete.

Diagnosis

The diagnosis of breech presentation can often be made by the Leopold examination (see Chapter 8), in which the fetal head may be palpated in the fundal region and the softer breech occupies the lower uterine segment above the symphysis pubis. Vaginal examination enables palpation of the fetal buttocks, anus, sacrum, and ischial tuberosi-

ties with a frank breech. With a complete breech, it is possible to palpate one or both feet alongside the fetal buttocks. Vaginal examination of an incomplete breech reveals one or both fetal feet as the presenting part(s).

The diagnosis may be facilitated by radiography or sonography. It may be easier to establish the type of breech presentation with an anteroposterior x-ray film of the maternal abdomen and pelvis. Sonography, however, has the advantage of being better suited for the detection of fetal anomalies, which must be ruled out in any patient with a breech presentation.

Management During Pregnancy

External cephalic version may be attempted when a breech presentation is diagnosed before the onset of labor and after 37 weeks gestation. This procedure involves the use of an intravenous tocolytic agent such as ritodrine to relax the uterus and transabdominal manipulation of the fetus under ultrasonic guidance. The aim of this undertaking is to elevate the breech out of the maternal pelvis while guiding the fetal head into the pelvis, thus attaining a vertex presentation. Version should not be carried out prior to 37 weeks gestation because of the tendency for the fetus subsequently to revert spontaneously to a breech presentation.

The success rate of external version is about 75 per cent. The procedure must be carried out in a hospital that is equipped to perform an emergency cesarean section, since the major risk is placental abruption or cord compression. The patient should have nothing by mouth for 8 hours prior to the version attempt in case emergency delivery is necessary with general anesthesia. Evidence of uteroplacental insufficiency, hypertension, oligohydramnios, or a history of previous uterine surgery is a contraindication to external cephalic version.

Mechanism of Labor

The mechanism of labor with a breech presentation differs markedly from that of a vertex presentation. Engagement and descent of the breech usually occur in one of the oblique diameters of the maternal pelvis. Once the posterior hip encounters the pelvic floor, internal rotation occurs to bring the anterior hip under the pubic arch. At this point, the bitrochanteric diameter occupies the anteroposterior diameter of the pelvic outlet.

After internal rotation, the anterior hip delivers, followed by the posterior hip, legs, and feet. Subsequent external rotation with the back rotating anteriorly brings the shoulders into the oblique diameter of the inlet. The shoulders then descend, and internal rotation occurs to bring them into the anteroposterior diameter of the pelvic outlet. After delivery of the shoulders, the fetal head enters the pelvis in a flexed position in one of the oblique diameters of the pelvic inlet. Internal rotation brings the posterior aspect of the neck under the symphysis, and the head then delivers in a flexed position.

Management During Labor

Vaginal Delivery

The intrapartum management of a breech presentation depends on the maternal pelvis, the type of breech, and the gestational age.

Table 20–1. CRITERIA FOR VAGINAL DELIVERY OF A BREECH PRESENTATION

Fetus must be in a frank or complete breech presentation

Gestational age must be at least 36 wk

Estimated fetal weight should be between 2500 and 3800 gm

Fetal head must be flexed

Maternal pelvis must be adequately large, as assessed by x-ray pelvimetry or tested by prior delivery of a reasonably large baby

There must be no other maternal or fetal indication for cesarean section

Anesthesiologist must be in attendance

Obstetrician must be experienced

Assistant must be scrubbed and prepared to guide the fetal head into the pelvis

The standard of care in most communities is to deliver all breech presentations routinely by cesarean section to avoid the increased perinatal morbidity and mortality that occur with vaginal delivery secondary to umbilical cord prolapse, birth asphyxia, and birth trauma. The concept of delivering all breeches by cesarean section, however, has been questioned by the Consensus Conference on Cesarean Childbirth. The incidence of umbilical cord prolapse with frank breech presentations approaches that for vertex presentations, so the management of the term frank breech is controversial.

Strict criteria for allowing a trial of labor and vaginal delivery of a term breech are summarized in Table 20–1. These are directed toward minimizing the possibility of umbilical cord prolapse, dystoria, birth trauma, and asphyxia.

The problems associated with a prolapsed cord can be minimized by continuous electronic fetal heart monitoring and the capability of a "crash" cesarean section. Sonography must be performed to exclude the presence of fetal anomalies. If a fetal anomaly is found that is incompatible with life, such as anencephaly, the patient should not be delivered by cesarean section. On the other hand, if an anomaly is found that would predispose the fetus to trauma if delivered vaginally, such as an omphalocele, delivery should be accomplished by cesarean section. Using these criteria, term frank and complete breeches may be delivered vaginally without affecting the perinatal mortality rate. There is a greater incidence of birth trauma, however, particularly brachial plexus injuries, in fetuses delivered vaginally, especially if the baby is large.

There are three types of vaginal breech delivery. *Spontaneous breech delivery* occurs when the fetus delivers spontaneously without any manipulation by the obstetrician other than that of supporting the fetus. With a *partial (or assisted) breech extraction,* the fetus is allowed to deliver spontaneously until the fetal umbilicus is at the introitus (i.e., the cord is compressed) at which point the remainder of the fetus is extracted. A *total breech extraction* occurs when the obstetrician extracts the entire body of the fetus. The preferred method of vaginal delivery is the partial breech extraction, although total breech extraction is often used for delivery of the second twin.

Partial Breech Extraction

Once the fetus has delivered spontaneously to the umbilicus (Fig. 20–2), the thumbs of the obstetrician are placed over the fetal sacrum and the fingers over the fetal hips. Gentle downward traction is exerted until the scapulas appear at the introitus. After delivery of the scapulas, the anterior axilla becomes visible, and, at this time, the shoulders are ready to deliver. By rotating the trunk, such that the bisacromial diameter is in the anteroposterior plane, the anterior shoulder and arm will usually deliver first. Subsequent rotation of the trunk in the opposite direction will facilitate delivery of the other shoulder. If the shoulders do not deliver by trunk rotation, the posterior arm and shoulder are delivered by splinting the fetal elbow with the fingers and sweeping the arm across the fetal chest. Subsequent gentle downward traction on the fetal trunk will then facilitate delivery of the other shoulder and arm. Occasionally, one or both arms are located around the back of the neck (nuchal arm). Delivery in this instance may be facilitated by rotation of the trunk through 180 degrees. Should rotation of the fetus fail to deliver the nuchal arm, it may have to be forcibly extracted, and fracture of the humerus or clavicle may result.

Once the shoulders have been delivered, the head is delivered using either the Mauriceau-Smellie-Veit maneuver or Piper forceps. With the Mauriceau-Smellie-Veit maneuver, the child is straddled over one forearm. The obstetrician places the index and ring fingers on the fetal maxilla and the middle finger in the mouth to maintain flexion of the head. The other hand is placed over the shoulders so that the middle finger presses upward on the occiput to aid flexion while the index and ring fingers apply traction to the shoulders. Employing this maneuver, the fetal neck is kept in a flexed position and delivery of the head is accomplished by gentle downward traction. Suprapubic pressure by an assistant will help to maintain flexion of the fetal head. Some obstetricians use Piper forceps routinely, since this method has been shown to effect delivery of the head with the least amount of trauma to the fetus.

Cesarean Section

Premature breeches are generally delivered by cesarean section because of the large disparity between the size of the fetal head and that of the fetal trunk, the head being much larger. Therefore, if labor and vaginal delivery occur, successively larger parts of the fetus deliver, with the largest part, the fetal head, delivering last. The fetal lower extremities, abdomen, and trunk may deliver through an incompletely dilated cervix, with the larger head becoming trapped against the cervix. When this occurs, the umbilical cord may be compressed in the birth canal. This may lead to fetal asphyxia, and birth trauma may occur in an attempt to deliver the head rapidly, which has no time to mold to the shape of the maternal pelvis.

With incomplete term breeches, delivery should be accomplished by cesarean section for two reasons. First, the incidence of umbilical cord prolapse is about 10 per cent for these types of breeches, as opposed to about 2 per cent for a frank breech. Second, the fetal lower extremities, abdomen, and trunk may deliver through an incompletely dilated

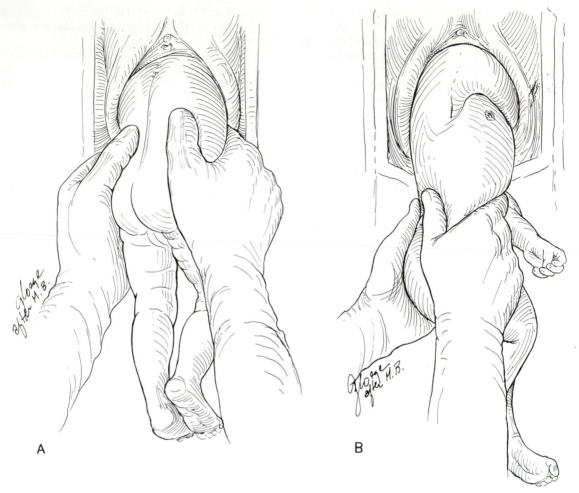

Figure 20–2. Partial breech extraction. *A,* After spontaneous delivery to the umbilicus, traction is applied to the infant's pelvis. When the scapulae are visible, rotation of the trunk allows delivery of the anterior shoulder. *B,* Delivery of the anterior shoulder by downward traction.

cervix, resulting in entrapment of the aftercoming head against the cervix.

Complications and Outcome

Perinatal morbidity and mortality are increased with breech presentation. The perinatal mortality of all breech fetuses is approximately 25 per 1000 live births, versus two to three for nonbreeches. When prematurity and multiple gestation are excluded, the perinatal mortality for breeches is still about four times that of nonbreeches. At least two series have shown, however, that when strict screening criteria are satisfied, breech mortality rates for vaginal delivery and cesarean section do not differ significantly.

Factors that contribute to the increased perinatal morbidity and mortality include lethal congenital anomalies, birth trauma, and birth anoxia. Birth anoxia usually results from compression of the umbilical cord secondary to cord prolapse during labor or entrapment of the aftercoming head during vaginal delivery. Birth trauma usually occurs with vaginal delivery as opposed to cesarean section and generally results from forceful traction being placed on the fetus. Fetal organs most likely to be injured are the

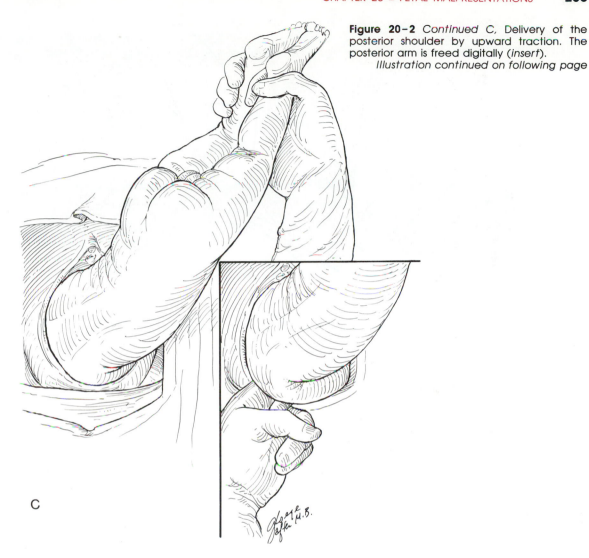

Figure 20–2 *Continued C,* Delivery of the posterior shoulder by upward traction. The posterior arm is freed digitally (*insert*).
Illustration continued on following page

C

brain, spinal cord, liver, adrenal glands, and spleen. Other sites of injury include the brachial plexus, pharynx, bladder, and sternocleidomastoid muscle. Maternal mortality and morbidity are increased with breech presentation secondary to the widespread use of cesarean section as the mode of delivery.

FACE PRESENTATION

Face presentation occurs when the fetal head is hyperextended such that the fetal face, between the chin and orbits, is the presenting part. The incidence is about one in 500 deliveries.

Etiology

Controversy exists as to the etiologic factors. Normally, the attitude of the fetal head is one of flexion because of the greater tone of the flexor muscles in the neck. It is generally agreed that high maternal parity may predispose to hyperextension of the fetal neck in that the pendulous maternal abdomen and unengaged fetal head allow the back of the fetus to sag forward in the same direction as

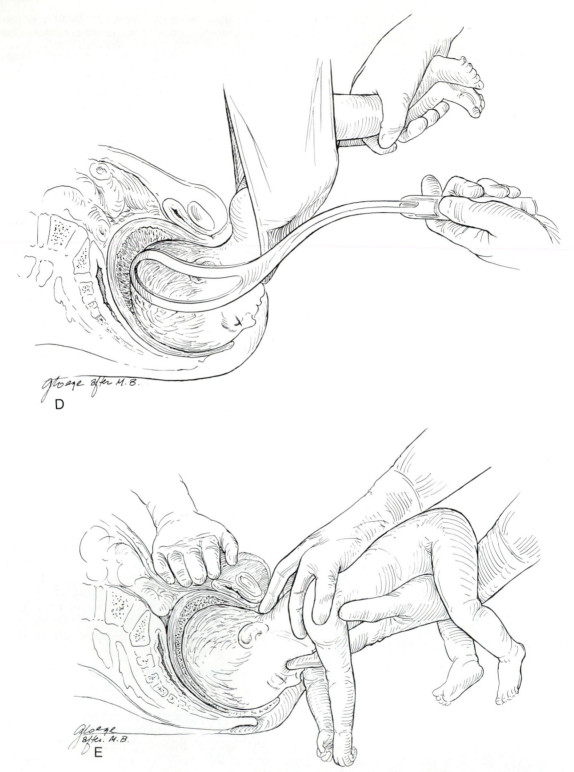

Figure 20–2 *Continued D,* Delivery of the aftercoming head using Piper forceps. *E,* Delivery of the aftercoming head using the Mauriceau-Smellie-Veit maneuver. Every effort is made to maintain flexion of the head.

the occiput. Other factors that may predispose to hyperextension of the fetal neck that are not universally agreed on include a contracted maternal pelvis and fetal macrosomia. Most authorities are of the opinion that the hyperextension is intrinsic to the fetus.

Diagnosis

The diagnosis of a face presentation may be made by Leopold examination, the fetal cephalic prominence lying on the same side as the spine with a deep groove between them. In reality, the diagnosis is usually made at the time of vaginal examination during labor with palpation of the fetal mouth, nose, malar bones, and orbital ridges. Such a presentation may be confirmed by sonography or radiography if sonography is not available. Since anencephalic fetuses in the cephalic presentation, by definition, present face first, anencephaly must be ruled out when a face presentation is suspected.

Mechanism of Labor

The position of the presenting face is classified according to the location of the fetal chin (mentum). Approximately 60 per cent of face presentations are mentoanterior at the time of diagnosis, whereas 15 per cent are mentotransverse and 25 per cent mentoposterior. The mechanism of labor with a face presentation is such that the submentobregmatic diameter presents into the maternal pelvis. This is the same length as the suboccipitobregmatic diameter that presents with vertex presentations (see Chapter 10). Labor occurs by internal rotation, which places the fetal chin under the symphysis with delivery occurring by subsequent flexion of the head (Fig. 20–3). The chin and mouth appear at the vulva initially, followed by the nose, eyes, and brow.

Management and Outcome

The intrapartum management of a face presentation is expectant, since about 75 per cent deliver by normal spontaneous delivery or low forceps. Vaginal delivery can occur only once the head rotates to a mentoanterior position. With a persistent mentoposterior position, vaginal delivery cannot occur because the mentum would have to deliver under the symphysis by extension, and the fetal neck is already hyperextended.

Approximately half of the mentoposterior presentations will spontaneously rotate to a mentoanterior position. The majority of mentotransverse presentations will also rotate spontaneously to a mentoanterior position. Face presentation is not a contraindication to augmentation of labor with pitocin.

Cesarean section is indicated when dilatation and descent do not progress despite adequate uterine activity, as occurs with persistent mentotransverse or mentoposterior positions. Midpelvic delivery by vacuum or forceps and maneuvers to attempt to convert the face presentation to a vertex presentation are contraindicated, since they result in increased perinatal morbidity and mortality. When delivered by spontaneous vaginal delivery or low forceps (Fig. 20–4), perinatal morbidity and mortality for face presentations are similar to those for vertex presentations.

BROW PRESENTATION

Brow presentation occurs when the presenting part of the fetus is between the facial orbits and anterior fontanelle (Fig. 20–5). This type of presentation arises as the result of extension of the fetal head such that it is midway between flexion (vertex presentation) and hyperextension (face presentation). The incidence is about one in 1400 deliveries. With a brow presentation, the presenting diameter is the supraoccipitomental, which is much longer than the presenting diameter for a face or a vertex presentation (see Chapter 10).

Etiology

The etiology is the same as that for face presentation. The brow presentation is usually unstable or transitional and probably occurs when the head is in the process of converting from a vertex to a face presentation or vice versa.

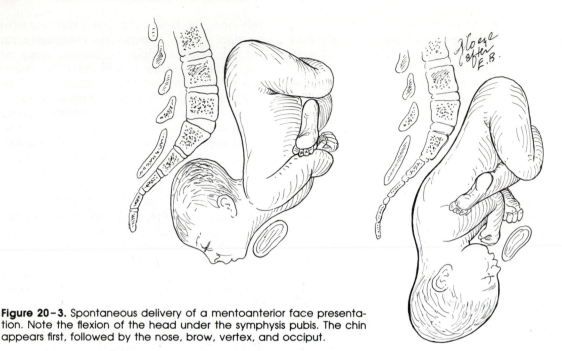

Figure 20–3. Spontaneous delivery of a mentoanterior face presentation. Note the flexion of the head under the symphysis pubis. The chin appears first, followed by the nose, brow, vertex, and occiput.

Diagnosis

The diagnosis of a brow presentation can be made by Leopold examination, with the examiner being able to palpate both the fetal chin and occiput. As with face presentation, the diagnosis is usually made by vaginal examination during labor by palpating the anterior fontanelle, orbital ridges, and eyes. The position of the presenting part is classified according to the location of the brow (frontum).

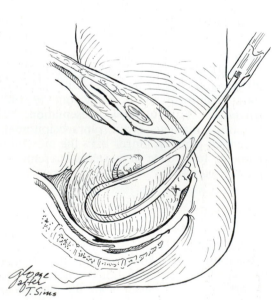

Figure 20–4. Simpson forceps applied to a mentoanterior face presentation.

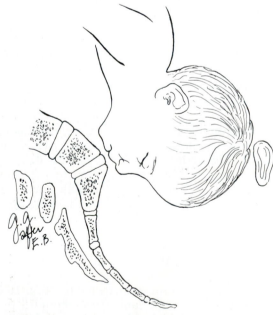

Figure 20–5. Brow presentation. Note the large presenting diameter (supraoccipitomental).

Management and Outcome

The intrapartum management is expectant. As mentioned previously, the brow presentation is an unstable one. Fifty to 75 per cent will convert to either a face presentation, through extension, or a vertex presentation, through flexion, and will subsequently deliver vaginally. With a persistent brow presentation, the large presenting diameter makes vaginal delivery impossible, unless the fetus is very small or the maternal pelvis very large, and delivery must be accomplished by cesarean section. There is an increased incidence of both prolonged labor (30 to 50 per cent) and dysfunctional labor (30 per cent). As with face presentations, midpelvic delivery and methods to convert the brow presentation to a vertex presentation are contraindicated. Perinatal morbidity and mortality are similar to those for vertex presentations.

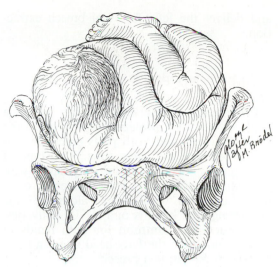

Figure 20–6. Shoulder presentation. Note the transverse lie of the fetus with the back down.

SHOULDER PRESENTATION

Shoulder (or acromion) presentation occurs when the long axis of the fetus is perpendicular or at an acute angle to the long axis of the mother, as occurs with a transverse or oblique lie (Fig. 20–6). The oblique lie is unstable and usually converts to a longitudinal or transverse lie. Shoulder presentation is rare and occurs with an incidence of 0.3 per cent.

The fetal head lies in either the right or left maternal iliac fossa. Radiographic or sonographic examination readily confirms the diagnosis. The diagnosis can, at times, be made by vaginal examination if enough dilatation of the cervix has occurred. In this situation, one may palpate the fetal ribs, scapula, and clavicle. With advanced labor, the shoulder becomes wedged into the maternal pelvis, and the fetal hand and arm not uncommonly prolapse into the vagina.

Etiology

Etiologic factors include unusual relaxation of the maternal abdominal wall (which results from high parity), prematurity, placenta previa, multiple gestation, hydramnios, and contracted maternal pelvis.

Management

With such a presentation, vaginal delivery is impossible unless the fetus is extremely small (that is, extremely immature), since the fetal head and trunk would have to enter the maternal pelvis at the same time. If the diagnosis is made prior to labor, external cephalic version may be successful. Otherwise, cesarean section must be performed. If the fetal feet occupy the fundal region, which occurs with a back down transverse lie, a vertical uterine incision is recommended to provide enough room for the operator to reach up inside the uterus to the fundus, grasp the feet,

Diagnosis

The diagnosis is readily made by Leopold examination, with no fetal pole detected at the fundus or above the pubic symphysis.

and deliver the fetus by total breech extraction.

COMPOUND PRESENTATION

Compound presentation occurs when a fetal extremity prolapses alongside the presenting part and both parts enter the maternal pelvis at the same time. This type of presentation occurs more frequently with premature gestations. The incidence of a hand or arm prolapsing alongside the presenting fetal head is one in 700 deliveries. It is much less common for both hands to present alongside the fetal head or for a hand to present alongside a breech.

The etiology is obscure, and the management of such a presentation is expectant. Usually, the prolapsed part of the fetus does not interfere with labor. If the arm prolapses, it is best to wait to see if it moves out of the way as the head descends. If it does not, the arm may be gently pushed upward while the head is simultaneously pushed downward by fundal pressure. If the complete extremity prolapses and the fetus then converts to a shoulder presentation, delivery must be accomplished by cesarean section.

SUGGESTED READING

Collea JV, Rabin SC, Weghorst GR, et al: The randomized management of term frank breech presentations: Vaginal delivery vs cesarean section. Am J Obstet Gynecol 131:186, 1978.

Cruikshank DP, Cruikshank JE: Face and brow presentation: A review. Clin Obstet Gynecol 24(2):333, 1981.

Cruikshank DP, White CA: Obstetric malpresentations: Twenty years' experience. Am J Obstet Gynecol 116:1097, 1973.

Gimovsky ML, Paul RH: Singleton breech presentation in labor. Am J Obstet Gynecol 143:733, 1982.

Gimovsky ML, Wallace RL, Schifrin BS, Paul RH: Randomized management of nonfrank breech presentation at term: A preliminary report. Am J Obstet Gynecol 146:34, 1983.

Shields JR, Schifrin BS: External cephalic version. In Nelson NM (ed): Current Therapy in Neonatal/Perinatal Medicine. 2nd ed. Philadelphia, BC Decker, 1990.

The Problem of Breech Presentation: Consensus Development Conference on Cesarean Childbirth. U.S. Public Health Service, National Institutes of Health, 1980, p. 367.

Twenty-one

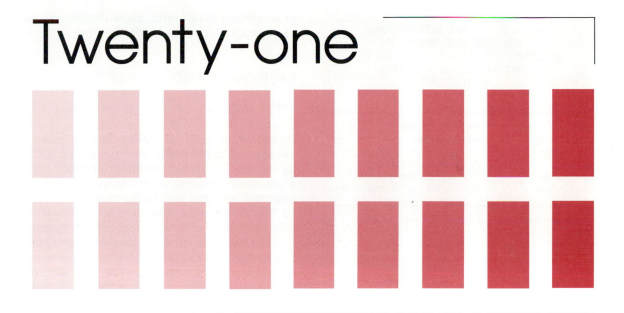

Multiple Gestation

JAMES R. SHIELDS AND ARNOLD L. MEDEARIS

Multiple gestation may be defined as any pregnancy in which two or more embryos or fetuses exist simultaneously. It is of utmost importance to recognize multiple gestation as a complication of pregnancy. The perinatal mortality and morbidity in multiple gestation exceed that of singleton gestations in a disproportionate manner, and maternal morbidity is increased. Although this chapter is devoted primarily to twin gestations, since they are the most common, the information presented also generally applies to pregnancies involving three or more fetuses.

ETIOLOGY AND CLASSIFICATION OF TWINNING

Multiple gestation may occur as the result of the division of a fertilized egg, fertilization of more than one egg by more than one sperm, or a combination of the two processes. The former process results in *monozy-* *gotic (identical) twins,* whereas the latter results in *dizygotic (fraternal) twins.* Since dizygotic twins arise from two fertilized eggs, they will always have two amnions and two chorions; the placentas may be either separate or fused, and the sexes may be different. With dizygotic twinning, the eggs may not be fertilized at the same time. *Superfecundation* may occur in which two ova are fertilized within a short period of time but not at the same coitus.

Monozygotic twins may arise from cleavage of a fertilized egg at various stages during embryogenesis, and the relationship of the fetal membranes depends on the time at which the embryo divides (Table 21–1). If division occurs within the first 72 hours of fertilization, before differentiation of the amnion and chorion, the result will be *diamnionic, dichorionic, monozygous twins* with either separate or fused placentas. If division occurs 4 to 8 days after ovulation, the chorion has already become differentiated, and

Table 21-1. THE RELATIONSHIP BETWEEN THE TIMING OF CLEAVAGE AND THE NATURE OF THE MEMBRANES IN TWIN GESTATIONS

TIME OF CLEAVAGE*	NATURE OF THE MEMBRANES
0–72 hr	Diamnionic, dichorionic
4–8 days	Diamnionic, monochorionic
9–12 days	Monoamnionic, monochorionic

*Time interval between ovulation and cleavage of the egg.

the result will be *diamnionic, monochorionic, monozygous twins.* If division occurs after 8 days, both amnion and chorion have differentiated, and the result will be *monoamnionic, monochorionic, monozygous twins.* Of all monozygotic twins, 70 per cent are monochorionic, and of these, the vast majority are diamnionic. The remaining 30 per cent are diamnionic, dichorionic (Fig. 21–1).

DETERMINATION OF ZYGOSITY

Obstetric ultrasonography may often allow for the prenatal determination of zygosity. Visualization of the amnion/chorion with high resolution and magnification as well as the fetal sex and number of placentas may lead to such a determination. After delivery of twins, an attempt should be made to confirm the zygosity. In 80 per cent of twins, this may be done relatively easily by determining the relationship of the fetal membranes, fetal sex, and major and minor blood groupings. Thirty per cent of twins will be of different sex and are, therefore, dizygotic. Twenty-three per cent will have monochorionic placentas and are, therefore, monozygotic. Twenty-seven per cent will have the same sex, dichorionic placentas, but different blood groupings and must be, therefore, dizygotic. Twenty per cent will have the same sex, dichorionic placentas, and identical blood groupings. For this latter group, further studies, such as human leukocyte antigen (HLA) typing or the acceptance or rejection of reciprocal skin grafts, allow determination of zygosity.

INCIDENCE AND EPIDEMIOLOGY

The frequency of multiple gestation is not constant throughout the world, but varies according to race, hereditary factors, maternal age, maternal parity, and the use of fertility agents. Dizygotic twinning increases with a maternal history of twinning, increasing maternal age, and increasing maternal parity. In North America, twinning occurs with a frequency of one in 90 gestations. In approximately one third of these twin gestations, the fetuses are monozygotic, or identical; the remaining two thirds are dizygotic, or fraternal. In contrast, twinning in western Nigeria occurs with a frequency of one in 22 gestations, the difference being due to a higher rate of dizygotic twinning. The incidence of multiple gestation with the use of clomiphene is about 10 per cent versus about 30 per cent following gonadotropin therapy.

Rates of multiple gestation are usually expressed as occurrences per births, as opposed to occurrences per conception. The actual rate per conception is difficult to analyze, since the abortion rate in twins is higher than that in singletons.

ABNORMALITIES OF THE TWINNING PROCESS

Abnormalities in the twinning process are common and may result in conjoined twins, placental vascular anastomoses, twin-twin transfusion syndrome, fetal malformations, and umbilical cord abnormalities. These abnormalities occur only in monochorionic (monozygotic) twins.

Conjoined Twins

If division of the embryo occurs after the embryonic disc has formed, that is, about 13 days after fertilization, cleavage of the embryo is incomplete and results in *conjoined ("Siamese") twins.* This is a very rare event, occurring once in 70,000 deliveries. Con-

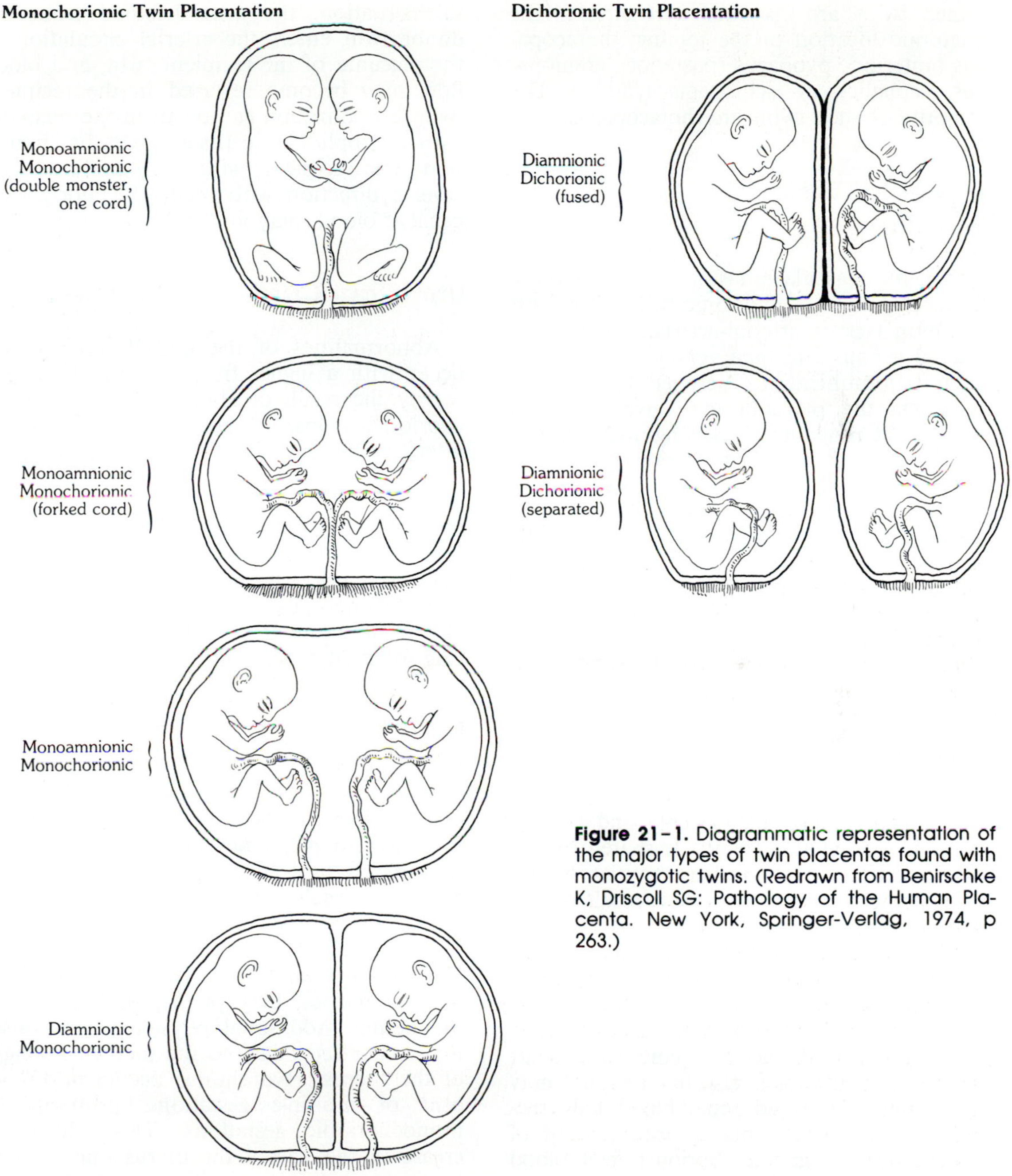

Monochorionic Twin Placentation

Dichorionic Twin Placentation

Monoamnionic
Monochorionic
(double monster,
one cord)

Monoamnionic
Monochorionic
(forked cord)

Monoamnionic
Monochorionic

Diamnionic
Monochorionic

Diamnionic
Dichorionic
(fused)

Diamnionic
Dichorionic
(separated)

Figure 21–1. Diagrammatic representation of the major types of twin placentas found with monozygotic twins. (Redrawn from Benirschke K, Driscoll SG: Pathology of the Human Placenta. New York, Springer-Verlag, 1974, p 263.)

joined twins are classified according to the anatomic location of the joining: thoracopagus (anterior), pyopagus (posterior), craniopagus (cephalic), or ischiopagus (caudal). The majority of such twins are thoracopagus.

Placental Vascular Anastomoses

Placental vascular anastomoses occur more frequently in monochorionic twins. The most common type is arterial-arterial, followed by arterial-venous and then venous-venous. Vascular communications between the two fetuses via the placenta may give rise to a number of problems, including abortion, hydramnios, twin-twin transfusion syndrome, and fetal malformations. The incidence of both minor and major congenital malformations in twins is twice that of singletons, the majority of malformations occurring in monochorionic twins.

Twin-Twin Transfusion Syndrome

The presence of arterial-venous anastomoses in the placenta of monochorionic twins will often lead to the twin-twin transfusion syndrome. Arterial blood from the donor twin enters the placenta and courses through a cotyledon, which is shared by the two twins. The blood then empties into a vein of the recipient twin. As a result of this chronic shunting, the donor twin develops hypovolemia, hypotension, anemia, microcardia, and growth retardation. The recipient twin may develop hypervolemia, hyperviscosity, thrombosis, hypertension, cardiomegaly, polycythemia, edema, and congestive heart failure. Hydramnios is also frequent and may result from increased renal blood flow secondary to hypervolemia or transudation of fluid across congested chorionic fetal blood vessels. The hyperperfused twin is prone to develop kernicterus during the neonatal period as a result of polycythemia and subsequent hyperbilirubinemia.

Fetal Malformations

Arterial-arterial placental anastomoses may result in a number of fetal malformations. In this situation, the arterial blood from the donor twin enters the arterial circulation in the placenta of the recipient twin, and blood flow may become reversed in the recipient twin. Embolization can occur in the recipient twin as trophoblastic tissue enters its circulation. The recipient twin, being perfused in a reverse direction with relatively poorly oxygenated blood, may fail to develop normally.

Umbilical Cord Abnormalities

Abnormalities of the umbilical cord also occur with a higher frequency in twins, primarily the result of abnormalities in monochorionic twins. Absence of one umbilical artery occurs in about 3 to 4 per cent of twins, as opposed to 0.5 to 1 per cent of singletons. The absence of one umbilical artery is significant because in 30 per cent of such cases, it is associated with other congenital anomalies (e.g., renal agenesis). Marginal and velamentous umbilical cord insertions also occur more frequently, the latter occurring in about 5 per cent of twins.

MATERNAL PHYSIOLOGIC RESPONSE

A number of normal maternal physiologic responses to pregnancy are exaggerated with multiple fetuses. On the average, multiple gestation results in a 500-ml increase in blood volume over that of a singleton. The increased blood volume, combined with the increased iron and folate requirements of additional fetuses, may predispose the mother to anemia. Additional physiologic responses may occur secondary to the increased weight of the uterus. Hydramnios occurs in 12 per cent of multiple gestations, primarily in monochorionic gestations. This added increase in the size of the uterus may lead to increasing respiratory difficulty as the overdistended uterus causes greater elevation of the diaphragm. The weight of the uterus may cause further compression of the great vessels, resulting in a more pronounced decrease in uterine blood flow secondary to aortic compression, supine hypotension, or both. Maternal edema and proteinuria are common. Greater compression of the ureters can also occur, leading to obstructive uropathy and renal failure. These severe complications are more common when acute hydramnios develops.

DIAGNOSIS

Historic factors such as a maternal family history of dizygotic twinning, the use of fertility drugs, a maternal sensation of feeling larger than with previous pregnancies, or a sensation of excessive fetal movements increase the suspicion of a multiple gestation. Physical signs include excessive weight gain, abdominal palpation of an excessive number of fetal parts, auscultation of two separate fetal heart rates that differ by more than 10 beats per minute, and rapid uterine growth. Most of the time, twinning will result in a fundal height that is 4 cm larger than expected for a singleton. This is referred to as a size/dates discrepancy.

When a multiple gestation is suspected, confirmation should be established by sonography. Separate gestational sacs may be seen as early as 6 weeks of gestation. After the tenth week, multiple fetal parts may be visualized.

The need for early diagnosis of multiple gestation cannot be overemphasized. In several studies, almost half of all twin gestations are not diagnosed until delivery of the first twin. Failure of early diagnosis leads to an increased incidence of intrauterine growth retardation and preterm labor, both of which increase the perinatal morbidity and mortality. In addition, there is an increased likelihood of maternal complications.

ANTEPARTUM MANAGEMENT

Intensive antepartum management serves to prolong gestation, increase birth weight, decrease perinatal morbidity and mortality, and decrease in the incidence of maternal complications. The complications of multiple gestation are shown in Table 21–2.

The patient should be seen weekly beginning in the mid-second trimester. The cervix should be assessed frequently, since multiple gestation may lead to early cervical effacement and dilatation. The patient should be examined for the development of nondependent edema, the urine routinely checked for

Table 21–2. COMPLICATIONS OF MULTIPLE GESTATIONS

MATERNAL	FETAL
Anemia	Hydramnios
Hypertension	Malpresentation
Premature labor	Placenta previa
Postpartum uterine atony	Abruptio placentae
Postpartum hemorrhage	Premature rupture of the membranes
Pre-eclampsia	Prematurity
	Umbilical cord prolapse
	Intrauterine growth retardation
	Congenital anomalies
	Increased perinatal morbidity
	Increased perinatal mortality

protein, and the blood pressure monitored closely. With multiple gestation, pregnancy-induced hypertension tends to occur more frequently, earlier, and more severely than with singletons. Dietary considerations must not be overlooked because there is an increased need for calories, iron, vitamins, and folate. The Institute of Medicine has recommended that the target (total) weight gain at term for women carrying twins should be 16 to 20.5 kg (35 to 45 lb).

The prevention of prematurity is of utmost importance. Many regimens have been developed, including bed rest, hospitalization, prophylactic β-sympathomimetic (tocolytic) agents, and cervical cerclage. Bed rest during the late second and third trimesters increases birth weight, probably by increasing uterine blood flow. Some studies have shown that bed rest also prolongs gestation and decreases perinatal mortality, whereas others have failed to demonstrate these additional benefits. Swedish studies have reported a perinatal mortality rate equal to that of singletons (0.6 per cent). Their patients were advised to undergo bed rest at home until the third trimester, when they were hospitalized for additional bed rest. They were subsequently discharged at 36 weeks, unless complications arose. Pregnancies were not usually permitted to go beyond 38 weeks gestation. In general, women with multiple gestations should not work and they should be encouraged to take rest periods three times per day.

Fetal surveillance is also crucial in decreasing perinatal morbidity and mortality. Routine sonography should be performed at monthly intervals beginning at 24 weeks to assess fetal growth, since twins have a tendency to suffer from intrauterine growth retardation (IUGR). IUGR may be concordant or discordant. Discordant is defined as a difference of 20 to 25 per cent between the twins. Assessment of fetal well-being by nonstress testing (NST) should be performed weekly beginning at 38 weeks, or earlier if the pregnancy is complicated by other factors, such as IUGR, discordant growth, hypertension, or hydramnios. If these complications develop, NST should be instigated immediately and the frequency increased to twice per week. The use of the contraction stress test to rule out uteroplacental insufficiency in the face of a nonreactive NST is contraindicated in multiple gestations, since these pregnancies are already predisposed to develop preterm labor.

INTRAPARTUM MANAGEMENT

Should preterm labor develop prior to 35 weeks, aggressive measures must be considered. These include treatment with tocolytic agents to arrest labor, assessment of fetal pulmonary maturity, and maternal administration of glucocorticoids when necessary to accelerate fetal lung maturation if the gestational age is less than 34 weeks. Care must be taken to avoid iatrogenic fluid overload. Table 21–3 provides a list of necessary prerequisites for the management of labor in pregnancies complicated by multiple gestation.

Vertex-Vertex Presentations

To choose the optimal method of delivery, the presentations of the fetuses must be accurately known. By convention, the presenting twin is designated as twin A and the second twin as twin B. All combinations of presentation are possible. Vertex-vertex occurs most frequently (50 per cent of the time), followed by vertex-breech, breech-vertex, and breech-breech.

For *vertex-vertex presentations,* labor is allowed as with a singleton vertex presentation.

Table 21–3. PREREQUISITES FOR THE INTRAPARTUM MANAGEMENT OF MULTIPLE GESTATIONS

A secondary or tertiary care center

A delivery room equipped for immediate cesarean section, if necessary

A well-functioning large-bore intravenous line (e.g., 16-gauge) to administer fluids and blood rapidly, if necessary

Two units of typed and cross-matched blood

The capability to monitor continuously the fetal heart rates simultaneously

An anesthesiologist who is immediately available to administer general anesthesia should intrauterine manipulation or cesarean section be necessary for delivery of the second twin

Two obstetricians scrubbed and gowned for the delivery, one of whom is skilled in intrauterine manipulation and delivery of the second twin

Imaging techniques, preferably sonography, for determining the precise presentations of the twins

Two pediatricians, one of whom is skilled in the immediate resuscitation of the newborn

An appropriate number of nurses to assist in the delivery and care of the newborn infants

Both fetal heart rates must be monitored continuously during labor. Oxytocin (Pitocin) is not contraindicated for dysfunctional labor, but should be administered in dilute solution with an infusion pump. Uterine contractions should be monitored with an intrauterine pressure catheter. After delivery of the first twin, the cord is immediately clamped, identified as twin A, and cut. Cord blood samples are not obtained until the second fetus has been delivered to prevent potential hemorrhage from the undelivered fetus through placental vascular anastomoses. A vaginal examination is then performed to assess the presentation and station of the second twin. If the second twin is still in a vertex presentation, labor is allowed to continue. The second fetal heart rate is continuously monitored. Should the uterine contractions become ineffective, oxytocin should be administered in a dilute solution and labor allowed to progress. When the vertex becomes fixed in the pelvis, amniotomy and placement of a fetal scalp electrode should be performed. Labor should be allowed to continue in anticipation of a spontaneous delivery, outlet forceps, or midpelvic delivery, if necessary.

Time Interval Between Twins

The optimal time interval between delivery of the first and second twin is 5 to 15 minutes. Delivery of the second twin before 5 minutes may reflect unnecessary intervention, resulting in birth trauma. Delivery after 30 minutes may result in uteroplacental insufficiency secondary to decreased uteroplacental blood flow that results from the reduction in intrauterine volume. In addition, a longer interval may result in fetal hemorrhage from the second twin as a result of premature separation of the placenta. A longer interval may be allowed only if the second twin is carefully monitored.

Postdelivery Procedures

After delivery of the second fetus, the cord blood samples are obtained and the placenta delivered. Care should be taken not to disrupt the relationship of the fetal membranes, since these will often reveal the nature of the twins. Following delivery of the placenta, the uterus should be vigorously massaged and oxytocin added to the intravenous solution to diminish the risk of postpartum atony and hemorrhage. These occur more frequently with multiple gestation, and the average intrapartum blood loss with twins is 500 ml more than with singletons.

Management of Other Presentations

Controversy exists as to the optimum mode of delivery of twins with a *vertex-breech* or *vertex-transverse presentation*. In inexperienced hands, routine cesarean section should be performed to avoid the potential birth trauma and asphyxia that may occur with internal podalic version and total breech extraction. With experienced obstetricians, the second twin can be safely delivered vaginally by breech extraction and maternal morbidity is decreased.

After delivery of the first twin, ultrasonography may be useful to determine the precise presentation of the second twin and the location of the fetal limbs. If it is oblique or transverse, external cephalic version and subsequent delivery as a vertex may be possible. Otherwise, breech extraction, with or without *internal podalic version,* is necessary.

If the second twin is to be delivered vaginally by breech extraction, general anesthesia with halothane to relax the uterus is required after delivery of the first twin, unless the patient has an adequate epidural anesthetic. The obstetrician reaches up into the uterus, identifies the fetal feet, and exerts gentle traction in a downward direction until the feet are at the introitus. If the fetal head is not in the fundus, it is simultaneously guided upward transabdominally by the other hand (i.e., internal podalic version). Once the feet are at the introitus, amniotomy is performed if the membranes have not already ruptured, and delivery is accomplished by total breech extraction. This procedure should not be performed in premature gestations of less than 34 weeks, since there is an increased risk of entrapment of the aftercoming head. Cesarean section should be used under such circumstances.

For *breech-vertex presentations,* cesarean section is indicated to avoid the phenomenon of interlocking twins as well as potential complications of a vaginal breech delivery. Interlocking of twins may occur when the first twin delivers partially and its chin interlocks with the neck and chin of the second twin. This occurs once in 800 twin deliveries. The result is disastrous, however, in that decapitation may be required to facilitate delivery of the first twin if attempts to transabdominally dislodge the second twin fail.

If the first twin presents as a complete or incomplete breech, cesarean section is indicated regardless of the presentation of the second twin, since these types of presentations are associated with a higher incidence of umbilical cord prolapse and entrapment of the aftercoming head. When the first twin is in a transverse lie, cesarean section is also indicated.

An exception to the aforementioned guidelines involves delivery of multiple gestations complicated by active preterm labor and fetal immaturity (e.g., gestational age less than 25

Table 21-4. CAUSES OF PERINATAL MORBIDITY AND MORTALITY IN TWINS

Respiratory distress syndrome
Birth trauma
Cerebral hemorrhage
Birth asphyxia
Birth anoxia
Congenital anomalies
Stillbirths
Prematurity

to 26 weeks). Because survival is poor at this gestational age, delivery by cesarean section should probably be avoided. Cesarean delivery does not improve fetal outcome and only exposes the mother to increased morbidity.

PERINATAL OUTCOME

Perinatal mortality and morbidity in twins greatly exceed those of singletons. The perinatal mortality rate in twin gestations (30 to 50 per 1000 live births) is approximately five times that of singletons.

Respiratory distress syndrome (RDS) secondary to *prematurity* accounts for approximately one half of the perinatal mortality in twins. The average duration of gestation in twins (35 weeks) is considerably less than that for singletons (39 weeks). Since birth asphyxia also predisposes the fetus to develop RDS, it is not surprising that second-born twins have twice the perinatal mortality of first-born twins. This may result from increased birth asphyxia associated with intrauterine manipulation during delivery of the second twin, uteroplacental insufficiency that occurs after the delivery of the first twin, or both conditions. Not only does the perinatal mortality rate increase with decreasing gestational age, it also increases after 40 weeks gestation.

Other factors that contribute to perinatal mortality and morbidity are listed in Table 21-4. Death secondary to *birth trauma* occurs four times more often with second-born twins and twice as often in first-born twins when compared with singletons. *Con-*genital anomalies and *stillbirths* account for about one third of the perinatal mortality rate. Stillbirths occur twice as frequently in twins as in singletons. *Cerebral hemorrhage, asphyxia,* and *anoxia* account for one tenth of the perinatal mortality rate.

The type of placentation also affects the perinatal mortality rate. The perinatal mortality rate for monochorionic twins (120 per 1000 live births) is about three times that for dichorionic twins. It is believed that this is secondary to an increased incidence of *hydramnios,* which occurs as a result of the *twin-twin transfusion syndrome.* Hydramnios results in a 40 per cent perinatal mortality rate as a result of an increase in prematurity and congenital anomalies. Also, monozygotic twins have a substantially increased incidence of pre-eclampsia. This explains why monozygotic twins have a 2.5 times greater perinatal mortality rate than dizygotics.

There is a fourfold increase in the incidence of *cerebral palsy* in twins and a greater incidence of *neonatal hypoglycemia. Low birth weight* (less than 2500 gm) occurs in over 50 per cent of twins and results from an increased incidence of prematurity and IUGR. The mean birth weight in twins is 2395 gm versus 3377 gm for singletons. IUGR tends to be asymmetric and usually begins in the early third trimester. Because of the twin-twin transfusion syndrome, monozygotics are affected more often than dizygotics. Discordance is not uncommon. Regarding postnatal growth, twins tend to be shorter and lighter than singletons of similar birth weight until the age of four.

Retained Dead Fetus Syndrome

It is not infrequent for one twin to die in utero at a time that is remote from term, with the pregnancy continuing and the remaining twin surviving (the retained dead fetus syndrome). Disseminated intravascular coagulopathy may develop in either the live fetus or the mother as a result of transfer of nonviable fetal material with thromboplastin-like activity into the circulation of the remaining twin or the mother. In this situation, the maternal platelet count and fibrinogen level should be checked once a week. The dead fetus becomes reabsorbed if the demise occurs prior to 12 weeks gestation. Beyond this time, the fetus shrinks, becomes dehydrated and flattened, and is recognized at the time of delivery of the live twin as a *fetus papyraceus* or *fetus compressus*.

MULTIPLE GESTATION WITH MORE THAN TWO FETUSES

The processes that result in monozygotic and dizygotic twinning may occur separately or in combination, giving rise to triplets, quadruplets, and higher order multiple gestations. The incidence of triplets is one in 8000 and of quadruplets one in 700,000 births. Prematurity increases as the number of fetuses increases. The average length of gestation is 33 weeks for triplets and 29 weeks for quadruplets. The mean birth weights for triplets and quadruplets are 1818 gm and 1395 gm, respectively. The mode of delivery depends on the gestational age and the presentation of the presenting fetus. If the gestational age is close to term, vaginal delivery may be accomplished, although many authorities believe that multiple gestations involving more than two fetuses should be delivered routinely by cesarean section to avoid birth trauma and asphyxia.

The problems with perinatal mortality and morbidity described for twins apply to multiple gestations with more than two fetuses, and they occur with greater frequency. The perinatal mortality rate for triplets is higher and is mainly due to problems associated with prematurity. The stillbirth rate for triplets is three times that of singletons. Quadruplets have a stillbirth rate four times that of singletons.

SUGGESTED READING

Bell D, Johansson D, McLean FH, Usher RH: Birth asphyxia, trauma and mortality in twins: Has cesarean section improved outcome? Am J Obstet Gynecol 154:235, 1986.

Carlson NJ: Discordant twin pregnancy: A challenging condition. Contemp Ob/Gyn, Aug. 1989.

D'Alton ME, Dudley DK: The ultrasonic prediction of chorionicity in twin gestation. Am J Obstet Gynecol 160:557, 1989.

Jones KL, Benirschke K: The developmental pathogenesis of structural defects: The contribution of monozygotic twins. Semin Perinatol 7(4):239, 1983.

Kovacs BW, Kirschbaum TH, Paul RH: Twin gestations: I. Antenatal care and complications. Obstet Gynecol 74:313, 1989.

Medearis AL, Jonas HS, Stockbauer JW, et al: Perinatal deaths in twin pregnancy. Am J Obstet Gynecol 134:421, 1979.

Persson PH, Grennert L, Gennser G, et al: On improved outcome of twin pregnancies. Acta Obstet Gynecol Scand 58:3, 1979.

Twenty-two

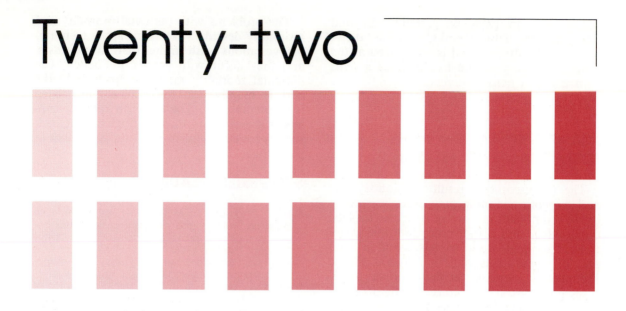

Identification and Management of Fetal Distress During Labor

KLAUS J. STAISCH

Intrapartum asphyxia is an infrequent cause of neonatal mortality and morbidity. Neurologic follow-up studies of infants who participated in randomized clinical trials on the value of electronic fetal monitoring point toward a prelabor etiology for most cerebral palsy and mental retardation. It appears that current applications and concepts of heart rate monitoring do not reduce neurologic abnormalities. The uncertainties that exist about the types of fetal surveillance during labor are discussed at the end of this chapter.

Intrapartum acidosis and hypoxia may occur in any pregnancy, but are more common in those defined as being at high risk during either the antepartum or intrapartum period. Unfortunately, currently available risk assessment profiles do not predict all instances of intrapartum fetal distress. On the basis of antepartum maternal history, physical examination, and laboratory data, 20 to 30 per cent of pregnancies may be designated high risk, and 50 per cent of perinatal morbidity and mortality occurs in this group. The other 50 per cent of perinatal morbidity and mortality occurs in pregnancies that are considered to be normal at the onset of labor. In spite of improved antenatal testing, labor must be considered a potentially hazardous period for every pregnancy.

METHODS OF MONITORING FETAL HEART RATE

Auscultation of Fetal Heart Rate

The time-honored technique of evaluating the fetus during labor has been auscultation of the fetal heart using a fetal stethoscope. However, if this technique is carried out during labor every 15 minutes for a duration of 30 seconds, only 3 per cent of the available rate information is obtained. Other limitations include the inability to listen to the fetal heart rate (FHR) during contractions, errors in counting the rate, and an inability to appreciate beat to beat variability. No well-designed study exists in the literature showing that fetal outcome is improved by periodic auscultation through a stethoscope. The presence of an FHR signifies fetal life and its absence denotes death, but there is no consistent relationship between the auscultated rate between contractions and the intermediate degrees of fetal distress.

Continuous Electronic Fetal Monitoring

Electronic fetal monitoring allows continuous reporting of the fetal heart rate and uterine contractions (FHR-UC) by means of a monitor that prints results on a 2-channel strip chart recorder. The uterine contraction represents a stress on the fetus, and the alteration in fetal heart rate correlates with fetal oxygenation. The FHR-UC record can be obtained using external transducers that are placed on the maternal abdomen. This technique is used in early labor.

Internal monitoring is carried out by placing a spiral electrode onto the fetal scalp to monitor heart rate and a plastic catheter transcervically into the amniotic cavity to monitor uterine contractions (Fig. 22–1). To carry out this technique, the fetal membranes must be ruptured, and the cervix must be dilated to at least 2 cm. Internal monitoring gives better FHR tracings because the rate is computed from the sharply defined R-wave peaks of the fetal electrocardiogram, whereas with the external technique, the rate is computed from the less precisely defined first heart sound obtained with an ultrasonic transducer. The internal uterine catheter allows precise measurement of the intensity of the contractions in millimeters of mercury, whereas the external tocotransducer measures only frequency and duration, not intensity.

In the clinical setting, internal and external techniques are often combined by using a scalp electrode for precise heart rate recording and the external tocotransducer for contractions. This approach minimizes possible side effects from invasive internal monitoring. With increasing evidence of the benefits derived from this technique, the concept of monitoring all patients is gaining support.

ETIOLOGY OF FETAL DISTRESS

The developing fetus presents a paradox. Its arterial blood oxygen tension is only 25 ± 5 mm Hg compared with adult values of about 100 mm Hg. The rate of oxygen consumption, however, is twice that of the adult per unit weight, and its oxygen reserve is only enough to meet its metabolic needs for 1 to 2 minutes. Blood flow from the maternal circulation, which supplies the fetus with oxygen through placental exchange of respiratory gases, is momentarily interrupted during a contraction. A normal fetus can withstand the stress of labor without suffering from hypoxia because sufficient oxygen exchange occurs during the interval between contractions.

Under normal circumstances, the FHR is determined by the atrial pacemaker. Modulation of the rate occurs physiologically through innervation of the heart by the vagus (decelerator) and sympathetic (accelerator) nerves. A fetus whose oxygen supply is marginal cannot tolerate the stress of contractions and will become hypoxic. Under hypoxic conditions, baroreceptors and chemoreceptors in the central circulation of the fetus influence the FHR by giving rise to contraction-related or "periodic" FHR changes. The hypoxia will also result in anaerobic metabolism. Pyruvate and lactic acid accumulate causing fetal acidosis. The degree of fetal acidosis can be measured by sampling blood from the presenting part. By definition, fetal distress occurs when the fetus is unable to maintain biochemical homeostasis as assessed

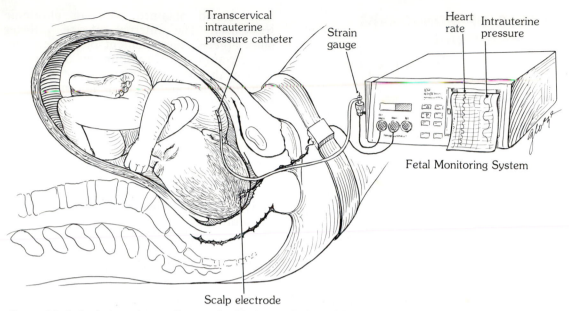

Figure 22-1. Technique for continuous electronic monitoring of fetal heart rate and uterine contractions.

by a fetal scalp blood pH of 7.25 or less. Clinical and experimental data indicate that fetal death occurs when 50 per cent or more of the transplacental oxygen exchange is interrupted.

Fetal oxygenation can be impaired at different anatomic locations within the utero-placental-fetal circulatory loop. For example, there may be impairment of oxygen transportation to the intervillous space as a result of maternal hypertension or anemia; oxygen diffusion may be impaired in the placenta because of infarction or abruption; or the oxygen content in the fetal blood may be impaired because of hemolytic anemia in Rh-isoimmunization. Figure 22-2 summarizes the clinical conditions that may be associated with fetal distress during labor.

FETAL HEART RATE PATTERNS

The assessment of the FHR depends on an evaluation of the baseline pattern and the periodic changes related to uterine contractions.

Baseline Assessment

This requires determination of the rate in beats per minute (BPM) and the variability.

Normal and abnormal rates are listed in Table 22-1. Baseline variability can be divided into short-term and long-term intervals. These are described as follows:

1. Short-term or beat to beat variability. This reflects the interval between either successive fetal electrocardiogram signals or mechanical events of the cardiac cycle. Normal short-term variability fluctuates between 5 and 25 BPM. Variability below 5 BPM is considered to be potentially abnormal. When associated with decelerations, a variability of less than 5 BPM usually indicates severe fetal distress.

2. Long-term variability. These fluctuations may be described in terms of the frequency and amplitude of change in the baseline rate. The normal long-term variability is 3 to 10 cycles per minute. Variability is physiologically decreased during the state of quiet sleep of the fetus, which usually lasts for about 25 minutes until transition occurs to another state.

Periodic Fetal Heart Rate Changes

These are changes in baseline FHR related to uterine contractions. The responses to

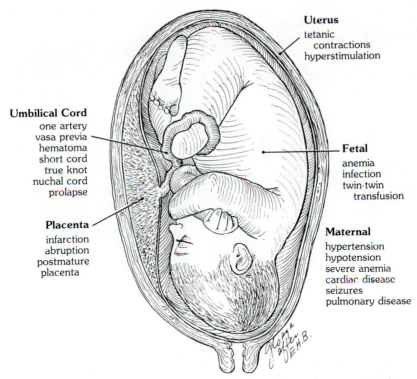

Uterus
tetanic
  contractions
hyperstimulation

Umbilical Cord
one artery
vasa previa
hematoma
short cord
true knot
nuchal cord
prolapse

Fetal
anemia
infection
twin-twin
  transfusion

Placenta
infarction
abruption
postmature
placenta

Maternal
hypertension
hypotension
severe anemia
cardiac disease
seizures
pulmonary disease

Figure 22–2. Clinical conditions associated with fetal distress in labor.

uterine contractions may be categorized as follows:

1. *No change.* The FHR maintains the same characteristics as in the preceding baseline FHR.
2. *Acceleration.* The FHR increases in response to uterine contractions. This is a normal response.
3. *Deceleration.* The FHR decreases in response to uterine contractions. Decelerations may be early, late, variable, or mixed. All except early decelerations are abnormal.

Types of Patterns

Early Deceleration (Head Compression). This pattern usually has an onset, maximum fall, and recovery that is coincident with the onset, peak, and end of the uterine contraction (Fig. 22–3). The nadir of the FHR coincides with the peak of the contraction. This pattern is seen when engagement of the fetal head has occurred. Early decelerations are not thought to be associated with fetal distress. The pressure on the fetal head leads to increased intracranial pressure that elicits a vagal response similar to the Valsalva maneuver in the adult. The vagal reflex can be abolished by the administration of atropine, but this approach is not used clinically.

Late Deceleration (Uteroplacental Insufficiency). This pattern has an onset, maximal decrease, and recovery that is shifted to the right in relation to the contraction (Fig. 22–4). The severity of late decelerations is graded

Table 22–1. BASELINE FETAL HEART RATES

RATE	BEATS PER MINUTE
Normal	120–160
Abnormal	
Tachycardia	>160
Bradycardia	<120

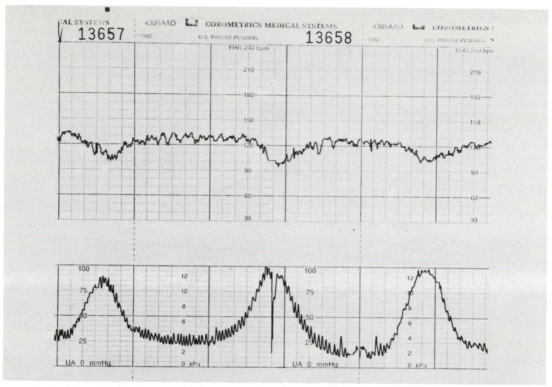

Figure 22–3. Early deceleration. Note that the deceleration starts and ends with the uterine contraction. Good beat to beat variability is demonstrated.

by the magnitude of the decrease in FHR at the nadir of the deceleration (Table 22–2). Fetal hypoxia and acidosis are usually more pronounced with severe decelerations. Late decelerations are generally associated with low scalp blood pH values and high base deficits, indicating metabolic acidosis from anaerobic metabolism. The partial pressure of carbon dioxide (P_{CO_2}) in the fetal blood is usually in the normal range, and the fetal blood oxygen partial pressure (P_{O_2}) is only slightly below normal because of the Bohr effect—the shift to the left of the oxygen dissociation curve caused by the acidosis. The P_{O_2} is, therefore, not a sensitive indicator for monitoring fetal compromise.

Variable Deceleration (Cord Compression). This pattern has a variable time of onset and a variable form and may be nonrepetitive. Variable decelerations are caused by umbilical cord compression. Partial or complete compression of the cord causes a sudden increase in blood pressure in the central circulation of the fetus. The bradycardia is mediated via baroreceptors. This reflex can be abolished or ameliorated by atropine (e.g., chemical vagotomy). This approach is not used clinically, however. Fetal blood gases indicate respiratory acidosis with a low pH and high P_{CO_2} values. When cord compression has been prolonged, hypoxia is also present, showing a picture of combined respiratory and metabolic acidosis in fetal blood gases.

The severity of variable decelerations is graded by their duration (Table 22–2). When the FHR falls below 80 BPM during the nadir of the deceleration, there is usually a loss of the P-wave in the fetal electrocardiogram, indicating a nodal rhythm or a second-degree heart block.

Combined or Mixed Patterns. These patterns may be difficult to define and may exhibit characteristics of any of the aforementioned patterns.

STRATEGIES FOR INTERVENTION

A normal FHR pattern on the electronic monitor indicates a greater than 95 per cent

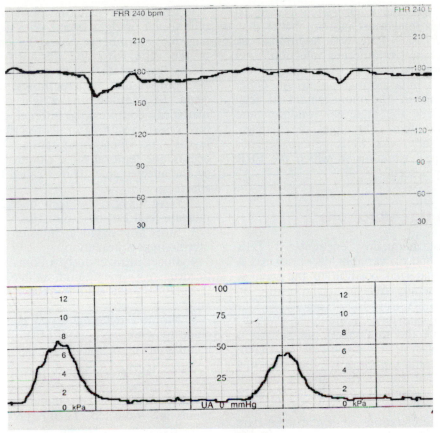

Figure 22–4. Late decelerations in a severely distressed fetus. Note the tachycardia and lack of beat to beat variability in addition to the late decelerations.

probability of fetal well-being. Abnormal patterns may occur, however, in the absence of fetal distress. The false-positive rate (i.e., good Apgar scores and normal fetal acid-base status in the presence of abnormal FHR patterns) is as high as 80 per cent. Therefore, electronic fetal monitoring is a screening rather than a diagnostic technique. Failure to appreciate this limitation may lead to inap-

propriate intervention and contribute to a high rate of cesarean deliveries.

Strategies for intervention always depend on the clinical circumstances in which fetal distress is seen. When abnormal FHR patterns are seen, the first step should be a search for the underlying cause. When the cause is identified, such as maternal hypotension, steps should be taken to correct the

Table 22–2. PRINCIPLES OF GRADING LATE AND VARIABLE DECELERATIONS

CRITERIA OF GRADING	MILD	MODERATE	SEVERE
Late deceleration: amplitude of drop in FHR	<15 BPM	15–45 BPM	>45 BPM
Variable deceleration: duration of deceleration	<30 sec duration	30–60 sec	>60 sec

Adapted from Kubli FW, Hon EH, Khazin AF, et al: Observations on heart rate and pH in the human fetus during labor. Am J Obstet Gynecol 104:1190, 1969.

problem. In general, a term-sized fetus tolerates ominous fetal heart patterns better than a preterm fetus. A fetus with additional risk factors, such as intrauterine infection from chorioamnionitis, may deteriorate sooner than a fetus in a normal parturient. Other considerations in the management of fetal distress include the maternal condition and the stage of labor. Therefore, the management of an abnormal FHR pattern depends on the clinical situation in which the FHR abnormality is seen.

Variable Decelerations

The most frequently encountered FHR pattern is that of variable decelerations. A change in maternal position to the right or left side generally relieves fetal pressure on the cord and abolishes the decelerations. One hundred per cent oxygen should be given by face mask to the mother. If the pattern is persistent, placing the mother in the Trendelenburg position or elevating the presenting part by vaginal examination may be tried. If an oxytocic infusion is running, it should be stopped.

Variable decelerations of severe degree are most frequently seen during the second stage of labor, with the patient pushing during uterine contractions. The safest intervention to deliver the fetus with cord compression is often low or outlet forceps. When progressive acidosis occurs, as determined by serial scalp blood pH determinations, cesarean section should be performed if vaginal delivery is not imminent. Another circumstance requiring immediate intervention is persistent bradycardia (prolonged bradycardia). This condition is encountered when the FHR falls to 60 to 90 BPM for more than 2 minutes. Prolonged bradycardia may be a final stage of fetal decompensation.

Late Decelerations

Late decelerations of the FHR are most commonly seen in pregnancies associated with uteroplacental insufficiency. The following steps are taken in rapid succession to alleviate fetal distress and to determine the underlying cause (Fig. 22–5):

1. Change the maternal position from supine to left or right lateral. The supine hypotension syndrome is caused by compression of the vena cava and aorta by the heavy uterus, leading to lowering of maternal cardiac output and underperfusion of the placenta. In addition, the weight of the term uterus can compress the internal and external iliac vessels, resulting in poor perfusion of the uterus and fetal bradycardia. When this occurs, the femoral pulse cannot be palpated on the affected side. This is called the Poseiro effect.

2. Give oxygen by face mask. This can increase fetal Po_2 by 5 mm Hg.

3. Stop any oxytocic infusion to exclude uterine hyperstimulation.

4. Inject intravenously a bolus of a tocolytic drug (e.g., magnesium sulfate, 2.0 gm or terbutaline, 0.25 mg) to relieve uterine tetany.

5. Monitor maternal blood pressure to exclude hypotensive episodes that can occur as a consequence of epidural analgesia.

When late decelerations persist for greater than 30 minutes despite the above-mentioned maneuvers, fetal scalp blood pH measurements are indicated. To interpret pH values properly, notation should be made by means of an event marker on the fetal monitor indicating the timing of the scalp blood sample.

Operative delivery for fetal distress is indicated when fetal acidosis is present (pH less than 7.2) or when late decelerations are persistent in early labor and the cervix is insufficiently dilated to allow blood sampling from the presenting part.

Fetal Tachycardia

As a baseline change, tachycardia is not a very good sign of fetal distress. In general, fetal tachycardia occurs to improve placental circulation when the fetus is stressed. Brief periods of tachycardia (15 to 30 minutes) are usually associated with excessive oxytocin (Pitocin) augmentation of labor, after which the heart rate returns to baseline when the augmentation is discontinued. Prolonged periods of tachycardia are usually associated with elevated maternal temperature or an

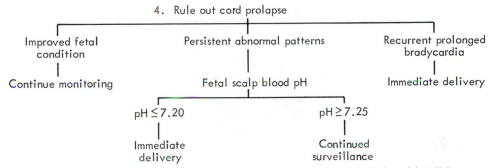

Figure 22–5. Algorithm for the management of an abnormal fetal heart tracing.

intrauterine infection, which should be ruled out. The acid-base status is usually normal.

MECONIUM

The presence of meconium in the amniotic fluid may be a sign of fetal distress. Classification of meconium into early and late passage facilitates a clearer understanding of its importance. Early passage occurs any time prior to rupture of the membranes and is classified as light or heavy, based on its color and viscosity. Light meconium is lightly stained amniotic fluid, yellow or greenish in color. Heavy meconium is dark green or black in color and usually thick and tenacious. Light passage is not associated with poor outcome. Heavy passage is associated with lower 1- and 5-minute Apgar scores and is associated with the risk of meconium aspiration. Late passage usually occurs during the second stage of labor, after clear amniotic fluid has been noted earlier. Late passage, which is most often heavy, is usually associated with some event (e.g., umbilical cord compression or uterine hypertonus) late in labor causing fetal distress. Since heavy meconium is associated with poor outcome, aggressive management of these patients is important. It has been suggested that amnioinfusion through the intrauterine pressure catheter dilutes meconium and lessens the risk from meconium aspiration before birth.

FETAL BLOOD SAMPLING

Fetal scalp blood sampling for pH determination is indicated when fetal distress is suggested by clinical parameters, such as heavy meconium, or by moderate to severely abnormal FHR patterns. Blood is obtained from the fetus by placing an amnioscope transvaginally against the fetal skull (Fig. 22–6). Cervical mucus is removed with cotton swabs. Silicone grease is applied to the skull for blood bead formation. A 2×2-mm lancet is used for a stab incision, and a drop of blood is aspirated into a heparinized glass capillary tube.

Fetal blood pH correctly predicts neonatal outcome 82 per cent of the time, as measured by the Apgar score. The false-positive rate is about 8 per cent, and the false-negative rate about 10 per cent. Determinations of P_{O_2} and P_{CO_2}, and base deficit from scalp blood are possible but not particularly useful clinically. A pH value can be obtained from a 7-cm column of blood in a collecting glass capillary tube (0.015 ml). For P_{O_2} and P_{CO_2} determinations, a 25-cm blood column is necessary. This requires a longer sampling time and often leads to clotting within the tube during collection. Clotted blood cannot

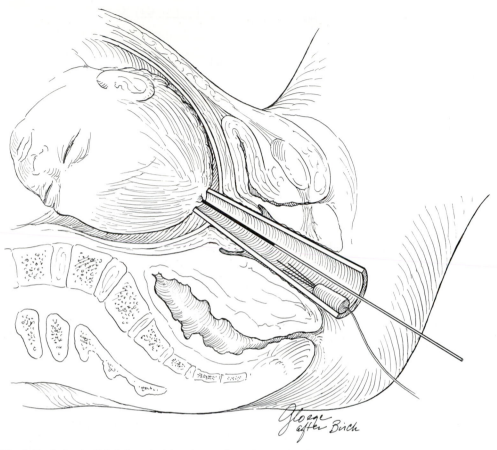

Figure 22–6. Technique of fetal scalp blood sampling via an amnioscope. After making a small stab incision in the fetal scalp, the blood is drawn off through a capillary tube.

be aspirated into the gas analyzer. Furthermore, Po_2 and Pco_2 do not correlate as well as pH with the Apgar score. Determination of base deficit can be helpful to differentiate between respiratory and metabolic acidosis.

It is good clinical practice to doubly clamp the umbilical cord after delivery to allow blood gas analysis from the umbilical artery and vein to evaluate the fetal condition at birth. This is particularly true in cases of fetal distress that lead to operative delivery. Evaluation of pH, Po_2, Pco_2, and base deficit in the cord blood, in addition to Apgar scores, gives valuable information to the pediatrician who assumes responsibility for the newborn. The normal range for these indices is given in Table 22–3.

Ultrasound Doppler velocimetry, for blood flow measurements in umbilical and fetal blood vessels, and percutaneous umbilical blood sampling have been used antepartum. Their usefulness for labor management is not yet determined.

Newborn cerebral dysfunction, manifested as seizures and attributable to true birth asphyxia, does not seem to occur unless the Apgar score at 5 minutes is 3 or less, the umbilical artery blood pH is less than 7.00, and resuscitation is necessary at birth. The impact of lesser degrees of asphyxia, as measured by the Apgar score and acid-base status at birth, remains unknown.

COMPLICATIONS OF FETAL MONITORING

The introduction of a catheter into the uterine cavity and application of a scalp electrode may cause a slight increase in the inci-

Table 22–3. NORMAL RANGES FOR FETAL SCALP AND CORD BLOOD INDICES

BLOOD	pH	PCO$_2$ (mm Hg)	PO$_2$ (mm Hg)	BASE DEFICIT (mEq/L)
Scalp Blood				
Early labor	7.34–7.38	43–57	20–24	(−0.2)–(0.4)
Active phase	7.34–7.40	36–54	20–24	(−2.0)–(0.0)
Complete cervical dilatation	7.26–7.42	36–60	20–24	(−3.3)–(−0.3)
Cord Blood				
Artery	7.22–7.34	32–64	14–22	(−7.8)–(−2.2)
Vein	7.29–7.41	25–53	23–35	(−6.2)–(−1.8)

Modified from Hobel CJ: Intrapartum clinical assessment of fetal distress. Am J Obstet Gynecol 110:336, 1971.

dence of maternal infection, but length of labor, rupture of the membranes, and the number of vaginal examinations are of much greater importance in this regard. The incidence of fetal scalp abscesses and soft tissue injuries from electrode applications is less than 5 per cent. Scalp abscesses are managed by opening the intradermal vesicle to allow for drainage. These small abscesses heal without the need for antibiotic therapy. Spread of the infection into adjacent tissues is rare.

The incidence of scalp abscesses from microblood sampling is less frequent than infection from electrode application. After fetal scalp blood sampling, a cotton swab should always be applied throughout the next uterine contraction and the puncture site inspected for hemostasis during the second contraction. If these precautions are followed, hemorrhage does not occur with scalp blood sampling.

CONTROVERSIES ABOUT FETAL MONITORING IN THE DIAGNOSIS AND TREATMENT OF FETAL DISTRESS

During the early 1970s, electronic FHR monitoring was developed to reduce the intrapartum death rate and to prevent neurologic damage in the newborn infant after studies supported the existence of a correlation between abnormal FHR patterns, fetal acidosis, and low Apgar scores at birth.

It was believed that with this objective technique, fetal hypoxia would be detectable in a timely fashion, allowing the decision to intervene in order to protect the fetus from the consequences of intrauterine oxygen deprivation. Retrospective reports even indicated that among electronically monitored fetuses at high risk, there were fewer intrapartum deaths than among fetuses at low risk who were monitored by intermittent ausculation.

Between 1976 and 1990, there were eight prospective, randomized trials of electronic fetal monitoring, involving a total of 17,756 fetuses. None of these prospective studies found any decrease in the rate of fetal death in utero nor in the incidence of low Apgar scores or fetal acidosis. In addition, there was no decrease in the incidence of neurologically abnormal newborns in the electronically monitored group.

The results of the prospective studies point toward a prelabor etiology for much of the neurologic morbidity. Perhaps the small proportion of neurologic deficits that do occur during labor cannot be prevented with current concepts and applications of FHR monitoring.

Before discontinuing the use of the fetal monitor, it must be realized that the randomized trials all had dedicated nurses for the ausculation group, a condition that is not present in many hospitals.

At the present time, it seems prudent to follow the recommendation of the American College of Obstetricians and Gynecologists. For high-risk patients, they advise using either continuous electronic fetal monitoring or intermittent ausculation every 15 minutes in the first stage and every 5 minutes in the second stage of labor, the same frequency as was used in the randomized trials. Although there are no research data to support the use of auscultation, the College recommends auscultation for low-risk patients every 30 minutes in the first stage of labor and every 15 minutes in the second stage until delivery is completed.

Until new concepts for monitoring are validated, the type of fetal monitoring needs to take into consideration the wishes of the informed patient, the capabilities of the nursing service to carry out monitoring, and the requirements of the physician managing the labor.

SUGGESTED READING

Bieniarz J, Maqueda E, Caldeyro-Barcia R: Compression of aorta by the uterus in late human pregnancy. I. Variations between femoral and brachial artery pressure with changes from hypertension to hypotension. Am J Obstet Gynecol 95:795, 1966.

Fleischman AR: Ethical dilemmas in labor management. In Cohen WR, Acker DB, Friedman EA (eds): Management of Labor. Rockville, MD, Aspen Publishers, 1989, p 551.

Gilstrap LC: Diagnosis of birth asphyxia on the basis of fetal pH, Apgar score, and newborn cerebral dysfunction. Am J Obstet Gynecol 161:825, 1989.

Hobel CJ: Intrapartum clinical assessment of fetal distress. Am J Obstet Gynecol 110:336, 1971.

Hobel CJ, Hyvarinen MA, Okada DM, et al: Prenatal and intrapartum high-risk screening. I. Prediction of the high-risk neonate. Am J Obstet Gynecol 117:1, 1973.

Hon EH: Atlas of Fetal Heart Rate Patterns. New Haven, CT, Harty Press, 1968.

Kubli FW: Observations on heart rate and pH in the human fetus during labor. Am J Obstet Gynecol 104:1190, 1969.

Martin CB: Physiology and clinical use of fetal heart rate variability. Clin Perinatol 9:339, 1982.

Meis PJ, Hall M III, Marshall JR, et al: Meconium passage: A new classification for risk assessment during labor. Am J Obstet Gynecol 131:509, 1978.

Modanlou H, Yeh S, Hon EH, et al: Umbilical cord pH, PO_2, PCO_2 associated with Apgar scores greater than 6 at 5 minutes. Am J Obstet Gynecol 117:943, 1973.

Parer JT: Fetal heart rate. In Creasy RK, Resnik R (eds): Maternal Fetal Medicine. Philadelphia, WB Saunders, 1989, p 314.

Shy KK: Effects of electronic fetal-heart-rate monitoring, as compared with periodic auscultation, on the neurologic development of premature infants. N Engl J Med 322:588, 1990.

Twenty-three

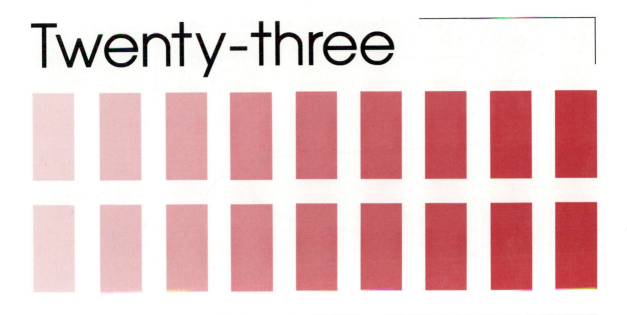

Dystocia

RICHARD A. BASHORE

Although the definition of dystocia is "difficult childbirth," the term is used interchangeably with *dysfunctional labor* and characterizes labor that does not progress normally. The problem may be caused by (1) ineffective uterine expulsive forces; (2) an abnormal lie, presentation, position, or fetal structure; or (3) disproportion between the size of the fetus and pelvis, resulting in mechanical interference with the passage of the fetus through the birth canal. It is important that the cause or causes of abnormal labor be determined as accurately as possible so that an effective and safe management plan may be developed.

The early part or latent phase of labor is involved with softening and effacement of the cervix but minimal dilatation. This is followed by a more rapid rate of cervical dilatation known as the active phase of labor, which is further divided into acceleration,

maximum slope, and deceleration phases. The descent of the fetal presenting part usually begins during the active phase of labor, then progresses at a more rapid rate toward the end of the active phase, and continues after the cervix is completely dilated. A useful method for assessing the progress of labor and detecting abnormalities in a timely manner is to plot the rate of cervical dilatation and descent of the fetal presenting part (Fig. 23–1).

Normal cervical dilatation and descent of the fetus take place in a progressive manner and occur within a well-defined time period. Dysfunctional labor occurs when rates of dilatation and descent exceed these time limits. The phase of labor when the abnormality occurs and the configuration of the abnormal labor curve may indicate the potential causes of the abnormal labor. Although the management of abnormal labor is not dictated by the

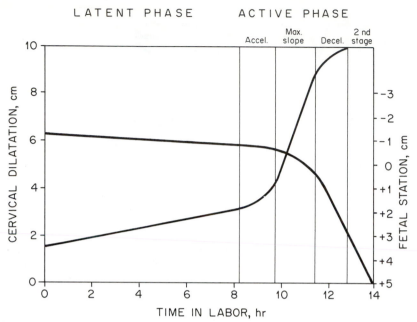

Figure 23-1. Graphic plot of cervical dilatation and descent of the fetal presenting part during labor. (Reprinted from Management of Labor by W.R. Cohen and E.A. Friedman (Eds.), p. 13, with permission of Aspen Publishers, Inc., © 1983.)

appearance of the labor curve, an appreciation of the underlying cause of the problem should suggest rational management plans.

ABNORMALITIES OF THE LATENT PHASE OF LABOR

The normal limits of the latent phase of labor extend up to 20 hours for nulliparous patients and to 14 hours for multiparas. A latent phase that exceeds these limits is considered prolonged (Fig. 23-2) and may be caused by hypertonic uterine contractions, premature or excessive use of sedatives or analgesics, or, less commonly, by hypotonic uterine contractions. Hypertonic contractions are ineffective and painful and are associated with increased uterine tone, whereas hypotonic contractions are usually less painful and are characterized by an easily indentable uterus during the contraction. Hypotonic contractions occur more frequently during the active phase of labor. A long, closed, firm cervix requires more time to efface and undergo early dilatation than does a soft, partially effaced cervix, but it is doubtful that a cervical factor alone will cause a prolonged latent phase. Some patients who appear to be developing a prolonged latent phase are shown eventually to be in false labor with no progressive dilatation of the cervix.

The identification of the cause or causes of a prolonged latent phase is usually not difficult. Palpation or recording of uterine contractions and observation of the patient over a period of time will usually suggest whether uterine activity is hypotonic or hypertonic or whether the patient is in false labor. The outcome of a prolonged latent phase is generally favorable for both the mother and the fetus, provided that no other abnormalities of labor subsequently occur.

Management

The management of a prolonged latent phase depends on the cause. A prolonged latent phase caused by premature or excessive use of sedation or analgesia usually resolves spontaneously after the effects of the medication have disappeared. Hypertonic activity responds erratically to oxytocin but will usually respond to a therapeutic rest with morphine sulfate or an equivalent drug.

Hypocontractile dysfunction usually responds well to an intravenous oxytocin infu-

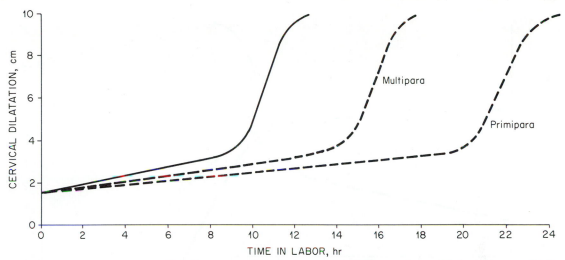

Figure 23-2. Normal cervical dilatation curve (—) and curves depicting prolonged latent phases of labor (---) for multiparous and primiparous patients. (Modified from Friedman EA: Labor: Clinical Evaluation and Management. 2nd ed. New York, Appleton-Century-Crofts, 1978, p 65.)

sion. One technique that has been recommended for stimulation of labor involves the addition of 10 units of oxytocin to 1000 ml of intravenous solution for a final concentration of 10 mU of oxytocin to each 1 ml of solution. An infusion of this solution is begun at a rate of between 0.5 to 1.0 mU per minute and is increased at approximately 50 per cent increments every 20 to 30 minutes until uterine contractions of the desired frequency and intensity are obtained. Alternatively, it has been suggested that the incremental increases should occur at intervals of up to 45 minutes, to permit additional time for the full clinical effect of the oxytocin to be realized.

Although for many years clinicians have considered artificial rupture of the membranes an effective method for management of a prolonged latent phase, this approach continues to be controversial. Additionally, this procedure, when undertaken during the latent phase of labor, carries with it the added risk of intrauterine infection if it does not result in improvement in the labor pattern.

ABNORMALITIES OF THE ACTIVE PHASE OF LABOR

When the cervix reaches a dilatation of approximately 3 to 4 cm, the rate of dilatation progresses more rapidly. Cervical dilatation of less than 1.2 cm per hour in nulliparas and 1.5 cm in multiparas constitutes a *protraction disorder of the active phase of labor*. During the latter part of the active phase, the fetal presenting part also descends more rapidly through the pelvis and continues to descend through the second stage of labor. A rate of descent of the presenting part of less than 1.0 cm per hour in nulliparas and 2.0 cm per hour in multiparas is considered to be a *protraction disorder of descent* (Fig. 23-3). If a period of 2 hours or more elapses during the active phase of labor without progress in cervical dilatation, an *arrest of dilatation* has occurred; a period of more than 1 hour without a change in station of the fetal presenting part is defined as an *arrest of descent* (Fig. 23-4).

The appearance of a protraction or an arrest disorder of dilatation or descent during the active phase of labor calls for a careful appraisal of the patient, since either disorder may signal cephalopelvic disproportion or an abnormality of fetal position. In the absence of cephalopelvic disproportion or fetal malposition, protraction or arrest disorders are usually caused by hypotonic uterine contractions, conduction anesthesia, or excessive sedation. With either disorder, the maternal pelvis should be evaluated, although whether x-ray pelvimetry is appropriate for this evaluation is controversial and is discussed later

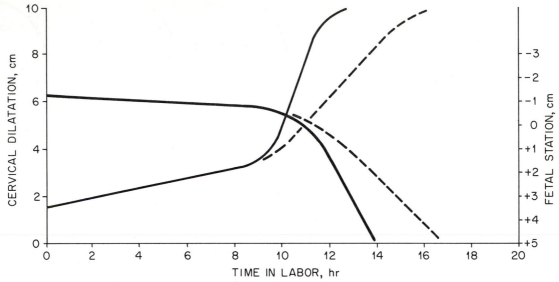

Figure 23–3. Normal dilatation and descent curves of labor (—) and curves depicting protracted dilatation and descent abnormalities of labor (---). (Modified from Friedman EA: Labor: Clinical Evaluation and Management. 2nd ed. New York, Appleton-Century-Crofts, 1978, p 65.)

under Dystocia Caused by Maternal Pelvic Abnormalities.

Management

Protraction disorders do *not* respond to oxytocic stimulation, therapeutic rest, or artificial rupture of the membranes. Patients with this disorder should be treated expectantly so long as the fetal heart rate remains satisfactory and labor continues to be progressive. A large percentage of patients with *arrest disorders* unrelated to cephalopelvic disproportion or fetal malposition *do* respond to oxytocic stimulation. If these disorders are related to oversedation, normal labor patterns will resume if the effect of the drug is allowed to wear off.

Dystocia Caused by Abnormal Presentation and Position

Presentations other than vertex and positions other than occipitoanterior are considered to be abnormal in the laboring patient. Disorders of the dilatation and descent phases of labor occur with increased frequency in cases of abnormal presentation or position because of the altered relationship between the presenting part of the fetus and the maternal pelvis. Fetal malpresentations are discussed further in Chapter 20.

Breech Presentation

The average rate of dilatation and descent for frank, complete, and footling breeches does not differ significantly from the average labor curves for a vertex presentation in either nulliparous or multiparous patients. Patients with a breech presentation, however, experience a greater likelihood of dysfunctional labor than do those with a vertex presentation, most frequently as a result of the presence of a large fetus.

As previously noted (see Chapter 20), fetuses in a breech presentation estimated to weigh less than 1500 gm or more than 3600 gm are usually delivered by elective cesarean section to reduce the incidence of neonatal morbidity and mortality caused by traumatic delivery. The management of patients allowed to labor with a breech presentation who subsequently develop a dysfunctional labor pattern is controversial. If the maternal pelvis is of normal size and configuration on

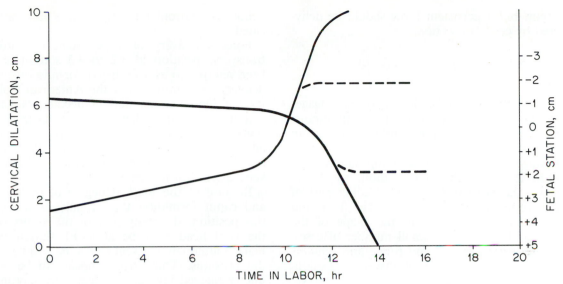

Figure 23–4. Normal dilatation and descent curves of labor (—) and curves depicting arrest disorders of dilatation and descent (- - -). (Modified from Friedman EA: Labor: Clinical Evaluation and Management. 2nd ed. New York, Appleton-Century-Crofts, 1978, p 66.)

the basis of x-ray pelvimetry, the question of the use of oxytocin arises on the assumption that the abnormal labor is the result of hypotonic uterine activity. Since there is an increase in fetal mortality when oxytocin is used to stimulate dysfunctional labor with a breech presentation, the presence of inadequate contractions may be confirmed with an intrauterine pressure catheter before initiating augmentation of labor. Even though the maternal pelvic measurements may be normal on x-ray pelvimetry, an arrest in labor may indicate fetopelvic disproportion as a result of the presence of a macrosomic infant whose weight has been underestimated.

Face Presentation

Face presentation occurs when complete deflexion of the fetal head occurs, resulting in substitution of the submentobregmatic diameter for the suboccipitobregmatic diameter as the largest portion of the head presenting to the maternal pelvis. Since these two diameters are approximately the same length (9.5 cm), however, progress in early labor for a face presentation is not significantly different from a vertex presentation, provided that there is no pelvic contraction. If the mentum is posterior, vaginal delivery of a term-sized fetus is impossible. Spontaneous rotation of

the head to mentum anterior, however, will occur in the majority of cases, but this may require some time to accomplish. Rotation by forceps is generally not advisable.

Because there is an increased incidence of cephalopelvic disproportion and fetal macrosomia associated with a face presentation, cesarean section, rather than oxytocic stimulation, is the wiser choice in the presence of dysfunctional labor.

Brow Presentation

Brow presentation results from incomplete deflexion of the fetal head with a resulting presentation approximately midway between a vertex and a face. The dilatation phase of labor is usually not significantly different from that for a vertex presentation, but the descent phase is typically prolonged because the brow presentation results in the supraoccipitomental diameter (13.5 cm) presenting to the maternal pelvis. Unless a brow presentation converts spontaneously to a vertex or a face, the head cannot deliver except when the fetus is unusually small or the pelvis extremely large. It is appropriate to permit a period of observation in the descent phase in the presence of a brow presentation to determine whether spontaneous conversion will occur, but a persistent brow should be delivered by cesarean section.

Persistent Occipitotransverse Position

The fetal head normally enters and engages in the maternal pelvis in an occipitotransverse position. It subsequently rotates to an occipitoanterior position or, in a small percentage of cases, to an occipitoposterior position. It is thought that rotation occurs because the head flexes as the leading part of the vertex encounters the pelvic floor and then rotates to adjust to the shape of the gynecoid pelvis. In a small number of cases, the head fails to flex and rotate and remains in a persistent occipitotransverse position. This position may be caused by cephalopelvic disproportion; altered pelvic architecture, such as in a patient with a platypelloid or android type pelvis; or a relaxed pelvic floor brought about by epidural anesthesia or multiparity.

The diagnosis of a persistent occipitotransverse position may be difficult at times, owing to the obscuring of suture lines and fontanelles by the excessive molding and caput formation that often accompany this abnormal position.

A persistent occipitotransverse position with arrest of descent for a period of 1 hour or more is known as *transverse arrest.* Arrest occurs because of the deflexion that accompanies the persistent occipitotransverse position, resulting in the larger occipitofrontal diameter (11 cm) becoming the presenting diameter. Until the head undergoes flexion and rotation, further descent cannot take place. Transverse arrest commonly occurs with the vertex at a +2 to +3 station.

The management of transverse arrest at a +2 to +3 station is complex for a number of reasons, among which is the fact that at these stations the widest part of the fetal head is at or above the level of the ischial spines. If the midpelvis is compromised, cesarean section delivery is indicated. If the pelvis is judged to be of normal size, oxytocin stimulation of labor may be appropriate if inadequate uterine contractions are thought to be the cause of the arrest. If the pelvis is of normal size and shape, manual or forceps rotation may be indicated. When the pelvis is of a platypelloid or android type, rotation is not indicated.

Forceps delivery of a persistent occipitotransverse position at +2 to +3 station has been referred to as a midpelvic or midforceps delivery. A committee of the American College of Obstetricians and Gynecologists has recommended that delivery from these stations be redefined as a low forceps. Eventually this recommendation may be adopted, but the complexities of management of transverse arrest will not change.

Because of the marked degree of molding and caput formation that usually occurs in this position, the bony part of the vertex of the fetal head may be at a +1 station or higher, although the scalp may be visible at the introitus. Thus, what appears to be an uncomplicated low forceps operation may instead become an inadvertent high midforceps procedure. One method for avoiding this mishap involves a clinical evaluation of the relationship between the fetal head and the sacrum. If the fetal head fills the hollow of the sacrum, the biparietal diameter is usually at or below the spines, and an attempt at forceps delivery is appropriate.

Persistent Occipitoposterior Position

In the majority of cases, the head rotates from occipitotransverse to occipitoanterior in its descent through the maternal pelvis as one of the cardinal movements of labor. Even if the head rotates to an occipitoposterior position, most fetuses will eventually rotate spontaneously during labor to occipitoanterior, leaving only a small percentage (5 to 10 per cent) of fetuses with a persistent occipitoposterior position.

The course of labor in the presence of a persistent occipitoposterior position is usually normal except for a tendency for the second stage to be prolonged (greater than 2 hours) and associated with more discomfort than is usual for the occipitoanterior position. If a normal fetal heart rate is demonstrated by fetal monitoring, observation of a prolonged second stage of labor is appropriate, provided that labor continues to be progressive.

Delivery of the head may occur spontaneously in the occipitoposterior position, but if the perineum provides undue resistance to delivery, a forceps-assisted delivery may be required. Forceps rotation of an occipitoposterior to an occipitoanterior position may be performed but should be approached with caution if there is an arrest of descent of the fetal head. As noted in the discussion of the persistent occipitotransverse position, the fetal head may become markedly molded with extensive caput formation, which may cause difficulty in diagnosing its correct station and position. Before performing a forceps rotation, it is important that the position of the fetal head be accurately determined and the pelvis be carefully evaluated, since the size and configuration of the maternal pelvis will influence the outcome of the operation. For instance, an attempt at forceps rotation in the presence of a narrow midpelvis would be inadvisable. Feeling for a fetal ear may help identify the position of the head.

Whatever the method chosen for vaginal delivery of the persistent occipitoposterior position, it is important that a wide mediolateral episiotomy be performed after application of forceps, to lessen the resistance of the outlet to the delivery of the fetal head.

Dystocia Caused by Abnormalities of Fetal Structure

Macrosomia and Shoulder Dystocia

A fetus weighing 4000 gm or more is above the 90th percentile of fetal weight for term pregnancy and is considered to be of excessive size. Macrosomia may result from genetic determinants, maternal diabetes, multiparity, or post-term gestation. In general, the larger the fetus, the longer the labor and the greater the incidence of midforceps operations and of shoulder dystocia. Also, the more the fetus exceeds 4000 gm, the higher the rate of perinatal mortality and morbidity resulting from birth trauma.

Even with the aid of sonographic techniques for the evaluation of fetal head and body size, an accurate estimate of fetal weight is elusive. Additionally, when the fetus is of excessive size, the occurrence of shoulder dystocia will depend on the size of the maternal pelvis in relationship to the size of the

fetus, a clinical correlation that is difficult to make. Although the mean duration of labor is prolonged for excessive-sized fetuses, it is not unusual to encounter unexpected shoulder dystocia after a labor that has been entirely normal up to the moment of delivery.

Because shoulder dystocia may occur unexpectedly, it is necessary to be familiar with methods for dealing with the problem. Shoulder dystocia is not overcome by traction on the fetal head but, instead, by one or more maneuvers designed to displace the anterior shoulder from behind the symphysis pubis. The first maneuver involves downward or lateral pressure with the hand over the maternal suprapubic region in an effort to guide the anterior shoulder under or away from the symphysis pubis. Next, the McRoberts maneuver may be tried. The maternal thighs are sharply flexed against the maternal abdomen to reduce the angle between the sacrum and spine, thus freeing the impacted shoulder. If this is not successful, pressure is applied with the operator's fingers against the scapula of the posterior shoulder in an attempt to rotate the posterior shoulder upward until it replaces the anterior shoulder. If this maneuver does not correct the problem, a hand is inserted into the vagina, the posterior arm is grasped and pulled across the chest, resulting in delivery of the posterior shoulder and displacement of the anterior shoulder from behind the symphysis pubis. Fracture of the humerus may result from this maneuver, but the bone heals quickly in the neonate. If none of these maneuvers is successful, one or both clavicles are fractured, preferably by pressure on the clavicle directed away from the pleural cavity to prevent traumatic puncture of the lungs. Excessive traction on the head may result in damage to the brachial plexus, with the possibility of a permanent Erb's palsy. The maneuvers described here to overcome shoulder dystocia may, however, themselves result in brachial plexus damage.

A maneuver has been described, which is attributed to Zavanelli, to manage shoulder dystocia not corrected successfully by the methods already described. In this procedure, the fetal head is manually returned to its prerestitution position then slowly replaced into the vagina by steady upward pressure against the head. Delivery is subsequently accomplished by cesarean section. A uterine relaxant may be required to carry out this procedure.

Developmental Abnormalities

Localized abnormalities of fetal anatomy may lead to dystocia. *Internal hydrocephalus* may cause enlargement of the fetal head to the extent that vaginal delivery is not possible. The diagnosis is usually made by ultrasonography performed because of the clinical suspicion of excessive enlargement of the fetal head, or it may appear as an unexpected finding on ultrasonography performed for other indications.

Several options are available for the delivery of the fetus with hydrocephalus. Excessive cerebrospinal fluid may be removed by inserting a needle directly into the ventricular space through the dilated cervix during labor, or fluid may be removed transabdominally with the aid of ultrasonic visualization of the fetal head before or during labor. Alternatively, the fetus may be delivered by cesarean section to avoid the risk of infection, which may result from transvaginal or transabdominal drainage. Intrauterine shunting of the fetal ventricular system into the amniotic fluid compartment is an experimental procedure, and it is unclear at this time whether the long-term results justify the procedure.

The accumulation of *ascitic fluid* in the fetal abdomen or *enlargement of fetal organs,* such as the bladder or liver, may result in unexpected dystocia after the fetal head is delivered. Rhesus disease and nonimmune *hydrops* are potential causes of these abnormalities, and, should they be present, careful ultrasonic evaluation before or during labor is indicated to identify excessive enlargement of the fetal abdomen. Ascitic fluid or urine from a massively enlarged bladder may be removed by transabdominal drainage with a needle before vaginal delivery. Cesarean section may be indicated if the fetal abdomen cannot be sufficiently decompressed.

A defect in the fetal lumbosacral vertebrae may result in the protrusion of a meningeal sac *(meningocele)* or a sac containing spinal cord *(meningomyelocele).* These defects are usually detected as a result of abnormal serum or amniotic fluid alpha-fetoprotein values or by ultrasonography. If the sac is large, abdominal delivery is advisable to avoid dystocia or rupture of the sac and potential infection. If the sac is small and covered by fetal skin, as reflected by a normal alpha-fetoprotein value, vaginal delivery may be appropriate.

Dystocia Caused by Maternal Pelvic Abnormalities

Cephalopelvic disproportion exists if the maternal bony pelvis is not of sufficient size and of appropriate shape to allow the passage of the fetal head. This problem may occur as a result of contraction of one of the planes of the pelvis. Relative cephalopelvic disproportion may exist if the fetal head is excessively large or if it is in an abnormal position, even though the pelvic measurements are within normal limits. Contraction of the maternal pelvis may occur at the level of the inlet or midpelvis, but contraction of the outlet is extremely unusual unless it is found in association with a midpelvic contraction. Normal and abnormal pelvic architecture are discussed in Chapter 10.

Cephalopelvic disproportion at the level of the pelvic inlet causes a failure of descent of the head, and engagement will not occur. The finding of an unengaged head in a nulliparous patient at the start of labor indicates an increased likelihood of cephalopelvic disproportion at the pelvic inlet, but an unengaged fetal head in a multiparous patient in labor is not an unusual occurrence. Relative cephalopelvic disproportion can occur in the multiparous patient (the "multip trap"), however, and should be kept in mind.

The management of a nulliparous patient with an unengaged fetal head in labor should begin with a careful clinical evaluation of the maternal pelvis. If the capacity of the inlet is normal, expectant management with observation of the labor pattern is appropriate. If uterine contractions are ineffective, oxytocic stimulation of labor may be considered.

The occurrence of cephalopelvic disproportion at the level of the midpelvis occurs more frequently than inlet dystocia because the capacity of the midpelvis is smaller than that of the inlet and also because deflection or positional abnormalities of the fetal head resulting in dystocia are more likely to occur at that level. As noted previously in this chapter, the occurrence of bony dystocia at the level of the midpelvis is usually indicated by an arrest of descent of the head at a +2 to +3 station. It has also been noted that with cephalopelvic disproportion and arrest of descent, application of the head to the cervix is poor, resulting in the loss of part of the force needed for cervical distention. Thus, cephalopelvic disproportion may be associated with an abnormal rate of cervical dilatation before an arrest of descent is apparent.

X-ray Pelvimetry

When the question of cephalopelvic disproportion arises, the use of x-ray pelvimetry as a tool for the evaluation of the maternal bony pelvis is controversial. Those opposed to this procedure indicate that the information obtained does not accurately predict which patients will require abdominal delivery because progress in labor with or without oxytocic stimulation is more useful in determining the route of delivery. The opponents also cite the potential hazards that may be associated with radiation exposure of the fetus.

Those favoring the use of x-ray pelvimetry point out that the procedure should be confined to a small group of patients with arrest of descent in whom clinical pelvimetry suggests disproportion and in whom a midpelvic operation is under consideration. They believe that if x-ray pelvimetry is obtained in labor at the point of dystocia, the information obtained will not only provide a precise evaluation of pelvic capacity and architecture, especially of the midpelvis, but also will indicate the true level of the vertex and allow diagnosis of any deflexion or positional abnormality of the fetal head. Based on this information, an ill-advised attempt at midforceps delivery may be avoided. The proponents also indicate that the radiation hazards associated with pelvimetry are more theoretical than real.

Computed tomography has been proposed as an alternative method for evaluation of pelvic capacity. If this approach proves to be practical, it would have obvious advantages over x-ray pelvimetry.

SUGGESTED READING

Acker DB, Sachs BP, Friedman EA: Risk factors for shoulder dystocia in the average-weight infant. Obstet Gynecol 67:614, 1986.

Bodmer B, Benjamin A, McLean FH, Usher RH: Has use of cesarean section reduced the risks of delivery in the preterm breech presentation? Am J Obstet Gynecol 154:244, 1986.

Brenner WE, Bruce RD, Hendricks CH: The characteristics and perils of breech presentation. Am J Obstet Gynecol 118:700, 1978.

Friedman EA: Labor: Clinical Evaluation and Management. 2nd ed. New York, Appleton-Century-Crofts, 1978.

Gonik B: An alternative maneuver for management of shoulder dystocia. Am J Obstet Gynecol 145:882, 1983.

Laube DW, Varner MW, Cruikshank DP: A prospective evaluation of x-ray pelvimetry. JAMA 246:2187, 1981.

Pritchard JA, MacDonald PC, Gant NF (eds): Williams Obstetrics. 17th ed. Norwalk, CT, Appleton-Century-Crofts, 1985, p 641.

Sandberg EC: The Zavanelli maneuver: A potentially revolutionary method for the resolution of shoulder dystocia. Am J Obstet Gynecol 152:479, 1985.

Twenty-four

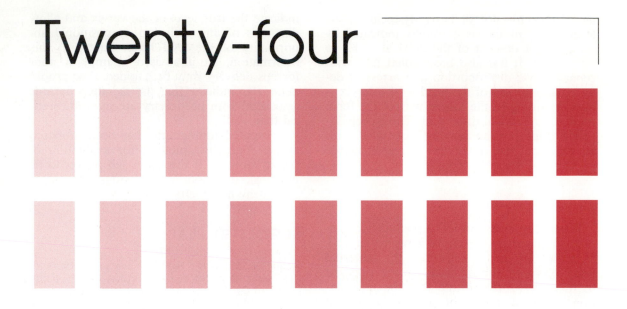

Preterm Labor and Premature Rupture of Membranes

ANNE D. M. GRAHAM

PRETERM LABOR

Preterm labor and delivery are major causes of perinatal morbidity and mortality. Although less than 10 per cent of all infants born in the United States are preterm, their contribution to neonatal morbidity and mortality ranges from 50 to 70 per cent. To decrease the medical and economic impact of preterm delivery, a major goal of obstetric care is not only to reduce the incidence of preterm deliveries but also to increase the gestational age of those infants whose preterm births are unavoidable.

Definition and Incidence

Preterm birth is defined as that occurring after 20 weeks and before 37 completed

weeks of gestation. Labor occurring between these gestational ages is defined as preterm labor. In older literature, a weight-based criterion was used, preterm birth being defined as birth of an infant weighing less than 2500 gm. The advantage of such a parameter is that it is absolute and easily obtained, whereas determination of gestational age is less precise. Since birth weight depends, however, not only on the length of gestation but also correlates with other characteristics of the mother and fetus that govern fetal growth, a weight-based criterion does not differentiate between those infants that are merely small for gestational age and those that are truly preterm.

The true incidence of preterm deliveries is difficult to delineate because of the errors of gestational age assessment and the use of birth weight to define preterm birth in most

270

Table 24–1. ETIOLOGY OF PRETERM LABOR AND DELIVERY

ETIOLOGY	PERCENT OF PRETERM LABOR
Idiopathic	50
Multiple gestation	10–15
Medical indications for induction	5–20
Uterine anomalies	5–15
Miscellaneous (infection, polyhy- dramnios, incompetent cervix)	5

studies. Although dependent on the population studied, the preterm delivery incidence averages about 7 per cent, but varies from a low of 5 per cent in some parts of western Europe to a reported 34 per cent in India.

Etiology and Risk Factors

The etiologic factors for preterm delivery are outlined in Table 24–1. In most cases, the cause is unknown. A variety of socioeconomic, psychosocial, and medical conditions have been found to carry an increased risk of delivering preterm.

Socioeconomic Factors. A higher incidence of preterm births among patients of low socioeconomic status is seen in a number of countries. In the United States, the incidence of preterm deliveries in the black population is twice as high as that in the white population. This factor cannot be viewed as a single entity but probably encompasses other characteristics of the population, such as access to and procurement of antenatal care and information. Other risk factors are shown in Table 8–5.

Medical and Obstetric Factors. When one preterm birth has occurred, the relative risk of preterm delivery in the next pregnancy is 3.9; the risk increases to 6.5 with two previous preterm deliveries. If only one of two previous deliveries was preterm, the relative risk for a subsequent preterm delivery is increased approximately twofold and is greater if the preterm delivery occurred in the second rather than the first pregnancy (2.5 versus 1.3).

Second-trimester abortions seem to carry an increased risk for subsequent preterm de-livery, especially if a previous preterm birth has also occurred. The risk associated with induced first-trimester abortions is controversial. Repeated spontaneous first-trimester abortions, however, do increase the risk.

Certain preterm births are unavoidable because of the need for medical intervention for maternal or fetal indications, such as severe pre-eclampsia or uncontrolled third-trimester bleeding associated with placenta previa or abruptio placentae. Iatrogenic preterm birth remains a problem because of elective induction of labor or cesarean section in a preterm pregnancy thought to be at term because of incorrect dating. This should decline with physician education and the trend toward trial of labor for patients who have had a previous cesarean section.

Other medical and obstetric factors associated with an increased risk of delivering preterm include bleeding in the first trimester, urinary tract infections, multiple gestation, uterine anomalies, polyhydramnios, and incompetent cervix.

Prevention

The principal means of decreasing the problem of prematurity are the identification of high-risk patients, to allow education and clinical assessment for preterm labor, and the recognition of preterm contractions early so that aggressive therapy can be instituted. To identify impending preterm labor, a number of mechanisms including home uterine monitoring can be used.

Diagnosis

The diagnosis of preterm labor should be based on the presence of regular uterine contractions in a preterm gestation associated with the cervical changes of either dilatation or effacement.

Management

Upon diagnosing preterm labor, a number of management decisions need to be addressed.

Provided that membranes are not ruptured and there is no contraindication to a vaginal examination, such as placenta previa, an initial assessment must be done to ascertain cervical length and dilatation and the station and nature of the presenting part. The patient should also be evaluated for the presence of any underlying correctable problem, such as a urinary tract infection. She should be placed in the lateral decubitus position, monitored for the presence and frequency of uterine activity, and re-examined for evidence of cervical change after an appropriate interval. During the period of observation, either oral or parenteral hydration should be carried out.

Approximately 20 per cent of patients will cease uterine contractions with adequate hydration or maternal sedation. These patients, however, remain at high risk for recurrent preterm labor.

Because of the role of cervical colonization and vaginal infection in the etiology of preterm labor and premature rupture of membranes, cultures should be taken for group B *Streptococcus, Chlamydia,* and possibly *Ureaplasma.* Whether or not prophylactic antibiotics should be administered pending the results of these cultures is controversial.

Once the diagnosis of preterm labor has been made, the following laboratory tests should be obtained: complete blood count, random blood glucose, serum electrolytes, urinalysis, and urine culture and sensitivity. If not previously performed, an ultrasonic examination of the fetus should be performed to assess fetal weight, to document presentation, and to rule out the presence of any accompanying congenital malformation. The test may also detect some underlying etiologic factor such as twins or uterine anomalies.

If the patient does not respond to bed rest and hydration, tocolytic therapy is instituted, provided that there are no contraindications. Measures implemented at 28 weeks should be more aggressive than those performed at 35 weeks. Similarly, a patient with advanced cervical dilatation on admission requires more aggressive management than one whose cervix is closed and minimally effaced.

Uterine Tocolytic Therapy

The physiologic events leading to the initiation of labor are discussed in Chapter 5. It is assumed that these events also occur in preterm labor. The pharmacologic agents presently being used all seem to inhibit the availability of calcium ions, but they may also exert a number of other effects. The agents currently used and their dosages are presented in Table 24–2.

Beta-Adrenergic Agonists. Uterine muscle has both alpha and beta-2-adrenergic receptors. α-Adrenergic stimulation causes contractions, whereas stimulation of the beta-2 receptors initiates myometrial relaxation.

β-Sympathomimetic agents act by the conversion of adenosine triphosphate (ATP) to cyclic adenosine monophosphate (cAMP). An increase of cAMP within the cell decreases the availability of free calcium ions by increasing their intracellular binding.

The β-adrenergic agents are structurally similar to the catecholamines and do have some beta activity, which therefore results in cardiac side effects. They are not as easily methylated as catecholamines and thus do not undergo first-pass hepatic degradation, so therapeutic levels can be reached with oral administration. They are eliminated by renal excretion, mostly in an unchanged form, although some conjugation occurs.

Parenteral administration achieves a quicker therapeutic level. The drug can be titrated to a dose at which uterine contractions cease, maternal pulse reaches 120 to 140 beats per minute, or side effects are poorly tolerated. Dosage is maintained at this level for 6 to 12 hours before weaning to oral therapy 30 minutes before the parenteral drug is discontinued. Strict attention must be paid to fluid balance in all patients, and blood glucose and serum potassium levels should be monitored more frequently in those patients who have diabetes or heart disease.

Ritodrine is presently the only agent approved by the Food and Drug Administration (FDA) for the treatment of preterm labor, although clinical trials for another β-agonist, hexoprenaline, are under way. Terbutaline and isoxsuprine have also been widely used in the United States. In Europe, salbutamol and orciprenaline have been tried. Terbutaline is used similarly to ritodrine. As with all β-agonists, the maternal pulse rate can be used as a guide to effective dosage.

After successful tocolysis, oral therapy is maintained until 37 weeks gestation. Patients who have preterm labor secondary to a treatable and reversible cause such as urinary tract

Table 24-2. UTERINE TOCOLYTIC AGENTS	

DRUG	DOSAGE

Ritodrine hydrochloride (Yutopar)	Solution: 150 mg ritodrine in 500 ml 5% dextrose (0.3 mg/ml); IV piggyback
	Parenteral:
	  Initial dose: 0.05–0.1 mg/min
	  Titrating dose: Increase by 0.05 mg q 10 min until contractions cease or unacceptable side effects occur; maximum dose is 0.35 mg/min or maternal pulse of 140 beats/min
	  Maintenance dose: 6 hr at maximum dose
	Oral: 10 mg 1/2 hr prior to discontinuing infusion. 10–20 mg q 2–4 hr; titrate dose and frequency to maintain maternal pulse of >100

Terbutaline sulfate (Brethine, Bricanyl)	Solution: 5 mg in 500 ml Ringer's lactate (10 μg/ml)
	Parenteral:
	  Initial dose: 10 μg/min IV piggyback or 0.25 mg SQ
	  Titrating dose: For infusion, increase by 10 μg/min q 20 min or SQ 0.25 mg q 3–6 hr until contractions cease, pulse rate becomes 120–140, or intolerable side effects occur
	  Maintenance dose: 1 hr at maximum dose with no contractions, then discontinue
	Oral: 2.5–5.0 mg q 4–6 hr; titrate frequency to pulse; begin 1/2 hr prior to discontinuing parenteral therapy

Magnesium sulfate	Solution: Initial solution contains 6 gm (12 ml of 50% MgSO$_4$) in 100 ml 5% dextrose; maintenance solution contains 10 gm (20 ml of 50% MgSO$_4$) in 500 ml 5% dextrose
	Parenteral:
	  Initial dose: 6 gm over 15–20 min
	  Titrating dose: 2 gm/hr until contractions cease; follow serum levels (5–7 mg/dl)
	  Maintenance dose: 1 gm/hr for 24–72 hr; may switch to oral β-agonist therapy before discontinuing

infection probably do not require continuous therapy, but there are no long-term studies to support this.

Although the β-adrenergic tocolytic agents are selected for their beta-2 specificity, they still possess some beta-1 activity. The presence of receptors in a number of organs results in a variety of side effects. Cardiovascular side effects are the most common and include an increase in heart rate, a rise in systolic pressure, and a decrease in diastolic pressure. Usually, mean arterial pressure remains the same, but the peripheral vasodilatation produced may cause profound hypotension in some patients. About 1 to 2 per cent of patients have chest pain secondary to myocardial ischemia, sometimes associated with arrhythmias or electrocardiographic changes.

A rare, more serious side effect is the development of pulmonary edema. A number of factors, both cardiogenic and noncardiogenic, may be involved. Prolonged maternal tachycardia, fluid retention secondary to decreased free water clearance, and increased myocardial work may contribute to cardiac failure. In addition, iatrogenic fluid overload contributes in some cases. Concurrent administration of glucocorticoids for pulmonary maturation may be a risk factor for the development of pulmonary edema.

β-Adrenergic stimulation causes increased liver and muscle glycogenolysis, resulting in an elevation of plasma glucose, and from muscle, increased lactic acid production. All patients treated with β-sympathomimetic agents are at risk for the development of hyperglycemia, but in a few reported cases, diabetic patients treated with these drugs have developed frank ketoacidosis. Circulating insulin rises secondary to the hyperglycemia, but a direct effect on pancreatic-adrenergic receptors contributes to the increase. Insulin drives potassium into the cells with resultant hypokalemia. Urinary excretion of potassium remains unchanged, indicating that total body potassium is adequate. Potassium replacement is not needed in otherwise healthy patients, since no adverse effects have been noted, even at levels as low as 2.3 mEq/dl. After several hours of drug administration, serum abnormalities tend to return to normal and are completely reversed by 24 hours.

Placental transfer of β-adrenergic agents does occur, but fetal effects, such as tachycardia, are delayed. At birth, fetal levels are the same or lower than those of maternal plasma. Hypoglycemia and hyperglycemia have been observed in infants born to mothers treated with β-adrenergic agonists.

Magnesium. Magnesium sulfate can be used as an effective uterine tocolytic and may be the drug of choice for patients with diabetes mellitus or heart disease. Magnesium acts at the cellular level by competing with calcium for entry into the cell at the time of depolarization. Successful competition results in an effective decrease of intracellular calcium ions, resulting in myometrial relaxation.

Although magnesium levels required for tocolysis have not been critically evaluated, it appears that the levels needed may be higher than those required for prevention of eclampsia. Levels from 5.5 to 7 mg/dl appear to be appropriate. These can be achieved using the dosage regimen outlined in Table 24–2. After the loading dose is given, a continuous infusion is maintained, and plasma levels should be determined until therapeutic levels are reached. The drug should be continued at therapeutic levels until contractions cease. Since magnesium is excreted by the kidneys, adjustments must be made in those patients with underlying renal disease and an abnormal creatinine clearance. Oral magnesium therapy has been successfully used in a number of patients, using a dosage of magnesium gluconate, 1 gm orally every 4 hours. Serum magnesium levels are not as high as those achieved with parenteral administration. Once successful tocolysis has been achieved with magnesium therapy, the patient is usually switched to either oral betamimetic agents, or if unsuccessful, a terbutaline pump.

A common minor side effect of magnesium therapy is a feeling of warmth and flushing on first administration. Respiratory depression is seen at magnesium levels of 12 to 15 mg/dl, and cardiac conduction defects and arrest are seen at higher levels.

In the fetus, plasma magnesium levels approach those of the mother, and a low plasma calcium may also be demonstrated. The neonate may show some loss of muscle tone and drowsiness resulting in a lower Apgar score. These effects are prolonged in the preterm neonate because of the decrease in renal clearance.

Long-term parenteral magnesium therapy has been used for control of preterm labor in selected patients. Although not well studied, an important side effect seems to be loss of calcium, leading in one reported case to osteoporosis and a vertebral fracture. The effect of fetal calcium metabolism has not been well studied, especially in terms of bone growth and calcification. It may be important in such patients to institute calcium therapy on a prophylactic basis.

Prostaglandin Synthetase Inhibitors. Prostaglandins induce myometrial contractions at all stages of gestation, both in vivo and in vitro. Because prostaglandins are locally synthesized and possess a relatively short halflife, prevention of their synthesis within the uterus could abort labor. Agents that inhibit prostaglandin synthetase are quite effective tocolytic agents. They can result, however, in oligohydramnios and premature closure of the fetal ductus, which in turn may lead to neonatal pulmonary hypertension and cardiac failure. Short-term usage may be fine, but if patients are placed on indomethacin, the fetus should be evaluated with ultrasonography for ductus arteriosus flow.

Prostaglandin synthetase inhibitors used for treatment of preterm labor include indomethacin (Indocin), aspirin, and flufenamic acid. Indomethacin is the most commonly used and can be administered both orally and rectally with some slight delay in absorption from rectal administration as compared with the oral route. Peak serum levels of indomethacin occur 1.5 to 2 hours after oral administration. Excretion of the intact drug occurs in maternal urine.

Transplacental transfer of the drug to the fetus occurs, and fetal levels approach those of the mother. In addition, about 90 per cent of the drug is protein bound in the neonate, which contributes to its prolonged half-life of

15 to 20 hours. An even longer half-life occurs in the preterm infant.

The side effects of these agents are related to their effect on the prostaglandin synthetase enzymes in other organ systems. Prostaglandins are important regulators of platelet aggregation, and inhibition of prostaglandin synthetase results in platelet dysfunction. Indomethacin induces a reversible effect that disappears when the drug is eliminated, but the dysfunction induced by aspirin is effective for the life of the platelet. Increased bleeding occurs during delivery and the postpartum period, especially in cases in which the drug is chronically administered. In addition, gastric irritation may occur.

During in utero existence, the pulmonary circulation is largely bypassed by the ductus arteriosus, which shunts 55 per cent of ventricular output to the descending aorta. Major changes in circulatory dynamics occur at the time of birth, during which conversion to a neonatal circulation results in closure of the ductus arteriosus, mediated in part by the high oxygen concentration and alterations in prostaglandin synthesis. It is thought that patency of the ductus during fetal life is maintained by local secretion of prostaglandins, and inhibition of synthesis will result in partial or complete closure of the ductus. Although closure is compatible with in utero existence, the resulting increase in blood flow to the pulmonary vasculature may induce hypertrophic changes in the smooth muscle of the pulmonary vessels that subsequently lead to the development of pulmonary hypertension in the neonate with all its coexistent cardiac and respiratory problems.

Calcium Channel Blockers. Nifedipine is an example of this class of drug. It has been shown both in vivo and in vitro to relax myometrial tissue. Clinical studies with calcium channel blockers have been very encouraging, and they may eventually replace the beta-mimetics. They can cause cardiovascular side effects, however, such as severe tachycardia and hypotension in both the mother and the neonate, and in animal studies they have been reported to cause hypoxia and fetal acidemia, leading to fetal death.

Efficacy of Tocolytic Therapy. Although the advent of tocolytic agents has failed to decrease the preterm incidence in large population studies, their use has shifted the distribution of births by gestational age to more prolonged gestations. There has also been an improvement in neonatal survival, decreased incidence of respiratory distress syndrome (RDS), and an increase in the birth weight of infants treated with these agents. Benefits do not accrue to infants older than 33 weeks' gestational age. All the β-sympathomimetic agents have similar efficacy and delay delivery for more than 72 hours in about 80 per cent of patients treated.

Magnesium is as effective as ritodrine. The prostaglandin synthetase inhibitors delay delivery in 80 to 90 per cent of patients for the 24 hours of treatment.

Antibiotic Therapy. A number of studies have advocated the use of antibiotic prophylaxis in patients with preterm labor. Such patients may have a higher incidence of subclinical chorioamnionitis than previously thought. In addition, it is believed that vaginal flora such as *Gardnerella vaginalis* may play a more important role in the initiation and continuation of preterm labor than previously realized.

Contraindications to Tocolytic Therapy. These include severe pre-eclampsia, severe bleeding from placenta previa or abruptio placentae, chorioamnionitis, intrauterine growth retardation, fetal anomalies incompatible with life, and fetal demise. Because of the low success rate, advanced cervical dilatation may also preclude tocolytic therapy, although therapy may delay delivery sufficiently for glucocorticoid administration to accelerate fetal lung maturity. All patients should be individualized, and if the patient is dilated 6 cm and contracting infrequently, it is advisable to employ tocolysis in order to administer glucocorticoid therapy.

Use of Hormones for Pulmonary Maturation

A number of hormones are effective in enhancing pulmonary maturity and decreasing the incidence of RDS. These include both glucocorticoids and thyroid releasing hormone (TRH).

Glucocorticoid administration to the mother is effective at less than 33 weeks gestation; the benefits derived seem to depend on a number of factors, including fetal sex (female infants benefit more than male) and ethnic group (black infants benefit more than white).

In contrast to glucocorticoids, thyroid hormones have been advocated to enhance pulmonary maturation in fetuses younger than 28 weeks of gestation. Because thyroid hormone does not effectively cross the placenta, TRH has been the most active agent used. It increases fetal thyroid hormone levels and therefore enhances lung maturation. Studies are currently underway to determine its true effectiveness, the duration of effectiveness, and the optimal gestational age for benefit.

Usually only about 10 per cent of patients in preterm labor qualify for treatment.

Labor and Delivery of the Preterm Infant

A certain number of patients will not respond to tocolytic therapy and will proceed to advanced labor and delivery of a preterm neonate. The goal in these patients is to conduct both labor and delivery in an optimal manner so as not to contribute to the morbidity or mortality of the preterm infant. All parameters for assessing gestational age and fetal weight must be considered in arriving at the best estimate of these parameters. With modern neonatal care, the lower limit of potential viability is 26 weeks or 600 gm, although multiple exceptions to these figures undoubtedly exist, so each case should be individualized.

Fetal heart rate patterns that are relatively innocuous in the term fetus may indicate a more ominous outcome for the preterm fetus. Continuous fetal heart monitoring and prompt attention to abnormal fetal heart rate patterns are extremely important. Acidosis at birth will adversely affect respiratory function by destroying surfactant and delaying its release.

Drugs administered to the mother usually pass to the fetus, and in the preterm fetus, hepatic enzyme degradation and renal excretion are immature, thereby resulting in a more prolonged drug effect.

If the fetus is presenting as a vertex, vaginal delivery is preferred, independent of gestational age, provided the fetal acidosis and delivery trauma are avoided. Use of outlet forceps and a large episiotomy to shorten the second stage are advocated.

Approximately 23 per cent of infants present as a breech at 28 weeks, compared with about 4 per cent at term. This presentation carries an increased risk of cord prolapse or compression. In addition, cervical entrapment of the aftercoming fetal head may occur at delivery because, prior to term, the head is proportionally larger than the buttocks. For the breech fetus estimated at less than 1500 gm, neonatal outcome is improved by cesarean section.

PREMATURE RUPTURE OF THE MEMBRANES

Definition and Incidence

Premature rupture of the membranes (PROM) is defined as amniorrhexis prior to the onset of labor at any stage of gestation. It has been suggested that the term *preterm premature rupture of the membranes* (PPROM) should be used to define those patients who are preterm with ruptured membranes, whether or not they have contractions.

Etiology and Risk Factors

The etiology of PROM remains unclear, but a variety of factors are purported to contribute to its occurrence, including vaginal and cervical infections, abnormal membrane physiology, incompetent cervix, and nutritional deficiencies of copper or ascorbic acid (vitamin C). The mechanisms by which these may act are as yet unexplained.

Diagnosis

Diagnosis of PROM is based on the history of vaginal loss of fluid and confirmation of amniotic fluid in the vagina. Episodic urinary incontinence, leukorrhea, or loss of the mucous plug must be ruled out. Management of the patient presenting with this history depends on the gestational age. For the patient not in labor, whether preterm or term, the examiner's hands should not be inserted into the vagina because of the risk of introducing infection and the usually long latency period from the time of examination until delivery. A sterile vaginal speculum examination should be performed to confirm the diagnosis, to assess cervical dilatation and length, and, if the patient is preterm, to obtain cervical cultures and amniotic fluid samples for pulmonary maturation tests.

On examination, pooling of amniotic fluid in the posterior vaginal fornix can usually be seen. A Valsalva maneuver or slight fundal pressure may expel fluid from the cervical os, which is diagnostic of PROM. Confirmation of the diagnosis can be made by (1) testing the fluid with nitrazine paper, which will turn blue in the presence of the alkaline amniotic fluid, and (2) placing a sample on a microscopic slide, air drying, and examining for ferning. False-positive nitrazine test results occur in the presence of alkaline urine, blood, or cervical mucus. In the presence of blood, which is usually seen in patients who are also in early labor, the pattern may appear to be skeletonized, and a distinct ferning may not be seen. As in the case of preterm labor with intact membranes, a complete ultrasonic examination should be carried out to rule out fetal anomalies and to assess gestational age and amniotic fluid volume.

Management

General Considerations

An intact amniotic sac serves as a mechanical barrier to infection, but in addition, amniotic fluid has some bacteriostatic properties that may play a role in preventing chorioamnionitis and fetal infections. Intact membranes are not an absolute barrier to infection, since bacterial colonization occurs in 10 per cent of patients in term labor with intact membranes and in up to 25 per cent of patients in preterm labor.

For preterm fetuses with PPROM, the risks associated with preterm delivery must be balanced against the risks of infection and sepsis that may make in utero existence even more problematic. For the mother, the risks are not only the development of chorioamnionitis, but also the possibility of failed induction in the presence of an unfavorable cervix, resulting in subsequent cesarean section.

Management is dictated to a large extent by the gestational age at the time of membrane rupture and the prevailing incidence of chorioamnionitis in the institution in which the patient is being managed. In addition, the quantity of amniotic fluid remaining after PPROM may be as important as gestational age in determining pregnancy outcome. In general, preterm delivery is a greater risk factor than infection.

Ultrasonic definition of oligohydramnios is not standardized. Subjective criteria include marked crowding of the fetal limbs and obvious lack of amniotic fluid. Objective criteria include (1) measurement of the vertical axis of amniotic fluid present in four quadrants, the total being called the *amniotic fluid index* (a value of less than 4 cm is considered abnormal), and (2) measurement of the largest vertical axis that does not contain umbilical cord. A value of less than 1 cm is consistent with oligohydramnios. The less than 1 cm rule has been most widely used and has been correlated with poor physical outcome when used as part of the biophysical profile.

Oligohydramnios associated with PPROM in the fetus at less than 24 weeks gestation may lead to the development of pulmonary hypoplasia. Factors that may be responsible include fetal crowding with thoracic compression, restriction of fetal breathing, and disturbances of pulmonary fluid production and flow. The duration of membrane rupture is an important consideration. Constraints placed on fetal movements in utero can also result in a variety of positional skeletal abnormalities, such as talipes equinovarus. The latter also depends on the duration of ruptured membranes.

If PROM occurs at 36 weeks or later and the cervix is favorable, labor should be induced after 4 to 6 hours if no spontaneous contractions occur. In the presence of an unfavorable cervix with no evidence of infection, it is reasonable to wait 24 hours prior to induction of labor to decrease the risk of failed induction and maternal febrile morbidity. The following discussion applies when premature membrane rupture occurs prior to 36 weeks gestational age.

Laboratory Tests

In addition to those obtained for the patient in preterm labor, sufficient amniotic fluid can usually be obtained from the vaginal pool for pulmonary maturation studies.

Because of the higher incidence of chorioamnionitis in association with PROM, amniotic fluid should also be sent for Gram stain and culture.

Conservative Expectant Management

Conservative expectant management applies to the care of those patients with PPROM who are observed with the expectation of prolonging gestation. Since the risk of infection appears to increase with the duration of membrane rupture, the goal of expectant management is to continue the pregnancy until the lung profile is mature (see under Tests of Pulmonary Maturity). Careful surveillance must be maintained to diagnose chorioamnionitis at an early enough stage to minimize fetal and maternal risks. In its fulminant state, chorioamnionitis is associated with a high maternal temperature and a tender, sometimes irritable uterus. In cases of subclinical infection, however, diagnosis and treatment may be delayed. A combination of factors should alert the clinician to the possibility of chorioamnionitis, including maternal temperature greater than 100.4°F (38°C) in the absence of any other site of infection, fetal tachycardia, and uterine irritability on nonstress testing.

The presence of bacteria by Gram stain or culture of amniotic fluid obtained at amniocentesis correlates with subsequent maternal infection in about 50 per cent of cases and neonatal sepsis in about 25 per cent. The presence of white blood cells alone in amniotic fluid is unreliable in predicting infection and should not be used as an indicator of chorioamnionitis. The decision to perform amniocentesis is based on the gestational age, the presence of early signs of infection, and the amount of fluid as seen by real-time ultrasonography.

Antibiotics should not be used routinely as prophylactic therapy for PPROM. They serve to mask maternal infection and may cause the development of resistant organisms. If group B streptococci are cultured from the cervix, however, penicillin G should be given in an attempt to eradicate the organism and lessen the chance of ascending infection, since neonatal infection is associated with a higher fetal mortality rate.

Management of Chorioamnionitis

Once chorioamnionitis is diagnosed, antibiotic therapy should be delayed only until appropriate cultures are taken. Ampicillin is still the drug of choice. In the penicillin-sensitive patient, cephalosporins may be indicated, noting the 12 per cent incidence of crossover sensitivity. Ampicillin is given either alone or in combination with a aminoglycoside and anaerobic coverage, depending on the severity of infection. Good results have also been obtained with third-generation cephalosporins. Once antibiotics have been started, labor should be induced. If the cervix is unfavorable with active chorioamnionitis and evidence of fetal involvement, it may be necessary to perform a cesarean section.

An important concern is the presence of active genital herpes in the presence of ruptured membranes. A site remote from the cervix and vagina is probably not associated with an increased risk of fetal infection, so the site of infection should be taken into consideration before recommending immediate abdominal delivery.

Tocolytic Therapy

The use of tocolytics to control preterm labor in patients with PROM is controversial. The arguments against their use are that they may mask evidence of maternal infection such as tachycardia, and contractions associated with the membrane rupture may be indicative of uterine infection. Arguments for their use are that PROM is sometimes initially associated with evidence of uterine contractions and time is gained for pulmonary maturation. In the presence of infection, tocolysis will usually be unsuccessful.

Use of Corticosteroids

There appears to be a decreased incidence of RDS in infants who are born after 16 hours of ruptured membranes when compared with infants of similar gestational age born without PROM. Use of corticosteroids is therefore not necessary and may lead to an increased incidence of neonatal and maternal infection.

Outpatient Management

After inpatient observation for a few days without any evidence of infection, outpatient management can be considered. To be eligible for such management, the patient should be reliable, fully informed regarding the risks involved, and prepared to participate in her own care. The fetus should be presenting as a vertex, and the cervix should be closed to minimize the chance of cord prolapse. At home, no coital activity should occur, and the patient must monitor her temperature at least four times per day. Instructions should be given to return immediately if the temperature exceeds 100°F (37.8°C).

The patient should be seen weekly, at which time her temperature is taken, non-stress testing is done, and the baseline fetal heart rate is evaluated. Ultrasonic evaluation of fetal growth and amniotic fluid volume should also be done every 2 weeks. Any patient with oligohydramnios is not a candidate for outpatient management.

Labor and Delivery

The same considerations discussed under preterm labor apply to patients with PROM. The decrease in amniotic fluid that is sometimes seen, however, can result in early cord compression and the presence of variable fetal heart decelerations. This is true of both vertex and breech presentations, and therefore there is a necessity for abdominal delivery in a large number of cases unless fluid replacement can be instituted by amnio-infusion.

TESTS OF PULMONARY MATURITY

By far, the major determinant of successful ex utero existence is the ability of the neonate to maintain successful oxygenation. Pulmonary maturation involves changes in pulmonary anatomy in addition to alterations of physiologic and biochemical parameters. Stages of anatomic pulmonary development include (1) an embryonic phase from 3 to 6 weeks; (2) a pseudoglandular phase from 7 to 17 weeks; (3) a canalicular phase from 18 to 24 weeks, during which capillary plexuses develop around the terminal bronchioles; and (4) the terminal sac phase that occurs at about 24 weeks, during which terminal bronchioles divide into three or four respiratory

bronchioles. Type II pneumocytes, important in surfactant synthesis, begin to proliferate during this phase.

Surfactant is required for successful lung function. Surfactant is a complex mixture of phospholipids, neutral lipids, proteins, carbohydrates, and salts that is important in decreasing alveolar surface tension, maintaining alveoli open at a low internal alveolar diameter, and decreasing intra-alveolar lung fluid. Synthesis takes place in the type II pneumocytes by incorporation of choline, and there appears to be significant recycling by resorption and secretion.

Initially, the important phospholipid was thought to be phosphatidylcholine (lecithin), but it is apparent that other components, such as phosphatidylinositol (PI) and phosphatidylglycerol (PG), are also important. These substances are produced and secreted in increasing amounts as gestation advances, and the continued egress of tracheal fluid into the amniotic fluid results in their increasing presence near term.

Measurement of these substances in the amniotic fluid obtained by amniocentesis allows prediction of the risk of development of RDS in the neonate. Lecithin levels increase rapidly after 35 weeks gestation, whereas sphingomyelin levels remain relatively constant after this gestational age. The lecithin and sphingomyelin concentrations are measured by thin-layer or high-pressure liquid chromatography and are expressed as the L/S ratio. The presence of blood or meconium in the amniotic fluid will affect the L/S ratio, meconium decreasing it and blood normalizing it to a value of 1.4.

About 2 per cent of infants with ratios equal to or greater than 2 develop RDS, compared with 60 per cent of infants with ratios less than 2. There is, therefore, a high false-negative rate associated with this test, and in the diabetic patient, a mature L/S ratio is not so reassuring.

Lung Profile

Using two-dimensional, thin-layer chromatography, both PG and PI can be measured. Along with the L/S ratio, these make up the lung profile. RDS is rare when the L/S ratio is greater than 2 and PG is present, whereas when the L/S ratio is less than 2 and no PG is present, over 90 per cent of infants develop RDS. If the L/S ratio is immature but PG is present, less than 5 per cent of infants will develop RDS. The lung profile offers a more reliable predictor of pulmonary maturity, especially in infants of diabetic mothers. Other advantages of using PG are that contamination with vaginal secretions or blood, as occurs in cases of ruptured membranes and vaginal pool sampling, does not interefere with the detection of PG.

The foam stability test provides an estimate of the surface-tension–lowering capacity of amniotic fluid. Ninety-five per cent ethanol is added to amniotic fluid to decrease the contribution to bubble formation of other surface-acting components, such as protein and bilirubin. The presence of bubbles is associated with less than a 1 per cent incidence of RDS. The Foam Stability Index (Beckman) is a commercially available test. In general, it is rapid, and if carried out according to specific directions, it can be used as the first test to assess lung maturity. Its false-positive and negative rates are higher than the L/S ratio and PG determinations.

SURFACTANT THERAPY

RDS in preterm infants is caused by a lack of suffcent surfactant or surface-tension–lowering properties in the lung fluid. Production of surfactant by type II pneumocytes may be induced by corticosteroids and TRH, but many premature infants still develop RDS. Several animal studies using installation of surfactant into the pulmonary tree immediately postpartum have shown dramatic improvements in lung mechanics and survival of the preterm infant. These studies have been confirmed in human trials, with all studies reporting a decrease in both the incidence and severity of RDS. Surfactant therapy is currently available for routine use.

SUGGESTED READING

Beall MH, Edgar BW, Paul RH, Smith-Wallace T: A comparison of ritodrine, terbutaline, and magnesium sulfate for the suppression of preterm labor. Am J Obstet Gynecol 153:854, 1985.

Benedetti TJ: Maternal complications of parenteral β-sympathomimetic therapy for premature labor. Am J Obstet Gynecol 145:1, 1983.

Depp R, Boehm JJ, Nosek JA, et al: Antenatal corticosteroids to prevent neonatal respiratory distress syndrome: Risk versus benefit considerations. Am J Obstet Gynecol 137:338, 1980.

Garite TJ, Freeman RK, Linzey EM, et al: Prospective randomized study of corticosteroids in the management of premature rupture of the membranes and the premature gestation. Am J Obstet Gynecol 141:508, 1981.

Hallman M, Kulovich M, Kirkpatrick E, et al: Phosphatidylinositol and phosphatidylglycerol in amniotic fluid: Indices of lung maturity. Am J Obstet Gynecol 125:613, 1976.

Lamont RF, Anthony F, Myatt L, et al: Production of prostaglandin E2 by human amnion in vitro in response to addition of media conditioned by microorganisms associated with chorioamnionitis and preterm labor. Am J Obstet Gynecol 162:819, 1990.

Nageotte MP: Prevention and treatment of preterm labor in twin gestation. Clin Obstet Gynecol 33:61, 1990.

Neibyl JR: Prostaglandin synthetase inhibitors. Semin Perinatol 5:274, 1981.

Ohlsson A, Wang E: An analysis of antenatal tests to detect infection in preterm premature rupture of the membranes. Am J Obstet Gynecol 162:809, 1990.

Papiernik E: Prediction of the preterm baby. Clin Obstet Gynecol 11:315, 1984.

Sachs BP: Intrapartum and delivery room management of the very low birthweight infant. Clin Perinatol 16:809, 1989.

Twenty-five

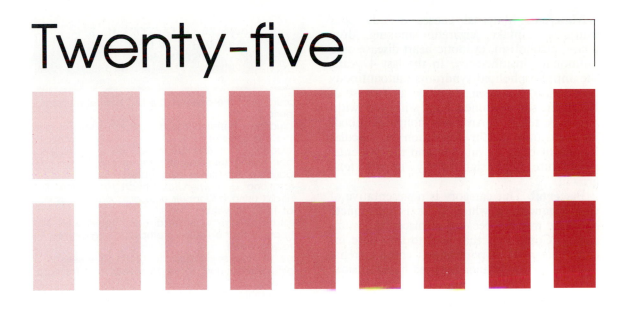

Intrauterine Growth Retardation, Intrauterine Fetal Demise, and Post-term Pregnancy

LEWIS A. HAMILTON, JR., AND CALVIN J. HOBEL

INTRAUTERINE GROWTH RETARDATION

Intrauterine growth retardation (IUGR) by definition occurs when the birth weight of a newborn infant is below the tenth percentile for a given gestational age. This condition is important because it identifies a group of small for dates infants who are at increased risk for perinatal morbidity and mortality. Growth-retarded fetuses are particularly prone to problems such as meconium aspira-tion, asphyxia, polycythemia, hypoglycemia, and mental retardation. Early recognition of growth retardation offers the opportunity to minimize the adverse effects of many of these complications.

Etiology

The etiologies of IUGR can be grouped into three main categories: maternal, placental, and fetal. Combinations of these are frequently found in pregnancies with IUGR.

Maternal. Maternal causes include poor nutritional intake, cigarette smoking, drug abuse, alcoholism, cyanotic heart disease, and pulmonary insufficiency. In the last 4 years, the antiphospholipid syndrome (autoantibody production) has been identified as a cause of IUGR in some women both with and without hypertension. Antiphospholipid antibodies contribute to the formation of vascular lesions in both the uterine and the placental vasculature that significantly impair fetal growth.

Placental. This category is representative of circumstances in which there is inadequate substrate transfer because of placental insufficiency. Conditions that lead to this state include essential hypertension, chronic renal disease, and pregnancy-induced hypertension. If the latter occurs late in pregnancy and is not accompanied by chronic vascular or renal disease, significant IUGR is unlikely to occur.

Fetal. In this case, inadequate substrate is used. Examples of fetal causes include intrauterine infection (listeriosis and TORCH agents) and congenital anomalies.

Clinical Manifestations

Two types of fetal growth retardation have been described: symmetrical and asymmetrical. In fetuses with symmetrical growth retardation, there is inadequate growth of both the head and the body. The head to abdominal circumference ratio may be normal, but the absolute growth rate is decreased. When asymmetrical growth retardation occurs, usually late in pregnancy, the brain is spared so that the head size is proportionally larger than the abdominal size. Symmetrical growth retardation is most commonly seen in association with intrauterine infections or congenital fetal anomalies.

Regardless of whether growth retardation is symmetrical or asymmetrical, all growth-retarded pregnancies result in small for gestational age fetuses, usually a smaller placenta, and usually a diminished amount of amniotic fluid.

Diagnosis

IUGR may go undiagnosed unless the obstetrician establishes the correct gestational

---

Table 25–1. FACTORS TO BE EVALUATED IN DATING A PREGNANCY

Accuracy of the date of the last normal menstrual period

Evaluation of uterine size on pelvic examination in the first trimester

Evaluation of uterine size in relation to gestational age during subsequent antenatal visits (concordance or size/dates discrepancy)

Gestational age when fetal heart tones were first heard using a Doppler ultrasonic device (usually at 12 to 14 weeks)

Gestational age when fetal heart tones were first heard with the DeLee stethoscope (generally 18 to 20 weeks)

Date of quickening (usually 18 to 20 weeks in a primigravida and 16 to 18 weeks in a multigravida)

Sonographic parameters—measurement of the biparietal diameter is most accurate for pregnancy dating between 16 and 20 weeks gestation

---

age of the fetus (Table 25–1), identifies high-risk factors from the obstetric database, and serially assesses fetal growth by fundal height or ultrasonography.

One of the most effective tools in diagnosing IUGR is sonographic evaluation of the fetal parameters. Since repeated sonographic assessments during pregnancy are not feasible in every patient, serial uterine fundal height measurements should serve as the primary screening tool. A more thorough sonographic assessment should be undertaken when (1) the fundal height lags more than 2 cm behind a well-established gestational age or (2) the mother has such high-risk conditions as pre-existing hypertension; chronic renal disease; advanced diabetes with vascular involvement; pre-eclampsia; viral disease; addiction to nicotine, alcohol, or hard drugs; or the presence of serum lupus anticoagulant or antiphospholipid antibodies.

At present, sonographic assessment is made primarily through serial determinations of six parameters: (1) fetal biparietal diameter (BPD), (2) head circumference, (3) abdominal circumference (Fig. 25–1), (4) head to body ratio, (5) femur length, and (6) calculated fetal weight. Quantitating the degree of IUGR is not well established. If the fetal measurements fall within the tenth to

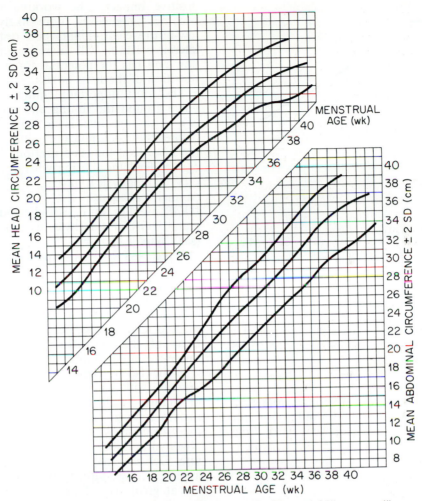

Figure 25-1. Mean head and abdominal circumferences with 5th and 95th percentile confidence limits between 16 and 40 weeks menstrual age. (Adapted from Campbell S, Griffin D, Roberts A, et al: Early prenatal diagnosis of abnormalities of the fetal head, spine, limbs, and abdominal organs. In Orlandi C, Polani PE, Bovicelli L (eds): Recent Advances in Prenatal Diagnosis: Proceedings of the First International Symposium on Recent Advances in Prenatal Diagnosis, Bologna, 15th–16th September, 1980. New York, Wiley, 1980.)

twenty-fifth percentile of growth curves, mild IUGR should be considered. When measurements fall below the tenth percentile, the fetus is considered to have moderate IUGR.

During advancing gestation, the head circumference remains greater than the abdominal circumference until approximately 34 weeks, at which point the ratio approaches 1 (Fig. 25–2). Following 34 weeks, the normal pregnancy is associated with an abdominal circumference that is greater than the head circumference. When asymmetrical growth retardation occurs, usually late in pregnancy, the BPD is essentially normal, whereas the

ratio of head to abdominal circumference is abnormal. With symmetrical growth retardation, the head to abdominal circumference ratio may be normal, but the absolute growth rate is decreased and estimated fetal weight is reduced.

From 50 to 90 per cent of infants with manifestations of IUGR at birth can be identified with serial prenatal ultrasonic scans. The accuracy depends on the quality of the assessments, the criteria used for diagnosis, and the effect of interventions applied when this diagnosis is made. For example, it is not unusual to observe an improvement in fetal

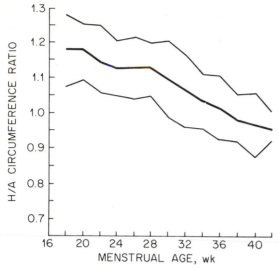

Figure 25–2. Graphic representation of the mean head to abdominal circumference ratios with 5th and 95th percentile confidence limits from 17 to 42 weeks menstrual age. (From Campbell S, Thomas A: Ultrasound measurement of the fetal head to abdominal circumference ratio in the assessment of growth retardation. Br J Obstet Gynaecol 84:165, 1977.)

growth after interventions such as work stoppage; bed rest; dietary modification; and curtailment of the use of tobacco, hard drugs, and alcohol.

Management

Prepregnancy. An important part of preventative medicine is to anticipate risks that can be modified before a woman becomes pregnant. Improving nutrition and stopping smoking are two approaches that should improve fetal growth in women who are underweight or who smoke or both. For women with antiphospholipid antibodies associated with the delivery of a prior IUGR infant, low-dose aspirin (81 mg/day) in early pregnancy may reduce the likelihood of recurrent IUGR.

Antepartum. Once a fetus has been identified as having decreased growth, the obstetrician should direct his or her efforts toward modifying any associated factors that can be changed. Because poor nutrition and smoking exert their main effects on birth weight in the latter half of pregnancy, cessation of smoking and improved nutrition can have a

positive impact. The working woman who becomes fatigued is more likely to have a low-birth-weight infant. Bed rest in the left lateral position will increase uterine blood flow and has the potential for improving the nutrition of the fetus at risk.

The most important clinical decisions revolve around the timing and mode of delivery. The objective is to expedite delivery before the occurrence of fetal compromise but after fetal lung maturation. This requires regular fetal monitoring with a nonstress test (NST), biophysical profile, and possibly an oxytocin challenge test (OCT). With mild IUGR, weekly testing is indicated; with moderate IUGR, testing twice a week is indicated (see Chapter 8).

If the NST is reactive or the OCT is negative and the amniotic fluid volume adequate, the pregnancy should be allowed to continue, since there are no data to support early delivery of these infants in the absence of documented fetal distress. Serial ultrasonic evaluations of fetal growth should be done at thrice-weekly intervals.

If the NST becomes nonreactive in conjunction with a positive OCT in the presence of mature fetal lungs (lecithin to sphingomyelin ratio greater than 2), interruption of the pregnancy is necessary. In the presence of oligohydramnios, amniocentesis may not be safe. Delivery may be recommended without assessing lung maturity because these fetuses are at great risk of asphyxia, and the stress associated with IUGR usually accelerates fetal pulmonary maturity.

Over the last several years, a series of studies has indicated that Doppler-derived umbilical artery systolic to diastolic ratios are abnormal in IUGR fetuses. Fetuses with growth retardation tend to have increased resistance to flow and to demonstrate low, absent, or reversed diastolic flow. This relatively simple noninvasive technique can be used to evaluate high-risk patients, but further research must be done comparing Doppler ultrasonography with established biophysical parameters before the role of this technique in the assessment and management of the growth retarded fetus can be clarified.

Labor and Delivery

During labor, these high-risk patients must be electronically monitored to detect the earliest evidence of fetal distress (see Chapter 22). The fetoplacental unit in these infants does not have the normal reserve. In the presence of recurrent abnormal fetal heart rate patterns, which are unresponsive to traditional treatment (lateral positioning and oxygen by mask), delivery must be expedited, usually by cesarean section.

A combined obstetric-neonatal team approach to delivery is mandatory because of the likelihood of neonatal asphyxia. Meconium aspiration can often be prevented by suctioning the oropharynx with the delivery of the head and by intubating and suctioning the trachea to clear it after delivery of the trunk (see Chapter 13).

After birth, the infant should be carefully examined to rule out the possibility of congenital anomalies and infections. The monitoring of blood glucose levels is important, since these fetuses do not have adequate hepatic glycogen stores, and hypoglycemia is a common finding. Hypothermia is not uncommon in these infants. Respiratory distress syndrome is more common in the presence of fetal distress, since fetal acidosis reduces surfactant synthesis and release.

Prognosis

The long-term prognosis for infants with IUGR must be assessed according to the varied etiologies of the growth retardation. If infants with chromosomal abnormalities, congenital anomalies, and infection are excluded, the outlook for these newborns is generally good.

INTRAUTERINE FETAL DEATH

Intrauterine fetal death (IUFD) is fetal demise after 20 weeks gestation but before the onset of labor. It complicates about 1 per cent of pregnancies. With the development of newer diagnostic and therapeutic modalities over the past 2 decades, the management of IUFD has shifted from watchful expectancy to a more active intervention.

Etiology

In more than 50 per cent of cases, the etiology of antepartum fetal death is not

Table 25-2. CAUSES OF FETAL DEATH

CAUSE	PERCENTAGE OF FETAL DEATHS
Placental and cord complications	10-20
Hypertensive diseases	5-20
Medical complications (including autoimmune disease)	5-10
Eythroblastosis fetalis	3-15
Congenital anomalies	5-10
Intrauterine infections (TORCH and *Listeria*)	5-10
Undetermined	50

known or cannot be determined. Associated causes are noted in Table 25-2 and include hypertensive diseases of pregnancy, diabetes mellitus, erythroblastosis fetalis, umbilical cord accidents, fetal congenital anomalies, fetal or maternal infections, fetomaternal hemorrhage, and antiphospholipid antibodies.

Diagnosis

Clinically, fetal death should be suspected when the patient reports the absence of fetal movements, particularly if the uterus is small for dates or if the fetal heart tones are not detected using a Doppler device. Since the placenta may continue to produce hCG, a positive pregnancy test does not exclude an IUFD.

Diagnostic confirmation has been greatly facilitated since the advent of ultrasonography. Real-time ultrasonography confirms the lack of fetal movement and absence of fetal cardiac activity. With the elapse of sufficient time, collapse of the fetal body with overlapping of cranial bones is discernible by x-ray film or ultrasonography. Although rarely indicated at the present time, the findings on abdominal x-ray examination are listed in Table 25-3.

Amniocentesis is rarely indicated to confirm the diagnosis of fetal death, but if performed it will show dark-brown, turbid fluid with markedly elevated levels of creatine phosphokinase.

Table 25–3. INDICATIONS OF FETAL DEATH ON ABDOMINAL X-RAY FILM

Gas in the cardiovascular system (occurs within 3 or 4 days)

Subsequent overlapping of the fetal skull bones (Spalding's sign) due to liquefaction of the brain

Marked curvature or angulation of the spine (following maceration of the spinous ligaments)

Management

Fetal demise between 13 and 28 weeks allows for two different approaches.

Watchful Expectancy. About 80 per cent of patients will experience the spontaneous onset of labor within 2 to 3 weeks of fetal demise. The patient's feeling of personal loss and guilt may create such anxiety, however, that this conservative approach may prove unacceptable. Thus, in general, the management of women who fail to go into labor spontaneously is active intervention by induction of labor.

Induction of Labor. Justifications for such intervention include the emotional burden on the patient associated with carrying a dead fetus, the slight possibility of intrauterine infection, and the 10 per cent risk of disseminated intravascular coagulation when a dead fetus is retained for more than 5 weeks.

Vaginal suppositories of prostaglandin E_2 (Prostin) have received the approval of the Food and Drug Administration (FDA) for use from the twelfth to the twenty-eighth week of gestation. Prostaglandins are very effective drugs with an overall success rate of 97 per cent. Although at least 50 per cent of patients receiving prostaglandins experience nausea and vomiting or diarrhea with temperature elevations, these side effects are transient. There have been reported cases of uterine rupture and cervical lacerations, but with properly selected patients, the drug is safe. The maximum recommended dose is a 20-mg suppository every 3 hours. Intravenous oxytocin is acceptable for induction of labor if the cervix is favorable.

After 28 weeks gestation, if the cervix is favorable for induction and there are no contraindications, oxytocin is the drug of choice. The use of prostaglandin E_2 suppositories at this gestational age is associated with an increased risk of uterine rupture, so a smaller dosage should be used. If the cervix is not favorable for induction, one or more laminaria tents placed into the cervical canal before oxytocin induction may enhance cervical ripening. Serial daily controlled infusions of oxytocin may be required to induce labor.

Monitoring of Coagulopathy. Regardless of the mode of therapy chosen, weekly fibrinogen levels should be monitored during the period of expectant management, along with a hematocrit and platelet count. If the fibrinogen level is decreasing, even a "normal" fibrinogen level of 300 mg/dl may be an early sign of consumptive coagulopathy in cases of fetal demise. An elevated prothrombin and partial thromboplastin time, the presence of fibrinogen-fibrin degradation products, and a decreased platelet count may clarify the diagnosis.

If laboratory evidence of mild disseminated intravascular coagulation is noted in the absence of bleeding, delivery by the most appropriate means is recommended. If the clotting defect is more severe or if there is evidence of bleeding, blood volume support or use of component therapy (cryoprecipitate or fresh frozen plasma) should be given prior to intervention.

Follow-up

Physician responsibilities do not end with delivery of the fetus. In addition to emotional support of the parents, a search should be undertaken to determine the cause of the intrauterine death. TORCH studies and cultures for *Listeria* are indicated. In addition, all women with a fetal demise should be tested for the presence of anticardiolipin antibodies. If congenital abnormalities are detected, fetal chromosomal studies and total body radiographs should be done, in addition to a complete autopsy. The autopsy report, when available, must be discussed in detail with both parents. In a stillborn fetus, the best tissue for a chromosomal analysis is the fascia lata, obtained from the lateral aspect of the thigh. The tissue can be stored in saline or Hanks' solution. A significant number of cases of IUFD are the result of fetomaternal hemorrhage, which can be detected by identifying fetal erythrocytes in maternal blood (Kleihauer-Betke test). Unfortunately, not a great deal of progress has been made in determining the etiology of the 50 per cent of fetal deaths listed as due to "unknown causes." If a fetal autopsy cannot be obtained, fetal blood studies should be attempted and occasionally a radiograph of the fetus can help identify congenital anomalies. Subsequent pregnancies occurring in a woman with a history of IUFD must be managed as high-risk cases.

POST-TERM PREGNANCY

The prolonged or post-term pregnancy is one that persists beyond 42 weeks (294 days) from the onset of the last normal menstrual period. Estimates of the incidence of post-term pregnancy range from 6 to 12 per cent of all pregnancies.

Perinatal mortality is two to three times higher in these prolonged gestations. Much of the increased risk to the fetus and neonate can be attributed to development of the fetal postmaturity (dysmaturity) syndrome. Occurring in 20 to 30 per cent of post-term pregnancies, this syndrome is related to the aging and infarction of the placenta, resulting in placental insufficiency with impaired oxygen diffusion and decreased transfer of nutrients to the fetus. If evidence of intrauterine hypoxia is present (such as meconium staining of the umbilical cord, fetal membranes, skin, and nails), perinatal mortality is even further increased.

The fetus with postmaturity syndrome typically has loss of subcutaneous fat, long fingernails, dry peeling skin, and abundant hair. The 70 to 80 per cent of postdate fetuses not affected by placental insufficiency continue to grow in utero, many to the point of macrosomia (birth weight greater than 4000 gm). This macrosomia often results in abnormal labor, shoulder dystocia, birth trauma, and an increased incidence of cesarean birth.

Etiology

The initiation of human labor is triggered by a complex of fetal and maternal factors (see Chapter 5). The cause of postdate pregnancy is unknown in most instances. Prolonged gestation is common in association with an anencephalic fetus and is probably linked to the lack of a fetal labor-initiating factor from the fetal adrenals, which are hypoplastic in anencephalics. Prolonged labor may also be rarely associated with placental sulfatase deficiency and extrauterine pregnancy.

Diagnosis

The diagnosis of post-term pregnancy is often difficult. The key to appropriate classification and subsequent successful perinatal management is the accurate dating of gestation. It is estimated that uncertain dates are present in 20 to 30 per cent of all pregnancies. The factors to be taken into consideration in attempting to distinguish a postdated pregnancy from a misdated pregnancy are shown in Table 25–1. If there is no concordance between at least two of the criteria listed, the patient is considered to have poor dates.

Management

Antepartum. The appropriate management of prolonged pregnancy revolves around identification of the low percentage of fetuses with postmaturity syndrome who are at risk of intrauterine hypoxia and fetal demise. Now that biophysical and biochemical tests of fetal well-being are available, there has been a movement toward individualization of the time of delivery for each patient. If the gestational age is firmly established at 42 weeks, the fetal head is well fixed in the pelvis, and the cervix is favorable, however, the patient should generally be induced.

The two clinical problems that remain are (1) patients with good dates at 42 weeks gestation with an unripe cervix and (2) patients with an uncertain gestational age seen for the first time with a possible or probable diagnosis of prolonged pregnancy.

In the first group of patients, a twice-weekly NST and the biophysical profile should be performed. The amniotic fluid index (AFI) is an important ultrasonic measurement that should also be used in the management of these patients. The AFI is the sum of the vertical dimensions (in centimeters) of amniotic fluid pockets in each of four quadrants of the gestational sac. Delivery is indicated if there is any indication of oligohydramnios (AFI ≤ 5) or if spontaneous fetal heart rate decelerations are found on the NST. As long as these parameters of fetal well-being are reassuring, labor need not be induced unless the cervix becomes favorable or the fetus is judged to be macrosomic. At 43 weeks gestation with firm dates, delivery should be considered by the appropriate route, regardless of other factors, in view of the increasing potential for perinatal morbidity and mortality.

When the patient presents very late in gestation for initial assessment with the label of prolonged pregnancy but the gestational age is in question, an expectant approach is often acceptable. The risk of intervention with the delivery of a preterm infant must be considered.

Intrapartum. Continuous electronic fetal monitoring must be employed during the induction of labor. The patient should be encouraged to stay on her left side. The fetal membranes should be ruptured as early as is feasible in the intrapartum period so that internal electrodes can be applied and the color of the amniotic fluid assessed. If electronic fetal monitoring suggests fetal distress, fetal acid-base status should be determined by fetal scalp blood sampling. If fetal acidosis is confirmed (pH less than 7.20), immediate delivery is indicated, usually by the cesarean route (see Chapter 22). If meconium is present, neonatal asphyxia should be anticipated, and the protocol outlined in Chapter 13 should be followed.

SUGGESTED READING

Bochkner CJ, Medearis AL, Ross MG, et al: The role of antepartum testing in the management of post term pregnancies with heavy meconium in early labor. Obstet Gynecol 69:903, 1987.

Brar HS, Platt LD: Reverse end-diastolic flow velocity on umbilical artery velocimetry in high-risk pregnancies: An ominous finding with adverse pregnancy outcome. Am J Obstet Gynecol 159:59, 1988.

Campbell S: Ultrasound measurement of the fetal head to abdominal circumference ratio in assessment of growth retardation. Br J Obstet Gynaecol 84:165, 1977.

Dyson DC, Millder PD, Armstrong MA: Management of prolonged pregnancy: Induction of labor versus antepartum fetal testing. Am J Obstet Gynecol 156:928, 1987.

El-Roery A, Myers SA, Gleicher N: The relationship between autoantibodies and intrauterine growth retardation in hypertensive disorders of pregnancy. Am J Obstet Gynecol 164:1253, 1991.

Fancourt R, Campbell S, Harvey DR, et al: Follow-up study of small-for-dates babies. Br Med J 1:1435, 1976.

Kockenour NK: Management of fetal demise. Clin Obstet Gynecol 30(2):322, 1987.

Lauersen NG, Cederqvist LL, Wilson KH: Management of intrauterine fetal death with prostaglandin E_2 vaginal suppositories. Am J Obstet Gynecol 137:753, 1980.

Leveno KJ, Quirk JG, Cunningham FG, et al: Prolonged pregnancy: Observations concerning the course of fetal distress. Am J Obstet Gynecol 150(5):465, 1984.

Liban E, Salzberger M: A prospective clinicopathological study of 1108 cases of antenatal fetal death. Isr J Med Sci 12:34, 1976.

Pitkin RM: Fetal death: Diagnosis and management. Am J Obstet Gynecol 157:583, 1987.

Platt LD, Manning FA, Murata Y, et al: Diagnosis of fetal death in utero by real-time ultrasound. Obstet Gynecol 55:191, 1980.

Rozenman D, Kessler I, Lancet M: Third trimester induction of labor with fetal death in utero. Surg Gynecol Obstet 151:497, 1980.

Southern EM, Gutknecht GD, Mohberg NR, et al: Vaginal prostaglandin E_2 in the management of fetal intrauterine death. Br J Obstet Gynaecol 85:437, 1978.

Wallenberg HCS, Rotmans N: Prevention of recurrent idiopathic fetal growth retardation by low-dose aspirin and dipyridamole. Am J Obstet Gynecol 157:1230, 1987.

Twenty-six

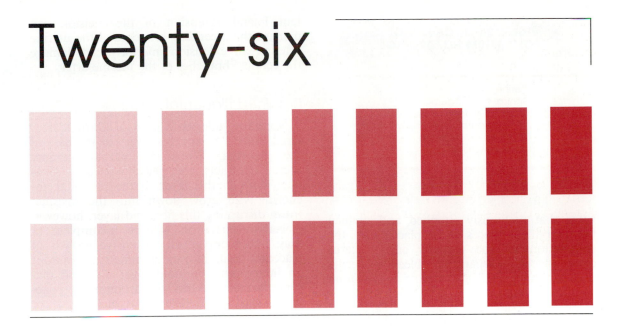

Postpartum Hemorrhage and Puerperal Sepsis

ROBERT H. HAYASHI

The three most common causes of maternal death are hemorrhage, infection, and hypertensive disease. In this chapter, the postpartum manifestations of two of these problems, hemorrhage and infection, are discussed. Both of these are associated not only with maternal mortality, but also with significant maternal morbidity and prolonged hospitalization.

POSTPARTUM HEMORRHAGE

Postpartum hemorrhage is defined as blood loss in excess of 500 ml at the time of vaginal delivery. There is normally a greater blood loss following delivery by cesarean section; therefore, blood loss in excess of 1000 ml is considered a postpartum hemorrhage in such patients. The excessive blood loss usually occurs in the immediate postpartum period but can occur slowly over the first 24 hours. Delayed postpartum hemorrhage can occasionally occur, the excessive bleeding commencing more than 24 hours after delivery. This is usually due to subinvolution of the uterus and disruption of the "placental site scab" several weeks postpartum or to the retention of placental fragments that separate several days after delivery. Postpartum hemorrhage occurs in about 4 per cent of deliveries.

Etiology

Most of the blood loss occurs from the myometrial spiral arterioles and decidual

Table 26–1. CAUSES OF POSTPARTUM HEMORRHAGE

Uterine atony
Genital tract trauma
Retained placental tissue
Low placental implantation
Coagulation disorders
Uterine inversion

veins that previously supplied and drained the intervillous spaces of the placenta. As the contractions of the partially empty uterus cause placental separation, bleeding occurs and continues until the uterine musculature contracts around the blood vessels and acts as a physiologic-anatomic ligature. Failure of the uterus to contract after placental separation (uterine atony) leads to excessive placental site bleeding. Other causes of postpartum hemorrhage are listed in Table 26–1.

Uterine Atony

The majority of postpartum hemorrhages (75 to 80 per cent) are due to uterine atony. The factors predisposing to postpartum uterine atony are shown in Table 26–2.

Genital Tract Trauma

Trauma during delivery is the second most common cause of postpartum hemorrhage. During vaginal delivery, lacerations of the cervix and vagina may occur spontaneously but are more common following the use of forceps or a vacuum extractor. The vascular beds in the genital tract are engorged during pregnancy, and bleeding can be profuse. Lacerations are particularly prone to occur over the perineal body, in the periurethral area, and over the ischial spines along the posterolateral aspects of the vagina. The cervix may lacerate at the two lateral angles while rapidly dilating in the first stage of labor. Apart from acute postpartum bleeding, neglected lacerations may cause substantial but slow blood loss over many hours. Uterine rupture may occasionally occur. At the time of delivery by low transverse cesarean section, an inadver-

tent lateral extension of the incision can damage the ascending branches of the uterine arteries; an extension inferiorly can damage the cervical branches of the uterine artery.

Retained Placental Tissue

Normally, there is a layer of fibrinoid material called "Nitabuch's layer" at the base of the placenta. When the partially empty uterus contracts, the placenta cleanly separates through this layer. If the placental anchoring villi grow down into the myometrium disrupting this fibrinoid layer, however, placental separation will be incomplete or may not occur at all. Extensive growth of placental tissue into the myometrium without an intervening fibrinoid layer is called placenta accreta. When the trophoblast penetrates the myometrium to the serosa or beyond, it is called placenta percreta. A complete placenta accreta will not cause bleeding because the placenta remains attached, but the partial type may cause profuse bleeding, as the normal part of the placenta separates and the myometrium cannot contract sufficiently to occlude the placental site vessels. In about half the patients with delayed postpartum hemorrhage, placental fragments are present when uterine curettage is performed.

Low Placental Implantation

Low implantation of the placenta can predispose to postpartum hemorrhage because the relative content of musculature in the

Table 26–2. FACTORS PREDISPOSING TO POSTPARTUM UTERINE ATONY

Overdistention of the uterus
  Multiple gestation
  Polyhydramnios
  Fetal macrosomia
Prolonged labor
Oxytocic augmentation of labor
Grandmultiparity (a parity of 5 or more)
Precipitous labor (one lasting less than 3 hr)
Magnesium sulfate treatment of pre-eclampsia
Chorioamnionitis

uterine wall decreases in the lower uterine segment, which may result in insufficient control of placental site bleeding.

Coagulation Disorders

Peripartal coagulation disorders are high-risk factors for postpartum hemorrhage but fortunately are quite rare. Patients with coagulation problems, such as occur with thrombotic thrombocytopenic purpura, amniotic fluid embolism, abruptio placentae, idiopathic thrombocytopenic purpura, or von Willebrand's disease, may develop postpartum hemorrhage because of their inability to form a stable blood clot in the placental site.

Patients with thrombotic thrombocytopenia have a rare syndrome of unknown etiology characterized by thrombocytopenic purpura, microangiopathic hemolytic anemia, transient and fluctuating neurologic signs, renal dysfunction, and a febrile course. In pregnancy, the disease is usually fatal. An amniotic fluid embolus is also rare and is associated with approximately an 80 per cent mortality. This syndrome is characterized by a fulminating consumption coagulopathy, intense bronchospasm, and vasomotor collapse. It is triggered by an intravascular infusion of a significant amount of amniotic fluid during a tumultuous or rapid labor in the presence of ruptured membranes. During the process of placental abruption (premature separation of the placenta), a small amount of amniotic fluid may leak into the vascular system, and the thromboplastin in the amniotic fluid may trigger a consumption coagulopathy without the other elements of a large amniotic fluid embolus. Patients with idiopathic thrombocytopenic purpura have platelets with abnormal function or a shortened life span. This causes thrombocytopenia and a bleeding tendency. Circulating antiplatelet antibodies of the IgG type may occasionally cross the placenta and result in fetal and neonatal thrombocytopenia as well. Von Willebrand's disease is an inherited coagulopathy characterized by a prolonged bleeding time due to factor VIII deficiency. During pregnancy, these patients are likely to have a decreased bleeding diathesis, since pregnancy elevates factor VIII levels. In the postpartum period, they are susceptible to immediate hemorrhage and also to delayed bleeding as the factor VIII levels fall.

Uterine Inversion

Uterine inversion is the "turning inside out" of the uterus in the third stage of labor. It is quite rare, occurring in only about one out of 20,000 pregnancies. Just after the second stage, the uterus is somewhat atonic, the cervix open, and the placenta attached. Improper management of the third stage can cause an iatrogenic uterine inversion. If the inexperienced physician exerts fundal pressure while pulling on the umbilical cord before complete placental separation (particularly with a fundal implantation of the placenta), uterine inversion may occur. As the fundus of the uterus moves through the vagina, the inversion exerts traction on peritoneal structures, which can elicit a profound vasovagal response. The resulting vasodilatation increases bleeding and the risk of hypovolemic shock. If the placenta is completely or partially separated, the uterine atony may cause profuse bleeding, which compounds the vasovagal shock.

OBSTETRIC SHOCK

An occasional patient may develop hypotension without significant external bleeding. This condition is called obstetric shock. The causes of obstetric shock include concealed hemorrhage, uterine inversion, and amniotic fluid embolism.

An improperly sutured episiotomy can lead to a concealed postpartum hemorrhage. If the first suture at the vaginal apex of the episiotomy incision does not incorporate the cut and retracted arterioles, they can continue to bleed, creating a hematoma that can dissect cephalad into the retroperitoneal space. This may cause shock, without external evidence of blood loss. A soft tissue hematoma, usually of the vulva, may occur following delivery in the absence of any laceration or episiotomy and may also contribute to occult blood loss.

Spontaneous uterine rupture during labor is rare (one in every 1900 deliveries) but usually results in significant intraperitoneal bleeding. Uterine rupture can also occur secondary to blunt abdominal trauma at the time of an automobile accident. A predisposing factor for uterine rupture is a uterine scar, particularly from a previous classic cesarean section.

Differential Diagnosis

Identification of the cause of postpartum hemorrhage or obstetric shock requires a systematic approach. The fundus of the uterus should be palpated through the abdominal wall to determine the presence or absence of uterine atony. In the rare case of uterine inversion, a crater-like depression is felt at the fundus. Next, a quick but thorough inspection of the vagina and cervix should be performed to ascertain whether any lacerations may be compounding the bleeding problem. Any uterine inversion or pelvic hematoma should be excluded during the pelvic examination. If the cause of bleeding has not been identified, manual exploration of the uterine cavity should be performed, if necessary under general anesthesia. With fingertips together, a gloved hand is slipped through the open cervix, and the endometrial surface is palpated carefully to identify any retained products of conception, uterine wall lacerations, or partial uterine inversion. If no cause for the bleeding is found, a coagulopathy must be sought.

MANAGEMENT OF POSTPARTUM HEMORRHAGE AND OBSTETRIC SHOCK

The first step toward good management is the identification of patients at risk for postpartum hemorrhage and the institution of prophylactic measures during labor to minimize the possibility of maternal mortality. Patients with any predisposing factors for postpartum hemorrhage, including a history of postpartum hemorrhage, should be screened for anemia and atypical antibodies to ensure that an adequate supply of type-specific blood is on hand in the blood bank. An intravenous infusion via a large-bore catheter should be commenced prior to delivery and blood held in the laboratory for possible cross-matching.

During the diagnostic work-up of an established hemorrhage, the patient's vital signs must be monitored closely. Four units of packed red blood cells must be typed and cross-matched, and intravenous crystalloids (such as normal saline or lactated Ringer's solution) infused to restore intravascular volume.

Uterine Atony

If uterine atony is determined to be the cause of the postpartum hemorrhage, a rapid continuous intravenous infusion of dilute oxytocin (40 to 80 units in 1 L of normal saline) should be given to increase uterine tone. If the uterus remains atonic and the placental site bleeding continues during the oxytocic infusion, ergonovine maleate or methylergonovine, 0.2 mg, may be given intramuscularly or as an intravenous bolus. The ergot drugs are contraindicated in patients with hypertension, since the pressor effect of the drug may increase blood pressure to dangerous levels.

Analogs of prostaglandin F_2-alpha given intramuscularly are quite effective in controlling postpartum hemorrhage caused by uterine atony. The 15-methyl analog (0.25 mg) has a more potent uterotonic effect and longer duration of action than the parent compound.

Failing these pharmacologic treatments, a bimanual compression and massage of the uterine corpus may control the bleeding and cause the uterus to contract. Although packing the uterine cavity is not widely practiced, it may occasionally control postpartum hemorrhage and obviate the need for surgical intervention. The vital signs, hematocrit, and fundal height should be monitored frequently while the packing is in place, since continued bleeding will not be initially evident through the packing.

Another approach that may be tried if bleeding persists is placement of the patient into an antigravity suit ("G" suit), which will, when inflated, compress the lower extremities and the abdominal cavity. Experience with this device in trauma patients has demonstrated good control of intra-abdominal bleeding. This approach may occasionally be used to temporize while the blood volume is being expanded and preparations are made for more definitive surgery.

Operative intervention is a last resort. If the patient has completed her childbearing, a supracervical abdominal hysterectomy is de-

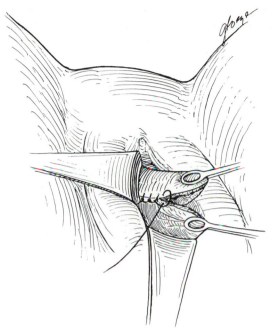

Figure 26-1. Suturing a cervical laceration. The first suture must be placed above the apex of the laceration.

finitive therapy for intractable postpartum hemorrhage caused by uterine atony. If reproductive potential is important to the patient, ligation of the uterine arteries adjacent to the uterus will lower the pulse pressure distal to the ligatures. This procedure is more successful in controlling uterine placental site hemorrhage and easier to perform than bilateral hypogastric artery ligation.

Genital Tract Trauma

When postpartum hemorrhage is related to genital tract trauma, surgical intervention is necessary. Repair of genital tract lacerations requires the implementation of an important principle: The first suture must be placed well above the apex of the laceration to incorporate any bleeding, retracted arterioles into the ligature. Repair of vaginal lacerations requires good light and good exposure, and the tissues should be approximated without dead space. A running lock suture technique is the most hemostatic. Cervical lacerations need not be sutured unless they are actively bleeding. Sponge-holding forceps may be used to pull the cervix down to the introitus to facilitate inspection and suturing (Fig. 26–

1). Large expanding hematomas of the genital tract require surgical evacuation of clots and a search for bleeding vessels that can be ligated. Stable hematomas can be observed and treated conservatively. A retroperitoneal hematoma generally begins in the pelvis. If the bleeding cannot be controlled from a vaginal approach, a laparotomy and bilateral hypogastric artery ligation may be necessary.

The intraoperative laceration of the ascending branch of the uterine artery during delivery through a low transverse cesarean section can be easily controlled by the placement of a large suture ligature through the myometrium and broad ligament below the level of the laceration. A uterine rupture usually necessitates subtotal or total abdominal hysterectomy, although small defects may be repaired.

Retained Products of Conception

When the placenta cannot be delivered in the usual manner, manual removal of the placenta is necessary (Fig. 26–2). This should be performed urgently if bleeding is profuse. Otherwise, it is reasonable to delay 30 minutes to await spontaneous separation. General anesthesia may be required. Following manual removal of the placenta or placental remnants, the uterus should be scraped with a large curette. Extensive placenta accreta usually necessitates hysterectomy.

Uterine Inversion

The management of a uterine inversion requires quick thinking. The patient rapidly goes into shock, and immediate intravascular volume expansion with intravenous crystalloids is required. An anesthesiologist should be summoned. When the patient's condition is stable, the partially separated placenta should be completely removed and an attempt made to replace the uterus by placing a cupped hand around the fundus and elevating it in the long axis of the vagina. If this is unsuccessful, a further attempt under halothane anesthesia should be made. Another approach would be to use a tocolytic drug such as terbutaline to relax the uterine mus-

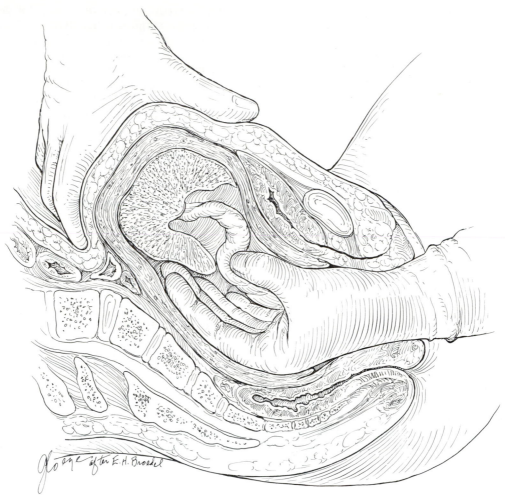

Figure 26–2. Manual removal of the placenta. The abdominal hand provides counterpressure on the uterine fundus against the shearing force of the fingers in the uterus.

cle tone. Once replaced, a dilute oxytocic infusion should be started to cause the uterus to contract before removing the intrauterine hand. Rarely, the uterus cannot be replaced from below, and a surgical procedure may be required. At laparotomy, a vertical incision should be made through the posterior portion of the cervix to incise the constriction ring and allow the fundus to be replaced into the peritoneal cavity. Suturing of the cervical incision will complete this procedure.

Amniotic Fluid Embolus

The principal objectives of treatment for amniotic fluid embolism are to support the respiratory system, correct the shock, and replace the coagulation factors. These necessitate immediate cardiopulmonary resuscitation, usually with mechanical ventilation; rapid volume expansion with an electrolyte solution; placement of a bladder catheter to monitor urine output; correction of the red cell deficit by transfusion with packed red blood cells; and reversal of the coagulopathy with the use of platelets, fibrinogen, and other blood components.

Coagulopathy

When postpartum hemorrhage is associated with a coagulopathy, the specific defect should be corrected by the infusion of blood

Table 26-3. BLOOD PRODUCTS USED TO CORRECT COAGULATION DEFECTS

BLOOD PRODUCT	VOLUME (ml) IN 1 UNIT*	EFFECT OF TRANSFUSION
Platelet concentrate	30–40	Increases platelet count by about 20,000 to 25,000
Cryoprecipitate	15–25	Supplies fibrinogen, factor VIII, and factor XIII (3 to 10 times more concentrated than the equivalent volume of fresh plasma)
Fresh frozen plasma	200	Supplies all factors except platelets (1 gm fibrinogen)
Packed red blood cells	200	Raises hematocrit 3 to 4%

* 1 unit = the quantity obtained from 1 unit (500 ml) of fresh whole blood.

products, as outlined in Table 26–3. Patients with thrombocytopenia require platelet concentrate infusions; those with von Willebrand's disease require fresh frozen plasma. A packed red cell infusion is given to a patient who has bled enough to drop the circulating red cell population sufficiently to compromise the delivery of oxygen to the tissues. Generally, a hematocrit of more than 25 per cent will suffice. Massive transfusions (greater than 3 L), especially with whole blood, will aggravate an already disturbed coagulation system by further depleting platelets and factors V and VIII. Thus, 1 unit of fresh frozen plasma should be given for every 2 units of blood after 6 units have been transfused.

PUERPERAL SEPSIS

Prior to the antiseptic and antibiotic era, puerperal sepsis was the overwhelming cause of maternal mortality and morbidity. Nearly 200 years ago, Alexander Gordon in Scotland observed that puerperal fever was transmitted from patient to patient, and about 50 years later, Ignaz Semmelweis in Vienna and Oliver Wendell Holmes in Boston independently concluded that it was the physician who transmitted the disease among puerperae. They proposed that simply washing hands between patient examinations would control the epidemics. Thus began the antiseptic era. Louis Pasteur later identified the hemolytic streptococcus as the pathogen.

Puerperal sepsis still accounts for significant postpartum maternal morbidity and mortality. Patients with a puerperal genital tract infection are susceptible to the development of septic shock, pelvic thrombophlebitis, and pelvic abscess. Possible sequelae include the impairment of future fertility, owing to tubal or endometrial damage or hysterectomy.

Following a vaginal delivery, approximately 6 or 7 per cent of puerperae demonstrate febrile morbidity, defined as a temperature of 100.4°F (38°C) or higher, occurring for more than two consecutive days (exclusive of the first postpartum day) during the first 10 postpartum days. Following primary cesarean section, the incidence of febrile morbidity is about twice that following vaginal delivery. The majority of these fevers are caused by endometritis.

Etiology

The pathophysiology of puerperal sepsis is closely related to the various microbial inhabitants of the vagina and cervix. The vaginal flora during gestation resembles that in the nonpregnant state (see Chapter 35), although there is a trend toward isolating more *Mycoplasma genitalis* and anaerobic streptococci in the last trimester. Potentially pathogenic organisms can be cultured from the vagina in approximately 80 per cent of pregnant women. These organisms include enterococci, hemolytic and nonhemolytic streptococci, anaerobic streptococci, enteric bacilli, pseudodiphtheria bacteria, and *Neisseria* species other than *N. gonorrhoeae*. Excessive overgrowth of these organisms during pregnancy is inhibited by the acidity of the vagina (pH 4 to 5), primarily as a result of the production of lactic acid by the lactobacilli.

The uterine cavity is normally free of bacteria during pregnancy. After parturition, the pH of the vagina changes from acidic to alkaline because of the neutralizing effect of the alkaline amniotic fluid, blood, and lochia as well as the decreased population of lactobacilli. This change in pH favors an increased growth of aerobic organisms. Approximately 48 hours postpartum, progressive necrosis of the endometrial and placental remnants produces a favorable intrauterine environment for the multiplication of anaerobic bacteria.

About 70 per cent of puerperal infections are caused by anaerobic organisms. Most of these are anaerobic cocci (*Peptostreptococcus, Peptococcus,* and *Streptococcus*), although mixed infections with *Bacteroides fragilis* are encountered in up to one third of cases. Of the aerobic organisms, *Escherichia coli* is the most common pathogen, followed by enterococci. Puerperal infection from clostridia is rare.

During the preantibiotic era, most patients with puerperal sepsis were infected by group A beta-hemolytic streptococci. These organisms are not normal inhabitants of the vaginal flora and originate from an outside source, such as the nasopharynx or skin of a carrier or infected individual. Today the incidence of this highly contagious and virulent organism is vastly reduced as a result of antiseptic techniques. Intrauterine infection with beta-hemolytic streptococci rapidly progresses to parametritis, peritonitis, and septicemia. The contagiousness of pyogenic streptococci demands precautionary measures, such as the screening of patients, hospital personnel, and visitors for overt and occult infections to avoid contamination of mothers or infants if a case is detected in the neonatal nursery.

Intrauterine staphylococcal infection is rare. This organism is frequently responsible for infection of perineal wounds and abdominal incisions. *Trichomonas vaginalis* and *Candida albicans* are frequent inhabitants of the vagina, but no connection with puerperal sepsis has been established. Mycoplasma organisms have been shown to contribute to puerperal endometritis.

Predisposing Factors

Predisposing factors to the development of a puerperal genital tract infection are shown in Table 26–4.

Table 26–4. FACTORS PREDISPOSING TO THE DEVELOPMENT OF PUERPERAL GENITAL TRACT INFECTION

Poor nutrition and hygiene
Anemia
Premature rupture of the membranes
Prolonged rupture of the membranes
Prolonged labor
Frequent vaginal examinations during labor
Cesarean section
Operative delivery
Cervical/vaginal lacerations
Manual removal of the placenta
Retained placental fragments or fetal membranes

After delivery, the placental site vessels are clotted off, and there is an exudation of lymph-like fluid along with massive numbers of neutrophils and other white cells to form the lochia. Vaginal microorganisms readily enter the uterine cavity and may become pathogenic at the placental site, depending on such variables as the size of the inoculum, the local pH, and the presence or absence of devitalized tissue. The latter may include tissue incorporated in the suture line of a cesarean section.

The normal body defense mechanisms usually prevent any progressive infection, but a breakdown of these defenses will allow the bacteria to invade the myometrium. Further invasion into the lymphatics of the parametrium can cause lymphangitis, pelvic cellulitis, and the possibility of widespread infection from septic emboli. An endomyoparametritis is a potentially life-threatening condition. It commonly begins with retention of secundines that block the normal lochial flow, allowing accumulation of intrauterine lochia that in turn changes the local pH and acts as a culture medium for bacterial growth. Unless normal lochial flow is established, bacterial invasion will progress.

Clinical Features

Puerperal infection manifests as rising fever and increasing uterine tenderness on postpartum day two or three. With the development of parametritis (pelvic cellulitis), the temperature elevation will be sustained, and the patient may develop signs of pelvic peritonitis. Erratic temperature fluctuations and severe chills suggest bacteremia and dissemination of septic emboli, with the particular likelihood of spread to the lungs.

When the usual relative pelvic venous stasis is combined with a large inoculum of pathogenic anaerobic bacteria, a pelvic vein thrombophlebitis is likely to develop, usually on the right side of the pelvis. The clinical picture of pelvic thrombophlebitis is characterized by a persistent spiking fever for 7 to 10 days after delivery, despite antibiotic therapy.

Diagnosis

Evaluation of a febrile postpartum patient should include a careful history and physical examination. Extrapelvic causes of fever, such as breast engorgement, mastitis, aspiration pneumonia, atelectasis, pyelonephritis, thrombophlebitis, or wound infection, should be excluded.

Although a pelvic examination is generally not helpful in diagnosing pelvic thrombophlebitis, occasionally, tender, thrombosed, and edematous ovarian, parauterine, or iliac veins may be palpated. This diagnosis is usually made by exclusion, however, and the prompt lysis of fever following commencement of heparin anticoagulant therapy.

Before the institution of antibiotic therapy for puerperal endometritis, two aerobic and anaerobic cultures should be obtained from the blood, endocervix, and uterine cavity, and a catheterized urine specimen should be obtained for culture. The antibiotic sensitivities from these cultures may be used to determine appropriate second-line drug therapy in the event of failure of the first-line drugs. Antibiotics should commence following diagnosis rather than waiting for culture results, which may take several days for anaerobic organisms.

Management

A febrile puerperal patient with cessation of lochial flow should undergo a pelvic examination and removal of any secundines that may be occluding the cervical os.

The antibiotic treatment of puerperal infection usually follows two major principles.

First, early antibiotic treatment should be instituted to confine, then eliminate, the infectious process. Second, the antibiotics should have anaerobic coverage because these organisms are involved in 70 per cent of puerperal infections. Antibiotics should be continued for at least 48 hours after the patient becomes afebrile. Anaerobic organisms especially require prolonged chemotherapy for elimination.

Broad-spectrum antibiotics, such as ampicillin and the cephalosporins, are effective first-line drugs for mild and moderate cases of puerperal infection. When the infection is moderate to severe, a penicillin-aminoglycoside combination has traditionally been used as first-line therapy. The major pelvic pathogen resistant to this combination, however, is *Bacteroides fragilis,* which is usually sensitive to either clindamycin or chloramphenicol. Therefore, the use of clindamycin with either an aminoglycoside or ampicillin should provide better first-line coverage.

When pelvic thrombophlebitis or thromboembolism is suspected or clinically diagnosed, heparin therapy should be instituted to increase the clotting time (Lee-White) or activated prothrombin time two to three times above normal. Only 2 to 3 weeks of anticoagulant therapy are needed for uncomplicated pelvic thrombophlebitis. Patients with femoral thrombophlebitis require 4 to 6 weeks of heparin therapy followed by the administration of oral anticoagulants for a few months.

If the patient does not respond to heparin therapy and the clinical course is one of unrelenting fever and pelvic tenderness, a diagnosis of pelvic abscess must be entertained. Diagnosis is made by pelvic examination and confirmed by pelvic ultrasonography or computed tomographic scan. The finding of a tender, pelvic parametrial mass suggests an abscess. Ultrasonography will confirm that the mass is fluid-filled rather than solid. The presence of a pelvic abscess demands surgical drainage.

SUGGESTED READING

Cunningham FG, Hauth JC, Strong JD, et al: Infectious morbidity following cesarean section. Obstet Gynecol 52:656, 1978.

Gibbs CE, Locke WE: Maternal deaths in Texas, 1969 to 1973. Report of 501 consecutive maternal deaths from Texas Medical Association Committee on Maternal Death. Am J Obstet Gynecol 126:687, 1976.

Gibbs RS: Postpartum endometritis. In Monif GR (ed): Infectious Diseases in Obstetrics and Gynecology. 2nd ed. Philadelphia, Harper & Row, 1982, p 377.

Hayashi RH, Castillo MS, Noah ML: Management of severe postpartum hemorrhage due to uterine atony using an analogue of prostaglandin F2 alpha. Obstet Gynecol 58:426, 1981.

Lucas WF: Postpartum hemorrhage. Clin Obstet Gynecol 23:637, 1980.

O'Leary JL, O'Leary JA: Uterine artery ligation for control of postcesarean section hemorrhage. Obstet Gynecol 43:849, 1974.

Schulman H: Use of anticoagulants in suspected pelvic infection. Clin Obstet Gynecol 12:240, 1969.

Sweet RL, Ledger WJ: Puerperal infectious morbidity: A two year review. Am J Obstet Gynecol 117:1093, 1973.

Twenty-seven

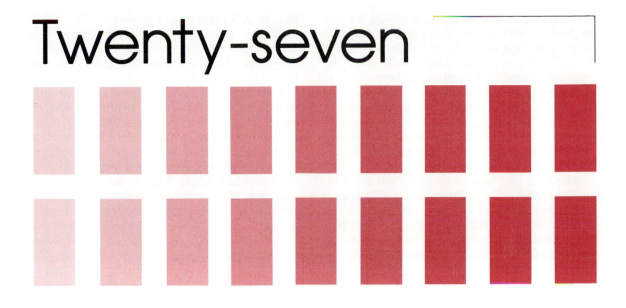

Rhesus Isoimmunization

KHALIL TABSH AND NANCY THEROUX

Rhesus (Rh) isoimmunization is an immunologic disorder that occurs in a pregnant, Rh-negative patient carrying an Rh-positive fetus. The immunologic system in the mother is stimulated to produce antibodies to the Rh antigen, which then cross the placenta and destroy fetal red blood cells.

PATHOPHYSIOLOGY

A person who lacks the specific Rh antigen on the surface of the red blood cells is called "Rh-negative," and an individual with the antigen is considered "Rh-positive." A number of antigens make up the Rh complex, including C, D, E, c, e, and other variants such as D^u antigen. Over 90 per cent of cases of Rh isoimmunization are due to D antigens. Therefore, this chapter is mainly limited to a discussion of the D antigen, although the same principles apply to any other antigen-antibody combination.

Among black Americans, 8 per cent are Rh-negative; among white Americans, about 13 per cent are Rh-negative. When Rh-negative patients are exposed to Rh antigen, they may become sensitized. Two mechanisms are proposed for this sensitization. The most likely mechanism is the occurrence of an undetected fetal to maternal hemorrhage during pregnancy. The other proposal is the "grandmother" theory. This theory suggests that an Rh-negative woman may have been sensitized from birth by receiving enough Rh-positive cells from her mother during her own delivery to produce an antibody response.

In general, two exposures to the Rh antigen are required to produce any significant sensitization, unless the first exposure is massive. The first exposure leads to primary sensitization, whereas the second causes an anamnestic response leading to the rapid production of immunoglobulins, which can cause a transfusion reaction or hemolytic disease of the fetus during pregnancy.

The initial response to exposure to Rh antigen is the production of IgM antibodies for a short period of time, followed by the production of IgG antibodies that are capable of crossing the placenta. If the fetus has the Rh antigen, these antibodies will coat the fetal red blood cells and cause hemolysis. If the hemolysis is mild, the fetus can compensate by increasing the rate of erythropoiesis to maintain its red cell mass. If the hemolysis is severe, it can lead to profound anemia, resulting in hydrops fetalis from congestive cardiac failure and intrauterine fetal death.

The fetal and maternal circulation are normally separated by the placental "barrier." Small hemorrhages can and do occur, however, in either direction across the intact placenta throughout pregnancy. With advancing gestational age, the incidence and size of these transplacental hemorrhages increase. Most immunizations occur at the time of delivery, and antibodies appear either during the postpartum period or following exposure to the antigen in the next pregnancy.

If a pattern of mild, moderate, or severe disease has been established with two or more previous pregnancies, the disease tends either to be of the same severity or to become progressively more severe with subsequent pregnancies. It is unusual for a woman to deliver a mildly affected infant following the previous delivery of a severely affected one. If a woman has a history of fetal hydrops with a previous pregnancy, the risk of hydrops with a subsequent pregnancy is about 90 per cent. Hydrops usually develops at the same time as or earlier than in the previous pregnancy.

INCIDENCE

Although transplacental hemorrhage is very common, the incidence of Rh immunization within 6 months of the delivery of the first Rh-positive, ABO-compatible infant is only about 8 per cent. In addition, the incidence of sensitization with the development of a secondary immune response in the next Rh-positive pregnancy is 8 per cent. Therefore, the overall risk of immunization following the first full-term, Rh-positive, ABO-compatible pregnancy is about 16 per cent. The risk of Rh sensitization following an ABO-incompatible, Rh-positive pregnancy is only about 2 per cent. The protection against immuniza-

tion in ABO-incompatible pregnancies is due to the destruction of the ABO-incompatible cells in the maternal circulation and the removal of the red blood cell debris by the liver.

Transplacental hemorrhage may occur after spontaneous or induced abortions. The incidence of immunization following spontaneous abortion is 3.5 per cent, whereas that following induced abortion is 5.5 per cent. The risk is low in the first 8 weeks but rises to significant levels by 12 weeks gestation. The risk of immunization following amniocentesis or ectopic pregnancy is less than 1 per cent.

RECOGNITION OF THE PREGNANCY AT RISK

A blood sample from every pregnant woman should be sent at the first prenatal visit for determination of the blood group and Rh type and for antibody screening. In Rh-negative patients, the blood group and Rh status of the father of the baby should be determined. If the father is Rh-positive, his Rh genotype and ABO status should be determined. This may be done by testing the father's red blood cells with the reagents available for the antigens D, E, C, e, and c. If he is homozygous for the D antigen, every fetus he fathers will be Rh-positive and could potentially be affected. If he is heterozygous, only half of his children will be affected. Thus, information regarding the zygosity of the father is of value only in absolutely predicting the presence or absence of the Rh antigen in the fetus if the father is homozygous.

The Rh-negative woman whose partner is Rh-positive and whose initial antibody screen is negative should subsequently have anti-D antibody titers checked at 28 to 30 weeks and again at 34 to 36 weeks. The risk of transplacental hemorrhage increases at the time of delivery, especially with cesarean section or manual removal of the placenta. At delivery, cord blood must be sent for determination of the fetal blood group, Rh type, and for a direct Coombs' test. If a transplacental hemorrhage of greater than 30 ml of blood is suspected, a Kleihauer-Betke test is helpful in determining the volume of the hemorrhage.

The D antigen is a mosaic and has several alleles. D^u antigen is an incomplete variant that may or may not react with anti-D antibodies. Some Rh-negative patients who are D^u-positive and deliver an Rh-positive (D-positive) infant may become sensitized to the D antigen.

Maternal Rh-Antibody Titer

Anti-D antibody titers generally provide limited information regarding the severity of fetal hemolysis in Rh disease. A relationship between titers and outcome has been observed only in the case of the first sensitized pregnancy when the initial antibody screen is negative.

Amniotic Fluid Spectrophotometry

Analysis of amniotic fluid remains the most frequently used method of gauging the severity of fetal hemolysis. A correlation exists between the amount of biliary pigment in the amniotic fluid and the severity of anemia in the fetus.

The source of bilirubin in the amniotic fluid is controversial. The most likely source is tracheal and pulmonary efflux; transudate from the umbilical and placental vessels, however, may contribute. Because the standard biochemical methods for estimation of serum bilirubin are not sensitive enough for the small concentrations found in the amniotic fluid, spectrophotometric analysis is the most widely used technique for estimating amniotic fluid bilirubin concentration.

Optical density readings are made over the 350 to 700 μ wavelength range, and the values are plotted on a semilogarithmic paper with wavelength as the linear coordinate and the optical density as the logarithmic coordinate (Fig. 27–1). The optical density deviation (ΔOD) at 450 μ from a baseline drawn between the optical density values at 365 and 550 μ measures the amniotic fluid unconjugated bilirubin level, which in turn correlates with the cord blood hemoglobin of the newborn at birth.

Bilirubin is oxidized to colorless pigments when exposed to light; therefore, the fluid should be protected from light. Heme pigments and meconium may cause falsely high spectrophotometric values.

Bilirubin is normally found in amniotic fluid in a concentration that gradually diminishes toward term. For predictive interpretation, Liley devised a spectrophotometric graph based on the correlation of cord blood hemoglobin concentrations at birth and the amniotic fluid change in optical density at 450 μ. Using this method, he was able to establish predictive zones for mild, moderate, and severe disease. The Liley chart (Fig. 27–2) can be used to determine the severity of the disease and the appropriate management at a given gestational age.

Technique of Amniocentesis

Ultrasonically guided amniocentesis carries very little risk to the fetus or mother and is the only appropriate method for obtaining an amniotic fluid specimen. An ultrasonic examination is performed to localize a pocket of amniotic fluid far enough away from the fetus and placenta to obtain a sample safely. A 20- or 22-gauge spinal needle is inserted, and 10 ml of fluid is aspirated. The fluid is transferred to a dark tube to prevent deterioration owing to light exposure and is sent for assessment of the ΔOD 450.

Ultrasonic Detection of Rh Sensitization

Serial ultrasonic examinations of a woman with a fetus at risk for hemolytic disease can be a useful adjunct to amniocentesis in confirming fetal well-being and determining the advent of fetal hydrops. The examination should include a routine fetal assessment plus a determination of placental size and thickness and hepatic size. Both the placenta and the fetal liver are enlarged with hydrops. Fetal hydrops is easily diagnosed by the characteristic appearance of one or more of the following: ascites, pleural effusion, pericardial effusion, or skin edema. Appearance of any of these factors during an ultrasonic examination eliminates the need for diagnostic amniocentesis and necessitates therapeutic intervention based on fetal gestational age.

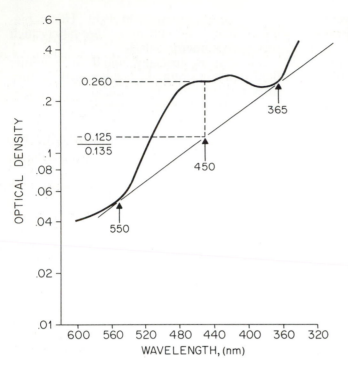

Figure 27–1. Plot of wavelength against optical density.

Percutaneous Umbilical Blood Sampling

Advances in fetal intervention techniques and the advent of high-resolution ultrasonography have made direct fetal blood sampling possible, and this has become the most accurate method for the diagnosis of fetal hemolytic disease. Fetal blood sampling can allow measurement of fetal hemoglobin, hematocrit, blood gases, pH, and bilirubin levels. The technique for fetal blood sampling is similar to that described for fetal intravenous transfusion discussed later in this chapter. The major drawback to this diagnostic procedure is that it requires expertise above and beyond that required for amniocentesis. The major risk is that of fetal exsanguination, but when performed by an experienced practitioner, the risk of this complication is only 0.5 per cent or less.

DETECTING FETOMATERNAL HEMORRHAGE

The Kleihauer-Betke test is dependent on the fact that adult hemoglobin is more read-

ily eluted through the cell membrane in the presence of acid than is fetal hemoglobin (HbF). The maternal blood is fixed on a slide with ethanol (80 per cent) and treated with a citrate phosphate buffer to remove the adult hemoglobin. After staining with hematoxylin and eosin, the fetal cells can readily be distinguished from the empty maternal cells. All cells are then counted, and an estimate of the extent of the fetal to maternal hemorrhage is made, based on the following equation:

$$\frac{\text{Number of fetal cells counted}}{\text{Number of maternal cells counted}}$$
$$= \frac{X^*}{\text{Estimated maternal blood volume (ml)}}$$

CLINICAL MANAGEMENT OF THE Rh-SENSITIZED PATIENT

Because single ΔOD 450 values are helpful only if they are very high (zone III) or very low (zone I), serial sampling of amniotic fluid is generally indicated. The severity of hemo-

---

* X = ml fetomaternal hemorrhage.

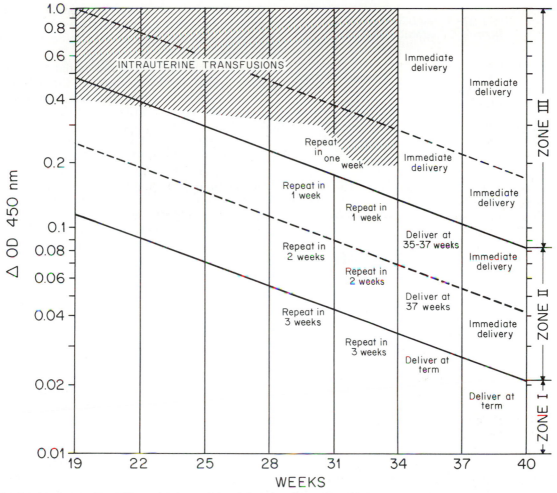

Figure 27-2. Modified Liley chart used to determine the appropriate management of the patient with isoimmunization.

lytic disease in the prior pregnancy provides an index for the timing of the first amniocentesis (Table 27-1). With serial sampling, one of three trends will emerge. Falling ΔOD 450 values are indicative of a fetus that is either unaffected (e.g., Rh-negative) or very mildly affected. No intervention is indicated in these patients. If the ΔOD 450 is either stable or rising, frequent ΔOD 450 determinations are necessary. If the ΔOD 450 enters zone II or III after 34 weeks, determination of fetal lung maturity and delivery are indicated. If this occurs prior to 34 weeks, however, delivery is best avoided because of the risk of complications from prematurity. In this case, intrauterine transfusion is the treatment of choice if the ΔOD 450 enters zone III. The amniotic fluid lecithin to sphingomyelin (L:S) ratio and phosphatidylglycerol levels (PG) play a key role in determining the optimal timing for delivery.

Intrauterine Transfusion

Intrauterine transfusion was introduced in 1963 and the technique has markedly changed the prognosis for severely affected fetuses between 20 and 32 weeks gestation. The goal is to inject fresh group O, Rh-negative packed red blood cells into the fetal peritoneal cavity or intravenously into the

Table 27–1. GUIDELINES FOR TIMING OF AMNIOCENTESIS

SEVERITY OF DISEASE IN PREVIOUS PREGNANCIES	TIMING OF FIRST AMNIOCENTESIS (WEEKS)
No disease	26–30
Mild-moderate: Delivery at 37–40 wk	20–28
Severe without death: Delivery at 34–37 wk	20–25
Severely affected neonate with hydrops or stillbirth	20–24

umbilical or hepatic veins. In addition to routine blood screening, the blood for transfusion is also irradiated, washed, and tested for cytomegalovirus. For intraperitoneal transfusions, the volume to be infused is based on the following formula:

$$\text{Volume} = [\text{Gestational age (weeks)} - 20] \times 10$$

For example, a 30-week fetus would require a 100-ml transfusion (30 weeks − 20 × 10 = 100 ml). For intravenous transfusions, most practitioners administer 30 to 50 ml of blood per kilogram of fetal body weight established by ultrasonic examination. Curare is usually injected directly into the fetal thigh with a 22-gauge spinal needle prior to beginning the transfusion to immobilize the fetus during the procedure.

Repeat transfusions are generally done at 1- to 3-week intervals. The final transfusion is performed at 32 weeks gestation, and in general, the fetus is delivered when the lungs are mature (by L:S ratio and PG) and the weight is more than 2000 gm. Cesarean section is performed because these very anemic fetuses do not tolerate the stress of labor well.

Fetal Intraperitoneal Transfusion. Intraperitoneal transfusions have been successfully used for 30 years. Red blood cells are absorbed via the subdiaphragmatic lymphatics and return via the right lymphatic duct into the fetal intravascular compartment. After transfusion, the absorption of blood may be monitored with serial transverse ultrasonic scans of the fetal abdomen. In nonhydroptic fetuses, the blood should be absorbed within 7 to 9 days. In the presence of hydrops, absorption may be slower but occasionally is quite rapid and may necessitate weekly transfusions with the removal of ascitic fluid, if present.

Under real-time ultrasonic guidance, a 20-gauge spinal needle is inserted through the mother's abdomen into the fetal peritoneal cavity. The correct positioning of the needle is determined by injection of a small amount of normal saline and carbon dioxide, which can be easily visualized with ultrasonography. The original technique involved injection of radiographic dye under fluoroscopy before the transfusion to confirm the position of the needle, but this is now rarely used. The red blood cells are slowly injected manually in 10-ml aliquots through an extension catheter attached to the spinal needle. If fetal bradycardia occurs at any time during the procedure, the transfusion is terminated.

Intravascular Transfusion. Because many fetuses do not present for transfusion until ascites is present, the technique of intravenous fetal transfusion has become increasingly popular. In addition, transfusion into the peritoneal cavity can result in fetal bradycardia or a pseudosinusoidal fetal heart rate pattern following the procedure because of compression at the site of insertion of the umbilical cord.

Under ultrasonic guidance, a 22-gauge spinal needle is inserted into the umbilical vein or the hepatic part of the umbilical portal venous system. If the umbilical vein is used, the preferred sites are the placental cord insertion site or a loop of umbilical cord. Correct placement of the needle is confirmed by injection of a small amount of normal saline that appears as turbulence when injected into the blood vessel. Intravenous transfusions are carried out more rapidly than intraperitoneal transfusions because the needle tip can easily become dislodged during the procedure. As soon as the fetal blood sample has been obtained and confirmed by the mean corpuscular volume, the transfusion is begun. As with intraperitoneal transfusion, the procedure is terminated if fetal bradycardia occurs.

Other Modes of Therapy

Administration of promethazine hydrochloride has been suggested based on animal studies that have shown that the drug inhibits the ability of fetal macrophages to bind Rh-positive blood cells, therefore decreasing the hemolytic process. The efficiency of this drug in humans is questionable. Maternal plasmapheresis may be helpful in severe erythroblastosis when intrauterine transfusions are not successful, but perinatal outcome with this technique has not been impressive. Phenobarbital has been used to induce fetal hepatic microsomal glucuronyltransferase activity, thereby increasing uptake and excretion of bilirubin by the liver. Treatment with phenobarbital is initiated 2 to 3 weeks before delivery.

PREVENTION OF RHESUS ISOIMMUNIZATION

Because Rh isoimmunization occurs in response to exposure of an Rh-negative mother to the Rh antigen, the mainstay for prevention is the avoidance of maternal exposure to the antigen. RH_O (D) immune globulin (anti-D gamma globulin) diminishes the availability of the Rh antigen to the maternal immune system, although the exact mechanism by which it prevents Rh-isoimmunization is not well understood.

RH_O (D) immune globulin is prepared from fractionated human plasma obtained from hyperreactive sensitized donors. The plasma is screened for hepatitis B surface antigen and anti HIV-1, the antibody to the acquired immunodeficiency syndrome (AIDS) virus. It is available in several dosage forms for intramuscular injection. Since the advent of its use in 1967, Rh immune globulin has dramatically reduced the incidence of Rh isoimmunization. Between 1970 and 1979, the incidence of hemolytic disease of the newborn in the United States fell 65 per cent.

Because the greatest risk for fetal to maternal hemorrhage occurs during labor and delivery, Rh immune globulin was initially administered only during the immediate postpartum period. This resulted in a 1 to 2 per cent failure rate, however, thought to be due to exposure of the mother to fetal red blood cells during the antepartum period. The indications for the use of Rh immune globulin have therefore been broadened to include any antepartum event (such as amniocentesis) that may increase the risk of transplacental hemorrhage. The routine prophylactic administration of Rh immune globulin at 28 weeks gestation is now the standard of care. This approach remains controversial for some practitioners because of concern about its cost-effectiveness and the safety of the volunteers who are used in the commercial production of the vaccine.

Indications for Administration of RH_O (D) Immune Globulin

The following provides a practical approach to the administration of Rh immune globulin to an Rh-negative patient with no Rh antibodies.

During a normal pregnancy, 300 μg Rh immune globulin is administered at 28 weeks gestation, following testing for sensitization with an indirect Coombs' test. A 300-μg dose is administered following amniocentesis at any gestational age. If a fetomaternal hemorrhage is suspected at any time during the pregnancy, a Kleihauer-Betke test should be performed. If positive, Rh immune globulin is administered in a dose of 10 μg/ml of fetal blood that entered the maternal circulation. Following an uncomplicated delivery, 300 μg Rh immune globulin is given within 72 hours. If a larger than normal fetal to maternal hemorrhage is suspected, such as may occur in patients with abruptio placentae or those requiring cesarean section or manual removal of the placenta, a Kleihauer-Betke determination should be performed after delivery and the appropriate dose of the Rh immune globulin determined.

Establishment of fetal circulation occurs at approximately 4 weeks gestation, and the presence of the RH_O (D) antigen has been demonstrated as early as 38 days following conception. Consequently, Rh isoimmunization can occur at any time during pregnancy, from the early first trimester on. Since fetal erythrocytes can be readily detected in the maternal blood following induced or spontaneous abortion, 50 μg Rh immune globulin should be given to all Rh-negative women following any type of abortion.

Fetal erythrocytes have been demonstrated in the maternal circulation following rupture of a tubal pregnancy. Consequently, Rh immune globulin should be given to an Rh-negative woman with an ectopic pregnancy. Since chorionic villi in gestational trophoblastic disease are avascular and devoid of fetal erythrocytes, Rh immune globulin is probably not necessary following molar pregnancy. At least one case of sensitization following a molar pregnancy, however, has been reported.

Whenever maternal exposure to fetal cells seems a possibility, it should be investigated. For example, fetal death of unknown etiology, unexplained newborn anemia, and antepartum bleeding may all be associated with fetal to maternal hemorrhage. If fetal cells are found in the maternal circulation, Rh immune globulin should be administered in a dose of 10 μg/ml of fetal blood entering the maternal circulation. There is controversy over whether or not a woman with D^u positive blood should receive Rh immune globulin after the delivery of an infant with D-positive blood. This is not done in the United States, and manufacturers do not list this condition as an indication.

IRREGULAR ANTIBODIES

Although the prophylactic use of immunoglobulins has led to a decline in the incidence of Rh isoimmunization, hemolytic disease of the newborn caused by antibodies produced by other red blood cell antigens (so-called irregular antibodies) has increased slightly. This is probably due to the wider use of blood transfusions. Approximately 2 per cent of cases of hemolytic disease of the newborn are due to irregular antibodies. The risk to the fetus depends on both the type of antibody (whether it is IgM or IgG) and the strength of the antibody. For example, the Kell antigen is capable of eliciting a strong IgG response that may cause neonatal disease similar to Rh hemolytic disease.

When an irregular antibody is detected in the maternal blood, the father should be checked for the presence of that antigen. If the father is negative for the antigen in question, no further investigations are necessary. If the father is antigen-positive, the antibody is IgG, and the titer is significant (greater than 1:8), amniotic fluid studies similar to

Table 27-2. HEMOLYTIC DISEASE DUE TO IRREGULAR ANTIBODIES

BLOOD GROUP SYSTEM	ANTIGEN	SEVERITY OF HEMOLYTIC DISEASE
Kell	K	Mild to severe (hydrops)
	k	Mild only
Duffy	Fy^a	Mild to severe (hydrops)
Kidd	Jk^a	Mild to severe
	Jk^b	Mild to severe
MNS_s	M	Mild to severe
	S	Mild to severe
	U	Mild to severe
Lutheran	Lu^a	Mild
	Lu^b	Mild
Diego	Di^a	Mild to severe
	Di^b	Mild
Public antigens	Yt^a	Moderate to severe
	Ge	Mild
	Co^a	Severe
Private antigens	Becker	Mild
	Biles	Moderate
	Good	Severe
	Heibel	Moderate
	Radin	Moderate
	Wright	Severe

Modified from Weinstein L: Irregular antibodies causing hemolytic disease of the newborn: A continuing problem. Clin Obstet Gynecol 25(2):321, 1982.

those performed in Rh disease must be carried out. A partial list of the common irregular antibodies that can lead to hemolytic disease of the newborn is shown in Table 27-2.

SUGGESTED READING

Berkowitz RL, Chitkara U, Wilkins IA, et al: Intravascular monitoring and management of erythroblastosis fetalis. Am J Obstet Gynecol 158:783, 1988.

Bevis DCA: Blood pigments and hemolytic disease of the newborn. J Obstet Gynecol Br Emp 63:68, 1956

Bowman JM: Suppression of Rh-isoimmunization. Obstet Gynecol 52:1, 1978.

Bowman JM: The management of Rh-isoimmunization. Obstet Gynecol 52:385, 1978.

Grannum P, Copel JA: Prevention of Rh-isoimmunization and treatment of the compromised fetus. Sem Perinatol 12:324, 1988.

Henry G, Wexler P, Robinson A: Rh-immune globulin after amniocentesis for genetic diagnosis. Obstet Gynecol 48:557, 1976.

Lawrence M: Diagnostic amniocentesis in early pregnancy. Br Med J 2(6080):191, 1977.

Liley AW: Errors in the assessment of hemolytic disease from amniotic fluid. Am J Obstet Gynecol 86:485, 1963.

Liley AW: Liquor amnii analysis in the management of pregnancy complicated by rhesus sensitization. Am J Obstet Gynecol 82:1359, 1961.

Weinstein L: Irregular antibodies causing hemolytic disease of the newborn: A continuing problem. Clin Obstet Gynecol 25:321, 1982.

White CA, Stedman CM, Frank S: Anti-D antibodies in D- and D^u positive women: A cause of hemolytic disease of the newborn. Am J Obstet Gynecol 145:1069, 1983.

Twenty-eight

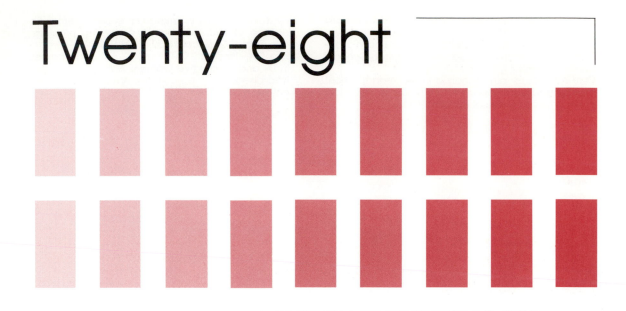

Operative Delivery

JOHN P. NEWNHAM AND CALVIN J. HOBEL

Changing patterns of obstetric care have significantly influenced the methods of operative delivery. During the first 60 years of the twentieth century, retreat from a difficult forceps delivery was labeled "obstetric cowardice," and cesarean section was considered the end point of failed obstetric care. In modern obstetric practice, abdominal delivery is readily resorted to when an operative vaginal delivery would be hazardous to mother, child, or both. Widespread improvements in anesthesia, surgical technique, antibiotics, and blood transfusion have decreased the morbidity and mortality from cesarean section, making it a relatively safe option. However, the type and time of operative intervention remain among the most important of the many decisions involved in modern obstetric practice. Current acceptance of the liberal use of cesarean section in no way obviates the need to acquire a full understanding of the mechanisms of normal child

birth and the principles of safe operative vaginal delivery.

CESAREAN SECTION

Cesarean section is defined as delivery of the fetus through incisions in the anterior abdominal and uterine walls. The origin of the term remains a matter of dispute. Claims by legend that Julius Caesar was delivered via this route are unlikely to be true, because his mother lived for many years after his birth in a time when the operation would almost certainly have been fatal. It is possible, however, that the name was derived from the Latin word caedere, meaning "to cut," or, possibly, from the Roman law lex Caesarea, whereby abdominal delivery of the fetus from a woman dying in late pregnancy was required in the hope of saving the child.

Survival following cesarean section was a rare event until 1882, when suturing the uterine incision was first suggested. Of the many subsequent milestones that further reduced the operative mortality, perhaps the most notable was the popularization of the transverse lower segment incision in the 1920s. This approach obviated the need to incise the thick muscular wall of the uterine corpus and excluded the uterine wound from the peritoneal cavity by placing the bladder flap over the lower segment incision.

Epidemiology

The rate of cesarean section deliveries in the United States has increased fourfold, from 5.5 per 100 births in 1970 to 22.7 per 100 births in 1985. The incidence of cesarean section in individual obstetric units is dependent on the patient population and physicians' attitudes. Currently, the rate ranges from 10 to 40 per cent of all births. It is generally agreed that the more liberal use of cesarean section has contributed to a decrease in the perinatal mortality rate.

Indications

The indications for cesarean section, singularly or in combination, are relative rather than absolute and can be classified as shown in Table 28–1. The most frequent indication for cesarean section is dystocia, which usually presents as "failure to progress" in labor. This problem may result from cephalopelvic disproportion, fetal malpresentation, or failure to induce labor. There are several maternal conditions in which only a short trial of labor is considered safe, including eclampsia, pre-eclampsia, diabetes mellitus, and cardiac disease. Previous classic cesarean section is an absolute indication for a repeat cesarean section. Certain cases of previous lower uterine segment cesarean section and previous myomectomy that did not involve the full thickness of the uterine wall are now considered suitable for a trial of vaginal delivery.

Cesarean section is the appropriate management for fetal distress in which vaginal delivery is not imminent. Many fetuses presenting by breech are best delivered by

TABLE 28–1. INDICATIONS FOR CESAREAN SECTION

TYPE	INDICATION
Maternal/Fetal	Dystocia
	Cephalopelvic disproportion
	Failed induction of labor
	Abnormal uterine action
Maternal	Maternal diseases
	Eclampsia/severe pre-eclampsia
	Diabetes mellitus
	Cardiac disease
	Cervical cancer
	Previous uterine surgery
	Classic cesarean section
	Previous uterine rupture
	Full-thickness myomectomy
	Obstruction to the birth canal
	Fibroids
	Ovarian tumors
Fetal	Fetal distress
	Cord prolapse
	Fetal malpresentations
	Breech, transverse lie, brow
Placental	Placenta previa
	Abruptio placentae

cesarean section, particularly those in whom the gestation is preterm.

Types of Operation

Classification of the types of cesarean section refers to the uterine incision rather than the skin incision. The operation is generally performed through a transverse incision in the lower segment of the uterus (Fig. 28–1). The advantages of this approach include a decreased chance of rupture of the scar in a subsequent pregnancy and a reduced risk of bleeding, peritonitis, paralytic ileus, and bowel adhesions.

An alternative approach is the classic operation that employs a vertical incision in the upper segment of the uterus. A vertical incision may be made in the lower segment, in which case the procedure is referred to as a low vertical cesarean, although the incision invariably extends into the upper segment of the uterus (Fig. 28–2).

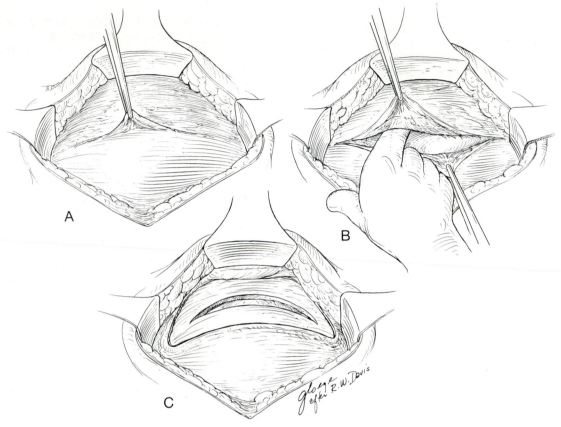

Figure 28–1. Lower transverse cesarean section. *A*, Loose uterovesical fold of peritoneum; *B*, separation of the bladder from the lower uterine segment, after incising the uterovesical fold; *C*, transverse incision through the lower uterine segment exposing the fetal membranes. Note the retraction of the bladder inferiorly.

Several indications for classic and low vertical cesarean section remain and are as follows:

1. When a preterm fetus presents by breech. In this circumstance, usually at 34 weeks gestation or less, the lower segment is still poorly formed, and a transverse incision may be too narrow to allow an atraumatic delivery of the fetus.
2. When the fetal lie is transverse and cannot be corrected to a longitudinal lie, particularly if the back is inferior and the membranes are ruptured. An extreme example is a shoulder presentation with the arm prolapsed down the vagina.
3. When access to the lower segment is restricted because of fibroids or, rarely, dense adhesions.

4. When hysterectomy will immediately follow the cesarean section.
5. When a postmortem cesarean section is done to attempt to rescue a live child from a dead mother.
6. When invasive cervical cancer is present.

Morbidity and Mortality

The risk of maternal death from cesarean section is four to six times greater than that from vaginal delivery. Problems related to the anesthetic are currently the major cause of mortality. The overall mortality rate from cesarean section is currently less than one in 1000, although the danger of the procedure itself may be approximately doubled by the

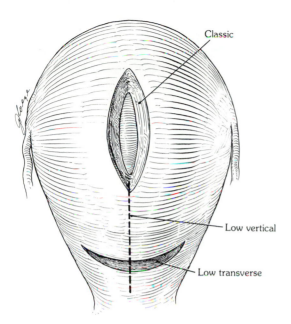

Figure 28-2. Types of cesarean section.

medical or obstetric complication that led to the operation.

The maternal complications of cesarean section include those of the normal postpartum period and those of any major surgical procedure. Important complications specific to cesarean section are:

1. Hemorrhage. Primary hemorrhage may occur from failure to achieve hemostasis at the site of the uterine incision or from uterine atony, which may follow prolonged labor.

2. Postoperative sepsis. The frequency of this complication is significantly greater when cesarean section is performed during labor or in the presence of intrauterine infection. Prophylactic antibiotics for 24 hours significantly reduce the incidence of this problem.

3. Injury to surrounding structures. The bowel, bladder, vessels within the broad ligament, and ureters are particularly liable to injury. Transient hematuria may result from overzealous use of the retractor in the region of the bladder wall.

Management of Subsequent Pregnancies

The mode of delivery of subsequent pregnancies relates specifically to the risk of uter-

ine rupture. The probability of this complication, if labor is allowed, is about 6 per cent for previous classic cesarean sections and about 1 per cent for previous transverse lower segment cesarean sections. Rupture of a classic scar can occur before the onset of contractions. Whenever the rupture occurs, it may result in a catastrophic hemorrhage, with extrusion of the fetus into the peritoneal cavity.

Lower uterine segment scars are situated mainly in fibrous tissue. Rupture before labor is rare. Moreover, while extension laterally into uterine vessels can occur, dehiscence with only mild to moderate hemorrhage is more common. The dehiscence may not be apparent until manual exploration of the lower segment is performed immediately postpartum.

Because of these considerations, repeat cesarean section before the onset of labor is mandatory in the presence of a classic scar. For lower segment scars, some obstetricians in the United States still adhere to the general dictum "once a cesarean, always a cesarean." Most patients with a history of a transverse lower segment cesarean section, however, are now allowed a trial labor. Contraindications to such a trial include inadequate pelvic dimensions, the presence of other medical or obstetric complications, and fetal macrosomia. In some institutions in the United States, women with a history of two or more lower segment cesarean sections are now allowed a trial of labor.

Cesarean Hysterectomy

On occasion, it may be appropriate to remove the uterus at the time of cesarean section. This option may be life-saving in cases of postpartum hemorrhage not responsive to more conservative therapy. Relative indications include cervical malignancy and severe damage to the uterus from rupture. Every effort to avoid hysterectomy should be made in those women who wish to retain their fertility.

OBSTETRIC FORCEPS

The obstetric forceps is a tool designed to provide traction, rotation, or both to the fetal

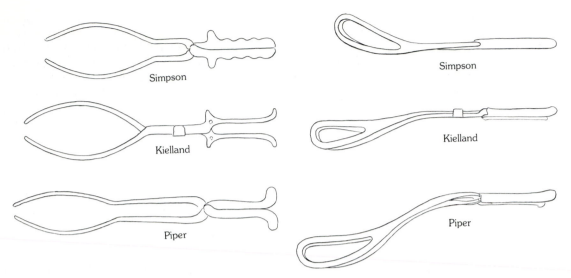

Figure 28-3. Types of obstetric forceps in common use.

head when the unaided expulsive efforts of the mother are insufficient to accomplish safe delivery. The first obstetric forceps was designed and used by the Chamberlen family in England during the seventeenth century. Widespread use of this instrument was not achieved in the United States until the early decades of the twentieth century.

Design of Instrument

The design of the obstetric forceps consists of two blades that are introduced separately into the vagina. The components of each blade are illustrated in Figure 28-3. All varieties of forceps have a cephalic curve designed to grasp the fetal head. Conventional forceps used for traction only (e.g., Simpson) have in addition a pelvic curve, which corresponds to the axis of the birth canal. Forceps designed for rotation of the fetal head, of which Kielland's is the most frequently used, are characterized by the absence of a pelvic curve.

Indications

The indications for forceps delivery are best classified as maternal, fetal, or both. The most frequent indication is delay in the second stage of labor, caused by either abnormal uterine action or failure of the head to rotate adequately. Maternal conditions such as hypertension, cardiac disorders, or pulmonary disease, in which strenuous pushing in the second stage of labor is considered hazardous, may be indications for forceps delivery. Fetal distress is a frequent indication, but there is no place for difficult and heroic vaginal procedures when the fetal condition is already compromised. Forceps may also be used to control the aftercoming head in a vaginal breech delivery and to assist delivery of the head at cesarean section.

Types of Forceps Application

Forceps operations may be classified according to the station and position of the presenting part at the time the forceps are applied. The American College of Obstetricians and Gynecologists has proposed the following classification:

1. Outlet forceps—the application of forceps when the scalp is visible at the introitus without separating the labia, the skull has reached the pelvic floor, the sagittal suture is in the anteroposterior diameter or in the right or left occiput anterior or posterior position, and the fetal head is at or on the perineum. According to this definition, rotation cannot exceed 45 degrees.

2. Low forceps—the application of forceps when the leading point of the skull is at station +2 or more. Low forceps have two subdivisions: rotation of 45 degrees or less and rotation of more than 45 degrees.

3. Mid forceps—the application of forceps when the head is engaged but the leading point of the skull is above station +2. Under no circumstances should forceps be applied to an unengaged presenting part.

Requirements for Forceps Delivery

To embark on forceps delivery, the following requirements must be fulfilled:

1. Delivery must be mechanically feasible. This is determined by clinical assessment of the level of the presenting part, the presence or absence of molding, and the adequacy of the maternal pelvis. Engagement of the fetal head is mandatory.

2. The presenting part must be suitable. There are only three presentations in which obstetric forceps may be used: vertex, face where the chin is anterior (mentoanterior), and the aftercoming head in a vaginal breech delivery.

3. There must be no doubt regarding the position of the fetal head.

4. Uterine contractions must be present. Second-stage uterine atony, fortunately uncommon, should be corrected by an oxytocin infusion before forceps delivery, not only because the uterine expulsive efforts are a vital component of delivery, but also because of the grave risk of immediate postpartum hemorrhage if atony persists.

5. The membranes must be ruptured. Intact membranes may retard descent of the presenting part, and their rupture may remove the apparent indication for the forceps.

6. The cervix must be fully dilated.

7. Anesthesia must be adequate. Although outlet forceps may be performed with pudendal nerve block and local infiltration, Kielland's forceps rotation usually requires epidural or spinal anesthesia.

8. The bladder must be empty. It is routine to drain the bladder by urinary catheterization before forceps delivery.

Complications

Maternal Complications. Forcible rotation or traction may result in trauma to maternal soft tissues, ranging from mild abrasions to severe lacerations. Structures most likely to be injured are the vagina, cervix, and uterus, and bleeding may be profuse. Severe lacerations are most common with a difficult rotation forceps.

Fetal Complications. Inappropriate application of forceps resulting in one blade overlying the fetal face will produce unsightly bruising. This can be expected to disappear within the first few days of life. The use of excessive force for traction or rotation, however, may cause serious injury to the fetal scalp, cranium, or underlying brain. The risk for neurologic damage is greatest when a difficult forceps procedure is used to deliver an already hypoxic fetus.

VACUUM EXTRACTION

The vacuum extractor is an instrument that employs a suction cup applied to the fetal head. Traction is applied to the cup to aid the mother's expulsive efforts. The method has the following advantages over forceps:

1. Unlike forceps, the vacuum extractor cup does not occupy space adjacent to the fetal head. Hence, delivery by this method generally requires a smaller episiotomy than that for a forceps delivery, and in multiparous women, the fetus can often be delivered over an intact perineum, a situation rarely achievable with forceps.

2. Delivery of occipitotransverse and posterior positions does not require forced rotation of the head. Rotation occurs spontaneously at the station best suited to the configuration of the fetal head and maternal pelvis.

3. With correct application of the cup, the vacuum extractor functions to reduce the diameter of the presenting part by flexing the head. The elliptical shape of the deflexed fetal head can be converted to the smaller and more circular diameter of the vertex by traction posteriorly on the head. This is achieved by correctly placing the cup in the midline,

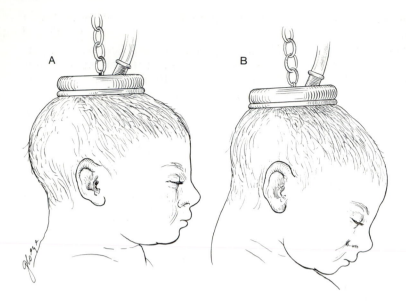

Figure 28–4. Application of the vacuum extractor. *A,* Incorrect application, which deflexes the fetal head, thereby increasing the presenting diameter; and *B,* correct application over the posterior fontanelle, which flexes the fetal head.

over the posterior fontanelle, as displayed in Figure 28–4.

4. Attempted delivery with the vacuum extractor in the presence of unrecognized disproportion will result in the loss of suction and failure of the procedure. In contrast, forceps will not dislodge during their inappropriate usage, and the unwary operator may proceed to inflict injury to the fetus, mother, or both by forcible and persistent traction.

Requirements for Vacuum Extraction

The requirements for the use of the vacuum extractor are the same as those previously outlined for forceps delivery, with the following exceptions:

1. While generally the cervix should be fully dilated, the vacuum extractor can be used, at times, in multiparous women in whom a small rim of cervix remains, provided that the rim will displace easily over the fetal head.

2. The vacuum extractor is contraindicated in preterm delivery, since the fetal head and scalp are prone to injury from the suction cup.

3. The vacuum extractor is suitable for all vertex presentations, but unlike forceps, it must never be used for delivery of fetuses presenting by the face or breech.

Complications

The most frequent complication resulting from the use of the vacuum extractor is vaginal laceration from entrapment of vaginal mucosa between the suction cup and fetal head. This problem can be avoided by digital examination of the entire circumference of the suction cup before initiation of the vacuum and traction. Fetal scalp injuries, including subaponeurotic hemorrhage and scalp lacerations, may result from prolonged use of the vacuum extractor. As a general rule, if traction on the suction cup during three contractions has not produced encouraging descent of the fetal head, the trial of vaginal delivery by vacuum extractor should be abandoned. If the cup is inadvertently placed on a face presentation, serious eye damage may occur.

CHOICE OF INSTRUMENT

Most obstetricians favor one of the two instruments, forceps or vacuum extractor, based on their experience, training, and general preference. Neither instrument is perfect, and neither is to be condemned. Perhaps of greatest importance is the operator's technical skill and judgment in preoperative evaluation.

SUGGESTED READING

Amirikia H, Zarewych B, Evans TN: Cesarean section: A 15 year review of changing incidence, indications, and risks. Am J Obstet Gynecol 140:81, 1981.

Bashore RA, Phillips WH, Brinkman CR: A comparison of the morbidity of midforceps and caesarian delivery. Am J Obstet Gynecol 162: 1428, 1990.

Bird GC: The use of the vacuum extractor. Clin Obstet Gynecol 9:641, 1982.

Bottoms SF, Rosen MG, Sokol RJ: The increase in the caesarean birth rate. N Engl J Med 302:559, 1980.

Broekhuizen FF, Washington JM, Johnson F, Hamilton PR: Vacuum extraction versus forceps delivery: Indications and complications, 1979 to 1984. Obstet Gynecol 69:338, 1987

Caesarean Childbirth: Report of a Consensus Development Conference. US Department of Health and Human Services. Bethesda, MD, NIH Publication No. 82-2067, Oct 1981.

Cardozo LD, Gibb DMF, Studd JWW, et al: Should we abandon Kielland's forceps? Br Med J 287:315, 1983.

Chalmers JA, Chalmers I: The obstetric vacuum extractor is the instrument of first choice for operative vaginal delivery. Br J Obstet Gynecol 96:505, 1989.

Cohn M, Barclay C, Fraser R, et al: A multicentre randomised trial comparing delivery with a silicone rubber cup and rigid metal vacuum extractor cups. Br J Obstet Gynaecol 96:545, 1989.

Committee on Obstetrics: Maternal and fetal medicine. The American College of Obstetrics and Gynecology: Obstetric Forceps # 71—August 1989.

Howie PW, Davey PG: Prophylactic antibiotics and caesarean section. Br Med J 300:2, 1990.

Lowe B: Fear of failure: A place for the trial of instrumental delivery. Br J Obstet Gynaecol 94:60, 1987.

Ophir E, Yagoda A, Rojansky N, Oettinger M: Trial of labor following caesarean section: Dilemma. Obstet Gynecol Surv 44:19, 1989.

Robertson PA, Laros Jr KR, Zhao R: Neonatal and maternal outcome in low-pelvic and midpelvic operative deliveries. Am J Obstet Gynecol 162:1436, 1990.

Ryden G: Vacuum extraction or forceps? (Editorial.) Br Med J, 292:75, 1986.

Taffel SM, Placek PJ, Liss T: Trends in the United States caesarean section rate and reasons for the 1980–85 rise. Am J Public Health 77:955, 1987.

Part 3

Gynecology

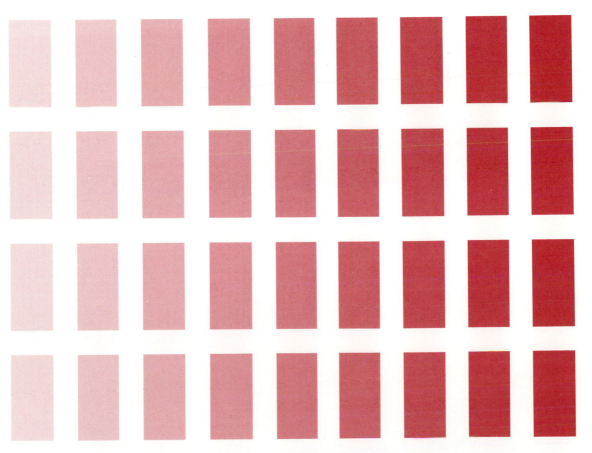

J. GEORGE MOORE — SUBEDITOR

Twenty-nine

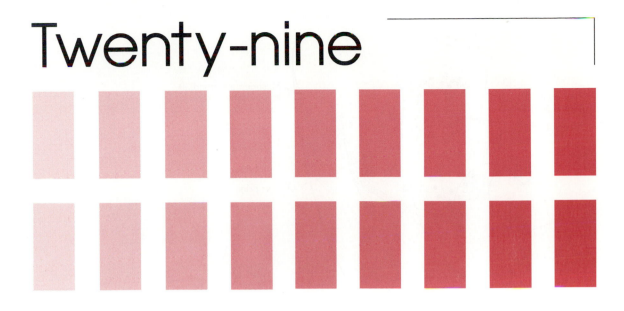

Embryology and Congenital Anomalies of the Female Genital System

WILLIAM A. GROWDON

A knowledge of the embryology of the female genital tract is critical to the understanding of anomalous development of female genital organs. This chapter discusses the normal embryologic development of the female reproductive system, congenital anomalies, and the clinical features and management of anomalous development.

NORMAL EMBRYOLOGIC DEVELOPMENT OF THE OVARY

The earliest event in gonadogenesis is noted at approximately 4 weeks gestational age,* when a thickening of the peritoneal, or coelomic, epithelium on the ventromedial surface of the urogenital ridge occurs. A bulging genital ridge is subsequently produced by rapid proliferation of the coelomic epithelium in an area that is medial, but parallel, to the mesonephric ridge. Prior to the fifth week, this indifferent gonad consists of germinal epithelium surrounding the internal blastema, a primordial mesenchymal cellular mass destined to become the ovarian

---

* Gestational ages are given in weeks from conception, which is approximately 2 weeks less than menstrual gestational age.

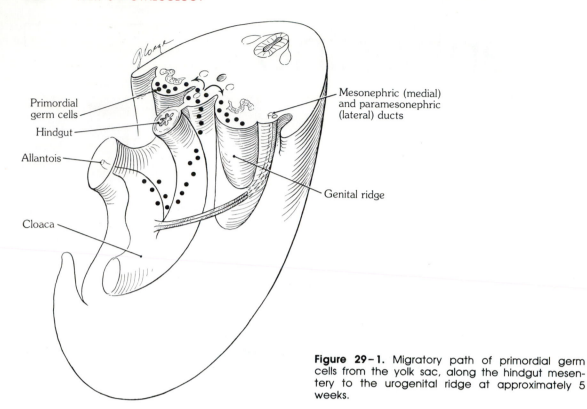

Primordial germ cells

Hindgut

Allantois

Cloaca

Mesonephric (medial) and paramesonephric (lateral) ducts

Genital ridge

Figure 29–1. Migratory path of primordial germ cells from the yolk sac, along the hindgut mesentery to the urogenital ridge at approximately 5 weeks.

medulla. After 5 weeks, projections from the germinal epithelium extend like spokes into the mesenchymal blastema to form primary sex cords. Soon thereafter in the seventh week, a testis can be identified histologically if the embryo has a Y chromosome. In the absence of a Y chromosome, definitive ovarian characteristics do not appear until somewhere between the twelfth and sixteenth weeks.

As early as 3 weeks gestation, large primordial germ cells appear intermixed with other cells in the endoderm of the yolk sac wall of the primitive hindgut. These germ-cell precursors migrate along the hindgut dorsal mesentery (Fig. 29–1) and are all contained in the mesenchyme of the urogenital ridge by 8 weeks gestation. Subsequent replication of these cells by mitotic division occurs, with maximal mitotic activity noted up to 20 weeks gestation and cessation noted by term. These oogonia, the end result of this germ-cell proliferation, are incorporated into the cortical sex cords of the genital ridge.

Histologically, the first evidence of follicles is seen at about 20 weeks, with germ cells surrounded by flattened cells derived from the cortical sex cords. These flattened cells are recognizable as granulosa cells of coelomic epithelial origin and theca cells of mesenchymal origin. The oogonia enter the prophase of the first meiotic division and are then called primary oocytes. It has been estimated that more than 2 million primary oocytes, or their precursors, are present at 20 weeks gestation age, but only about 300,000 primordial follicles are present by 7 years of age.

Regression of the primary sex cords in the medulla produces the rete ovarii, which are found histologically in the hilus of the ovary along with another testicular analog called Leydig cells that are thought to be derived from mesenchyme. Vestiges of the rete ovarii and of the degenerating mesonephros may also be noted, at times, in the mesovarium or mesosalpinx. Structural homologues in males and females are shown in Table 29–1.

INTERNAL GENITAL DEVELOPMENT

The upper vagina, cervix, uterus, and fallopian tubes are formed from the parameso-

Table 29–1. STRUCTURAL HOMOLOGUES IN MALES AND FEMALES

PRIMORDIA	FEMALE	MALE	MAJOR DETERMINANT FACTORS
Gonadal			
Germ cells	Oogonia	Spermatogonia	Sex chromosomes
Coelomic epithelium	Granulosa cells	Sertoli cells	
Mesenchyme	Theca cells	Leydig cells	
Mesonephros	Rete ovarii	Rete testis	
Ductal			
Paramesonephric (müllerian)	Fallopian tubes Uterus Part of vagina	Testis hydatid	Absence of Y chromosome
Mesonephric (wolffian)	Gartner's duct	Vas deferens Seminal vesicles	Testosterone Müllerian inhibiting factor
Mesonephric tubules	Epoöphoron Paroöphoron	Epididymis Efferent ducts	
External Genitalia			
Urogenital sinus	Vaginal contribution Skene's glands Bartholin's glands	Prostate Bulbourethral glands Prostatic utricle	Presence or absence of testosterone, dehydrotestosterone, and 5-alpha reductase enzyme
Genital tubercle	Clitoris	Penis	
Urogenital folds	Labia minora	Corpora spongiosa	
Genital folds	Labia majora	Scrotum	

nephric (müllerian) ducts. Although human embryos, whether male or female, possess both paired paramesonephric and mesonephric (wolffian) ducts, the absence of Y chromosomal influence leads to the development of the paramesonephric system with total regression of the mesonephric system. With a Y chromosome present, a testis is formed and müllerian inhibiting substance is produced, creating the reverse situation.

Mesonephric duct development occurs in each urogenital ridge between weeks 2 and 4 and is thought to influence the growth and development of the paramesonephric ducts. The mesonephric ducts terminate caudally by opening into the urogenital sinus. First evidence of each paramesonephric duct is seen at 6 weeks gestation as a groove in the coelomic epithelium of the paired urogenital ridges, lateral to the cranial pole of the mesonephric duct. Each paramesonephric duct opens into the coelomic cavity cranially at a point destined to become a tubal ostium. Coursing caudally at first, parallel to the developing mesonephric duct, the blind distal end of each paramesonephric duct eventually crosses dorsal to the mesonephric duct, and the two ducts approximate in the midline. The two paramesonephric ducts fuse terminally at the urogenital septum, forming the uterovaginal primordium. The distal point of fusion is known as the müllerian tubercle (Müller's tubercle) and can be seen protruding into the urogenital sinus dorsally in embryos of 9 to 10 weeks gestation (Fig. 29–2). Later dissolution of the septum between the fused paramesonephric ducts leads to the development of a single uterine fundus, cervix, and, according to some investigators, the upper vagina.

Degeneration of the mesonephric ducts is progressive from 10 to 16 weeks in the female fetus, although vestigial remnants of the latter may be noted in the adult (Gartner's duct cyst, paroöphoron, epoöphoron) (Fig. 29–3). The myometrium and endometrial stroma are derived from adjacent mesenchyme; the glandular epithelium of the fallopian tubes, uterus, and cervix is derived from the paramesonephric duct.

Solid vaginal plate formation and lengthening occur from the twelfth through the

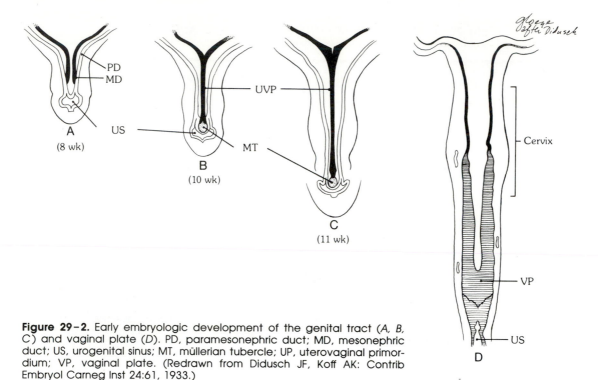

Figure 29-2. Early embryologic development of the genital tract (*A, B, C*) and vaginal plate (*D*). PD, paramesonephric duct; MD, mesonephric duct; US, urogenital sinus; MT, müllerian tubercle; UP, uterovaginal primordium; VP, vaginal plate. (Redrawn from Didusch JF, Koff AK: Contrib Embryol Carneg Inst 24:61, 1933.)

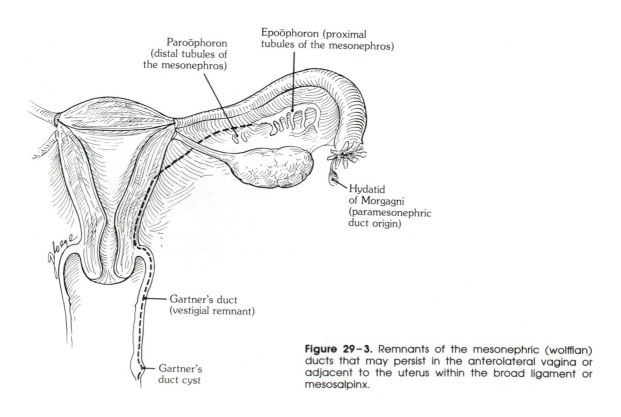

Figure 29-3. Remnants of the mesonephric (wolffian) ducts that may persist in the anterolateral vagina or adjacent to the uterus within the broad ligament or mesosalpinx.

Figure 29–4. Development of the external female genitalia. *A,* Indifferent stage (approximately 7 weeks); *B,* approximately 10 weeks; *C,* approximately 12 weeks.

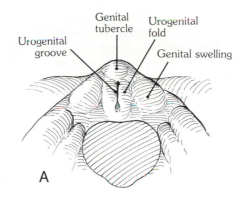

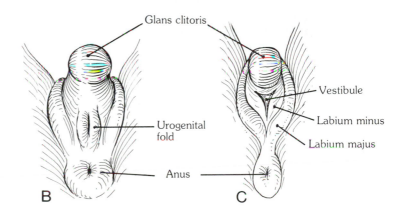

twentieth week, followed by caudad to cephalad canalization, which is usually completed in utero. There is controversy surrounding the relative contribution of the urogenital sinus and paramesonephric ducts to the development of the vagina, and it is uncertain whether the whole of the vaginal plate is formed secondary to growth of the endoderm of the urogenital sinus or whether the upper vagina is formed from the paramesonephric ducts.

EXTERNAL GENITAL DEVELOPMENT

Prior to the seventh week of development, the appearance of the external genital area is the same in males and females. Elongation of the genital tubercle into a phallus with a clearly defined terminal glans portion is noted in the seventh week, and gross inspection at this time may lead to faulty sexual identification. Ventrally and caudally, the urogenital membrane, made up of both endo-

dermal and ectodermal cells, further differentiates into the genital folds laterally and the urogenital folds centrally. The lateral genital folds develop into the labia majora, while the urogenital folds develop subsequently into the labia minora and prepuce of the clitoris.

The external genitalia of the fetus are readily distinguishable as female at approximately 12 weeks (Fig. 29–4). In the male, the urethral ostium is located conspicuously on the elongated phallus by this time and is smaller, owing to urogenital fold fusion dorsally, producing a prominent raphe from the anus to the urethral ostium. In the female, the hymen is usually perforated by the time delivery occurs.

ABNORMAL DEVELOPMENT OF THE OVARIES

Abnormal embryologic development of the ovaries is uncommon. Congenital duplication or absence of ovarian tissue may occur, and even ectopic ovarian tissue and supernumerary ovaries have been described. Although rare, the sexual bipotentiality noted in embryologic development can progress without the usual regression of one system, producing an ovotestis with subsequent intersex problems.

Genetic chromosomal disorders, such as Turner's syndrome (45 XO), are associated with a lack of normal gonadal development, as evidenced by the rudimentary streaked ovaries that are a hallmark of the disorder. Although this is nature's evidence that two X chromosomes are required for normal ovarian development, testicular predominance occurs with the addition of the Y chromosome, even in the face of multiple X chromosomes. Such predominance is seen in Klinefelter's syndrome (47 XXY), in which testicular development occurs embryologically. This is due to the structural gene believed to be contributed by the Y chromosome, which ensures the presence of H-Y histocompatibility antigen on all cells containing a Y chromosome. Since both male and female gonadal cells have H-Y antigen receptors believed to be contributed by the X chromosome, only the male H-Y antigen contribution will cause testicular development from antigen-receptor interaction.

ANOMALIES OF THE PARAMESONEPHRIC DUCTS AND UROGENITAL SINUS

Anomalies of the fallopian tubes, uterus, cervix, and vagina are uncommon. Although the exact etiology of these malformations is unknown, the three most commonly accepted theories for their occurrence are teratogenesis, genetic inheritance, and multifactorial expression.

Many variations and combinations of anomalies occur. Lack of development (agenesis), incomplete development (hypoplasia), incomplete canalization (atresia), completely separate development, and variations of extent and level of fusion categorize these anomalies.

Fallopian Tube Anomalies

Isolated anomalies of the fallopian tubes, the end result of abnormal development of

the proximal unfused portions of the paramesonephric ducts, are rare. Aplasia or atresia, usually of the distal ampullary segment, is most commonly unilateral in the presence of otherwise normal development. Bilateral aplasia is noted in some cases of uterine and vaginal agenesis.

Complete duplication of the fallopian tubes is rarely seen, but distal duplication and accessory ostia are relatively common. Because ovarian development is independent, the ipsilateral ovary of the involved aplastic or atretic side is usually normal in appearance and laterally placed near the pelvic brim.

Anomalies of the Uterine Fundus and Cervix

The most common anomalies are the result of malfusion of the paramesonephric ducts, with lesser or greater degrees of septation. Figure 29–5 shows variations of uterine development and indicates that communications can exist between dual systems at several levels. The genital tract may be obstructed at any level, although minute sinuses exist in some cases despite a lack of an obvious communication.

In müllerian agenesis, there is a complete lack of development of the paramesonephric system. Except for the fimbriated end, there is usually incomplete development of fallopian tubes, associated with absence of the uterus, cervix, and most of the vagina (Fig. 29–6). This condition occurs in an otherwise normal karyotypic and phenotypic female.

Vaginal Anomalies

The more common anomalies of the vagina include imperforate hymen, longitudinal and transverse vaginal septa, partial development (vaginal atresia), double vagina, and absence of the vagina.

Imperforate hymen represents the least of these canalization abnormalities, occurring at the site of vaginal plate formation in its contact with the urogenital sinus. After birth, a bulging, membrane-like structure may be noticed in the vestibule, usually blocking egress of mucus (Fig. 29–7). A similar anomaly, the transverse vaginal septum, is

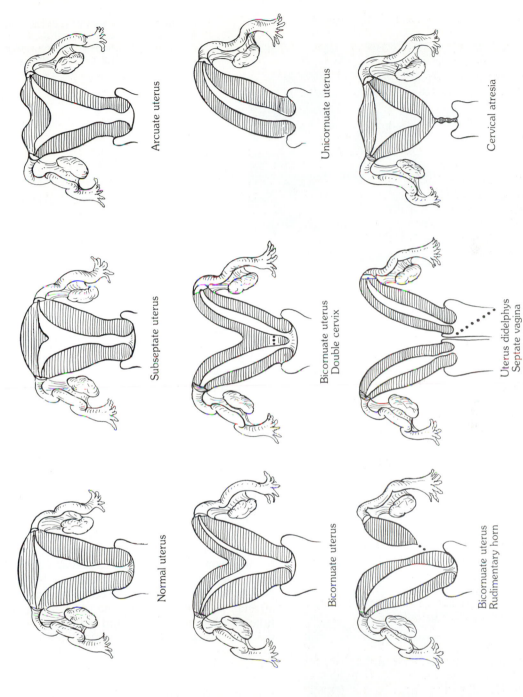

Figure 29–5. Variations in uterine development. The dots (. . .) represent potential sites of communication or obstruction.

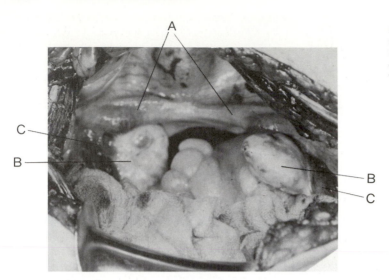

Figure 29–6. Internal genitalia in müllerian agenesis. Note the (A) bilateral nonfunctioning fibromuscular cords, (B) normal ovaries, and (C) fimbriae.

most commonly found at the junction of the upper and middle third of the vagina. At times, a transverse vaginal septum will have a sinus tract leading to recognition only when intercourse is later impeded. Patients with an imperforate hymen or transverse vaginal septum usually have normal development of the upper paramesonephric system.

Atresia of the vagina generally represents a more substantial lack of canalization at the caudal or cranial end of the vaginal plate. If cranially placed, the upper vagina and cervix may be atretic, with the uterine fundus and fallopian tubes unaffected.

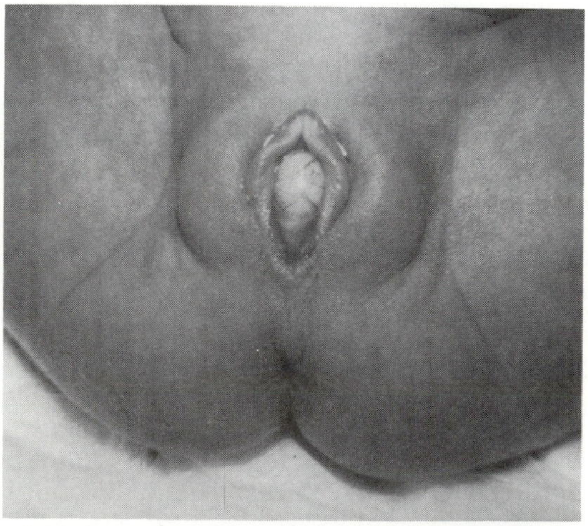

A midline longitudinal septum may be present, creating a double vagina. The longitudinal septum may be only partially present at various levels in the upper and middle vagina, either in the midline or deviated to one side. Additionally, a longitudinal septum may attach to the lateral vaginal wall creating a blind vaginal pouch with or without a communicating sinus tract. These septa are usually associated with a double cervix and one of the various duplication anomalies of the uterine fundus, although a normal upper tract may be present.

Vaginal agenesis represents the most extreme case of vaginal anomaly, with total absence of the vagina and usually absence of the uterus and fallopian tubes—that is, müllerian agenesis or the Rokitansky-Kuster-Hauser syndrome. Isolated complete vaginal atresia with normal uterine and fallopian tube development is rare and is thought to be the end result of isolated vaginal plate malformation.

Concurrent Urinary Anomalies

It is generally accepted that the laterally placed paramesonephric ducts are guided in their development by the mesonephric system. The complex interaction of the three nephric systems and the urogenital sinus is not completely understood. It is quite com-

Figure 29–7. Neonate with a bulging introital mass, the tense imperforate hymen blocking the egress of mucus from the vagina (mucocolpos). (Courtesy of Dr. Eric Fonkalsrud, Department of Surgery, UCLA Medical Center, Los Angeles, CA.)

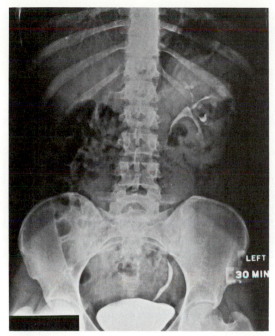

Figure 29–8. Intravenous pyelogram demonstrating ipsilateral renal agenesis in a woman with uterus didelphys and a blind right vaginal pouch.

mon for an anomaly in one system, however, to be associated with anomalies in the other. Urinary tract abnormalities are uncommon in the face of completely separate but normal development of the paramesonephric ducts, as occurs with uterus didelphys with a double vagina. Where partial unilateral development occurs, however, as in the case of a hypoplastic rudimentary horn, a high incidence of unilateral renal anomalies exists, most commonly an absence of the ipsilateral kidney. Uterus didelphys, with one of two vaginas existing as a blind pouch, is associated with renal agenesis on the side of the pouch in 100 per cent of reported cases. In patients with complete müllerian agenesis, other urinary tract anomalies may be present, such as pelvic kidneys, horseshoe kidney, and duplication of the collecting system (Fig. 29–8). In women found to have unilateral renal agenesis, approximately 50 per cent have associated genital tract anomalies.

INTERSEXUAL DEVELOPMENT

Problems of sexual identification may be present at birth, or they may not become apparent until later, particularly at puberty. The conditions may be classified as female or male pseudohermaphroditism or true hermaphroditism.

When ambiguous genitalia are present at birth, the problem of sexual assignment arises. Caution, sensitivity, and the avoidance of hasty decisions and confusing terminology should be the rule when dealing with anxious parents and relatives. Careful physical examination, pelvic ultrasonography, hormonal studies, examination of a buccal smear for sex chromatin, karyotyping, and consultation with colleagues may be necessary before the sex of rearing is assigned. The assignment of sex will determine the need for any corrective surgery or hormonal manipulation and the manner in which the parents rear the child. These factors are all critical to the child's proper gender identification.

Female Pseudohermaphroditism

Female pseudohermaphroditism is due to masculinization occurring in utero, the infant presenting with ambiguous genitalia. Masculinization of the genetically female fetus occurs secondary to the endogenous hormonal milieu, as in congenital adrenal hyperplasia, or as a result of exogenous hormonal ingestion by the mother, usually in the form of androgenic progestins. Tumors of the ovary or adrenal gland, which produce androgens, may also rarely cause this problem.

Enlargement of the clitoris is the most conspicuous abnormality. There are also various degrees of fusion of the labioscrotal folds, producing a hypospadiac urethral meatus and a malpositioned vaginal orifice (Fig. 29–9). Internal genital development is normal. Congenital adrenal hyperplasia is discussed in Chapter 49.

Male Pseudohermaphroditism

When the genetic sex is male (46 XY), there may be complete external phenotypic development along female lines. This occurs in the testicular feminization syndrome (androgen insensitivity syndrome), a genetic ab-

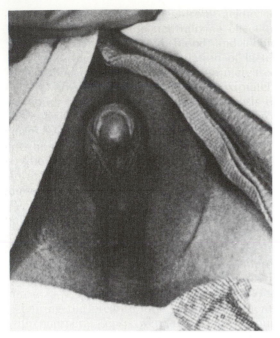

Figure 29–9. Ambiguous genitalia in a patient with congenital adrenal hyperplasia. This female exhibited clitoromegaly, hypospadias, and obscure vaginal orifice.

normality most commonly inherited as an X-linked recessive disorder. Secondary sexual characteristics appear at puberty along normal female lines, and the disorder is generally not recognized until menarche has failed to occur. Testes are usually undescended and located in the inguinal canals or labial areas. External genitalia are generally normal on examination, with the exception of scanty or absent pubic hair. Sufficient vaginal development to allow adequate coital activity is present in many cases. The gonads have normal testicular histology, and serum testosterone levels are normal. Because of a genetic deficiency of androgen receptors, however, the external genital development is along female lines. Müllerian inhibiting substance is produced, which is the reason for the lack of müllerian duct development.

Male pseudohermaphrodites may occur with varying degrees of virilization and varying degrees of müllerian development. These result most commonly from genetic mosaicism, such as 45 XO/46 XY. Many factors must be taken into account in the determination of gender role in these cases, and a full discussion of this problem is beyond the scope of this book.

True Hermaphroditism

In true hermaphroditism, which is rare, dual gonadal development occurs, either in the form of an ovotestis or as a separate ovary and testis. Although some of these cases represent mosaics of normal female and male chromosomal complement, the usual chromosomal pattern is 46 XX. Most true hermaphrodites have some degree of both female and male development internally and externally. The extent to which masculinization occurs depends on the relative amount of testicular tissue and its relative contribution of testosterone. Confirmation of the diagnosis requires laparotomy.

CLINICAL IMPLICATIONS OF FEMALE GENITAL ANOMALIES

Many anomalies of the female genital tract go unrecognized prior to puberty and, more specifically, menarche. Others, such as unilateral paramesonephric development along normal lines or uterus didelphys, may produce no signs and symptoms and go unrecognized throughout life.

Symptoms

The more usual complaints associated with female genital anomalies are listed in Table 29–2. Many of the anomalies present with symptoms caused by the collection of blood generated by a functioning endometrium. An imperforate hymen may present as a bluish membrane bulging at the vestibule. Cyclic abdominal pain after puberty associated with the presence of a pelvic mass may represent a hematocolpos, hematometra, or hematosalpinx. These disorders are produced by the collection of blood above various levels of obstruction resulting from vaginal atresia, longitudinal septa with obstruction, transverse septa with obstruction, or, rarely, isolated cervical atresia. A rudimentary uterine horn with functioning endometrium may

Table 29-2. SYMPTOMS AND SIGNS ASSOCIATED WITH FEMALE GENITAL ANOMALIES

SYMPTOMS

Primary amenorrhea	Leakage with tampon in place
Dyspareunia	Irregular vaginal bleeding
Dysmenorrhea	Habitual abortion
Cyclic pelvic pain	Spontaneous second-trimester abortion
Inability to achieve penile penetration	Premature labor
Infertility	Postpartum hemorrhage

SIGNS

Vaginal mass (hematocolpos, mucocolpos, Gartner's duct cyst)	Absent uterus/cervix
	Absent/short vagina
Abdominal mass (hematosalpinx, hematometra)	Ambiguous genitalia
	Absent pubic hair
	Fetal malpresentation
	Retained placenta

produce a hematometra. The symptom complex is quite variable. Some patients may have significant collections of blood in the genital tract with spillage into the peritoneal cavity yet have minimal signs and symptoms. The extent of vaginal or uterine distention may be sufficient to occlude the ureter, either at the pelvic brim or lower in its retroperitoneal course. Flank pain may then be the most prominent symptom leading to discovery of the abnormality.

If a small sinus tract is present in a vaginal septum, it will allow the egress of a small amount of darkish blood or, if bacterial contamination has occurred, foul odorous vaginal secretions. This may delay the diagnosis by allowing decompression of a noncommunicating vagina. With vaginal agenesis, vaginal atresia, or a noncommunicating transverse vaginal septum, primary amenorrhea will occur. When a communicating double vagina is present, patients may complain of menstrual soiling, despite the placement of one vaginal tampon.

Sexual dysfunction may be the presenting complaint with genital tract anomalies. Inability to achieve penile penetration may lead to the diagnosis of testicular feminization, imperforate hymen, transverse vaginal sep-

tum, or vaginal agenesis. With vaginal duplication, there is generally no problem with sexual activity.

Physical Examination

Careful examination of the external genitalia, digital exploration of the vagina, and a bimanual examination through the rectum should be performed. In the case of vaginal agenesis, the gonads may or may not be palpable, but there are usually no palpable midline structures, since the uterus is absent in most cases. The erroneous diagnosis of a vaginal wall cyst, such as a Gartner's duct cyst, may be made in the presence of a noncommunicating lateral vagina. Pelvic masses should not be mistaken for distended internal genital organs caused by distal obstruction without excluding the possibility of a pelvic kidney.

Investigations

Many diagnostic tools may be of use in detecting genitourinary anomalies. Sonography may elucidate internal anatomy, although it should be used only as an adjunct to careful history and physical examination, since the information obtained may be nonspecific. An intravenous pyelogram will elucidate unexpected anomalous urinary tract development. A hysterosalpingogram will elucidate uterine and tubal architecture (Fig. 29-10). Hysteroscopy, using low-molecular-weight dextran as a distending medium in the uterus, has been used for the diagnosis and treatment of intrauterine anomalies, such as small septa. Magnetic resonance imaging is also emerging as a useful noninvasive diagnostic tool. Although limited availability, cost, and the problems inherent in a lengthy immobilizing procedure are drawbacks, more precise anatomic definition may be obtained by this technique. In difficult cases, examination under anesthesia combined with laparoscopic visualization of internal anatomy may be helpful, especially in the face of noncommunicating duplication anomalies.

Treatment

Many genital tract anomalies require no treatment. An imperforate hymen or trans-

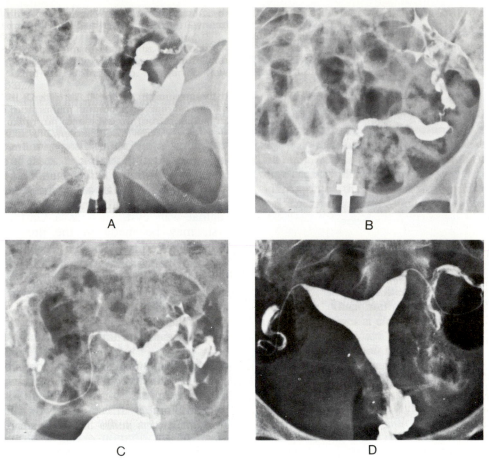

Figure 29–10. Hysterosalpingograms showing (*A*) uterus didelphys, (*B*) unicornuate uterus, (*C*) bicornuate uterus, and (*D*) arcuate uterus. (Courtesy of Dr. Marvin Weiner, Department of Radiological Sciences, UCLA Medical Center, Los Angeles, CA.)

verse vaginal septum requires excision of the obstructing tissue to remove the obstruction. In a patient with vaginal agenesis, creation of a neovagina using a split-thickness skin graft is required. In a patient with a uterine anomaly, the reproductive function should be tested prior to surgical manipulation; should a septum in the uterine fundus be identified as a factor contributing to habitual abortion, however, it may be surgically excised. Favorable pregnancy rates have been noted after some unification procedures, although delivery by cesarean section is necessary to prevent rupture of the uterus. In a phenotypic female with a Y chromosome, localization and removal of the gonadal tissue and subsequent hormonal management are necessary,

since neoplastic transformation commonly occurs in these gonads.

SUGGESTED READING

Arey LB: The genital system. In Arey LB (ed): Developmental Anatomy. Philadelphia, WB Saunders, 1974, p 315.

Buttram VC Jr, Gibbons WE: Müllerian anomalies: A proposed classification (an analysis of 144 cases). Fertil Steril 32:40, 1979.

Davies J: Human Developmental Anatomy. New York, Ronald Press, 1963, p 177.

Fedele L, Dorta M, Brioschi D, et al: Magnetic resonance imaging in Mayer-Rokitansky-Kuster-Hauser syndrome. Obstet Gynecol 76:593, 1990

Gilman J: The development of the gonads in man, with a consideration of the role of fetal endocrines and the histogenesis of ovarian tumors. Contrib Embryol Carneg Inst 32:84, 1948.

Gilsanz V, Cleveland RH, Reid BS: Duplication of the mullerian duct and genitourinary malformation. Radiology 144:793, 1982.

Hamilton WJ, Mossman HW: Urogenital system. In Hamilton WJ, Mossman HW (eds): Human Embryology. Baltimore, Williams & Wilkins, 1972, p 377.

Jones HW Jr, Scott WW: Genital Anomalies and Related Disorders. Baltimore, Williams & Wilkins, 1971.

Koff AK: Development of the vagina in the human fetus. Contrib Embryol Carneg Inst 24:61, 1933.

Rock JA, Jones HW Jr: The double uterus associated with obstructed hemivagina and ipsilateral renal agenesis. Am J Obstet Gynecol 138:339, 1980.

Spaulding MH: The development of the external genitalia in the human embryo. Contrib Embryol Carneg Inst 13:67, 1921.

Speroff L, Glass RH, Kase NG: Normal and abnormal sexual development. In Speroff L, Glass R (eds): Clinical Gynecologic Endocrinology and Infertility. 4th ed. Baltimore, Williams & Wilkins, 1989, p 379.

Ulfelder H, Robboy S: The embryological development of the human vagina. Am J Obstet Gynecol 126:769, 1976.

Valdes C, Srini M, Malinak LR: Ultrasound evaluation of female genital tract anomalies: A review of 64 cases. Am J Obstet Gynecol 149:285, 1984.

Witschi E: Migration of the germ cells of human embryos from the yolk sac to the primitive gonadal folds. Contrib Embryol Carneg Inst 32:69, 1948.

Thirty

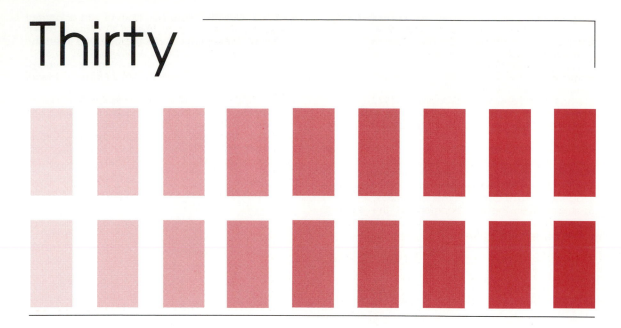

Dysmenorrhea and Premenstrual Syndrome

JOHN A. EDEN

Many cultures believed that menstruation was controlled by the moon and that menstrual fluid was toxic. In modern times, it has been shown that menstrual fluid contains substances that enhance uterine contractions. These substances have been shown to be prostaglandins.

Painful menstruation or dysmenorrhea may be primary or secondary to organic pelvic disease (Table 30–1). Premenstrual syndrome (PMS) is a collection of symptoms that occur at the same time of the menstrual cycle, most often 7 to 10 days before menstruation. Both dysmenorrhea and PMS are common and distressing problems that can have an impact on a woman's well-being and productivity.

About 50 per cent of menstruating women are affected by dysmenorrhea, and 10 per cent have severe symptoms necessitating bed rest. Women with dysmenorrhea have more days off work and do less well at school than unaffected women. The peak age incidence is 20 to 24 years.

DYSMENORRHEA

Pathophysiology

Primary dysmenorrhea is a feature of ovulatory cycles and usually appears within 6 to 12 months of the menarche. The etiology of primary dysmenorrhea has been attributed to uterine contractions or ischemia, psychological factors, and cervical factors. Psychological factors may alter the perception of pain but are not unique to the problem of dysmenor-

Table 30-1. ETIOLOGY OF DYSMENORRHEA
Primary dysmenorrhea
Secondary dysmenorrhea
Endometriosis
Pelvic inflammation
Adenomyosis
Fibroids
Intrauterine contraceptive device
Uterine polyps
Uterine malformations
Cervical stenosis
Pelvic congestion syndrome

Table 30-2. FEATURES OF PRIMARY DYSMENORRHEA
Initial onset
90% experience symptoms within 2 yr of menarche
Duration and type of pain
Dysmenorrhea begins a few hours before or just after the onset of menstruation and usually lasts 48-72 hr
Pain is described as cramp-like and is usually strongest over the lower abdomen and may radiate to the back or inner thigh
Associated symptoms
Nausea and vomiting
Fatigue
Diarrhea
Lower backache
Headache
Pelvic findings
Normal

rhea. There is no convincing evidence of cervical stenosis in patients with dysmenorrhea, so there is no basis for incriminating these latter two factors as major contributors to the problem of primary dysmenorrhea.

Women with dysmenorrhea have increased uterine activity, which may manifest as increased resting tone, increased contractility, increased frequency of contractions, or incoordinate action. Prostaglandins are C20 hydrocarbons with a cyclopentane ring and are produced by microsomal enzymes (prostaglandin synthetase) from arachidonic acid. Prostaglandins are released as a consequence of endometrial cell lysis with labilization of lysosomes and release of enzymes, which break down cell membranes.

The evidence that prostaglandins are involved in primary dysmenorrhea is convincing. Menstrual fluid from women with dysmenorrhea has higher than normal levels of prostaglandins (especially $PGF_{2\alpha}$ and PGE_2), and these levels can be reduced to below normal with nonsteroidal anti-inflammatory drugs (NSAIDs), which are effective treatments. Infusions of $PGF_{2\alpha}$ or PGE_2 reproduce the discomfort and many of the associated symptoms (Table 30-2). Secretory endometrium contains much more prostaglandin than proliferative endometrium. Anovulatory endometrium (without progesterone) contains little prostaglandin and these menses are usually painless.

Figure 30-1 summarizes the relationships amongst endometrial cell wall breakdown, prostaglandin synthesis, uterine contractions, ischemia, and pain.

Clinical Features

Clinical features are summarized in Table 30-2. Cramping usually begins a few hours before the onset of bleeding and may persist for hours or days. It is localized to the lower abdomen and may radiate to the thighs and lower back. The pain may be associated with altered bowel habits, nausea, tiredness, dizziness, and headache.

Treatment

NSAIDs are highly effective in the treatment of primary dysmenorrhea (Table 30-3). Typical examples include ibuprofen (400 mg every 6 hours), naproxen sodium (275 mg every 6 hours), and mefenamic acid (500 mg every 8 hours). Oral contraceptive pills (OCP) reduce menstrual flow and inhibit ovulation and are also effective therapy for primary dysmenorrhea. Some patients may benefit from using both oral contraceptive pills and NSAIDs.

Resistant cases may occasionally respond to tocolytic agents such as salbutamol or a calcium blocker such as nifedipine, progestogens (especially medroxyprogesterone acetate or dydrogesterone), psychotherapy, or hypno-

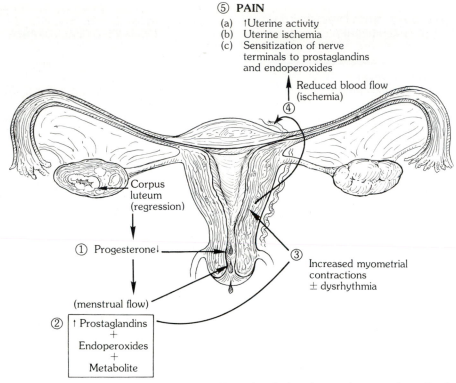

⑤ **PAIN**
(a) ↑Uterine activity
(b) Uterine ischemia
(c) Sensitization of nerve terminals to prostaglandins and endoperoxides

Reduced blood flow (ischemia)
④

Corpus luteum (regression)

① Progesterone↓

③ Increased myometrial contractions ± dysrhythmia

(menstrual flow)

② ↑ Prostaglandins
+
Endoperoxides
+
Metabolite

Figure 30-1. Postulated mechanism in the generation of pain in primary dysmenorrhea. Factors affecting central nervous perception of pain are not depicted. (Reprinted with permission from Dawood MY: Hormones, prostaglandins and dysmenorrhea. In Dawood MY (ed): Dysmenorrhea. Baltimore, Williams and Wilkins, 1981.)

therapy. Presacral neurectomy is rarely performed today.

If a patient fails to respond to combined OCP and NSAID therapy, the diagnosis of primary dysmenorrhea should be questioned and consideration given to a secondary cause. Laparoscopy and hysteroscopy with curettage should be performed to exclude pelvic disease.

SECONDARY DYSMENORRHEA

Pathophysiology

The mechanism of pain in secondary dysmenorrhea is not well understood, but may also involve prostaglandins.

Clinical Features

Clinical features are summarized in Table 30-4. In general, secondary dysmenorrhea is not limited to the menses, is less related to the first day of flow, develops in older women (thirties or forties), and may be associated with other symptoms (dyspareunia, infertility, abnormal bleeding).

Treatment

Management consists of the treatment of the underlying disease. Specific treatments are discussed in the relevant chapters.

PREMENSTRUAL SYNDROME

Definition and History

Hippocrates was the first to describe menstrual symptoms when he wrote: "Shivering, lassitude and heaviness of the head denoted the onset of menstruation . . . mistiness of

Table 30-3. TREATMENT OF PRIMARY DYSMENORRHEA
General measures
Reassurance and explanation
Medical measures
NSAIDs
Oral contraceptive pills
Progestogens
Tocolytics
Analgesics
Surgical measures (avoid)
Dilatation and curettage
Presacral neurectomy
Uterosacral ligament section
Other measures
Psychotherapy
Hypnotherapy
Transcutaneous nerve stimulators

vision is resolved by menstruation." In 1873, Maudsley noted that "the monthly activity of the ovaries which marks the advent of puberty in women has a notable effect upon the mind and body; wherefore it may become an important cause of mental and physical derangement."

Table 30-4. FEATURES OF SECONDARY DYSMENORRHEA

Endometriosis
  Pain extends to premenstrual or postmenstrual phase or may be continuous. May also have deep dyspareunia, premenstrual spotting, and tender pelvic nodules (especially on the uterosacral ligaments). Onset is normally in the twenties and thirties
Pelvic inflammation
  Initially pain may be menstrual, but often with each cycle it extends into the premenstrual phase. May have intermenstrual bleeding, dyspareunia, and pelvic tenderness
Fibroids, adenomyosis
  Dysmenorrhea is associated with a dull pelvic dragging sensation. Uterus is generally clinically enlarged and may be mildly tender
Ovarian cysts
  Should be clinically evident
Pelvic congestion
  A dull ill-defined pelvic ache usually worse premenstrually, relieved by menses. Often a history of sexual problems

The premenstrual problems suffered by women were formally described by Frank in 1931, and the term *PMS* was first used by Greene and Dalton in 1953. In modern times, the term *ovarian cycle syndrome* was coined by John Studd, which better describes the syndrome, as many symptoms also occur around the time of ovulation.

One useful definition of PMS is that of Magos: "distressing physical, psychological and behavioural symptoms not caused by organic disease which regularly recur during the same phase of the menstrual cycle, and which significantly regress or disappear during the remainder of the cycle." About 5 to 10 per cent of women suffer from severe PMS that interferes with daily life.

Pathophysiology

The etiology of PMS is unknown. A number of theories have been proposed to explain the syndrome, and these are listed in Table 30-5. The noncontroversial facts about the premenstrual syndrome are shown in Table 30-6.

Severe PMS may result from cyclical ovarian activity altering a central mechanism, which then erodes a woman's ability to cope with adverse psychological factors. This may explain why anovulatory drugs or psychotherapy often help these patients. Drug treat-

Table 30-5. ETIOLOGY OF PREMENSTRUAL SYNDROME— PROPOSED HYPOTHESES

Abnormal secretion of estrogen
Progesterone excess or deficiency
Excess or deficiency of cortisone, androgens, or prolactin
Antidiuretic hormone excess
Abnormality of endogenous opiates or melatonin secretion
Deficiencies of vitamins A, B_1, B_6 or minerals such as magnesium
Reactive hypoglycemia
Hormone allergy
Prostaglandin excess or deficiency
Menstrual toxin
Psychological, social, evolutionary, and genetic factors

Table 30–6. PREMENSTRUAL SYNDROME—THE NONCONTROVERSIAL FACTS

Most healthy women report some adverse symptoms prior to menses

The syndrome is associated with ovulation and does not occur before puberty, during pregnancy, or after the menopause. It does not occur in women who are anovulatory

Menstruation itself is incidental, as cyclic symptoms continue after hysterectomy if the ovaries are preserved

Extensive metabolic and psychological studies have failed to find a specific abnormality

Table 30–8. CONFIRMATORY EVIDENCE OF PREMENSTRUAL SYNDROME

Positive family history
Onset after menarche (often after 20 yr)
Worsening with age (35–45 yr)
Well-being during pregnancy
Positive menstrual diary (symptoms occur and regress at the same time of the cycle)
Improvement with drugs that inhibit ovulation

ments should aim to suppress the cyclic ovarian activity. Psychotherapy helps the woman cope with or resolve the problems being aggravated by PMS.

Clinical Features

Clinical features may be divided conveniently into physical, psychological, and behavioral. The most common symptoms are shown in Table 30–7.

Physical symptoms include abdominal bloating, edema and weight gain, headache, breast tenderness and swelling, pelvic ache, altered bowel habits, and reduced coordination. Psychological symptoms include irritability; anxiety; depression; an alteration in sleep, appetite, and libido; and tiredness. Behavioral changes include absenteeism, prone-ness to accidents, and possibly criminal behavior or suicide.

Diagnosis

The diagnosis is made by taking a history, performing an examination, and carrying out any appropriate investigations to exclude organic disease. Supportive evidence for PMS is shown in Table 30–8. Symptoms do not usually start with the first period and often get worse as the woman gets older. After 35 years, they may blend into early menopausal symptoms. There is an association among postnatal depression, menopausal depression, and PMS.

A menstrual diary is a useful aid in making the diagnosis. Important symptoms should be recorded and scored from none (0), through mild (+) to severe (+++). Weight should be recorded each day, and the record should be kept as simple as possible (no more than five symptoms). If a particular symptom occurs regularly at the same time of the cycle and is not present during the rest of the cycle, this is confirmatory evidence of PMS.

Table 30–7. MOST COMMON SYMPTOMS ASSOCIATED WITH PREMENSTRUAL SYNDROME

Feeling swollen
Weight gain
Loss of efficiency
Irritability
Difficulty concentrating
Tiredness
Mood swings
Depression

Treatment

There is a significant placebo effect from any drug used in this condition, and it can account for half the therapeutic effect. Pyridoxine and oil of primrose are often prescribed, but there is no evidence that these are superior to a placebo. The usual dose of pyridoxine used is 50 to 100 mg a day. Doses exceeding 1000 mg daily have been associated with peripheral nerve toxicity. Diuretics, especially spironolactone, 25 to 50 mg daily, can be used for fluid retention symptoms. Bromocriptine is effective for mastalgia but is expensive and has many side effects. Despite a paucity of controlled trials, progesterone by injection or suppository is often used when other conservative measures have failed. Some women will obtain relief of symptoms from an oral contraceptive pill or progestins, such as medroxyprogesterone acetate.

Psychological methods such as relaxation tapes, hypnotherapy, and psychotherapy are also useful. Diet is important. Women who suffer from sore breasts often obtain relief by reducing coffee and tea intake and embarking on a diet low in fat and high in complex carbohydrate. Reducing salt intake may help with fluid retention.

If a woman with severe PMS is having a hysterectomy to manage a problem such as large uterine fibroids, careful consideration should be given to removing the ovaries and giving estrogen replacement immediately after the operation. If the ovaries are conserved, the cyclic symptoms may continue and even worsen.

CONCLUSIONS

Dysmenorrhea and PMS are common complaints that cause considerable disruption to a woman's life. The key to appropriate management is an accurate history and examination. The main therapeutic agents used include oral contraceptive pills, NSAIDs, and progestogens.

SUGGESTED READING

Anderson ABM, Gillebaud J, Haynes PJ, et al: Reduction of menstrual blood loss by prostaglandin synthetase inhibitors. Lancet 1:774, 1976.

Chan WY, Fuchs F, Powell AM: Effects of naproxen sodium on menstrual prostaglandins and primary dysmenorrhea. Obstet Gynecol 61:285, 1983.

Dawood MY: Dysmenorrhea and prostaglandins. In Gold JJ, Josimovich JB (eds): Gynecologic Endocrinology. 4th ed. New York, Plenum, 1987, pp 405–422.

Frank RT: The hormonal causes of premenstrual tension. Arch Neurol Psychiatry 26:1053, 1931.

Greene R, Dalton K: The premenstrual syndrome. Br Med J 1:1007, 1953.

Khoo SK, Munro C, Battistutta D. Evening primrose and treatment of premenstrual syndrome. Med J Aust 153:189, 1990.

Magos A, Studd JWW: The premenstrual syndrome —a review. In Studd JWW, Whitehead MI (eds): The Menopause. Oxford, Blackwell Scientific Publications, 1988, pp 271–288.

O'Brien PM, Craven D, Selby C, et al: Treatment of the premenstrual syndrome by spironolactone. Br J Obstet Gynaecol 86:142, 1979.

Pickles VR, Hall WJ, Best FA, et al: Prostaglandins in endometrium and menstrual fluid from normal and dysmenorrheic subjects. J Obstet Gynaecol Br Commonw 72:185, 1965.

Smith S, Schiff I: The premenstrual syndrome—diagnosis and management. Fertil Steril 52(4):527, 1989.

West CP: Inhibition of ovulation with oral progestins —effectiveness in premenstrual syndrome. Eur J Obstet Gynecol Reprod Bio 34:119, 1990.

Thirty-one

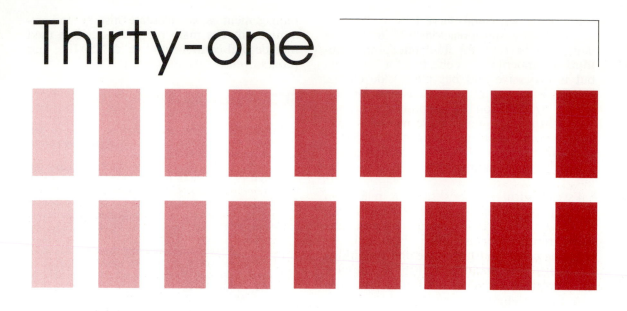

Benign Lesions of the Vulva, Vagina, and Cervix

THOMAS B. LEBHERZ

Vulvovaginal disease is among the 10 leading disorders encountered by family practitioners. Diagnosis is often delayed because most lesions produce pruritus and irritation, and there is a tendency for physicians to treat the symptoms without clinical examination. It is important to establish a specific diagnosis before initiating any therapy.

BENIGN VULVAR DISEASE

Medical History

In a patient with vulvar itching or irritation, it is important to inquire about general medical conditions that may have vulvar manifestations, such as diabetes mellitus, Crohn's disease, atopy, and psoriasis or other skin diseases. Urinary incontinence or chronic diarrhea may result in secondary vulvar reactions. Inquiry should be made about the use of soaps, perfumes, deodorants, and nylon or tight-fitting clothing because these are known to be potential causes of vulvar irritation, especially in a patient with an atopic history. Previous therapeutic measures should be ascertained and the patient's response to such medications determined.

Physical Examination

Careful inspection of the entire vulva under a good light is of utmost importance. Many lesions of the vulva are small and subtle. A simple hand-held magnifying lens, a "poor man's colposcope," aids naked eye in-

Table 31–1. CLASSIFICATION OF BENIGN LESIONS OF THE VULVA

Inflammatory vulvar dermatoses
   Intertrigo
   Secondary irritative vulvitis
   Hidradenitis suppurativa
   Fox-Fordyce disease
   Diabetic vulvitis
   Vestibular adenitis
   Behçet's disease
   Crohn's disease
   Insect Bites

Vulvar dystrophies
   Hyperplastic dystrophy
   Lichen sclerosus
   Mixed dystrophy

Benign cysts and tumors
   Cysts—Bartholin's, sebaceous
   Solid tumors—hidradenoma, nevus, fibroma, hemangioma

Dermatoses not unique to the vulva
   Psoriasis
   Acanthosis nigricans

spection. A photograph taken at the initial and subsequent visits can be helpful to follow the natural course of the disease.

Diagnosis

Definitive diagnosis of lower genital tract lesions requires biopsy. In the Navy, there is a saying: "If it doesn't move, paint it." With vulvar and vaginal lesions, a similar statement might be: "If there is a gross lesion, biopsy it." On the vulva, some local anesthesia with 1 per cent xylocaine, preferably with the addition of one in 200,000 epinephrine, is necessary for biopsy. The Keyes cutaneous biopsy punch or a newer disposable punch biopsy instrument can be used. If the patient complains of vulvar pruritus and there is no discrete vulvar lesion and no evidence of vaginitis, Collin's test or colposcopy may aid in localizing the best biopsy site. These tests are discussed in Chapter 56.

Classification

Benign lesions of the vulva do not lend themselves to a completely satisfactory classification. Table 31–1 subdivides them into four categories: (1) inflammatory vulvar dermatoses, (2) vulvar dystrophies, (3) benign cysts and tumors, and (4) dermatoses not unique to the vulva.

Inflammatory Vulvar Dermatoses

Intertrigo. This term refers to an inflammatory eruption in body folds brought about by apposition of moist skin surfaces with consequent chafing. In the genital area, this problem is commonly seen in the genito-crural folds and inner thighs. Predisposing factors are obesity, occlusive clothing, and sweating. The skin may be fiery red with a malodorous oozing from secondary infection with bacteria or with *Candida albicans.* The affected areas are not sharply defined.

Management consists of correcting the secondary invaders, such as the *C. albicans,* with an appropriate imidazole preparation. An antiseptic or antibiotic may be helpful for bacterial infection, and a steroid cream is often efficacious for controlling local itching. It is most important to keep the area dry and to educate the patient regarding basic personal hygiene.

Secondary Irritative Vulvitis. This condition presents as a nonspecific reddened area with itching and burning. A careful history may reveal the use of a specific irritant, such as deodorant spray or synthetic underclothes.

In recent publications, including the Bulletin of the Federal Food and Drug Administration, latex has been elucidated as an allergen. Because this material is so commonly used in contraception, pessaries for pelvic relaxation, and gloves for examination, this factor must be strongly considered when evaluating vulvitis.

Physical examination may reveal redness and marked edema. There may be ulceration or even frank necrosis if the condition has been present long enough. Biopsy of these lesions reveals only evidence of chronic inflammatory dermatitis. At the initial visit, it is important to rule out the presence of a diffuse *Candida* infection, which can mimic secondary irritative vulvitis.

Management consists of having the patient stop using all deodorants, perfumes, scented soaps, colored toilet paper, detergents, and clothing softeners. She should be advised to use loose-fitting cotton underclothing. If the condition is severe, she may be advised to refrain from wearing tight pants, to wash in a shower, and to dry the affected area with a hair dryer rather than a towel. The simplest and most effective dusting powder is cornstarch, which causes no allergic response. Topical use of hydrocortisone 1 per cent for 3 to 4 weeks may be prescribed to help settle the inflammatory response.

Vulvar Papillomatosis (Human Papilloma Viral [HPV] Vulvitis). This entity was described by Growdon and Lebherz in 1985. The condition is a common cause of vulvar burning and dyspareunia. The dyspareunia is an initial burning or pain with intromission, and this burning continues for 24 to 48 hours after intercourse. Most patients have been seen numerous times by other physicians and practitioners, and the condition is usually misdiagnosed as nonspecific vulvitis, chronic yeast infection, or a psychosexual problem. The problem tends to occur in the 16- to 35-year-old age group but has been observed in patients as old as 60. The patient may notice a roughened surface at the introitus.

Examination of the introitus or vestibule of the vulva reveals small papillary growths, which are tear drop and fern frond in appearance and are better seen with a magnifying glass or colposcope. Application of 3 per cent acetic acid solution causes the lesion to be more evident. The lesions are usually found on the lower half of the introitus but may involve the entire introitus, sometimes extending to the urethral meatus and outer third of the urethra.

Diagnosis is confirmed by biopsy. Classically, this condition is described as papillary squamous epithelium with evidence of inflammation, koilocytosis, and hyperplastic dystrophy. Special staining reveals evidence of a viral involvement 25 per cent of the time. Newer techniques of DNA probing have incriminated HPV but not 100 per cent of the time.

Treatment consists of evaluation of the male for a similar lesion (e.g., penitis) and destruction of the papillomas with laser or chemical cautery. We prefer 40 to 60 per cent trichloroacetic acid application, and this is accomplished three to four times at 10- to 14-day intervals.

Hidradenitis Suppurativa. This is a chronic disease that results from blockage and subsequent infection of the apocrine glands, which are present in the hair-bearing areas of the vulva. The cause is unknown, and patients may have the same disorder in their axillae. Once the process begins, it usually progresses slowly until all the hair-bearing areas of the vulva are involved. Initially, the patient presents with itching and burning and a skin abscess that opens and drains. Recurrent abscesses develop that coalesce and are extremely painful and tender. Eventually, the vulva becomes a mass of scar tissue, with chronically draining abscesses and sinus tracts. Biopsy allows definitive diagnosis, differentiating it from the chronic granulomatous vulvar infections.

Treatment consists of sitz baths, incision, drainage, and appropriate systemic and topical antibiotics. The patient should be cautioned not to wear tight-fitting underclothing or jeans. The use of oral contraceptives has been suggested to decrease the glandular secretions. Prolonged use of tetracycline can help prevent recurrent infections. If the disease process persists despite local treatment and prolonged antibiotic prophylaxis, partial or total vulvectomy with or without skin grafting may be necessary.

Fox-Fordyce Disease. This disease occurs almost exclusively in women during reproductive years. It may affect the vulva, axilla, or both. It is a disorder in which the apocrine sweat gland openings become plugged with keratin. Intense itching occurs as apocrine secretions leak through the dilated ducts. The skin changes are subtle, consisting of multiple, tiny, flesh-colored papules without erythema or induration. The intensity of itching correlates inversely with the level of estrogen during the menstrual cycle, and remissions are frequently noted in pregnancy. High estrogen oral contraceptives reduce apocrine activity and may produce sustained remissions. Topical medications for acne and topical estrogens may also be helpful.

Diabetic Vulvitis. Diabetic vulvitis (Fig. 31–1) is initiated by an infection with *C. albicans,* but the distinctive features continue long after the fungus has been eliminated. Diabetics are particularly prone to infection with this organism, so in patients with repeated candidiasis, blood glucose evaluation is indicated.

The symptoms of diabetic vulvitis include chronic pruritus, irritation, burning, dyspareunia, and dysuria. Grossly, the lesion tends

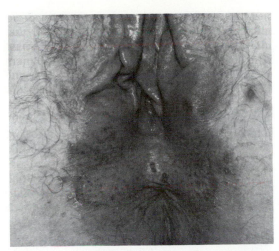

Figure 31–1. Diabetic vulvitis. Note the extensive perineal and perianal involvement.

to be widespread, involving the inner thighs, perianal area, mons pubis, and the rest of the vulvovaginal tissues. Tissue edema is always present, and the involved skin exhibits a typical livid color variously described as intensely red, beefy, or port wine. White patches representing active *Candida* infections may be seen in the vestibule. Diagnosis can be made by cutaneous scrapings, which, in a potassium hydroxide (KOH) suspension, reveal pseudohyphae. For confirmation, the organism may be cultured using Nickerson's or Sabouraud's medium.

Effective treatment requires strict control of the diabetes. Local measures consist of control of *C. albicans* with vaginal and vulvar applications of clotrimazole (Gyne-Lotrimin) or miconazole (Monistat). Cutaneous painting with 1 per cent aqueous gentian violet weekly for 3 weeks is helpful. An oral imidazole preparation helps decrease the gastrointestinal reservoir of organisms, which is a source of reinfection. Patients should be advised to use only cotton under clothing, to launder bed sheets daily, to change underclothing frequently, and to rinse the vulva with saline or tap water after voiding.

Vestibular Adenitis. The minor vestibular glands are mucus-secreting glands with a short duct composed of transitional and squamous epithelium that connects the gland with the vestibular skin. The duct openings are difficult to see. There are usually between 2 and 20 such glands. For reasons that are not clear, these glands may become inflamed.

Clinically, affected patients present with a complaint of introital discomfort and dyspareunia. The discomfort may be described as burning. Gross examination may be unrewarding, but careful study with a magnifying glass or colposcope reveals tiny erythematous foci with mild edema surrounding the gland openings. Frequently, the hymen is constricted, firm, and tender to palpation. Dysuria is often an associated symptom.

Treatment with topical antibiotic or hormone creams is usually disappointing. Laser therapy may be used to destroy the gland-bearing area to a depth of 1 to 2 mm. Alternatively, the involved vestibular tissue may be excised and the defect primarily repaired.

Behçet's Disease. This is a rare condition characterized by oral and genital ulcerations with associated ocular inflammation. The oral lesions appear like aphthous ulcers, whereas the genital lesions are more destructive and result in a scarred, fenestrated vulva. The etiology is unknown, but an autoimmune basis has been postulated. Bacterial and viral smears and cultures are negative, and biopsy is unrewarding. Diagnosis is made on the basis of the concurrence of oral and ocular involvement, the recurrent nature of the disease, and the exclusion of other specific entities, such as syphilis or Crohn's disease. No specific treatment is known. Remissions may occur with high estrogen oral contraceptives.

Crohn's Disease. Although Crohn's disease is considered primarily a disorder of the gastrointestinal tract, vulvar ulcers precede intestinal ulceration in 25 per cent of patients. Typically, the ulcers are slit-like with prominent edema. They have been described as "knife-cut" ulcers. Draining sinuses and fistulas may also occur. Biopsy is helpful but not absolutely diagnostic. Steroid therapy is necessary for advanced cases, and occasionally surgical excision of vulvar lesions is required.

Insect Bites. Two insects in particular are peculiar to the vulva: *Phthirus pubis,* the crab louse, and *Sarcoptes scabiei,* an itch mite. The organisms are usually transmitted through sexual contact, although they may be acquired by infected bedding and toilet seats.

Pruritus, particularly of the mons, is the most common complaint. Generally, the patient has identified the causative organism and presents for prompt treatment. Diagnosis can be suggested by seeing specks of "ground pepper" (excreta) on the skin. Nits or louse eggs may be attached to the hair shafts. A hand-held magnifying glass or colposcope is most helpful in identifying the organism. Closer identification can be made microscopically.

Treatment of both disorders requires at least two applications of the gamma isomer of benzene hexachloride (Kwell). Proper washing and heat drying of clothing and bed sheets is important. With scabies, all family members should be treated at the same time.

Vulvar Dystrophies

A variety of terms have been applied to disorders of vulvar epithelial growth and nutrition that produce a number of nonspecific gross changes. Such terms included leukoplakia, lichen sclerosus et atrophicus, sclerotic dermatosis, atrophic and hyperplastic vulvitis, and kraurosis vulvae. The International Society for the Study of Vulvar Diseases has recommended the classification of vulvar dystrophies shown in Table 31–1. The malignant potential of the vulvar dystrophies is less than 5 per cent, the patient at particular risk being the one with cellular atypia on initial biopsy.

Hyperplastic Dystrophy. This disease is primarily seen in postmenopausal women but may occur during the reproductive years. The most common symptom is pruritus. The surface of the lesion appears thickened and hyperkeratotic, and there may be evidence of scratching. The lesions tend to be discrete but may be symmetrical and multiple. Toluidine blue–directed biopsies are necessary to make the diagnosis and to evaluate the presence of atypia or even malignancy. This lesion is often seen coexisting with vulvar carcinoma, but in patients followed prospectively, malignancy has developed in less than 2 per cent of cases.

Treatment is quite specific, consisting of local applications of a fluorinated corticosteroid ointment three times a day for 6 weeks. Typically, the lesion totally disappears. If a new lesion recurs, it must be managed as a new case with repeat biopsy and an additional 6 weeks of treatment with topical steroids.

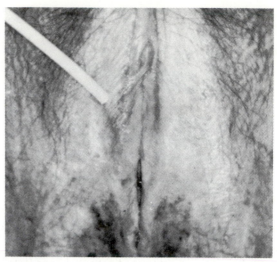

Figure 31–2. Lichen sclerosus. Note the symmetrical distribution of the atrophic changes, the very small labia minora, and flattened labia majora.

Lichen Sclerosus. Lichen sclerosus (Fig. 31–2) is the most common of all white lesions of the vulva. It is characterized by pruritus, dyspareunia, and burning. It may occur at any age but is most common in postmenopausal women. The lesions characteristically present with a diminution of subepithelial fat such that the vulvar architecture is atrophic, with small, even absent, labia minora, thin labia majora, and sometimes phimosis of the prepuce. The epithelium is pale with a shiny, crinkled surface, often with fissures and excoriation. The changes tend to be symmetrical and often coexist with perianal and perineal lesions that produce a butterfly pattern. Definitive diagnosis can be made only by biopsy, preferably directed by toluidine blue staining to detect areas of atypia. Malignancy associated with this lesion is rare but has been reported.

Treatment consists of a 2 per cent testosterone cream. This should be in a petrolatum base and applied twice daily for 3 weeks, then once daily for 3 weeks. A maintenance course of once daily or once every other day is continued, depending on the patient's needs. The patient must be cautioned concerning absorption of testosterone, which will occur and may produce defeminizing or masculinizing side effects. Treatment must be continued indefinitely, since the testosterone allows the patient to live with the disease rather than curing it. Approximately 80 per cent of patients have a satisfactory response. Laser therapy and vulvectomy have been used. Recurrences are common following surgical treatment, however, so close follow-up is necessary.

Mixed Dystrophy. As the name suggests, this lesion consists of hypoplastic and hyperplastic areas. It accounts for about 20 per cent of vulvar dystrophy cases. Atypia occurs somewhat more frequently in this lesion than in pure hyperplastic dystrophies. Symptoms consist of burning, pruritus, and dyspareunia. The lesion appears as areas of piled-up keratinized white epithelium along with patches of pale, thin, shiny, wrinkled epithelium. Diagnosis requires toluidine blue–directed biopsy, and multiple biopsies are necessary to exclude focal areas of atypia. Treatment consists of a fluorinated corticosteroid ointment three times daily for 6 weeks and then 2 per cent testosterone ointment three times daily for 6 weeks. Testosterone ointment should then be continued indefinitely. Areas of severe atypia may best be treated by local excision.

Cysts

Bartholin's Cyst. A Bartholin's cyst is the most common vulvar tumor. It presents as a swelling posterolaterally in the introitus, usually unilaterally. The cyst is usually about 2 cm in diameter but may be up to 8 cm. It contains sterile mucus when punctured, and, except for the enlargement, it is usually asymptomatic. Secondary infection sometimes occurs, producing a Bartholin's abscess. Treatment is by marsupialization of the gland to create a fistulous tract between the cyst or duct wall and the skin.

Sebaceous Cysts. These occur at all ages and are especially common in black women. They present as single or multiple firm, yellowish cysts in the vulvar hair-bearing skin. The contents have the typical odor of sebaceous material. No specific treatment is indicated unless infection occurs or a cyst becomes too large.

Solid Tumors

Hidradenoma. This is an unusual lesion, een mainly in women in their late twenties

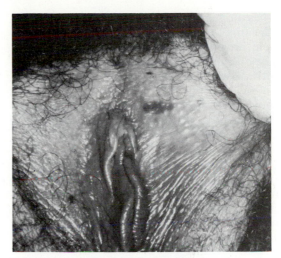

Figure 31–3. Multiple pigmented nevi on the vulva.

and thirties, that originates from the apocrine sweat glands. Hidradenomas are usually solitary and start as a small cyst-like lesion on a labium or interlabial sulcus. Initially, the overlying skin may appear umbilicated, but as the tumor enlarges, the covering epithelium becomes necrotic, leaving a central area of ulceration. Diagnosis and treatment are accomplished by excisional biopsy, which can usually be done in the office. The hidradenoma is never malignant, although histologically the papillary nature of the tumor may initially suggest an adenocarcinoma.

Nevus. Pigmented nevi occur on the vulva as they do elsewhere, but junctional activity, which carries a risk for subsequent malignant transformation, is more common in this location (Fig. 31–3). They may appear in a wide variety of colors. Excisional biopsy should be performed on all pigmented lesions on the vulva so that tissue can be sent for pathologic evaluation. These lesions should never be treated by cryosurgery or laser therapy.

Fibroma. Fibromas of the vulva are uncommon and when present are usually fibromyomas or fibrolipomas. They occasionally grow to a huge size. Neurofibromas may develop on the vulva as a manifestation of von Recklinghausen's disease. These lesions should be surgically removed if they cause a problem to the patient.

Hemangioma. The vulva may be the site of congenital hemangiomas. In the adult, three types of hemangiomata occur on the vulva. The small cherry angiomata are usually multiple and are less than 2 to 3 mm in size. They begin to appear during the fourth or fifth decade and are generally asymptomatic, unless bleeding occurs with trauma. As a rule, no treatment is required. Angiokeratomas measure about 5 mm in diameter and are also frequently multiple. Pyogenic granulomas usually arise on the labia during pregnancy. They are the largest of the adult vulvar hemangiomas, and although some regression may occur postpartum, wide excision is usually necessary to prevent recurrence.

Dermatoses Not Unique to the Vulva

Psoriasis. Psoriasis often involves the genital area. It is usually evident on the outer aspects of the labia majora and the genitocrural area but can involve the entire vulva. Frequently, there is evidence of psoriasis elsewhere. The silver scaling associated with psoriasis in other areas is rarely present in the sheltered genitocrural area, so clinical diagnosis may be difficult. Biopsy of the lesion allows definitive diagnosis, since the histologic picture is characteristic.

Treatment initially with a fluorinated corticosteroid is usually justified, and the initial response may be satisfactory. Chronic persistence and recurrence are common, however. Usually this problem is referred to a dermatologist.

Acanthosis Nigricans. This is a rare dermatologic problem that commonly involves skin folds, such as the axillae and genitocrural areas. Three variants of the disease have been described:

1. A "malignant" variety, itself a benign condition, which accompanies an internal adenocarcinoma, most commonly of the gastrointestinal tract. It spontaneously regresses with successful treatment of the bowel cancer.

2. A "benign" variety that may occur at birth, but that occurs more often in early childhood and, occasionally, in adulthood. After puberty, the lesion usually regresses.

3. Pseudoacanthosis nigricans, which develops most often in darkly pigmented persons and is invariably accompanied by marked obesity. The lesion usually disappears as the patient loses weight.

No specific treatment is available. When the malignant variety is present, a search must be made for an underlying adenocarcinoma.

VAGINA

Inclusion Cysts

These are common lesions that result from an infolding of vaginal epithelium. They are usually associated with lacerations from childbirth or surgery, particularly episiotomy. The cysts are usually asymptomatic and need not be removed.

Endometriosis

Endometriosis may occur in the upper one third of the vagina. It presents as cysts, often steel gray or black, that may bleed slightly at the time of the menses. These lesions are most common in the posterior fornix, where they usually represent an extension of endometriosis from the cul-de-sac peritoneum into the rectovaginal septum. Endometriotic cysts are usually 3 to 10 mm in size and, if punctured, are found to contain a thick, dark chocolate material. Diagnosis is made by biopsy. The lesions can be excised. If other endometriosis exists, it should be treated appropriately (see Chapter 34).

Gartner's Duct Cysts

These are usually benign cysts resulting from remnants of the wolffian duct. Rarely, a primary carcinoma of a Gartner's duct cyst can occur. These cysts may develop anywhere from the top of the broad ligament down to the middle one third of the vagina and are usually situated laterally. The cysts usually produce no symptoms and are diagnosed on routine pelvic examination. Unless the cyst is symptomatic, it should not be removed. Transvaginal excision may be necessary for large, symptomatic cysts.

Urethral Diverticulum

Urethral diverticuli are small sacs that can be palpated adjacent to the urethra. They arise from obstructed, infected periurethral glands that discharge into the urethra. The abscess lining becomes epithelialized, with the ultimate formation of a diverticulum. Diagnosis can usually be made by visualizing the opening into the urethral floor on urethroscopy; however, sometimes the openings are so small they can be missed. A pressure urethrogram is the ideal method of confirming the diagnosis. Urethral diverticuli can cause recurrent urethral infection, dribbling of urine, dyspareunia, and dysuria. Surgical correction is required if they are symptomatic.

CERVIX

Columnar Eversion

Columnar eversion is the most commonly seen lesion on the cervix (Fig. 31–4). Also erroneously called an "erosion," it represents a protrusion of the endocervical glandular tissue and is a physiologic process, not a disease. It is seen at birth, in patients on the oral contraceptive pill, and during pregnancy. In each of these situations, it is associated with hormonal changes that cause hypertrophy and hyperplasia of the endocervical glands. Because of lack of space in the endocervical canal, the glands must protrude beyond the external os. Columnar eversion may be associated with an increase in nonirritating vaginal discharge (leukorrhea). The diagnosis can be confirmed with colposcopy, and usually no treatment is required. Cessation of pregnancy or discontinuation of the pill is followed by gradual columnar inversion. Any remaining eversion will become covered with squamous epithelium through the process of squamous metaplasia.

Nonspecific Chronic Cervicitis

Nonspecific chronic cervicitis is a common problem. The numerous endocervical glands make the cervix prone to persistent infec-

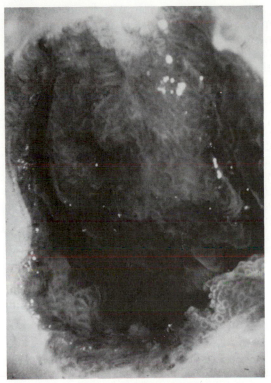

Figure 31–4. Columnar eversion. Note the transverse external os with columnar epithelium extending onto the ectocervix, particularly anteriorly.

tions, and puerperal lacerations are often a contributing factor in the pathogenesis of the condition. The infection may be caused by any of the organisms found in the vagina, especially staphylococci and streptococci. Chlamydial organisms may also be involved.

Clinically, the most prominent symptom is leukorrhea, which may be whitish or mucopurulent. Lower abdominal discomfort and dyspareunia may also occur. Speculum examination may reveal a chronically infected columnar eversion, and retention cysts of the cervical glands (nabothian follicles) may be present. If the usual causes of vaginitis have been ruled out—that is, *Gardnerella vaginalis, Trichomonas hominis,* or *C. albicans* —further culture or monoclonal immunofluorescent stains for *Chlamydia* should be considered. In all cases, a Papanicolaou smear should be performed, and, if the endocervix is red or ulcerated, colposcopy, with or without biopsy, is necessary to exclude malignancy.

If *Chlamydia* is found, appropriate treatment with tetracycline, erythromycin, or trimethoprim should be used. If no specific cause is found, treatment with cryosurgery or electrocautery can be carried out if the symptoms are troublesome.

Cervical Polyp

The cervical polyp is a localized proliferation of cervical mucosa that presents as a soft, red, friable, usually pedunculated lesion. It may occasionally be sessile. It is generally only a few millimeters in diameter but may reach several centimeters. The vascularity, ulceration, and secondary infection explain the bleeding produced by these small lesions. Although the incidence of malignancy is very low, both squamous and adenocarcinoma can develop in these polyps.

Treatment consists of removal in the office, usually by twisting the polyp off and curetting the base. All tissue must be sent for pathologic examination.

SUGGESTED READING

American College of Obstetricians and Gynecologists: Vulvar Dystrophies. ACOG Technical Bulletin No. 139. Washington, DC, January 1990.

Friedrich EG Jr: Vulvar dystrophy. Clin Obstet Gynecol 28:178, 1985.

Goetsch MF: Vulvar vestibulitis: Prevalence and historic features in a general gynecologic practice population. J Obstet Gynecol 164:1609, 1991.

James DG: Silk route disease (Behçet's disease). West J Med 148:433, 1988.

Lewis SH, Richard RM: Recognizing vulvar nonneoplastic epithelial disorders. Contemp Obstet Gynecol 33:13, 1989.

Thomas MRH, Ridley CM, McGibbon DH, et al: Lichen sclerosus et atrophicus and autoimmunity: A study of 350 women. Br J Derm 118:41, 1988.

Woodruff JD, Friedrich EG Jr: The vestibule. Clin Obstet Gynecol 28:134, 1985.

Thirty-two

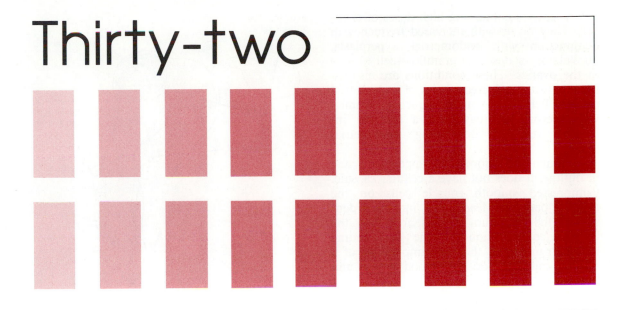

Benign Diseases of the Uterus

J. GEORGE MOORE

Benign diseases of the uterus are commonly encountered in gynecologic practice. In this chapter, uterine leiomyomas, endometrial hyperplasia, and endometrial polyps are discussed.

UTERINE LEIOMYOMA

Uterine leiomyomas ("fibroids") are smooth muscle tumors of the uterus. Twenty per cent of women develop uterine fibroids by 40 years of age, and they constitute the most common indication for major surgery in women. They cause serious complications of pregnancy, confuse the management of the menopause, and mask the diagnosis of more serious gynecologic neoplasms. Fibroids have the potential to grow to an enormous size. Their malignant potential is minimal, and the overwhelming majority cause no symp-toms and require no treatment other than careful observation.

Pathogenesis

The etiology of uterine leiomyomas remains unclear. Most likely, they develop from uterine smooth muscle cells, although they may be derived from connective tissue cells by a process of metaplasia or from smooth muscle cells of uterine arteries. There is an increased incidence and an increased rate of growth in black women.

Uterine leiomyomas are distinctly estrogen dependent. They rarely develop before the menarche and seldom develop or enlarge past the menopause unless stimulated by exogenous estrogens. The neoplasms enlarge with alarming speed and may attain a huge size during pregnancy or when exposed to oral contraceptives containing high doses of estrogen. They occur with increased frequency in conjunction with endometrial hyperplasia, anovulatory states, and granulosa-cell tumors of the ovaries. These conditions are also associated with an increased risk of endometrial cancer. Perhaps as a consequence, women with uterine myomas have a fourfold increased risk of developing endometrial cancer.

Although the leiomyoma appears discrete in outline, it does not have a cellular capsule. Compressed smooth muscle cells on the tumor's periphery lead to an increased density of the reticulum in this area, and the layered configuration of the surrounding myometrium gives the false impression of a cellular capsule. Very few blood vessels and lymphatics traverse the pseudocapsule, leading to degenerative changes as the tumors enlarge. The most commonly observed degenerative change is that of hyaline acellularity, in which the fibrous and muscle tissues are replaced with hyaline tissue. If the hyaline tissue breaks down from a further reduction in blood supply, cystic degeneration may occur. Calcification may occur in degenerated fibroids, particularly after the menopause, and is responsible for the term *womb stones.* Fatty degeneration may also occur but is rare. During pregnancy, about half of all fibroids undergo red or carneous degeneration caused by hemorrhage into the tumor. Sarcomatous degeneration occurs in less than one per 1000 fibroids.

Classification

Leiomyomas may occupy various positions in the uterine corpus and are generally described as submucous, intramural, and subserous (Fig. 32–1). They can also occur in the cervix, between the leaves of the broad ligament (intraligamentous), and in the various supporting ligaments of the uterus. As these neoplasms develop, most are intramural (Fig. 32–2); they may grow toward the endometrial cavity, however, to occupy a submucous position or grow toward the serous surface of the uterus and become subserous myomas. They may migrate further, eventually protruding through the endometrium or the serosa and becoming pedunculated. Occasionally, they become attached to the omentum or the bowel mesentery and lose their connection with the serosal surface of the uterus, develop an omental or mesenteric blood supply, and thus become parasitic myomas. Some submucous leiomyomas become pedunculated in the endometrial cavity, project through the cervix, and present as a leiomyomatous polyp, usually with an associated endometritis.

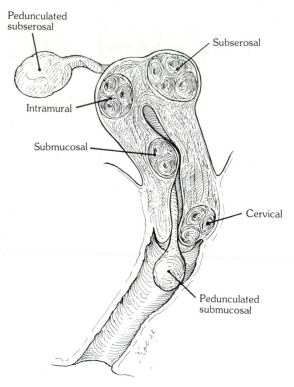

Figure 32–1. Uterine leiomyomata in various anatomic locations, as noted in the text.

Symptoms

The majority of uterine leiomyomas are asymptomatic. Occasionally, the patient may become aware of a lower abdominal mass if it protrudes above the symphysis pubis. Quite often the development of discomfort comes on insidiously, and the symptoms are difficult for a patient to define. She may complain of pelvic pressure, congestion, bloating, or a feeling of heaviness in the lower abdomen. She may note frequency of urination or

Figure 32–2. Multiple leiomyomata uteri. Note that the right ovarian ligament (A) extends from the posterior aspect of the uterine corpus. Clamps are on the uterine arteries and the cervix is parous.

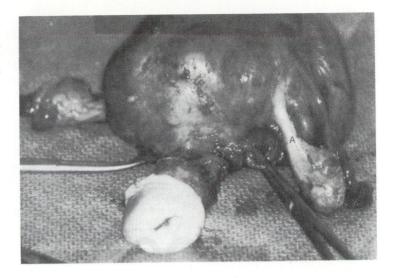

even urinary retention and hydronephrosis as the bladder and tumor compete for space within the pelvis.

Menorrhagia may be associated with intramural tumors and metrorrhagia may be associated with submucous myomas ulcerating through the endometrial lining. Blood loss occurring over a long period of time may result in anemia, weakness, dypsnea, and even congestive heart failure. The menorrhagia is related to the enlargement of the endometrial cavity and the greater surface area of endometrium, which will slough at the time of menstruation. Also, the presence of large leiomyomas brings about a greater blood supply to the uterus, and the process of menstruation therewith becomes more hemorrhagic.

Pain is generally not a feature, but severe pain associated with red degeneration within a fibroid (acute infarction) is not uncommon during pregnancy. Also, pressure pains may occur in the lower abdomen and pelvis if a myomatous uterus becomes incarcerated within the pelvis. Dyspareunia is also common in this situation. There is a substantially increased incidence of secondary dysmenorrhea in women with uterine myomas.

Although many women with uterine myomas become pregnant and carry their pregnancies to term, these lesions are associated with an increased incidence of infertility. A submucous leiomyoma may interfere with the implantation of the blastocyst or bring about an early abortion. Large leiomyomas may interfere with the growth of the developing fetus, resulting in intrauterine growth retardation. Tumors occurring in the lower uterine segment may cause dystocia and necessitate delivery by cesarean section. Low-lying uterine myomas, however, usually soften remarkably and rise from the pelvis as the lower uterine segment elongates during the course of labor, allowing the presenting part to enter the pelvis.

Signs

Very large fibroids can be palpated abdominally. Those smaller than a 12- to 14-week gestation are usually confined to the pelvis. The bladder should be emptied before examination to avoid the confusion of urinary retention. Bimanual vaginal examination reveals a firm, irregularly enlarged uterus with smoothly rounded or bosselated protrusions from the uterine wall. The tumors are almost always nontender. Their consistency may vary from rock hard, as in the case of a calcified postmenopausal leiomyoma, to soft or even cystic, as in the case of cystic degeneration of the tumor. Generally, the myomatous masses are in the midline and follow the contour of the uterus. Sometimes a large portion of the tumor lies in the lateral aspect of the pelvis and may be indistinguishable from an adnexal mass. Often the presence of a leiomyoma precludes a proper evaluation of the adnexae. If the mass moves with the cervix, it is suggestive of a leiomyoma.

Multiple large leiomyomas may enlarge the uterus to a size greater than that of a term pregnancy. Such large tumors contain huge reservoirs of blood, which may lead to cardiovascular instability during changes of body position or at the time of operation. Bruits similar to the uterine souffle of pregnancy may be heard and felt over these large masses.

Differential Diagnosis

The most common differential diagnoses are an ovarian neoplasm, a tubo-ovarian inflammatory mass, or a diverticular inflammatory mass. A complete blood count, urinalysis, sedimentation rate, and stool guaiac test may be helpful in this differential diagnosis. A barium enema can exclude diverticular disease. An intravenous pyelogram or computed tomographic scan may exclude the rare pelvic kidney or a retroperitoneal tumor, the latter being suggested by medial displacement of the ureter. A flat film of the abdomen and pelvis or pelvic ultrasonography may reveal characteristic calcification or other patterns suggestive of a leiomyoma. Ultrasonography will delineate the lesions and identify normal ovaries apart from the leiomyomata, thus aiding in the differential diagnosis if there is any uncertainty (Fig. 32–3).

It is occasionally impossible to distinguish between a moderate-sized asymptomatic uterine leiomyoma occupying a lateral pelvic position and a solid ovarian tumor. Often the innocent leiomyoma can be identified at laparoscopy, and laparotomy can be avoided.

In women beyond the age of 35, carcinoma of the endometrium and uterine myomas may coexist and cause abnormal bleeding. In such patients, a fractional curettage is an essential part of the diagnostic work-up.

Treatment

The recommended management for most uterine leiomyomas is prudent observation. If treatment is indicated and future reproductive capability is desired, myomectomy may be performed by either operative hysteroscopy (if the myoma is small and in a submucous position) or laparotomy. Hysterectomy is indicated in a symptomatic patient if reproductive capability is not important to the patient. Occasionally, uterine curettage will control menometrorrhagia. The GnRH agonists have been effectively used to reduce the size of myomata, to enhance fertility, and to reduce blood loss during surgery. The main indications for definitive treatment of a uterine leiomyoma are listed in Table 32–1.

Surgical Treatment

Probably the most common indication for surgical intervention is abnormal uterine bleeding, and it is mandatory that a fractional dilatation and curettage (D & C) be performed initially to rule out endometrial carcinoma. Even when submucous leiomyomata are detected at the time of endometrial curettage, the patient may have no further abnormal uterine bleeding. If the D & C is effective and if the adnexae can be evaluated sufficiently, the patient can avoid major surgery.

In dealing with moderate sized uterine myomas that are only mildly symptomatic, a relatively young woman is more likely to require surgical treatment (beyond a D & C) than a perimenopausal woman. In the latter case, the menopause may soon bring about an abatement of symptoms and shrinkage of the myomatous uterus, whereas the uterine myomas of the young woman will probably continue to grow with the estrogen stimulation of normal ovarian function. If the patient is close to the menopause and represents a very poor surgical risk, irradiation castration may be considered, reluctantly, as definitive therapy if disabling bleeding recurs following a D & C.

Pain may be the single indication for definitive treatment of uterine leiomyomas. Pelvic pain or pressure, low back pain, dyspareunia, secondary dysmenorrhea, or the discomfort associated with a pedunculated leiomyoma coming through the cervical os are all legitimate indications for myomectomy or, in most cases, hysterectomy. In younger women who still desire childbearing, the method of treatment may be a uterine

Figure 32–3. Pelvic sonogram showing uterine myomas pressing against the full urinary bladder.

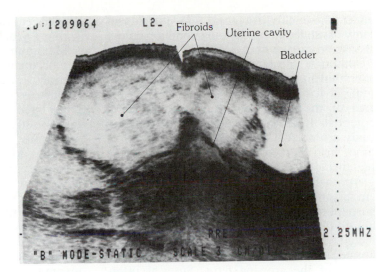

myomectomy, either by the vaginal approach, if it is a pedunculated submucous leiomyoma, or by the abdominal approach, if it is an intramural, subserous, or pedunculated fibroid. There should be a definite reason for myomectomy rather than hysterectomy, since the transabdominal myomectomy is more difficult to manage, results in more blood loss, and has a higher morbidity rate. Also, up to 25 per cent of patients require a subsequent operation because of recurrence following myomectomy.

Inability to evaluate the adnexae is probably the most important indication for surgery in large asymptomatic leiomyomas. There is no greater tragedy than finding advanced ovarian carcinoma in a patient who has been followed over a period of time for uterine fibroids. When the uterus is greater than the size of a 12-week gestation or when it has been displaced out of the pelvis into the abdomen, palpation of the ovaries on bimanual examination is virtually impossible. Although periodic ultrasonography may identify the ovaries, it is generally advisable to elect abdominal hysterectomy if the uterus is larger than the size of a 12-week gestation (three times the normal size).

In a patient 45 years of age or older, both tubes and ovaries are usually resected when a hysterectomy is done for myomas, but this requires adequate discussion with the patient preoperatively. If the patient has a pedunculated submucous leiomyoma projecting through the cervix, a prior vaginal myomectomy is indicated initially to facilitate the hysterectomy and to avoid contamination of the peritoneal cavity with the infected, pedunculated lesion.

Approximately 5 per cent of uterine leiomyomas are characterized by urinary tract abnormalities. Acute or chronic urinary retention, ureteral compression, hydronephrosis, and urgency or frequency of urination are definite indications for surgery. Occasionally, a period of urinary decompression and normalization of blood urea nitrogen levels is necessary prior to surgery.

When not associated with estrogen administration, extremely rapid growth of a uterine myoma during the menstrual years or any growth in a leiomyoma following the menopause represents an important indication for surgery. Although rare, the possibility of a sarcoma developing in a leiomyoma is real

Table 32–1. SURGICAL INTERVENTION IN A PATIENT WITH A UTERINE LEIOMYOMA

Abnormal uterine bleeding causing anemia
Severe pelvic pain or secondary dysmenorrhea
Inability to evaluate the adnexae (usually because fibroid is 12 weeks size)
Urinary tract symptoms (frequency or urinary retention)
Growth of the myoma following menopause
Infertility
Rapid increase in size

under these circumstances, and a hysterectomy and bilateral salpingo-oophorectomy should be carried out.

Although most uterine myomas do not affect fertility, any distortion of the endometrial cavity or compression of the isthmic area of the tube may decrease the fertility potential. If all other features of the fertility study are normal and if a sufficient period of time has elapsed, transabdominal uterine myomectomy for infertility is indicated.

Approximately 10 per cent of women who are pregnant with uterine fibroids must be hospitalized for complications relating to the fibroid during pregnancy. Such complications include early abortion, acute infarction of the fibroid, and interference with the proper nutrition of the growing fetus. Surgical intervention should be avoided during pregnancy, but interval myomectomy or hysterectomy following the pregnancy may be necessary.

Before any surgical procedure, efforts should be made to suppress menorrhagia with progestogens, and oral iron should be administered. If difficult surgery is expected, as in the case of a large cervical myoma, at least 2 units of blood should be secured from the patient over a 4- to 6-week period so that an autologous transfusion of packed red blood cells may be given intraoperatively if necessary.

Medical Management

Over the past decade GnRH agonists have been used largely as an adjunct to surgery in the management of uterine myomas. When used preoperatively for 8 to 12 weeks, they have been shown to relieve pain, decrease the size of the myomas, reduce bleeding, allow time for the correction of anemia, and reduce intraoperative blood loss at hysterectomy and especially myomectomy. The reduction in tumor and uterine size may be sufficient to allow the hysterectomy to be done vaginally rather than abdominally. GnRH analogues include naferelin acetate, which is given by nasal spray, 200 μg twice daily, and Depot Lupron, which is given intramuscularly, 7.5 mg every 28 days.

Several reports have demonstrated the usefulness of GnRH agonists in infertility patients with relatively small myomas. After a course of GnRH agonist therapy, as many as 48 per cent of such patients become pregnant within a year of cessation of treatment.

Maximum reduction in tumor size generally occurs within 12 weeks of GnRH agonist therapy. The effect is temporary and the tumors as well as their blood supply tend to grow back following the cessation of treatment, although the control of untoward symptoms can persist for as long as 6 months. Medical therapy for symptomatic myomas can be used in patients close to the menopause to avoid surgical management until the menopause allows a permanent reduction in tumor size.

Following therapy with GnRH analogs, pathologists have noted problems in interpreting the apparent increase in cellularity of the myoma. The therapy apparently does not decrease the number of cells in the tumor, but they are compressed into a smaller volume.

HYPERPLASIA OF THE ENDOMETRIUM

Endometrial hyperplasia represents an overabundant growth of the endometrium, generally caused by persistently high levels of estrogens, unopposed by progesterone. Endometrial hyperplasia is prone to develop in the years immediately following the menarche and in the years immediately prior to the menopause — periods when ovulation may be infrequent. It also commonly occurs in association with polycystic sclerotic ovaries and estrogen-producing tumors, such as granulosa-theca cell tumors. Endometrial hyperplasia is also associated with obesity because of the peripheral conversion of androstenedione to estrone in peripheral tissues, especially in postmenopausal women.

Histologic Variants

Cystic Glandular Hyperplasia. The simplest form of endometrial hyperplasia is cystic glandular hyperplasia, which microscopically is referred to as the "Swiss cheese" pattern (Fig. 32–4). Both the epithelial cells lining the glands and the stromal cells participate in the hyperplastic growth, and there

Figure 32–4. Cystic hyperplasia of the endometrium showing dilated cystic glands lined by tall columnar cells and active endometrial stromal proliferation.

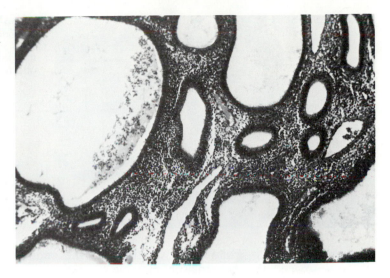

are abundant mitotic figures. Cystic glandular hyperplasia may be an early precursor of endometrial cancer. Cystic hyperplasia of the endometrium may be confused with cystic involution of the endometrium, which normally occurs postmenopausally and is not a hyperplastic condition. A variety of microscopic pictures can be seen with cystic hyperplasia, and the hyperplastic areas may be seen only focally. Both secretory and proliferative endometrial patterns are found in endometrial hyperplasia.

Adenomatous Hyperplasia. Adenomatous hyperplasia of the endometrium represents a hyperplastic condition in which the glands are not cystic and the stroma does not necessarily participate in the hyperplastic reaction. This condition represents an active proliferation of the glandular epithelium so that the glands are often crowded in a back to back manner with no intervening stroma (Fig. 32–5). Adenomatous endometrial hyperplasia represents the next step in the transition toward endometrial cancer, and the two diseases may coexist. When the cellular growth lining the endometrial glands becomes atypical with piling up of the epithelial cells and cellular atypia, the condition is referred to as adenomatous hyperplasia with cytologic atypia. This process may eventually progress to carcinoma in situ. The more cellular proliferation and cytologic atypia there is in the adenomatous areas, the greater is the chance of endometrial cancer developing. It is estimated that at least 20 per cent of patients with adenomatous hyperplasia eventually develop endometrial cancer.

Diagnosis

Generally, the diagnosis of endometrial hyperplasia is suspected on the basis of either postmenopausal bleeding or the prolongation or irregularity of menstrual bleeding. Frequently, clots are passed, and the blood loss is sufficient to cause anemia. In the initial stages of estrogen stimulation, there may be a period of amenorrhea, during which endometrial growth takes place, that is eventually followed by prolonged bleeding. Occasionally, the uterus is enlarged, both by the mass of endometrium and also by the growth of the myometrium in response to persistent estrogen stimulation. The diagnosis can be made by endometrial biopsy, but except in a woman under 30 years of age, D & C is usually necessary to exclude endometrial carcinoma.

Treatment

The treatment of endometrial hyperplasia depends on the age of the patient and the histologic variety of the lesion. In a young woman with simple cystic hyperplasia, effective treatment involves the use of progestogens on a cyclic basis—usually medroxyprogesterone acetate (Provera), 10 mg daily for

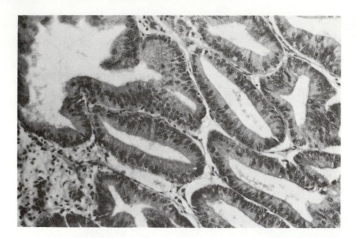

Figure 32–5. Adenomatous hyperplasia of the endometrium showing crowded glands with scanty interglandular stroma. Note the tall columnar cells lining the glands and focal multilayering.

10 days each month. Following cessation of the progestogen, the hyperplastic endometrium is shed. Occasionally, it may be necessary to add estrogens to the cyclic progestogen therapy to prevent "breakthrough" bleeding. A more convenient approach to treatment is to put the patient on oral contraceptives. If the bleeding is very heavy or if the progestogen is unsuccessful, it may be necessary to carry out a D & C for therapeutic purposes.

If cystic hyperplasia is found at D & C in an older woman, no further treatment may be necessary. If the bleeding recurs, however, cyclic progestogens or even hysterectomy may be in order.

If adenomatous hyperplasia is found at any age, especially if there is cellular atypia, there are two alternatives. One is to administer cyclic progestogens for a period of 3 or 6 months and then resample the endometrium. The other alternative is to perform a hysterectomy, probably vaginal, to preclude the later development of an endometrial cancer. The older the patient and the more atypical the adenomatous hyperplasia, the more likely is the subsequent development of endometrial cancer. The constitutional factors that increase the risk for endometrial cancer should also be taken into consideration in deciding whether to perform hysterectomy. The nulliparous, obese, diabetic woman in her fifties is at greatest risk, so early hysterectomy may be indicated in such cases.

ENDOMETRIAL POLYPS

Endometrial polyps represent a gross clinical diagnosis. A polyp arising in the area of the endometrium may take the form of a myoma, a carcinoma, a carcinosarcoma, or merely a polypoid endometrial hyperplasia. Hysteroscopy affords an accurate gross diagnosis, but the pathologic diagnosis can be made only on histologic examination.

Approximately 5 per cent of endometrial polyps are associated with malignancy, mostly in postmenopausal women. Most endometrial polyps are made up of benign endometrial tissue and a fair number are asymptomatic. Most, however, are associated with abnormal bleeding (particularly intermenstrual or postmenopausal bleeding), especially if they are large enough to protrude through the cervical os. Both the diagnosis and the treatment should take the form of a fractional D & C with the use of endometrial polyp forceps. Endometrial polyps may be missed at D & C not done in association with hysteroscopy.

SUGGESTED READING

Babaknia A, Rock JA, Jones HW Jr: Pregnancy success following abdominal myomectomy for infertility. Fertil Steril 30:644, 1978.

Baggish MS, Sze EHM, Morgan G: Hysteroscopic treatment of submucosal myomata uteri. J Gynecol Surg 5:27, 1989.

Conn PM, Crowley WF: GnRH and its analogues. N Engl J Med 324:95 1991.

Friedman AJ, Rein MD, Harrison-Atlas D, et al: Leuprolide acetate depot treatment before myomectomy. Fertil Steril 52:728, 1989.

Katz VL, Dotters DJ, Droegemueller W: Complications of uterine leiomyomas in pregnancy. Obstet Gynecol 73:593, 1989.

Kurman RJ, Kaminski RP, Norris HJ: The behavior of endometrial hyperplasia. A long term study of "untreated" patients. Cancer 56:403, 1985.

Huang SJ, Amparo EG, Fu YS: Endometrial hyperplasia: Classification and behavior. Surg Pathol 1:215, 1988.

Lumsden MA, West CP, Hawkins RA, et al: The binding of steroids to myometrium and leiomyomata (fibroids) in women treated with the gonadotropin releasing hormone agonist Zoladex (ICI 118630). J Endocrinol 12:389, 1989.

Maheux R: Treatment of uterine leiomyomata: Past, present and future. Horm Res 32:(suppl 1):125, 1989.

Mattingly RF, Thompson JD (eds): Te Linde's Operative Gynecology. Philadelphia, JB Lippincott, 1985.

Norris HJ, Tavassoli FA, Kurman RJ: Endometrial hyperplasia and carcinoma. Diagnostic considerations. Am J Surg Pathol 7:839, 1983.

Pettersson B, Adami HD, Lindren, A et al: Endometrial polyps and hyperplasia as risk factors for endometrial carcinoma. Acta Obstet Gynecol Scand 64:653, 1985.

Williams IA, Shaw RW: Effect of Naferelin on uterine fibroids. Eur J Obstet Gynecol Reprod Biol 34:111, 1990.

Thirty-three

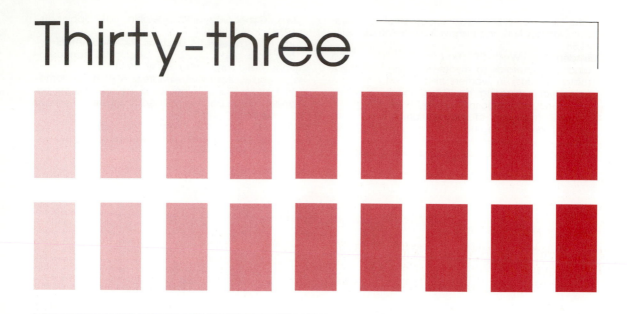

Benign Tumors of the Ovaries and Fallopian Tubes

J. GEORGE MOORE

The human ovary has a striking propensity to develop a wide variety of tumors, the majority of which are benign. Indeed, most ovarian tumors are non-neoplastic. As indicated in Table 33–1, ovarian tumors may be functional, inflammatory, metaplastic, or neoplastic. During the menstruating years, 70 per cent of noninflammatory ovarian tumors are functional. The remainder are neoplastic (20 per cent) or endometriomas (10 per cent).

Ovarian neoplasms have a higher malignancy rate than other pelvic tumors, the overall incidence being about 15 per cent. After the menopause, about half of all ovarian tumors are malignant, whereas during infancy and childhood, 10 per cent are malignant. Malignant ovarian tumors are discussed in Chapter 55. The management of ovarian tumors, whether functional, benign,

or malignant, involves difficult decisions that may affect a woman's hormonal status and fertility. Only functional and benign neoplastic tumors are considered in this chapter.

FUNCTIONAL OVARIAN TUMORS

Pathogenesis

If the ovarian follicle fails to rupture in the course of follicular development and ovulation, a follicular cyst lined by one or more layers of granulosa cells may develop. Similarly, a lutein cyst may develop if the corpus luteum becomes cystic or hemorrhagic (hemorrhagic corpus luteum) and fails to regress normally after 14 days.

356

Table 33–1. DIFFERENTIAL DIAGNOSIS OF OVARIAN TUMORS

PATHOGENESIS	SPECIFIC TYPE
Functional	Follicular cysts Lutein cysts Polycystic sclerotic ovaries
Inflammatory	Neisserian salpingo-oophoritis Pyogenic oophoritis—puerperal, abortal, or IUD-related Granulomatous oophoritis
Metaplastic	Endometriosis
Neoplastic	Premenarchal years—10% are malignant Menstruating years—15% are malignant Postmenopausal years—50% are malignant

Other specific types of lutein cysts may occur with abnormally high serum levels of human chorionic gonadotropin (hCG). Theca-lutein cysts may develop in association with the high levels of hCG present in patients with a hydatidiform mole or choriocarcinoma. Patients undergoing ovulation induction with gonadotropins or clomiphene may also develop theca-lutein cysts. These cysts are usually bilateral, may become quite large (10 to 15 cm), and characteristically regress as the gonadotropin level falls.

A luteoma of pregnancy takes the form of extensive luteinization of ovarian theca cells, purportedly from prolonged chorionic gonadotropin stimulation during pregnancy. They may be associated with multiple pregnancy or hydramnios, and they cause maternal virilization as well as abnormal genitalia in the female fetus. Although ovarian enlargement may be impressive, surgical resection is not indicated, and regression takes place postpartum.

Polycystic ovarian syndrome, a functional disorder generally associated with oligomenorrhea, anovulation, and elevated testosterone levels, is considered in Chapters 48 and 49.

Clinical Features

An ovarian follicular cyst is usually asymptomatic, unilocular ("simple"), and seldom more than 6 to 8 cm in diameter. It generally regresses during the subsequent menstrual cycle. Generally, a lutein cyst is larger than a follicular cyst, is apt to be more firm or even solid in consistency, and is more likely to cause pain or signs of peritoneal irritation. It is also more likely to cause delay in the upcoming period and some alteration of the next menstrual cycle. Occasionally, a functional ovarian cyst can twist on its pedicle and become infarcted, causing pain, tenderness, and rebound tenderness as well as a moderate leukocytosis. Rupture of a functional cyst may produce acute lower abdominal pain and tenderness, and, occasionally, a significant hemoperitoneum may occur.

Diagnosis

The presumptive diagnosis of a functional ovarian tumor is usually made when a 4- to 8-cm cystic adnexal mass is noted on bimanual examination; it is confirmed when the lesion regresses following the next menstrual period. Generally, the cyst is mobile, unilateral, and not associated with ascites. On rare occasions, the mass may exceed 8 cm and be quite tender to palpation. Occasionally, hemorrhagic lutein cysts may have a solid rather than a cystic consistency. A pelvic ultrasound study will confirm the cystic nature of the mass but cannot differentiate between a functional or neoplastic lesion. If the patient has delayed menses, abnormal uterine bleeding, or twisting of the cyst on its pedicle with infarction, the differential diagnosis must include ectopic pregnancy, salpingo-oophoritis, or torsion of a neoplastic cyst. Benign cystic teratomas not uncommonly twist and infarct. In these instances, a pregnancy test, erythro-

Table 33–2. MANAGEMENT OF A CYSTIC ADNEXAL MASS

AGE	SIZE OF CYST	MANAGEMENT
Premenarchal	>2 cm	Exploratory laparotomy
Reproductive age	<6 cm	Observe for 6 wk
	6–8 cm	Observe if unilocular; explore if multilocular or solid on ultrasonography
	>8 cm	Exploratory laparotomy
Postmenopausal	Palpable	Exploratory laparotomy

cyte sedimentation rate, and ultrasonic evaluation are generally helpful.

Management

If the patient is in her reproductive years and the adnexal cyst is less than 6 cm in diameter, it is appropriate to wait and examine the patient again after her next menses, perhaps with the prescription of an oral contraceptive to suppress gonadotropin levels (Table 33–2). If the cystic mass is between 6 and 8 cm, or if it is fixed or feels solid, a pelvic ultrasound study may be obtained to ensure that it is unilocular. If the mass is painful, multilocular, or partially solid, surgical exploration is in order. When the patient is in her forties, the chances of an ovarian neoplasm are increased, and observational delays must be undertaken with caution.

If the lesion does not fulfill the requirements for observation, surgical exploration may be indicated. Laparoscopy is generally not helpful in differentiating between a functional and a neoplastic ovarian cyst but aspiration of a unilocular cyst and cytologic examination of the fluid may be in order. A laparotomy may be necessary to allow resection of the cyst from the ovary (ovarian cystectomy) so that it can be examined histologically. There has been a tendency for some gynecologists to perform laparoscopic resection of apparently benign ovarian tumors. With this approach, there is some potential for tumor dissemination and treatment delay if the tumor ultimately proves to be malignant, and this practice should be discouraged.

Table 33–3 demonstrates the outcome of a fairly large series of patients with a cystic adnexal mass in their reproductive years who were started on gonadotropin suppression at the time of diagnosis then followed for 6 weeks. Spontaneous regression (confirming the functional nature of the cyst) occurred in approximately 70 per cent of patients, 16 per cent had neoplastic ovarian cysts, and 10 per cent had endometriosis. Nine per cent of the neoplastic cysts (1.4 per cent of the total series) were malignant.

NEOPLASTIC OVARIAN TUMORS

Ovarian neoplasms, as noted in Table 55–3, may be divided by cell type of origin into three main groups: epithelial, stromal, and germ-cell. Taken as a group, the epithelial tumors are by far the most common type, although the single most common benign ovarian neoplasm is the benign cystic teratoma (dermoid cyst), a germ-cell tumor. Mixed tumors, as the name implies, are derived from more than one ovarian cell type. The distribution of the various types of ovarian neoplasms surgically removed in a large metropolitan area is shown in Table 33–4.

Epithelial Ovarian Neoplasms

These tumors are believed to be derived from the mesothelial cells lining the peritoneal cavity; similar tumors occasionally arise from the mesothelium lining the pleural cavity. Since all müllerian structures are derived from the special mesothelium of the gonadal ridge and ultimately differentiate into several different histologic tissues (cervical epithe-

Table 33-3. ADNEXAL CYSTS OBSERVED FOR 6 WEEKS IN 286 PATIENTS AGED 16 TO 48 YEARS*

TYPE OF CYST	NUMBER OF PATIENTS	PERCENTAGE
Regressed under observation	205	72
Required exploratory laparotomy	81	28
Ovarian neoplasms	46	16
Benign epithelial	32	
Benign teratoma	9	
Malignant epithelial	4	
Dysgerminoma	1	
Endometriosis	28	10
Paraovarian cyst	4	1.4
Hydrosalpinx	3	1
Functional cysts	0	0

*Adapted from Spanos WJ: Preoperative hormonal therapy of cystic adnexal masses. Am J Obstet Gynecol 116:551, 1973.

lium, endometrium, ciliated endosalpinx as well as the serous ovarian surface), it is reasonable to postulate that the ovarian mesothelial cells retain the capability to change by metaplasia into any of these müllerian types of epithelium. Thus, the mucinous ovarian neoplasm cytologically resembles the endocervical epithelium (Fig. 33–1*A*), the endometrioid ovarian neoplasm resembles the endometrium, and, occasionally, ovarian tumors are made up of what appears to be ciliated endosalpingial tissue. The most common ovarian tumors retain their serous cell type and are termed *serous cystadenomas* (Fig. 33–1*B*).

Each of the epithelial (more accurately, mesothelial) ovarian neoplasms has characteristic clinical and histologic features. The

Table 33-4. INCIDENCE OF PRIMARY OVARIAN NEOPLASMS IN THE DENVER METROPOLITAN AREA*

TYPE OF OVARIAN NEOPLASMA	NUMBER	PERCENTAGE
Benign cystic teratoma	103	26.5
Serous cystadenoma/cystadenofibroma	72	18.5
Mucinous cystadenoma/cystadenofibroma	48	12.5
Fibroma	39	10.0
Serous carcinoma	26	6.7
Endometrioid carcinoma	14	3.6
Mixed carcinoma	12	3.1
Serous borderline tumor	12	3.1
Brenner tumor, benign	11	2.8
Thecoma	11	2.8
Clear cell carcinoma	8	2.1
Mucinous carcinoma	6	1.6
Mucinous borderline tumor	6	1.6
Immature teratoma	3	0.8
Other	18	4.7

* Adapted from Katsube Y, Berg JW, Silverberg SG: Epidemiologic pathology of ovarian tumors: A histopathologic review of primary ovarian neoplasms diagnosed in the Denver Standard metropolitan statistical area, July 1–December 31, 1969 and July 1–December 31, 1979. Int J Gynecol Pathol 1:5, 1982.

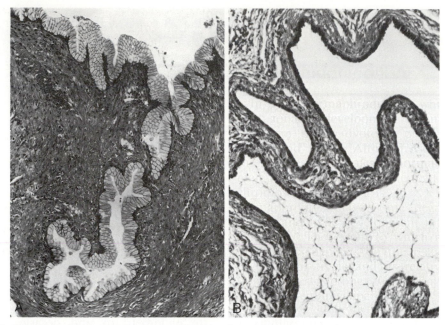

Figure 33–1. Histologic differences between (A) a benign mucinous cystadenoma and (B) a benign serous cystadenoma. Note the smaller cuboidal cells and focal cilia lining the serous tumor, and the taller columnar cells with basal nuclei and abundant mucin lining the mucinous tumor.

serous tumors are bilateral in about 10 per cent of cases. Of all serous tumors, about 70 per cent are benign, 5 to 10 per cent have borderline malignant potential, and 20 to 25 per cent are malignant. Serous cystadenomas tend to be multilocular (Fig. 33–2), although small unilocular serous cystomas are not uncommon. Histologically, serous tumors characteristically form psammoma bodies (from the Greek *psammos,* meaning sand), which are calcific, concentric concretions. Psammoma bodies occur occasionally in benign serous neoplasms and frequently in serous cystadenocarcinomas. Papillary patterns are also common.

The mucinous (formerly, pseudomucinous) neoplasms of the ovary can attain a huge size, often filling the entire pelvis and abdo-

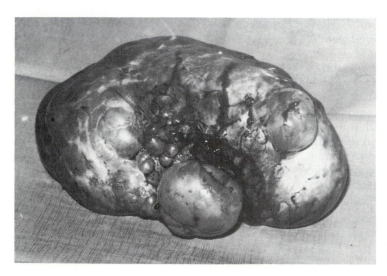

Figure 33–2. Gross appearance of a multilocular serous cystadenoma.

Figure 33–3. Huge mucinous cystadenoma filling the entire pelvis and abdomen.

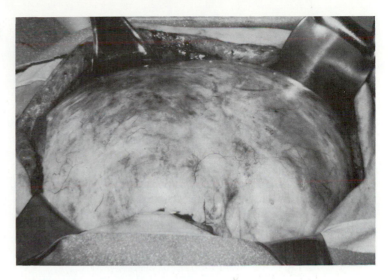

men (Fig. 33–3). They are often multilocular, and benign mucinous tumors are bilateral in less than 10 per cent of cases. About 85 per cent of mucinous tumors are benign. Rarely, a benign mucinous tumor may be complicated by pseudomyxoma peritonei. Mucinous tumors are sometimes associated with a mucocele of the appendix.

Endometrioid neoplasms may be malignant (endometrioid carcinoma). Benign endometrial tumors of the ovary most commonly take the form of endometriomas, which are not neoplasms in the strictest sense. Endometriosis is much more common than are benign endometrioid tumors. Benign endometrioid neoplasms of the ovary are not associated with endometrial stroma and do not demonstrate the extensive, but generally superficial, invasive characteristics of endometriosis. The distinction between benign endometrioid neoplasia and endometriosis in the ovary is not conceptually clear.

The Brenner tumor is a solid ovarian neoplasm, usually benign, with a large fibrotic component that encases epithelioid cells, which resemble transitional cells. In about one third of cases, they are associated with mucinous epithelial elements.

Sex Cord-Stromal Ovarian Neoplasms

These tumors include fibromas, granulosa-theca cell tumors, and Sertoli-Leydig cell tumors. Combinations of the latter two types are termed *gynandroblastomas.*

The tumors in this category are derived from the sex cords and specialized stroma of the developing gonad. As noted in Chapter 29, the embryologic origins of granulosa and theca cells as well as their counterparts in the testes the Sertoli and Leydig cells are from cells that make up the specialized gonadal stroma. If the ultimate differentiation of cell types occurring in the tumor is feminine, the neoplasm becomes a granulosa-cell tumor, a theca-cell tumor, or, as in most instances, a mixed granulosa-theca cell tumor. Those neoplasms containing cells that take on a masculine differentiation (far less common) become Sertoli-Leydig cell tumors. The fibroma represents the stromal cell neoplasm developing from mature fibroblasts in the ovarian stroma.

The granulosa-theca cell neoplasms as well as their androgenic counterparts are generally referred to as functioning (not functional) ovarian tumors. They occur in any age group, from birth on, and their functioning characteristics are responsible for a variety of associated signs and symptoms. The granulosa-theca cell tumors promote feminizing signs and symptoms, such as precocious puberty, precocious thelarche, or premenarchal uterine bleeding during infancy and childhood menorrhagia (or amenorrhea) and endometrial hyperplasia (or even endometrial cancer), breast tenderness, and fluid retention in the menstruating years; and postmenopau-

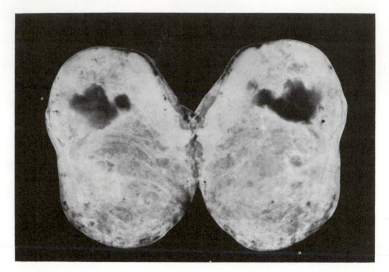

Figure 33–4. Ovarian fibroma that was removed from a patient with ascites and a right pleural effusion (Meigs' syndrome). Note the whorled appearance on the cut section and the area of cystic degeneration.

sal bleeding in older women. In contrast, the less frequent Sertoli-Leydig cell tumors are responsible for virilizing effects, such as hirsutism, recession of the frontal hairline, deepening of the voice, clitoromegaly, and change in body habitus to a muscular build. Fifteen per cent of these tumors have no such endocrinologic clinical effects. Except for the pure thecoma, these tumors have malignant potential and are discussed further in Chapter 55.

The ovarian fibroma is nonfunctioning, does not secrete steroids, and takes the form of a firm, rounded, smooth-surfaced tumor made up of interlacing bundles of fibrocytes (Fig. 33–4). It is glistening white on cut surface, as opposed to the soft yellow appearance of the granulosa-theca cell or hilus cell tumor. Occasionally, this tumor is associated with ascites. The transudation of this ascitic fluid through the transdiaphragmatic lymphatics into the right pleural cavity may result in Meigs' syndrome (ascites and right hydrothorax in association with an ovarian fibroma). The ovarian fibroma may be associated with theca-cell elements as a fibrothecoma.

Germ-Cell Tumors

Germ-cell neoplasms can occur at any age. They make up about 60 per cent of ovarian neoplasms occurring in infants and children.

Benign Cystic Teratoma. As noted previously, the most common ovarian neoplasm is the benign cystic teratoma, a germ-cell tumor that can take on a great variety of forms with virtually all adult tissues being represented. Fifteen to 20 per cent are bilateral. The benign cystic teratoma, commonly referred to as a dermoid cyst (Fig. 33–5), is composed primarily of skin and the dermal appendages, including sweat and sebaceous glands, hair follicles, and teeth. Because of the oily secretion of the sebaceous glands, the desquamated squamous cells, the presence of hair, and the presence of a dermoid tubercle (of Rokitansky), which often contains a hard, well-formed tooth, the dermoid cyst has a characteristic gross appearance (Figs. 33–6 and 33–7).

Other tissue components commonly found in benign cystic teratomas include brain, bronchus, thyroid, cartilage, intestine, bone, and carcinoid cells. As opposed to similar tissues found in a malignant immature teratoma, the tissues making up the benign (mature) teratoma are all of an adult, well-differentiated form.

Benign cystic teratomas can be found in the retroperitoneal area of the pelvis or upper abdomen, in the mediastinum, and even in the pineal body. Since primary sex (germ) cells originate in early embryonic life near the hindgut in the region of the yolk sac and allantois and migrate along the base of the mesentery to the gonadal ridge on either side

Figure 33–5. Histologic appearance of a dermoid cyst. Note the (A) keratinized squamous epithelium, (B) hair follicle, and (C) sebaceous glands.

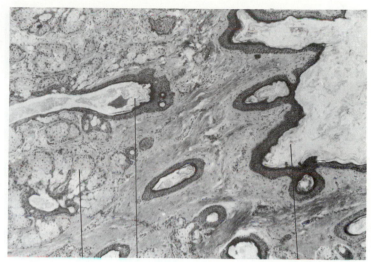

Sebaceous gland   Hair follicle   Keratinizing squamous epithelium

of the midline (see Chapter 29), it is postulated that some such cells go astray in their migration.

Mixed Ovarian Neoplasms

The most common ovarian tumor in which the neoplastic elements are composed of more than one cell type is the cystadenofibroma or the fibrocystadenoma. These tumors generally take their characteristics from the epithelial component, although they tend to be more solid than the epithelial ovarian neoplasms.

The gonadoblastoma is a tumor composed of cells resembling those of a dysgerminoma and others resembling granulosa and Sertoli cells. Characteristically, calcific concretions are a prominent feature of this neoplasm. Almost all patients with a gonadoblastoma have dysgenetic gonads (see Chapter 48), and a Y chromosome has been detected in over 90 per cent of cases investigated. Although the gonadoblastoma is initially benign, about half of these tumors may predispose to the

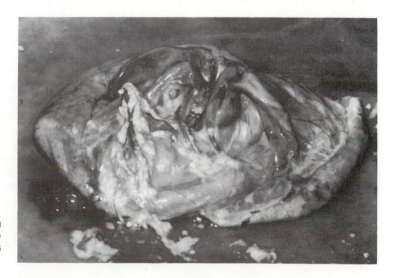

Figure 33–6. Gross appearance of a dermoid cyst cut open. Note the presence of hair and sebaceous material.

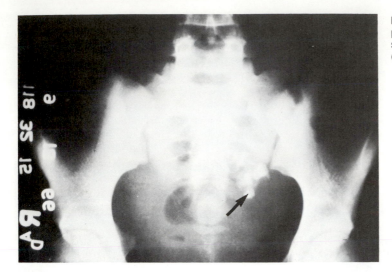

Figure 33–7. Pelvic x-ray film of a patient with a benign dermoid cyst showing the presence of teeth (*arrow*).

development of dysgerminomas or other malignant germ-cell tumors.

Diagnosis of Benign Ovarian Tumors

Symptoms

The clinical features of benign ovarian tumors are often deceptive and nonspecific. Except for the functioning ovarian neoplasms, most benign ovarian tumors are asymptomatic unless they undergo torsion or rupture. They usually enlarge very slowly, so that an increase in abdominal girth or pressure on surrounding organs is not perceived until the later stages of growth. Any pelvic pain is generally mild and intermittent, unless the tumor twists on its pedicle, when infarction may induce severe pain and tenderness. Torsion of an adnexal mass is often associated with "reverse renal colic," the pain originating in the iliac fossa and radiating to the flank. Nausea and vomiting are common. Peritoneal irritation from an infarcted tumor may cause radiation of pain in the distribution of the ilioinguinal and genitofemoral nerves (inguinal area, anterior thigh, and inner portion of the external genitalia).

On rare occasions, an ovarian cyst may rupture spontaneously from internal hemorrhage or intracystic pressure, resulting in pain and peritoneal irritation. A cyst may also rupture occasionally during or following a bimanual pelvic examination. Depending on the cystic contents, pain of varying degrees of severity can result. The escape of thin serous fluid without hemorrhage may evoke little pain or tenderness, but the oily contents of a dermoid cyst or the thick mucinous fluid of a mucinous cystadenoma may be irritating to both the parietal and the visceral peritoneum, with the development of severe pain and tenderness and the subsequent formation of troublesome intra-abdominal adhesions.

Signs

Bimanual pelvic examination generally indicates the presence of the tumor in the pelvis; if it has risen into the abdomen, however, this examination may be unremarkable. If the tumor is large enough, it may be delineated by abdominal palpation.

In contrast to the findings in a patient with ascites, percussion of the abdomen in a patient with a large ovarian cyst reveals dullness anteriorly with tympany in the flanks as the bowel is displaced laterally by the tumor. Shifting dullness suggests ascites.

If the tumor undergoes torsion and infarcts or ruptures, signs of peritoneal irritation may be present. Occasionally, the patient is initially seen after complete infarction has occurred and the peritoneal irritation has pro-

Table 33–5. ULTRASOUND SCORING SYSTEM FOR ADNEXAL MASSES*

Clear cyst and smooth borders	1
Clear cyst with slightly irregular border; cyst with smooth walls but low-level echoes (i.e., endometrioma)	2
Cyst with low-level echoes with slightly irregular border but no nodularity (i.e., endometrioma); clear cyst in postmenopausal patient	3
Equivocal, nonspecific ultrasound appearance: solid ovarian enlargement or small cyst with irregular borders and internal echoes (hemorrhagic cyst or benign ovarian tumor)	4–6
Multiseptated or irregular cystic mass consistent in appearance with ovarian tumor (7 = less nodularity, 8–9 = more nodularity)	7–9
Pelvic mass as above, with ascites	10

* 1 = benign; 10 = malignant.
Modified from Finkler NJ, Benacerraf B, Lavin PT, et al: Comparison of CA 125, clinical impression, and ultrasound in the preoperative evaluation of ovarian masses. Reprinted with permission from The American College of Obstetricians and Gynecologists (Obstetrics and Gynecology, 1988, 72, p. 659).

gressed to the point of abdominal rigidity. Paralytic ileus may also be present.

Investigations

Pelvic ultrasonography may be helpful if the tumor is indistinguishable from a functional cyst (size 4 to 8 cm, cystic to palpation). The malignant potential of an ovarian tumor may be evaluated with the ultrasound scoring system shown in Table 33–5. A score of 7 or more is strongly suggestive of a malignant mass. A lower abdominal or pelvic x-ray film will identify calcified structures and may show an encapsulated cyst of low-density fluid (see Fig. 33–7).

The serum CA 125 titer often helps to distinguish between benign and malignant masses, particularly in a postmenopausal patient. When clinical evaluation, pelvic ultrasonography, and the CA 125 titer all suggest malignancy, the positive predictive value of the combination approaches 100 per cent in postmenopausal women. Such patients should be referred to a gynecologic oncologist for laparotomy.

Laparoscopy is helpful in distinguishing between a uterine myoma, a quiescent hydrosalpinx, and an ovarian tumor, but it will not distinguish between a functional cyst, a benign neoplasm, or an encapsulated malignant ovarian neoplasm. Occasionally, laparoscopy may identify endometriosis on the surface of the ovary. It cannot identify unequivocally, however, that an ovarian endometrioma is not an ovarian neoplasm. Cystic ovarian tumors should be biopsied or aspirated through the laparoscope only with caution because of the likelihood of spilling contents around the peritoneal cavity. In general, laparotomy is preferable to laparoscopy in the evaluation of an adnexal mass.

Management of Ovarian Neoplasms

No ovarian neoplasm should be assumed to be benign until proved so by surgical exploration and microscopic examination. The indications for exploratory laparotomy in a patient with a pelvic mass have been discussed under functional tumors. If laparotomy is indicated, any ascitic fluid should be collected on opening the peritoneal cavity and sent for cytologic examination. Peritoneal washings should be obtained from the pelvis, both paracolic gutters, and both hemidiaphragms (see Chapter 55).

The definitive treatment will depend on the type of neoplasm, the patient's age, and her desire for future childbearing. A frozen section histologic diagnosis should be obtained intraoperatively.

Epithelial Ovarian Neoplasms. Epithelial ovarian neoplasms are generally treated by unilateral salpingo-oophorectomy. The contralateral ovary must be carefully inspected or a wedge biopsy must be performed to ensure that it is free of tumor. Because of the possible coexistence of an appendiceal mucocele with a mucinous cystadenoma, appendectomy is also indicated in such patients. If the patient is over 40 years of age, a total abdominal hysterectomy and bilateral salpingo-oophorectomy are appropriate. This is especially true if the tumor is a serous cystadenoma, since the incidence of bilaterality and malignancy are higher in serous tumors.

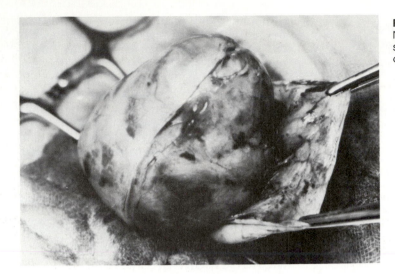

Figure 33–8. Ovarian cystectomy. Note the stretched-out ovarian tissue being separated from the cystic ovarian tumor.

If the patient is young and nulliparous, the ovarian neoplasm is unilocular, and there are no excrescences within the cyst, an ovarian cystectomy with preservation of the ovary may be performed (Fig. 33–8).

Stromal-Cell Neoplasms. Stromal-cell neoplasms of the ovary are generally treated by salpingo-oophorectomy when future pregnancies are a consideration. Ovarian fibromas, even when associated with ascites and right hydrothorax, are almost always benign and might even be treated by resection from the ovary in a young woman. After 40 years of age, total abdominal hysterectomy and bilateral salpingo-oophorectomy may be elected.

Germ-Cell Tumors. Cystic teratomas ("dermoids") can be treated by ovarian cystectomy (Fig. 33–8) if future childbearing is desired. Since 15 to 20 per cent are bilateral, the contralateral ovary should be carefully evaluated, any cysts resected, and the ovary bivalved if it is enlarged. Bivalve incision or wedge-resection of the opposite ovary is not recommended as a routine procedure, as it may cause adhesions and subsequent infertility. In a patient with a gonadoblastoma, dysgenetic ovaries are usually present, necessitating bilateral salpingo-oophorectomy, particularly in the presence of a Y chromosome. With the possibility of embryo transfer now becoming available to these patients, the uterus should be left in situ if future childbearing is desired, even if both ovaries are removed.

BENIGN TUMORS OF THE FALLOPIAN TUBES

Most benign lesions of the fallopian tubes are inflammatory (hydrosalpinx or pyosalpinx), and benign neoplasms of the oviducts are rare. Although the tubes, uterine corpus, and uterine cervix are from the same müllerian anlage, the tubes, unlike the uterus, have less tendency toward neoplastic transformation.

As might be expected, those tubal neoplasms that do occur are epithelial adenomas and polyps, myomas from the tubal musculature, inclusion cysts from the mesothelium, or angiomas from the tubal vasculature.

It is quite difficult to differentiate a tubal neoplasm from other adnexal masses on examination, and generally, operative exploration is necessary to confirm the diagnosis. Salpingectomy represents the definitive treatment, although if pathologic evaluation confirms the benign nature of the neoplasm, normal portions of the tube may be preserved for fertility reasons in selected instances.

PARAOVARIAN NEOPLASMS

As the name *paraovarian* implies (beside the ovary), paraovarian neoplasms are generally located within the broad ligament between the tube and the ovary. These tumors are generally small compared with ovarian cysts, measuring less than 8 cm, and, histologically, most appear to be derived from paramesonephric (müllerian) structures or occasionally from mesonephric (wolffian) remnants. Although the malignancy rate is not great (less than 10 per cent), it is necessary to resect the cystic mass (generally with the ipsilateral tube) to obtain a pathologic assessment.

SUGGESTED READING

Beck RP, Latour JPA: Review of 1019 benign ovarian neoplasms. Obstet Gynecol 16:479, 1960.

Finkler NJ, Benacerraf B, Lavin PT, et al: Comparison of serum CA 125, clinical impression, and ultrasound in the preoperative evaluation of ovarian masses. Obstet Gynecol 72:659, 1988.

Genadry R, Parmley T, Woodruff JD: The origin and clinical behavior of the paraovarian tumor. Am J Obstet Gynecol 129:873, 1977.

Katsube Y, Berg JW, Silverberg SG: Epidemiologic pathology of ovarian tumors: A histopathologic review of primary ovarian neoplasms diagnosed in the Denver Standard metropolitan statistical area, July 1–December 31, 1969 and July 1–December 31, 1979. Int J Pathol 1:3, 1982.

Limber GK, King RE, Silverberg SG: Pseudomyxoma peritonei: A report of ten cases. Ann Surg 178:587, 1973.

O'Connell GT, Ryan E, Murphy J et al: Predictive value of CA 125 for ovarian carcinoma in patients presenting with pelvic masses. Obstet Gynecol 70:930, 1987.

Scully RE: Tumors of the Ovary and Maldeveloped Gonads. Atlas of Tumor Pathology. 2nd series, fasc. 16. Washington, DC, Armed Forces Institute of Pathology, 1979.

Spanos WJ: Preoperative hormonal therapy of cystic adnexal masses. Am J Obstet Gynecol 116:551, 1973.

Thirty-four

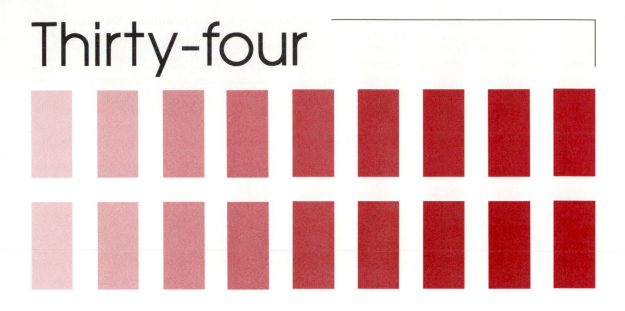

Endometriosis and Adenomyosis

J. GEORGE MOORE

Endometriosis and adenomyosis are benign conditions in which endometrial glands and stroma are found beyond the endometrium.

ENDOMETRIOSIS

Endometriosis is a benign condition in which endometrial glands and stroma are present outside the endometrial cavity, usually in the ovary or on the pelvic peritoneum. It assumes great importance in gynecology because of its frequency, distressing symptomatology, association with infertility, and potential for invasion of adjacent organ systems, such as the gastrointestinal or urinary tracts. In addition, endometriosis often presents a difficult diagnostic problem, and

few gynecologic conditions require such difficult surgical dissections.

Incidence

The exact incidence of endometriosis is not known, but it is estimated that more than 15 per cent of women have some degree of the disease. It is noted in about 20 per cent of gynecologic laparotomies, and of these it is an unexpected finding in approximately one half of cases.

Characteristically, endometriosis occurs in high-achieving nulliparous women with a type A personality. Less frequently, it is seen in minority ethnic patients on indigent hospital services. Generally, endometriosis is initiated in the third decade of life, becomes clinically apparent in the thirties, and regresses after the menopause. It may, on occasion, occur in infancy, childhood, or adolescence, but at these early ages it is almost always associated with obstructive genital anomalies. Although endometriosis should regress following the menopause, if estrogens are not prescribed, the scarifying involution may result in obstructive problems, especially in the gastrointestinal and urinary tracts.

Pathogenesis

Three main theories for the development of endometriosis have been proposed.

1. The lymphatic spread theory of Halban suggests that endometrial tissues are taken up into the lymphatics draining the uterus and are transported to the various pelvic sites where the tissue grows ectopically. Endometrial tissue has been found in pelvic lymphatics in up to 20 per cent of patients with the disease.

2. The müllerian metaplasia theory of Meyer proposes that endometriosis results from the metaplastic transformation of peritoneal mesothelium into endometrium under the influence of certain unidentified stimuli.

3. The retrograde menstruation theory of Sampson proposes that endometrial fragments transported through the fallopian tubes at the time of menstruation implant and grow in various intra-abdominal sites. Endometrial tissue normally shed at the time of menstruation is viable and capable of growth in vivo or in vitro.

To explain some rare examples of endometriosis in distant sites, such as the forehead or axilla, it is necessary to postulate hematogenous spread. Quite probably, all of these postulated mechanisms play a role in the development of endometriosis, and no single mechanism explains all cases.

Sites of Occurrence

Endometriosis occurs most commonly in the ovaries, the broad ligament, the peritoneal surfaces of the cul-de-sac including the uterosacral ligaments and posterior cervix,

and in the rectovaginal septum (Fig. 34–1). Quite frequently, the rectosigmoid colon is involved, as is the appendix and the vesico-uterine fold of peritoneum. Endometriosis is occasionally seen in laparotomy scars, developing especially after cesarean sections or myomectomies when the endometrial cavity has been entered. In spite of the great variety of sites, 60 per cent of patients with endometriosis have ovarian involvement.

Pathology

Characteristically, an endometrioma of the ovary forms a small cyst. It is filled with thick, chocolate-colored fluid that sometimes has the black color and tarry consistency of crankcase oil. This characteristic fluid represents aged, hemolyzed blood and desquamated endometrium. Usually, endometrial glands and stroma are present in the cyst wall. Sometimes, however, the pressure of the enclosed fluid destroys the endometrial lining of the endometrioma, leaving only a fibrotic cyst wall infiltrated with large numbers of hemosiderin-laden macrophages. Since corpus luteum cysts can give this same picture, pathologists are sometimes reluctant to diagnose endometriosis in the absence of endometrial glands and stroma in the cyst wall. Instead, they characterize the picture as, "consistent with endometriosis".

Most often, the ovarian endometrioma is tightly adherent to the posterior leaf of the broad ligament bound by dense, intractable adhesions. Occasionally, an ovarian endometrioma may reach dimensions as large as 20 cm in diameter. Most instances of ovarian endometriosis are bilateral, and there is usually involvement of parietal and visceral peritoneal surfaces. When endometriosis involves the peritoneal surfaces, it appears as flat, brownish discolorations, often referred to as "powder burns" or, if they are raised and bluish in color, as "mulberry spots." The tissues surrounding these lesions are puckered and scarred as a result of fibrosis. Frequently, the rectosigmoid colon becomes tightly bound by dense endometriotic adhesions to the posterior wall of the lower uterine segment and cervix, resulting in fixed retroversion of the uterus.

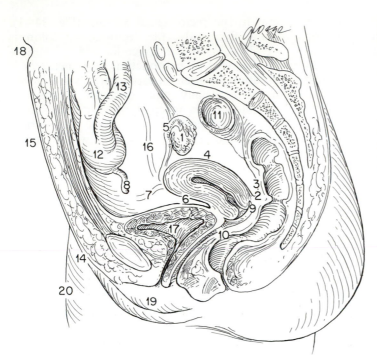

Figure 34-1. Common sites of endometriosis in decreasing order of frequency: (1) ovary, (2) cul-de-sac, (3) uterosacral ligaments, (4) broad ligaments, (5) fallopian tubes, (6) uterovesical fold, (7) round ligaments, (8) vermiform appendix, (9) vagina, (10) rectovaginal septum, (11) rectosigmoid colon, (12) cecum, (13) ileum, (14) inguinal canals, (15) abdominal scars, (16) ureters, (17) urinary bladder, (18) umbilicus, (19) vulva, and (20) peripheral sites.

Staging

Heretofore, the extent of endometriosis has been described anecdotally in each case. The American Fertility Society has employed a staging protocol in an attempt to correlate fertility potential with a quantified stage of endometriosis. The staging is based on the allocation of points depending on the sites and extent of disease (Table 34-1).

Symptoms

The characteristic triad of symptoms associated with endometriosis is dysmenorrhea, dyspareunia, and dyschezia. Generally, secondary dysmenorrhea first appears or worsens in the late twenties or early thirties. If the endometriosis is associated with obstructive genital anomalies, severe dysmenorrhea may commence at menarche.

Dyspareunia is generally associated with deep penetration and occurs mainly when the cul-de-sac, uterosacral ligaments, and portions of the posterior vaginal fornix are involved. Endometriomata in these sites are usually exquisitely tender to touch.

Dyschezia is experienced with uterosacral, cul-de-sac, and rectosigmoid colon involve-

ment. As the stool passes between the uterosacral ligaments, the characteristic dyschezia is experienced. This symptom is highly characteristic and is much more common with endometriosis than with chronic salpingo-oophoritis, a condition that is often confused with endometriosis. Premenstrual and postmenstrual spotting is a characteristic symptom of endometriosis. Menorrhagia is uncommon, the amount of menstrual flow usually diminishing with endometriosis. If the ovarian capsule is involved with endometriosis, ovulatory pain and midcycle vaginal bleeding often become a problem. Rarely, as other organ systems are involved, menstrual hematochezia, hematuria, and other forms of vicarious menstruation become evident.

The nature of pelvic pain caused by endometriosis is variable. It has been stated that the degree of pain varies inversely with the extent of the disease. Minimal endometriosis in the cul-de-sac is generally much more painful than a huge endometrioma within the ovary that is expanding freely into the abdominal cavity.

Infertility as a symptom of endometriosis is difficult to understand completely and even more difficult to quantify. Although approximately 10 per cent of "normal" couples are infertile, some 30 to 40 per cent of couples

Table 34-1.

**THE AMERICAN FERTILITY SOCIETY
REVISED CLASSIFICATION OF ENDOMETRIOSIS**

Patient's Name _____   Date _____

Stage I (Minimal)   - 1-5
Stage II (Mild)   - 6-15
Stage III (Moderate) - 16-40
Stage IV (Severe)   - >40
Total _____

Laparoscopy _____ Laparotomy _____ Photography _____
Recommended Treatment _____
_____
Prognosis _____

	ENDOMETRIOSIS	<1cm	1-3cm	>3cm
PERITONEUM	Superficial	1	2	4
	Deep	2	4	6
OVARY	R Superficial	1	2	4
	Deep	4	16	20
	L Superficial	1	2	4
	Deep	4	16	20

	POSTERIOR CULDESAC OBLITERATION	Partial	Complete
		4	40

	ADHESIONS	<1/3 Enclosure	1/3-2/3 Enclosure	>2/3 Enclosure
OVARY	R Filmy	1	2	4
	Dense	4	8	16
	L Filmy	1	2	4
	Dense	4	8	16
TUBE	R Filmy	1	2	4
	Dense	4*	8*	16
	L Filmy	1	2	4
	Dense	4*	8*	16

*If the fimbriated end of the fallopian tube is completely enclosed, change the point assignment to 16.

From the American Fertility Society: Revised American Fertility Society classification of endometriosis 1985. Fertil Steril 43:351, 1985. Reproduced with permission of the publisher.

are infertile if the female presents with endometriosis. The condition is found in 40 to 50 per cent of women who undergo surgery for infertility. Several mechanisms have been postulated to explain the association between endometriosis and infertility, and these are discussed in Chapter 51.

Signs

Endometriosis presents with a wide variety of signs varying from the presence of a small, exquisitely tender nodule in the cul-de-sac or on the uterosacral ligaments to a huge, relatively nontender, cystic abdominal mass. Occasionally, a small tender mulberry spot may be seen in the posterior fornix of the vagina.

Characteristically, a tender, fixed adnexal mass is appreciated on bimanual examination. The uterus is retroverted in a substantial number of women surgically explored for endometriosis. Frequently, no signs at all are appreciated on physical examination. The characteristic sharp, firm, exquisitely tender "barb" (from barbed wire) felt in the uterosacral ligament is the diagnostic sine qua non of endometriosis.

Differential Diagnosis

The main differential diagnoses confused with endometriosis are (1) chronic pelvic inflammatory disease or recurrent acute salpingitis, (2) hemorrhagic corpus luteum, (3) benign or malignant ovarian neoplasm, and, occasionally, (4) ectopic pregnancy.

Diagnosis

The diagnosis of endometriosis should be suspected in an afebrile patient with the characteristic symptom triad of endometriosis, a firm, fixed, tender adnexal mass, and tender nodularity in the cul-de-sac and uterosacral ligaments. This diagnosis is even more likely if the leukocyte count and erythrocyte sedimentation rate are normal. The serum CA-125 level is frequently elevated. An ultrasonic evaluation may indicate an adnexal mass of complex echogenicity. The definitive diagnosis is generally made by the characteristic gross and histologic findings at laparoscopy or laparotomy.

Management

The management of endometriosis depends on certain key considerations: (1) the certainty of the diagnosis, (2) the severity of the symptoms, (3) the extent of the disease, (4) the desire for future fertility, (5) the age of the patient, and (6) the threat to the gastrointestinal or urinary tracts or both.

Surgical Resection

Large (6 to 20 cm) endometriomata are amenable to surgical resection only. If the patient is in her forties, the preferred treatment is a total abdominal hysterectomy (TAH) and bilateral salpingo-oophorectomy (BSO), even if the disease is entirely resectable. Under such circumstances, the patient is quite likely to develop disconcerting menopausal symptoms, but these may be safely controlled with estrogen and progestin therapy with little risk of recurrence of the endometriosis. A woman in her middle or late thirties might optimally be treated by resection of the endometriosis from the ovaries and TAH. With reflux menstruation eliminated by the hysterectomy, endometriosis seldom recurs. If fertility is desired, conservative surgery must be considered. Even if removal of the tubes and ovaries are required, leaving the uterus may now be a consideration because embryo transfer to a hormonally pre-pared uterus has been successfully carried out.

In the late twenties and early thirties, especially with future fertility desired, the patient with fairly extensive endometriosis might well be treated by (1) resecting the endometriomata; (2) lysing tubal adhesions, with or without presacral neurectomy (to relieve dysmenorrhea); (3) suspending the uterus (to preclude the fixed retroversion of the uterine fundus into the cul-de-sac by endometriotic adhesions); and (4) removing the appendix (because the appendix is a likely sight for endometriosis, even when it appears grossly normal). Following the surgical resection of endometriosis, 50 to 60 per cent of patients become pregnant, usually in the first 2 years following surgery. With severe endometriosis, either preoperative or postoperative therapy with danazol or a gonadotropin-releasing hormone (GnRH) agonist appears to improve substantially the chance of subsequent fertility. Approximately 15 per cent of patients treated by such conservative surgery will require reoperation at a later date.

If endometriosis involves the cul-de-sac or uterosacral ligaments, the proximity to the ureter, bladder, and sigmoid colon must be considered. In the course of follow-up, an intravenous pyelogram, colonoscopy, or barium enema should be used to evaluate the spread to these organ systems. Rarely endometriosis may obstruct the ureter (Fig. 34–2). This is not an entirely benign disease, since 25 per cent of kidneys are lost when endometriosis blocks the ureter. Obstruction of the rectosigmoid and even obstruction of the small intestine may require resection of the involved intestinal segment. If endometriosis involves the full thickness of the urinary or intestinal tract, TAH and BSO are generally indicated, unless future childbearing is critically desired.

Electrocautery or laser treatment of small foci of endometriosis at the time of laparoscopy is appropriate to relieve pelvic pain. Resection of even small foci of endometriosis improves the cellular milieu of peritoneal fluid to improve fertility (Surrey and Halme, 1990).

Medical Therapy

If endometriosis is minimal in extent and the symptoms are tolerable, no treatment is

Figure 34–2. Endometriosis obstructing the ureter. Note the disease invading (A) the surrounding ureteric muscle and (B) the lumen of the ureter. This patient had a 2-cm focus of endometriosis confined to the lateral portion of the cardinal ligament with no intraperitoneal involvement.

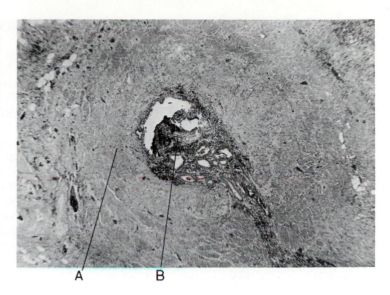

necessary, but the patient should be observed at 6-month intervals. The use of medroxyprogesterone acetate (Provera) or a combined estrogen and progestin oral contraceptive on a cyclic basis may inhibit the growth of endometriosis, since this treatment effects an "exhaustion atrophy" of the normally placed or ectopic endometrium. If the disease is minimal and symptoms are incapacitating or if infertility is a problem, the endometriosis may be treated by a pseudopregnancy regimen, using either escalating continuous doses of combined oral contraceptives or progestin only (medroxyprogesterone acetate, up to 30 mg daily, or norethindrone acetate, 5 to 15 mg daily) over a period of 6 to 9 months. Although most cases treated with pseudopregnancy result in temporary relief of symptoms and up to 40 per cent may become pregnant following cessation of treatment, this regimen is poorly tolerated by most patients, and the endometriosis generally redevelops following cessation of treatment. Continuous progestin may be more effective than continuous oral contraceptives.

Danazol, an androgen dervative, may also be used in a "pseudomenopause" regimen to suppress symptoms of endometriosis if fertility is not a present concern. It is given over a period of 6 to 9 months, and a dose of 100 to 800 mg daily may be necessary to suppress menstruation. Through its weak androgenic properties, danazol decreases the plasma levels of sex hormine binding globulin, and the increase of free testosterone can bring about hirsutism and acne. At 3 years after cessation of therapy, 40 per cent of patients have had recurrence. After a full course of danazol therapy, use of a cyclic oral contraceptive may help to delay or prevent recurrence. Whenever a palpable endometrioma is present, the likelihood of a complete response to medical therapy is small.

Endometriosis may be treated with a gonadotropin-releasing hormone (GnRH) agonist that effects a temporary medical castration, thereby bringing about a marked, albeit temporary, regression of endometriosis. Side effects of treatment and expense restrict long-term use. Two such agonists are presently available. nafarelin acetate (Synarel) is used as a nasal spray in a dose of 200 μg twice daily. Leuprolide acetate (Depot Lupron) is marketed in 7.5-mg single-dose vials with the agonist encased in timed-release microspheres. It is injected intramuscularly every 28 or 60 days. Both Lupron and Nafarelin are as effective as danazol without the androgenic side effects. Treatment of women with endometriosis usually produces relief of pain and involution of implants. About 50 per cent of infertile patients will conceive within 12 months of discontinuing the treatment. Use of GnRH agonists for gross endometriomas is generally not recommended except for infertility trials or as a presurgical adjuvant.

The disadvantages of these agonists are related to cost, hot flushes, vaginal dryness, and calcium loss from trabecular bone. The latter side effect can be counteracted with the concurrent administration of a progestogen without seriously decreasing the effectiveness of the GnRH agonist. It has been noted that GnRH agonists reduce the CA 125 level in patients with endometriosis and the level rises again after discontinuation of treatment. The long-term effects on endometriosis and its effect on large endometriomas have not been evaluated.

Prevention of Endometriosis

Whenever severe dysmenorrhea occurs in a young patient, the possibility of varying degrees of obstruction to the menstrual flow must be considered. The possibility of a blind uterine horn in a bicornuate uterus or an obstructing uterine or vaginal septum should be kept in mind. In more than half the patients who are noted to develop endometriosis during childhood and adolescence, varying degrees of genital tract obstruction may be found. Cervical dilatation to allow an easier egress of menstrual blood in patients with severe degrees of dysmenorrhea may be helpful in rare instances but is not generally recommended.

Whenever a congenital abnormality of the urinary or intestinal tract is detected, the genital tract should be investigated for an obstructive lesion. Infants with genital tract obstruction have been noted to develop endometriosis even in the first year of life.

ADENOMYOSIS

Adenomyosis is defined as the extension of endometrial glands and stroma into the uterine musculature. It is generally accepted that about 15 per cent of women develop varying degrees of adenomyosis in their late thirties and early forties. Originally, adenomyosis was referred to as endometriosis interna (as opposed to endometriosis externa), but these terms have become archaic. About 15 per cent of patients with adenomyosis have associated endometriosis. The basal layers of the endometrium extend in continuity to sites within the myometrium and generally do not participate in the proliferative and secretory cycles induced by the ovary.

Pathology

Generally, the uterus grossly is diffusely enlarged with a thickened myometrium containing characteristic glandular irregularities (Fig. 34–3). The endometrial cavity is also enlarged, consistent with the increased myometrium. Histologically, the extent of the process varies a great deal from superficial extension into the underlying myometrium to extension throughout the myometrium, occasionally with penetration of the peritoneal surface of the uterus. Occasionally, the adenomyosis may be confined to one portion of the myometrium and take the form of a fairly well-circumscribed adenomyoma. Contrary to the picture in a uterine myoma, no distinct capsular margin can be detected on cut section between the adenomyoma and the surrounding myometrium. Stromal adenomyosis (endometrial stromatosis) is considered to be a variant of adenomyosis in which the endometrium spreading into the myometrium is made up entirely of endometrial stroma without glands and may merge into a low-grade stromal sarcoma.

Symptoms

Typical symptoms of adenomyosis are severe secondary dysmenorrhea and menorrhagia. The menorrhagia is consistent with the enlarged surface area of the endometrial cavity and the increased volume of sloughed endometrium. The dysmenorrhea is of the colicky type. Many patients are asymptomatic. In about 30 to 40 per cent of patients with adenomyosis, the disease is a surprise pathologic finding in a patient without menorrhagia, dysmenorrhea, or uterine enlargement. Occasionally, in a patient with a large adenomyoma, pressure on the bladder or rectum may create a problem.

Signs

On pelvic examination, the uterus is symmetrically enlarged. Occasionally, it may enlarge asymmetrically and make it impossible to distinguish this condition from that of a myomatous uterus. The consistency of the

Figure 34–3. *A,* Grossly enlarged uterus with markedly thickened myometrium containing adenomyosis. *B,* Microscopic view of adenomyosis extending deep into the myometrium. Note the presence of both endometrial glands and stroma.

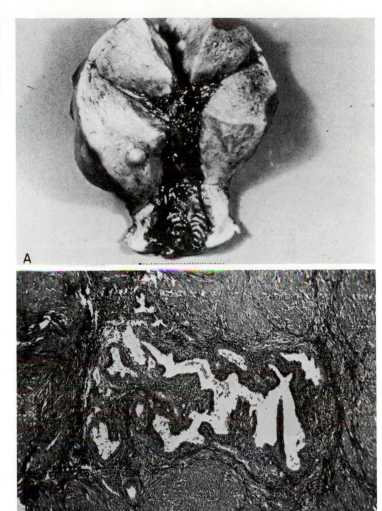

enlarged adenomyomatous uterus is generally softer than that of a uterine myoma.

Treatment

The treatment of adenomyosis depends entirely on the symptoms and the possibility of other diagnoses. Any menorrhagia should be investigated by fractional dilatation and curettage to rule out endometrial cancer, but if menorrhagia and dysmenorrhea are not a problem, palliative treatment only is indicated. If the menorrhagia is severe and recurrent following a dilatation and curettage or if the dysmenorrhea is disabling, the use of a GnRH agonist may provide relief. Total abdominal or vaginal hysterectomy, however, may be indicated. The ovaries should be preserved if they are normal, unless the patient is over 45 years of age.

SUGGESTED READING

Adamson G: Diagnosis and clinical presentation of endometriosis. Am J Obstet Gynecol 162:568, 1990.

American Fertility Society classification of endometriosis. Fertil Steril 43:351, 1985.

Ansbacher P: Treatment of endometriosis with danazol. Am J Obstet Gynecol 121:283, 1975.

Cedars MI, Lu JK, Meldrum DR, Judd HL: Treatment of endometriosis with a long-acting gonadotropin-releasing hormone agonist plus medroxyprogesterone acetate. Obstet Gynecol 75:641, 1990.

Henzl MR: GnRH agonists in the management of endometriosis. Clin Obstet Gynecol 31:840, 1988.

Meldrum DR, Pardridge WM, Karow WG, et al: Hormonal effects of danazol and medical oophorectomy in endometriosis: Enigmas in diagnosis and management. Obstet Gynecol 62:480, 1983.

Moore JG, Buvstock MA, Growdon WA: The clinical implications of retroperitoneal endometriosis. Am J Obstet Gynecol 158:1291, 1988.

Pittaway DE: CA-125 in women with endometriosis. Obstet Gynecol Clin North Am 16:237, 1989.

Ranney B: Endometriosis I: Conservative operations. Am J Obstet Gynecol 107:743, 1970.

Ranney B: Endometriosis II: Complete operations. Am J Obstet Gynecol 109:1137, 1971.

Ranney B: The prevention, palliation, and treatment of endometriosis. Am J Obstet Gynecol 123:778, 1975.

Surrey ES, Halme J: Effect of peritoneal fluid from endometriosis patients on endometrial proliferation in vitro. Obstet Gynecol 76:792, 1990.

Thirty-five

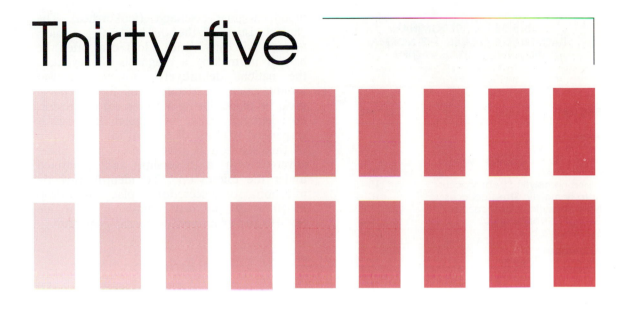

Vaginal and Vulvar Infections

JOHN GUNNING

Vaginal discharge and vulvar irritation are common symptoms, and their evaluation and management form a significant proportion of office gynecologic practice. Some vaginal secretions are always present, although the amount varies with the hormonal status of the patient. This chapter discusses the differentiation between physiologic and pathologic vaginal discharges and outlines the management of patients with a variety of vulvovaginal infections.

NORMAL PHYSIOLOGY AND BACTERIOLOGY OF THE VAGINA

The vagina is lined by nonkeratinized stratified squamous epithelium, and its character is influenced by estrogen and progesterone. At birth, the vagina of the newborn is colonized initially by anaerobic and aerobic bacteria acquired during passage through the birth canal. The epithelium of the vagina at this time is rich in glycogen as a result of the influence of placental and maternal estrogens. This results in a low pH (3.7 to 6.3), which permits survival and growth of the colonizing organisms. Shortly after birth, available estrogen decreases, and the epithelium becomes thin, atrophic, and largely devoid of glycogen. The pH rises to between 6 and 8. Acidophilic organisms no longer have a selective advantage, and the predominant flora become gram-positive cocci and bacilli.

With the onset of puberty, the vagina becomes estrogenized again, and the glycogen content increases. Lactobacilli (Doderlein's bacilli) predominate in the healthy estrogenized vagina and are responsible for the breakdown of glycogen to lactic acid, which results in a vaginal pH of between 3.5 and 4.5. A wide variety of aerobic and anaerobic bacteria can be cultured from the normal vagina (Table 35–1). Most women harbor three to eight types of bacteria at any given time. It is usually under nonphysiologic conditions that

Table 35–1. PREDOMINANT BACTERIAL FLORA IN THE NORMAL PREMENOPAUSAL VAGINA

BACTERIA	PERCENTAGE RANGE
Aerobes	
Lactobacillus	70–90
Staphylococcus epidermidis	30–60
Diphtheroids	30–60
Alpha-hemolytic *Streptococcus*	15–50
Beta-hemolytic *Streptococcus*	10–20
Nonhemolytic *Streptococcus*	5–30
Group D *Streptococcus*	10–40
Escherichia coli	20–25
Anaerobes	
Bacteroides fragilis	5–15
Bacteroides species	1–40
Peptococcus	5–60
Peptostreptococcus	5–40
Clostridium	5–15
Veillonella	10–15

organisms colonize in sufficient numbers to produce pathologic states.

Physiologic Vaginal Secretions

Vaginal secretions consist of cervical mucus (the major component); endometrial and oviductal fluid exudates from the sebaceous, sweat, Bartholin's, and Skene's glands; a transudate from the vaginal squamous epithelium together with exfoliated squamous cells; and metabolic products of the microflora. These secretions are composed of proteins, polysaccharides, acids, amino acids, enzymes, enzyme inhibitors, and immunoglobulins. The exact function of many of these chemicals is poorly understood at the present time. There is a physiologic increase in vaginal secretion during pregnancy and at the midcycle. Postmenopausally, vaginal secretions are markedly decreased, and dyspareunia may result.

Investigation of Vaginal Discharge

Patients with vaginal or vulvar infections frequently present complaining of a non-bloody vaginal discharge (leukorrhea). The characteristics of the discharge (e.g., color, texture, viscosity, and odor) can often be helpful in making a diagnosis. To evaluate the patient definitively, however, a wet mount smear preparation of the discharge must be made. Using a cotton tip applicator, an adequate sample of vaginal discharge is suspended in 2 ml of normal saline. A drop of this solution is placed on a glass slide, covered with a coverslip, and examined under the microscope. To identify mycotic infections, some secretion is placed in a drop of 10 to 20 per cent potassium hydroxide (KOH) and examined in the same manner.

CLINICAL CONDITIONS

Trichomonas Vaginitis

Trichomonas vaginitis is caused by the protozoan flagellate *Trichomonas vaginalis*, which is capable of living only in the female vagina and male urethra and is generally transmitted by sexual intercourse.

Clinical Features. Twenty-five per cent of patients harboring trichomonads are asymptomatic. Symptoms may vary from mild to severe and include vaginal discharge, vaginal and vulvar pruritus and burning, frequency of urination, and dyspareunia. The discharge is thin, bubbly, and pale greenish or grayish in color and has a pH of 5 to 6.5 (Table 35–2). The organism ferments carbohydrates, producing a gas with a rancid odor and causing a frothy appearing discharge. There frequently is erythema and edema of the vulva and vagina. Petechiae or strawberry patches on the vaginal mucosa and cervix are seen in approximately 10 per cent of patients harboring trichomonads.

Diagnosis. The diagnosis is made by identifying the organism in a wet mount smear preparation. The organism is pear-shaped and motile, with obvious flagella that propel it through the saline. It is smaller than an epithelial cell and larger than a white cell. Culture techniques confirm the diagnosis, but these are seldom necessary.

Management. The treatment is specific and consists of oral metronidazole (Flagyl) in either a single 2-gm dose or a 250-mg dose three times daily for 5 to 7 days. The single 2-gm dose may not be as effective as the

Table 35-2. DIFFERENTIAL DIAGNOSIS AND TREATMENT OF VAGINITIS

DESCRIPTION	TRICHOMONIASIS	CANDIDIASIS	BACTERIAL VAGINOSIS	HERPES
Discharge				
Amount	2 to 4	0 to 3	2 to 4	0 to 2
Color	Yellow-green	White-curdy	Gray	Mucoid
Odor	1	0	2 to 3	0
Frothy	1	0	1	0
pH	5 to 6.5	4 to 5	5 to 5.5	Variable
Symptoms				
Pruritus	0 to 4	2 to 4	0	0 to 1
Burning	0 to 1	1 to 2	0	2 to 4
Physical Examination				
Erythema	1 to 4	2 to 4	0	2 to 4
Edema	1 to 2	2 to 4	0	0 to 3
Petechiae	1	0	0	0
Ulcers	0	0	0	1 to 3
Wet Mount				
Clue Cells	0	0	1	0
Leukocytes	4	2	0 to 1	0 to 2

Key: 0 = none; 4 = severe.

longer treatment but facilitates patient compliance. The side effects of metronidazole include mild nausea, occasional vomiting, and a metallic taste. Since the drug acts like disulfiram (Antabuse), the patient should abstain from alcohol during treatment. Treatment failures are usually related to reinfection, and, therefore, the consort should be treated concurrently. Metronidazole should not be given during the first trimester of pregnancy because of its possible teratogenicity. During the first trimester, a 1-week course of clotrimazole (Gyne-Lotrimin) vaginal suppositories or cream applied at bedtime is usually sufficient to alleviate symptoms. Aci-Jel vaginal jelly may also be used for symptomatic relief.

Candida Vulvovaginitis

Candidiasis is caused predominantly by the yeast organism *Candida albicans*. The incidence of non-*albicans* infections, however, has increased over the last decade from 10 per cent to as much as 25 per cent in some areas. The main non-*albicans* organisms are *Candida glabrata* and *Candida tropicalis*. High-risk factors for developing candidiasis are pregnancy, diabetes mellitus, oral contraceptive use, and recent antibiotic use.

Clinical Features. Approximately 20 per cent of women harboring a *Candida* infection are asymptomatic. Symptoms, which frequently begin in the premenstrual phase of the cycle, include vaginal discharge, vulvar pruritus and burning, and dyspareunia. The discharge has a "cottage cheese" appearance with a pH of about 4.5. The vagina and vulva may be exquisitely tender with marked erythema and edema.

Diagnosis. The diagnosis is made by identifying the hyphae and spores of *C. albicans* in a KOH wet mount preparation (Fig. 35–1). When necessary, a culture for diagnosis may be performed using Nickerson's or Sabouraud's medium. Latex agglutination tests are available and may be useful for non-albicans strains, since they do not have the pseudohyphae seen with *C. albicans*.

Management. The standard antifungal agents are the polyenes (candicidin and nystatin), the imidazoles (miconazole, clotrimazole, butoconazole), and the oral preparation, ketoconazole. A more recently introduced, very effective antifungal agent is the triazole terconazole. Generally, treatment is with miconazole nitrate (Monistat) vaginal suppositories or cream inserted at bedtime for 7 to

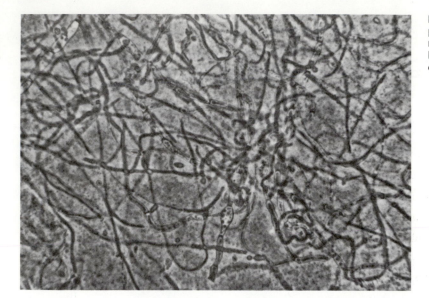

Figure 35–1. KOH wet mount preparation under high-power magnification showing fiber-like mycelia of *Candida albicans.*

14 days. There are several alternatives including clotrimazole (Gyne-Lotrimin) vaginal suppositories or cream used nightly for 7 to 14 days or butoconazole nitrate (Femstat) vaginal cream nightly for 3 days. Terconazole suppositories (80 mg) or 0.4 per cent terconazole cream, which is minimally absorbed, appear to be very effective for treating resistant infections. Coinfection with *Trichomonas vaginalis* is not unusual, and, if present, treatment for both is recommended.

Bacterial Vaginosis

Bacterial vaginosis (formerly called nonspecific vaginitis or *Gardnerella* vaginitis) is a sexually transmitted disease caused by a gram-negative bacillus, *Gardnerella (Haemophilus) vaginalis,* in the presence of anaerobic bacteria, such as *Bacteroides* and *Peptococcus* species. The combination of these bacteria produces the pathologic state.

Clinical Features. The most common symptom is a very profuse malodorous discharge. Itching or burning occurs in less than 20 per cent of patients in contrast to trichomoniasis and candidiasis. The discharge is thin and grayish appearing with a pH of 5.0 to 5.5. It may or may not have a distinctive odor. There is seldom evidence of vaginal or vulvar irritation. The addition of 10 to 20 per cent KOH to the discharge releases amines that produce a fishy odor.

Diagnosis. The diagnosis is made by preparing a saline wet mount and identifying characteristic clue cells, epithelial cells with numerous bacilli clinging to their surface (Fig. 35–2). There are very few white blood cells present, which also helps distinguish it from trichomoniasis and candidiasis. The presence of clue cells without clinical features is not significant.

Management. Metronidazole (Flagyl) is effective against both *Gardnerella vaginalis* and the anaerobic bacteria associated with it. A dose of 500 mg twice daily for 7 days is almost 100 per cent curative. Alternatives that are not nearly as effective are ampicillin, 500 mg four times daily for 7 days, or tetracycline, 500 mg four times daily for 7 days. The patient's sexual partner should be treated in the same manner. Treatment for the common types of vaginitis is summarized in Table 35–3.

Condylomata Acuminata

Condylomata acuminata occur as papillomatous lesions on the vulva and may involve the vagina or cervix. The lesions may be small and discrete or large and cauliflower-like. They usually present as multiple small lesions, which have been called "venereal

Figure 35–2. Saline wet mount showing clue cells of bacterial vaginosis. Note the clear background.

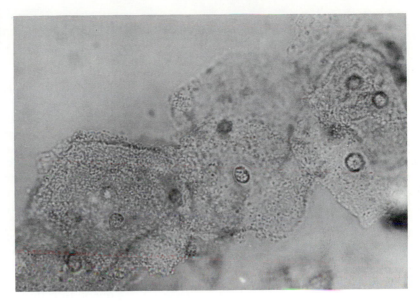

warts," and often occur in association with *Trichomonas vaginitis* and bacterial vaginosis.

The etiologic agent is the human papilloma virus, which is a member of the papovavirus group. It is transmitted by direct contact, usually sexual, and the lesions are much more profuse in patients who are pregnant, diabetic, on oral contraceptives, or on immunosuppressant therapy. Although the virus of the genital wart and that of the usual skin lesion appear similar under electron microscopy, they are antigenically different, subtypes 6 and 11 being responsible for genital warts.

Management. The first line of treatment for small isolated lesions on the vulva is weekly applications of 25 per cent trichloracetic acid. Podophyllin is sometimes used, but there is some question about its mutagenic effects. Care must be taken to protect the surrounding normal skin. If after 4 to 6 weeks of treatment the lesions persist or recur, other forms of desiccation may be used, such as cryosurgery, electrocautery treatment, or laser therapy. Occasionally, surgical extirpation is necessary. If biopsy or surgical excision is performed, the pathologist should be notified if podophyllin has been applied within the last 6 weeks, since this drug causes metaphase arrest, and its use can result in occasional bizarre mitoses, vacuolar degeneration, cellular necrosis, and an in-

flammatory response. These changes may be confused with malignancy. Podophyllin treatment should be avoided during pregnancy or if pregnancy is suspected, since maternal death, fetal death, and premature labor have been reported following its use.

In rare instances in which the warts are totally resistant or disseminated, such as seen in immunosuppressed patients, dinitrochlorobenzene (DNCB) sensitization followed by DNCB ointment application may be helpful. Spontaneous regression may occur, particularly if the lesions have appeared and grown rapidly during pregnancy. If the vagina is markedly involved during pregnancy, cesarean section should be considered as the method of delivery because of the possibility of extensive lacerations and the difficulty of suturing the wound edges.

Molluscum Contagiosum

Molluscum contagiosum is an epithelial proliferative process caused by a mildly contagious, growth-stimulating virus. The infection is transmitted by direct and indirect contact. Most patients with this disorder have no symptoms except occasional mild pruritus. Examination reveals multiple nodules varying in size from a pinhead to 1 cm in diameter on the vulva and perineal skin. The

Table 35–3. UNITED STATES PUBLIC HEALTH SERVICE RECOMMENDATIONS FOR FIRST-LINE THERAPY OF SEXUALLY TRANSMITTED DISEASES, 1989

HERPES SIMPLEX
First Episode — Recommended Regimen
Acyclovir 200 mg orally 5 times a day for 7 – 10 days or until clinical resolution occurs

Recurrent Episodes
Acyclovir 200 mg orally 5 times a day for 5 days
or
Acyclovir 800 mg orally 2 times a day for 5 days

Daily Suppressive Therapy
Acyclovir 200 mg orally 2 to 5 times a day
or
Acyclovir 400 mg orally 2 times a day

BACTERIAL VAGINOSIS
Recommended Regimen
Metronidazole 500 mg orally 2 times a day for 7 days

CANDIDIASIS
Recommended Regimens
Miconazole nitrate (vaginal suppository 200 mg), intravaginally at bedtime for 3 days
or
Clotrimazole (vaginal tablets 200 mg), intravaginally at bedtime for 3 days
or
Butaconazole (2% cream, 5 gm), intravaginally at bedtime for 3 days
or
Teraconazole 80 mg suppository or 0.4% cream, intravaginally at bedtime for 3 days.

TRICHOMONIASIS
Recommended Regimen
Metronidazole 2 g orally in a single dose

LYMPHOGRANULOMA VENEREUM
Recommended Regimen
Doxycycline 100 mg orally 2 times a day for 21 days

CHANCROID
Recommended Regimen
Erythromycin base 500 mg orally 4 times a day for 7 days
or
Ceftriaxone 250 mg intramuscularly in a single dose

typical lesion is a dome-shaped, reddish to yellow papule with an umbilicated center.

Treatment is to express the caseous content from each lesion manually, followed by an application of carbonic acid, trichloroacetic acid, or silver nitrate. An alternative method of therapy involves removing the papules with a small dermal curette and electrodesiccating the base.

Herpes Genitalis

Herpes genitalis is a venereal disease caused by the herpes simplex virus type II in 90 per cent of cases and herpes simplex virus type I in 10 per cent of cases. Both are DNA viruses. The symptoms of primary herpes infection usually appear within 3 to 7 days of exposure. The infection may be asymptomatic, since there are a number of patients who have antibodies against type II virus with no prior history of infection. Patients who have had oral herpes (type I virus) may have a degree of protection against subsequent infections with genital herpes (type II virus).

Clinical Features. In patients who become symptomatic, prodromal symptoms, such as mild paresthesia and burning in the perineal area, may be experienced before lesions become visible. The initial lesions may cause severe vulvar pain and exquisite tenderness. If the urethra or bladder mucosa is infected, urination may be extremely painful, and occasionally urinary retention occurs. Patients with primary infections usually have inguinal lymphadenopathy, generalized malaise, and a low-grade fever.

Physical findings depend on the stage of the lesions at presentation. The first manifestations are clear vesicles that involve the labia majora, labia minora, perineal skin, and vestibule of the vulva. The vagina and ectocervical mucosa may be involved. Lesions that primarily involve the vagina and ectocervix are usually asymptomatic. The vesicles rupture within 1 to 7 days and form ulcers. The ulcers are shallow but painful, and frequently each is surrounded by a red areola. Several small lesions may coalesce to form a large ulcer, the surface of which may become secondarily infected and necrotic. Small ulcers generally heal in 7 to 10 days. If superinfection is extensive, they may last for up to 6 weeks. When healing occurs, there is no residual scarring or ulceration.

Diagnosis. The diagnosis is made by the typical appearance of the vesicles and ulcers and the clinical syndrome. A cytologic smear of the ulcer base and cervix can confirm the diagnosis if it shows classic multinucleated cells with acidophilic intranuclear inclusion bodies. The false-negative rate is high, however. The definitive diagnosis is made by culture using Hanks' medium. It is important that the culture be taken of fluid from ruptured vesicles or that an ulcer be debrided and material taken from its base. False-negative cultures are frequent unless these precautions are observed.

Recurrence. About 30 per cent of patients who have had primary herpes develop recurrences. The virus migrates up nerve fibers to the dorsal root ganglia, where it usually remains dormant. A recurrence may be precipitated by an episode of stress, menstruation, or an upper respiratory illness. When recurrence occurs, the virus travels down the nerve fiber to the previously affected area. The resultant lesions are similar to those seen in the primary infection, although usually smaller. Local symptoms are generally of shorter duration, lesser severity, and seldom accompanied by systemic manifestations or inguinal lymphadenopathy.

Pregnancy. Genital infection during pregnancy secondary to herpes simplex virus types I and II is discussed in Chapter 16.

Management. A large number of therapeutic procedures have been recommended for herpes infections, but at the present time no effective treatment is available. Measures such as hot sitz baths and diluted Burow's solution may afford symptomatic relief. A Foley catheter may occasionally be required if voiding is difficult and painful. Acyclovir ointment, 5 per cent, which is an acyclic purine analog, may shorten the course of the initial attack and shorten the length of viral shedding if applied very early in the infection. This ointment regimen does not prevent recurrent infection, however, or have any impact on the time course of recurrent episodes. The frequency and severity of recurrent episodes may be helped by taking acyclovir tablets, 200 mg five times a day for 7 to 10 days or until clinical resolution occurs. Parenteral acyclovir is available for patients with severe disease and for immunocompromised patients with life-threatening infections.

Patients should be advised to abstain from sexual contact while lesions are present. If the infection is their first, they should continue to abstain until they become culture-negative, since prolonged viral shedding may occur in such cases. The risk of transmission during the asymptomatic period is unclear.

Syphilis

Syphilis is a sexually transmitted disease caused by *Treponema pallidum,* a motile anaerobic spirochete that invades intact moist mucosa.

Clinical Features. The vulva is the most frequent entry site in the female. About 10 to 60 days after inoculation, a chancre appears on the vulva, vagina, or cervix, heralding the stage of primary syphilis. The chancre is a firm, completely painless lesion with a punched out base and rolled edges. Painless inguinal lymphadenopathy usually occurs.

Diagnosis. The diagnosis is made by identifying the spirochete on dark-field microscopy of material scraped from the base of the chancre. If untreated, the chancre will heal spontaneously in 3 to 9 weeks. A serologic test for syphilis will be negative at this time but should be obtained for baseline documentation.

About 8 weeks after infection, or 3 to 6 weeks after the chancre appears, the patient usually develops systemic manifestations of secondary syphilis, including such symptoms as malaise, headache, anorexia, and a generalized maculopapular skin rash. At this time, the patient may develop condylomata lata on the vulva, perianal region, and upper thighs; these are broad exophytic excrescences that ulcerate and are highly contagious. Dark-field examination of material from these lesions reveals numerous spirochetes. Serologic tests for syphilis are generally positive at this stage.

If primary or secondary syphilis is not treated, the patient is at risk to develop tertiary syphilis, which may involve any organ system of the body. A rare manifestation is a gumma of the vulva, which appears as a nodule that enlarges, ulcerates, and becomes necrotic.

Management. Treatment of primary and secondary syphilis is benzathine penicillin G, 2.4 million units intramuscularly. An alternative is tetracycline, 500 mg orally four times daily for 15 days. For tertiary syphilis, the penicillin is given weekly for 3 weeks or the tetracycline is given for 30 days. Erythromycin, 500 mg orally four times daily for 15 days, can be used during pregnancy, if the patient is allergic to penicillin.

Chancroid

Chancroid is a highly contagious, sexually transmitted disease caused by the bacillus *Haemophilus ducreyi*. The disease is seen only in a few areas of the United States and occurs most frequently in tropical and subtropical climates.

Symptoms of vulvar pain and tenderness at the site of a small papule occur 3 to 5 days after exposure. The papule rapidly ulcerates and autoinoculation of adjacent areas may occur. The ulcers have a grayish base, a foul odor, and are very painful to the touch. Regional lymphadenopathy and subsequent bubo formation with suppuration frequently occur if the disease is not treated. Massive tissue destruction of the vulva and perineum may also occur if not treated.

The diagnosis is best documented by Gram's stain, culture, and biopsy. All three tests are needed, since the false-negative rate for each individual test is high.

The treatment for this disease is erythromycin, 500 mg orally four times daily for 7 days, or ceftriaxone, 250 mg intramuscularly in a single dose. An alternative is trimethoprim/sulfamethoxazole, 160/800 mg orally twice daily for 10 days.

Lymphogranuloma Venereum

Lymphogranuloma venereum is a venereal disease caused by *Chlamydia trachomatis* serotypes L-1, L-2, and L-3. *Chlamydia* organisms are obligatory intracellular parasites that are bacteria-like and definitely not viruses. Other serotypes cause psittacosis, trachoma, inclusion conjunctivitis, nongonococcal urethritis, salpingitis, and pneumonia of newborns. The disease is relatively uncommon in the United States and affects males 20 times more frequently than females.

Clinical Features. One to 4 weeks after the onset of infection, nonspecific symptoms, such as generalized malaise, headaches, and fever, may accompany the development of a papule, which subsequently develops into a painless vulvovaginal ulcer. This stage may not be clinically apparent but is followed about 1 month later by adenitis. Inguinal buboes develop frequently in males but are uncommon in females. In females, direct lymphatic spread occurs to the deep nodes around the anus and rectum. Occasionally, lymphatic involvement may be minimal, and spontaneous regression may occur. More often there is chronic progressive disease causing ulceration, elephantiasis, sinus tract formation, rectovaginal fistulas, abscesses, and secondary infection of the vulva and rectum. Rectal stenosis secondary to scarring may occur.

Diagnosis. The diagnosis is not easily made on the basis of history and physical examination. Biopsy examination is nonspecific and nondiagnostic. Complement fixation and microimmunofluorescence serologic tests for antibodies to *Chlamydia* (Frei test) are most helpful. Biological false-positive Venereal Disease Research Laboratory (VDRL) tests occur in about 20 per cent of patients.

Management. Treatment is tetracycline or erythromycin, 500 mg four times daily for 2 to 3 weeks. Alternative drugs are doxycycline, 100 mg twice daily for at least 3 weeks, or sulfamethoxazole, 1 gm twice daily for 3 weeks.

Granuloma Inguinale

Granuloma inguinale is caused by the bacterium *Donovania granulomatis*. It is uncommonly seen in the United States and occurs predominately in the black population.

Clinical Features. The condition begins with the appearance of a papule on the external genitalia approximately 1 to 12 weeks following initial contact. The papule rapidly ulcerates, and the ulcers are characterized by irregular borders and a beefy red granular base. The beginning papule and ulcer inoculate multiple adjacent sites. Progressively, there may be involvement of the perineum, perianal area, vagina, and cervix. The ulcers are painless. True bubo formation does not occur, although there may be some inguinal lymphadenopathy. As the ulcers become secondarily infected, fibrosis, scarring, depigmentation, and keloid formation characterize the advanced stage of the disease. Progressive fibrosis may lead to vaginal stenosis and elephantiasis, the latter secondary to lymphatic obstruction.

Diagnosis. The diagnosis is made by demonstrating Donovan bodies in tissue smears stained with Giemsa or Wright's stain. The Donovan body is an encapsulated bipolar staining bacterium with a reddish color found within the large mononuclear cells.

Management. Treatment is tetracycline in doses of 500 mg every 6 hours for 10 to 21 days. Healing should be expected within a period of 6 weeks. In cases that are unresponsive to this regimen, a longer course of treatment may be necessary.

TOXIC SHOCK SYNDROME

Toxic shock syndrome is a rare, potentially fatal, multisystem condition that is associated with strains of staphylococci capable of producing toxins, including an epidermal exfoliative toxin. The syndrome was originally described in children but has been recognized more recently in women, especially those under 30 years of age who are menstruating and using vaginal tampons. Toxic shock syndrome has also been noted rarely in association with other articles placed vaginally, such as diaphragms, sponges, and cervical caps, and may also be seen rarely in patients with postoperative wound infections, including infected episiotomies in the postpartum period. The clinical symptoms include a sudden high fever, flu-like symptoms (sore throat, headache, and especially diarrhea), erythroderma, signs of multisystemic failure, and refractory hypotension. Exfoliation of the palmar and plantar surfaces of the hands and feet as well as other skin surfaces usually occurs 1 to 2 weeks after the onset of the illness. Early recognition of the disease is of hallmark importance, for many of the deaths associated with this syndrome have occurred in patients who had been diagnosed incorrectly as having other potentially less dangerous illnesses such as allergic reactions, gastritis, or flu.

Management

Potential sources of infection such as foreign bodies or wound debris should be removed, along with extensive wound debridement and adequate hydration. Antibiotics specifically directed toward penicillinase-resistant *Staphylococcus aureus* should be used immediately. If steroids are begun within 72 hours, there appears to be a significant reduction in the severity of the overall illness and the duration of fever, but the use of steroids in this disease remains controversial.

Prognosis

If adequate supportive therapy is instituted early, full recovery can usually be expected. Multiple recurrences have been described in individual patients, although usually only one episode is encountered.

Prophylaxis

Tampons should be changed frequently during heavy flow or moderate flow days. Any objects designed for intravaginal use, especially the vaginal sponge, should be used with the knowledge that there is a potential for toxic shock syndrome, so patients should be informed of some of the clinical manifestations. Should any signs or symptoms of toxic shock syndrome occur, the patient should immediately remove the intravaginal product and seek emergency medical attention.

SUGGESTED READING

Bartlett JG, Moon NE, Goldstein PR, et al: Cervical and vaginal bacterial flora: Ecologic niches in the female lower genital tract. Am J Obstet Gynecol 130:658, 1978.

Davis JP, Chesney PJ, Wand PJ, et al: Toxic shock syndrome. N Engl J Med 303:1429, 1980.

Gardner HL: *Haemophilus vaginalis* vaginitis after twenty-five years. Am J Obstet Gynecol 137:385, 1980.

Hammill H, Kaufman RH: Vaginal candidiasis: Tailoring the treatment. The Female Patient 14:49, 1989.

Kutzer E, Oittner R, Leodolter S, Brammer KW: A comparison of fluconazole and ketoconazole in the oral treatment of vaginal candidiasis: Report of a double-blind multicentre study. Eur J Obstet Gynecol Reprod Biol 29:305, 1988.

Mehta P: Vaginal flora: A dynamic ecosystem. J Reprod Med 27:455, 1982.

Sikat P, Heemstra J, Ranney B, et al: Metronidazole chemotherapy for *Trichomonas vaginalis* infections. JAMA 182:904, 1980.

Sobel JD: Recurrent vulvovaginal candidiasis. N Engl J Med 315:1455, 1986.

Spiegel CA, Amsel R, Eschenbach D, et al: Anaerobic bacteria in nonspecific vaginitis. N Engl J Med 303:601, 1980.

Toxic shock syndrome update. FDA Drug Bulletin 10(3):17, 1980.

Weaver CH, Mengel MB: Bacterial vaginosis. J Fam Pract 27:207, 1988.

Thirty-six

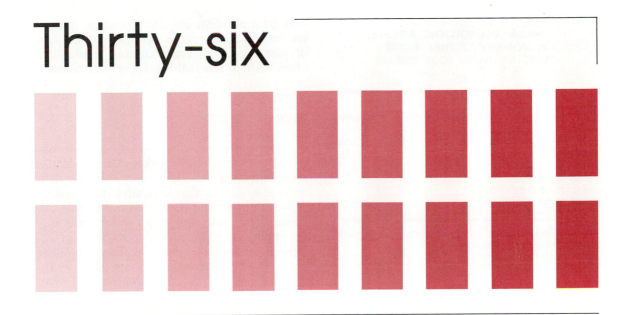

Pelvic Inflammatory Disease

LARRY C. FORD AND HUNTER A. HAMMILL

Pelvic inflammatory disease (PID) comprises a spectrum of inflammatory disorders of the upper genital tract, including endometritis, salpingitis, tubo-ovarian abscess, and pelvic peritonitis.

Infections of the female reproductive organs are a major cause of morbidity in gynecologic patients. Fortunately, new concepts regarding etiology and management are evolving. A better understanding of the bacteria involved in these infections is now available, and the continued proliferation of newer, broader-spectrum antibiotics has made successful therapy more feasible, particularly for early infections. In this chapter, PID occurring in nonpregnant patients is discussed and is divided into salpingo-oophoritis and tubo-ovarian abscess.

SALPINGO-OOPHORITIS

In the past, salpingo-oophoritis was considered to be either gonococcal or nongonococ-cal. More recently, it has been shown that many bacterial species may be involved.

Etiology

Apart from *Neisseria gonorrhoeae,* a variety of other microorganisms have been isolated from surgically obtained specimens of patients with acute salpingitis (Table 36–1). Whether these agents are pathogenic or are merely colonizing the tubes is a question that is not completely resolved, but current evidence favors a multibacterial etiology. Sexual activity is responsible for spreading the organisms, and usually numerous bacteria are transmitted. For example, *N. gonorrhoeae* may be passed, together with *Chlamydia, Mycoplasma,* and herpes simplex type II virus.

Acute PID sometimes may be exacerbated by menses, sexual intercourse, strenuous

Table 36–1. ETIOLOGIC AGENTS IN NONGESTATIONAL ACUTE PELVIC INFLAMMATORY DISEASE

Neisseria gonorrhoeae
Anaerobic bacteria (*Bacteroides* and gram-positive cocci)
Facultative gram-negative rods (such as *Escherichia coli*)
Chlamydia trachomatis
Mycoplasma hominis
Ureaplasma urealyticum
Actinomyces israelii

Note: In the individual patient, it is often impossible to differentiate among these agents.
Information obtained from Sexually Transmitted Diseases, Treatment Guidelines: 1989. US Department of Health and Human Services, Centers for Disease Control. MMWR 38(suppl): No. 5–8.

physical activity, and even a pelvic examination. The relationship to the menstrual period has been postulated to be due to the breakdown of the antibacterial barrier of cervical mucus, allowing infectious agents present in the lower genital tract to ascend to the upper tract. The potential pathogens may also 'cling' to sperm and be carried to the upper genital tract to potentiate infections.

A special situation is the presence of a nonvenereally transmitted infection in the presence of an intrauterine device (IUD). Such infections may be unilateral, and *Actinomyces israelii* may sometimes be isolated, especially if the IUD has been present for several years.

Clinical Features

The diagnosis of acute salpingo-oophoritis is made frequently but often inappropriately. The patient usually presents with lower quadrant pain, which is frequently bilateral. She may have recently started her menses. Occasionally, presenting symptoms may be nausea, dysuria, and a purulent vaginal discharge. On physical examination, the patient is usually febrile and has a tachycardia and a normal blood pressure. There is generalized lower abdominal tenderness without palpable masses. On speculum examination, there may be a purulent cervical discharge. Bimanual examination reveals cervical motion tenderness and bilateral adnexal tenderness, often without adnexal masses or induration.

Investigations

A *complete blood count* should be obtained. A neutrophil leukocytosis indicates acute infection. An elevated *erythrocyte sedimentation rate* is also indicative of infection. A *urinalysis* should be carried out to rule out urinary tract infection. A *pregnancy test* may be important if there is a possibility of ectopic pregnancy. A *cervical culture* should be obtained. The presence of gram-negative intracellular diplococci (*N. gonorrhoeae*) on a cervical smear is helpful in making the diagnosis.

Secondary diagnostic tests include *culdocentesis* and *pelvic ultrasonography*. Culdocentesis involves inserting an 18- or 20-gauge needle through the posterior vaginal fornix into the cul-de-sac. A mass in the cul-de-sac is a contraindication to the procedure. If purulent or serous material is obtained, it should be Gram stained and cultures for aerobes, anaerobes, and *N. gonorrhoeae* obtained. Pelvic ultrasonography is useful to define an adnexal mass, especially if an ectopic pregnancy is being considered.

The Infectious Disease Society for Obstetrics and Gynecology has suggested that certain criteria be present before the diagnosis of acute salpingo-oophoritis is made. These are shown in Table 36–2.

Differential Diagnosis

The differential diagnosis must include acute appendicitis, urinary tract infection, adnexal torsion, endometriosis, bleeding corpus luteum, and ectopic pregnancy.

The only definitive method of establishing the diagnosis of acute salpingo-oophoritis is by laparoscopy or laparotomy. Although not necessary for most patients, laparoscopy is strongly advised in those in whom the diagnosis is not clinically apparent or in whom the response to antibiotic therapy is inappropriate.

Table 36-2. CRITERIA FOR DIAGNOSIS OF ACUTE SALPINGO-OOPHORITIS*

Abdominal tenderness
Cervical motion tenderness
Adnexal tenderness

These should be accompanied by at least one of the following:

Elevated erythrocyte sedimentation rate
Leukocytosis
Purulent cervical discharge (defined as greater than 6 WBC/hpf)†
Purulent fluid obtained at culdocentesis
Oral temperature greater than 100.4°F (38°C)

* As outlined by the Infectious Disease Society for Obstetrics and Gynecology.
† White blood cells/high-power field.

Treatment

Drug Therapy

A variety of chemotherapeutic agents are used in the management of patients with PID, and the choice of agents is somewhat empirical (Table 36–3). An overview of the agents that are of most value follows.

Penicillins. When penicillin first became available, most organisms, including the enteric and anaerobic organisms, were sensitive to it. The use and abuse of penicillin and other antibiotics, however, have resulted in many organisms becoming resistant to drugs to which they were once sensitive. Because penicillin was among the first antibiotics to be isolated, it has seen the most number of "generations" or derivatives.

Of the first-generation penicillins, penicillin G is the model. These first-generation drugs are indicated for the therapy of syphilis and most streptococcal infections. In doses greater than 15 million units per day, the drug has some activity against nonpenicillinase-producing anaerobic bacteria. Most *Proteus* and *Pseudomonas* species, however, as well as many of the enteric organisms, are now resistant.

Second-generation penicillins, such as ampicillin and amoxicillin, have the advantage of oral as well as parenteral administration. They are also inactivated by penicillinase-producing bacteria. Amoxicillin, the hydroxy derivative of ampicillin, has increased gastrointestinal absorption and causes less gastrointestinal irritation. Second-generation penicillins have greater activity against enteric organisms but less anaerobic coverage, since they are active only in doses greater than 12 gm per day.

Of the third-generation penicillins, carbenicillin and ticarcillin are commonly used. Their advantage includes some enhanced anaerobic and enteric coverage. In particular, *Pseudomonas* coverage is enhanced. A disadvantage is the high sodium load, especially with carbenicillin.

Currently, two fourth-generation penicillins have been approved by the Food and Drug Administration (FDA) for use in the United States: piperacillin and mezlocillin. Their sodium loads are much lower than those of the third-generation drugs. The anaerobic spectrum is excellent, as is the enteric coverage. For example, mezlocillin covers greater than 90 per cent of *Clostridium* species and has pseudomonal and enteric coverage comparable to the aminoglycosides but without eighth cranial nerve toxicity.

Cephalosporins. The first-generation cephalosporins, such as cephalothin, cover many strains of the gram-positive cocci and *Escherichia coli*. The disadvantage of all first-generation cephalosporins is weak to absent enterococcal and anaerobic coverage.

The second-generation cephalosporins, such as cefoxitin, cefotetan and cefamandole,

Table 36-3. RATIONALE FOR SELECTION OF ANTIMICROBIALS FOR ACUTE PELVIC INFLAMMATORY DISEASE

Treatment of choice is not established
No single agent is active against the entire spectrum of pathogens
Several antimicrobial combinations provide a broad spectrum of activity against the major pathogens in vitro, but many have not been adequately evaluated for clinical efficacy in PID.

Information obtained from Sexually Transmitted Diseases, Treatment Guidelines: 1982. US Department of Health and Human Services, Centers for Disease Control. MMWR 31(suppl):33S, 1982.

differ in their in vitro spectrum. The enteric coverage of cefamandole is better than that of cefoxitin, whereas the antianaerobic activity of cefoxitin and cefotetan is clearly superior to that of cefamandole. Cefotetan has a longer half-life and hence needs less frequent dosage.

The role of third-generation cephalosporins, such as moxalactam, cefoperazone, ceftazidime, and cefotaxime, is limited in obstetrics and gynecology. Their purported advantages include enhanced in vitro anaerobic coverage over the first-generation cephalosporins and increased *Pseudomonas* coverage. They have, as yet, an unproved role as monotherapy for serious pelvic infections. The addition of a third-generation cephalosporin to a standard therapy combination, such as an aminoglycoside and clindamycin or an aminoglycoside plus a penicillin and chloramphenicol, adds nothing to the bacterial coverage. They also have no proved advantage over cefoxitin or cefotetan for prophylaxis.

Imipenem/cilastin is a potent, broad-spectrum antibacterial agent with superb anaerobic as well as enteric coverage, which can usually be used as a single agent for serious gynecologic infections.

Metronidazole. Metronidazole (Flagyl) covers many anaerobic bacteria but has no aerobic coverage, with the exception of *Gardnerella vaginalis.* Therefore, when used for therapy of serious infections, the drug must always be used in combination with other antibiotics, usually an aminoglycoside and frequently also a penicillin or cephalosporin.

Side effects can include an unpleasant metallic taste in the mouth and, rarely, reversible leukopenia. The drug is related to disulfiram (Antabuse), so there are severe untoward reactions with concomitant ethanol ingestion. Metronidazole has been shown to be mutagenic by the Salmonella Mammalian Microsome (Ames) Test and, therefore, should be avoided during pregnancy.

Clindamycin. Clindamycin is a member of the macrolide family, which also includes erythromycin. The drug has excellent activity against anaerobic organisms and aerobic gram-positive cocci but weaker activity against enteric bacteria. Therefore, it is usually combined with an aminoglycoside for the treatment of severe infections.

Diarrhea occurs in 5 to 10 per cent of patients. Although widely publicized, true pseudomembranous enterocolitis, which is caused by *Clostridium difficile,* is rare. In fact, ampicillin, because of its very broad usage, causes more cases per year of pseudomembranous enterocolitis than does clindamycin. If a patient develops diarrhea while taking clindamycin, urgent investigations should include (1) stool cultures for *C. difficile* using selective media that can give results in 12 hours and (2) serum antibody titers to *C. difficile* toxin. If either result is positive or if these tests cannot be performed rapidly, the clindamycin should be stopped.

Clindamycin combined with an aminoglycoside is a very effective treatment for most patients with severe pelvic infections.

Tetracycline. Tetracyclines have long been used for the outpatient treatment of PID. The advantages of these drugs include oral absorption, reasonable aerobic and anaerobic coverage, and chlamydial coverage. All tetracyclines are absolutely contraindicated in patients who are or might be pregnant because of their damaging effect on the fetal teeth.

There are two generations of tetracyclines. Second-generation drugs, which include minocycline and doxycycline, have some *in vitro* advantages over first-generation tetracyclines — in particular, better anaerobic coverage. The main advantage of the second-generation drugs is their higher compliance rate because of the once or twice daily dosage. In addition, minocycline has some antifungal activity; hence the incidence of superinfections with yeast is lower than with simple tetracycline.

Chloramphenicol. Chloramphenicol diffuses well into tissues after oral or parenteral administration and has excellent anaerobic and aerobic coverage. A rare side effect is idiosyncratic, irreversible aplastic anemia. The true incidence of this complication is probably less than one in 100,000 cases. There is a dose-dependent reversible bone marrow depression, primarily of the leukocyte series. The drug is not used routinely as first-line therapy, mainly for medicolegal reasons. If the patient is in septic shock, however, chloramphenicol should be added to the usual combination of antibiotics.

Aminoglycosides. The aminoglycosides, such as gentamicin, amikacin, and tobramycin, have excellent activity against enteric

Table 36–4. OUTPATIENT TREATMENT OPTIONS FOR ACUTE PELVIC INFLAMMATORY DISEASE

Cefoxitin 2.0 gm intramuscularly, with probenecid, 1.0 gm orally

or

Ceftriaxone 250 mg intramuscularly

or

Equivalent cephalosporin

plus

Doxycycline 100 mg orally 2 times daily for 10–14 days

Information obtained from Sexually Transmitted Diseases, Treatment Guidelines: 1989. US Department of Health and Human Services, Centers for Disease Control. MMWR 38(suppl):No. 5–8.

organisms, but they have no anaerobic activity. Therefore, aminoglycosides should never be used as single agents to treat PID.

Renal toxicity is the most common complication of aminoglycoside administration, and particular caution is necessary if the patient has had previous exposure to another nephrotoxin, such as cis-platinum. It is important to obtain blood urea nitrogen, serum creatinine, and, sometimes, creatinine clearance levels prior to the administration of aminoglycosides. In addition, therapeutic levels should be maintained by monitoring "peak" and "trough" levels of the drug in the serum. These levels should be attained on the second or third day of therapy and every other day thereafter. Tobramycin appears to have the least renal toxicity, so it should be used if there is any impairment of renal function.

Eighth cranial nerve toxicity, both auditory and vestibular, is also a complication associated with aminoglycosides. It is seldom seen in gynecologic infections, however, because treatment courses rarely exceed 10 days. Neuromuscular blockade is a rare complication.

Outpatient Management

When the symptoms are mild, particularly with recurrent episodes of PID, outpatient treatment may be sufficient, as shown in Table 36–4. Strict pelvic rest (no sexual ac-

tivity, no douching, no tampons) is necessary, and bed rest should be advised while there is fever or systemic symptoms.

The second-generation tetracyclines have better gonococcal coverage (including penicillinase-producing gonococci), reasonable aerobic and anaerobic coverage, and chlamydial coverage. Minocycline has been approved by the FDA for both male and female chlamydial infections.

Oral penicillins, including oral penicillin VK, ampicillin, amoxicillin, and carbenicillin, have poor activity against the mixed infections. In addition, although they have some activity against gonococci if given in high enough dosages, they have no antichlamydial activity. Oral cephalosporins have no antianaerobic activity. Like the penicillins, they do have antigonococcal coverage.

Sexual partners should be examined and treated promptly with a regimen effective against uncomplicated gonococcal and chlamydial infection. The patient should be re-evaluated clinically in 48 to 72 hours, and those not responding well should be hospitalized. A repeat culture should be taken to ensure cure. If the patient has an IUD in situ, it should be removed soon after antimicrobial therapy has been initiated.

Treatment of Uncomplicated Gonorrhea

The treatment of uncomplicated gonorrhea, which is usually diagnosed on a routine cervical culture or by a history of recently diagnosed gonorrhea in a sexual partner, is complicated by the following: (1) the increasing incidence of penicillinase-producing N. gonorrhoeae, (2) the emergence of tetracycline-resistant gonococci in some geographic areas, and (3) the high frequency of coexisting chlamydial infection, which has been documented in up to 45 per cent of patients with gonorrhea for whom adequate chlamydial cultures have been undertaken. Regimens recommended by the United States Department of Health and Human Services are shown in Table 36–5.

Generally, patients with gonorrhea should be treated simultaneously with antibiotics effective against both C. trachomatis and N. gonorrhoeae. The FDA has approved norfloxin, 800 mg in a single oral dose. The

Table 36-5. GONOCOCCAL INFECTIONS: TREATMENT OF ADULTS

Recommended regimen for uncomplicated urethral, endocervical, or rectal infections.
Norofloxin 800 mg orally once or ceftriaxone 250 mg intramuscularly once
                    plus
Doxycycline 100 mg orally 2 times a day for 7 days

Comment: Some authorities prefer a dose of 125 mg ceftriaxone intramuscularly because it is less expensive and can be given in a volume of only 0.5 ml, which is more easily administered in the deltoid muscle. The 250 mg dose is recommended, however, because it may delay the emergence of ceftriaxone-resistant strains. At this time, both doses appear highly effective for mucosal gonorrhea at all sites.

Information obtained from Sexually Transmitted Diseases, Treatment Guidelines: 1989. US Department of Health and Human Services, Centers for Disease Control. MMWR 38(suppl):No. 5-8.

advantages include activity against penicillinase-producing *N. gonorrhoeae.*

Inpatient Therapy

Patients with acute PID, especially the first episode, generally benefit from early hospitalization and intensive therapy. The indications for hospitalization are shown in Table 36-6.

Empiric therapy, based on probable etiologic agents, should be commenced immediately after the diagnosis is made. Cervical and vaginal cultures are not helpful as a basis for the selection of antibiotic agents. Even if

Table 36-6. HOSPITALIZATION OF WOMEN WITH ACUTE SALPINGO-OOPHORITIS

The diagnosis is uncertain
Surgical emergencies, such as appendicitis and ectopic pregnancy, must be excluded
Pelvic abscess is suspected
Severe illness precludes outpatient management
Patient is pregnant
Patient is unable to follow or tolerate an outpatient regimen
Patient has failed to respond to outpatient therapy
Clinical follow-up after 48-72 hr of antibiotic treatment cannot be arranged

Information obtained from Sexually Transmitted Diseases, Treatment Guidelines: 1982. US Department of Health and Human Services, Centers for Disease Control. MMWR 31(suppl):335, 1982.

Table 36-7. RECOMMENDED REGIMEN FOR INPATIENT TREATMENT OF PELVIC INFLAMMATORY DISEASE

Cefoxitin 2.0 gm IV every 6 hr
                    or
Cefotetan 2.0 gm IV every 12 hr
                    plus
Doxycycline 100 mg every 12 hr orally or IV

This regimen is given for at least 48 hr after the patient clinically improves. Doxycycline 100 mg orally 2 times a day is taken after the patient is discharged from the hospital, to complete a total of 10-14 days of therapy

Alternative Regimen
Clindamycin 900 mg IV every 8 hr
                    plus
Loading dose of gentamicin 2.0 mg/kg IV followed by a maintenance dose of 1.5 mg/kg IV every 8 hr

This regimen is given for at least 48 hr after the patient improves, following which the patient is discharged on doxycycline 100 mg orally twice daily to complete a total of 10-14 days of therapy

Imipenem/cilastatin 500 mg IV every 8 hr

This regimen is given for at least 48 hr after the patient clinically improves. Doxycycline 100 mg orally twice a day is taken after the patient is discharged from the hospital to complete a total of 10-14 days of therapy

cultures are obtained at laparoscopy or laparotomy, placed immediately in anaerobic transport devices, and rushed to the laboratory, it takes at least 3 days for the identification of anaerobic organisms and even longer to obtain antibiotic sensitivities. In view of the spectrum of bacteria known to be involved in the pathogenesis of PID, it is always desirable to cover anaerobic organisms shown in Table 36-1. Regimens recommended by the United States Department of Health and Human Services are shown in Table 36-7. Continuation of doxycycline for 10 to 14 days is important for the eradication of possible *C. trachomatis* infection.

TUBO-OVARIAN ABSCESS

Clinical Features

Patients with an acute tubo-ovarian abscess are usually very ill with severe pelvic and lower abdominal pain, high fever, prostration, nausea and vomiting, and possible septic shock.

Physical examination reveals a rapid pulse and a fever that may be up to 103°F (39.5°C). Abdominal examination reveals marked tenderness, muscular rigidity, occasionally a mass arising from the pelvis, and often rebound tenderness. Speculum examination should be performed to obtain a cervical smear for Gram staining as well as aerobic, anaerobic, and gonococcal cultures. Digital pelvic examination is usually very difficult because of extreme adnexal tenderness. An adnexal mass may be appreciated. On rectal examination, it is usually easier to feel a pelvic mass, which may be pointing into the cul-de-sac.

Differential Diagnosis

In the presence of severe lower abdominal pain, fever, leukocytosis, and a tender adnexal mass, the differential diagnosis must include the following disorders.

Septic Incomplete Abortion. Although illegal abortions are now much less common than in earlier years, this possibility should be kept in mind, particularly since uterine rupture and virulent organisms such as *Clostridium perfringens* may be involved.

Acute Appendicitis. The pain of acute appendicitis typically commences in the periumbilical region and subsequently localizes to the right lower quadrant. If the appendix perforates, with resultant peritonitis or appendiceal abscess formation, differentiation may be impossible without a laparotomy.

Diverticular Abscess. Particularly if the mass is on the left side of the pelvis, diverticular abscess should be considered. Usually the patient will have a history of previous episodes of diverticulitis, and a barium enema will reveal the typical features.

Adnexal Torsion. This problem is more likely if an ovarian cyst or hydrosalpinx is present. It may cause necrosis and rupture, closely simulating a tubo-ovarian abscess clinically. Fever and leukocytosis are usually much less impressive, but laparotomy is required if torsion appears likely.

Other Diagnoses. Other possible differential diagnoses include perforated peptic ulcer, pancreatitis, and mesenteric artery thrombosis.

Treatment

Patients with tubo-ovarian abscess should be treated with bed rest in the hospital, adequate oral and intravenous fluids, analgesics, and systemic antibiotics. Clindamycin plus an aminoglycoside are usually used or imipenem/cilastin. Even large abscesses may resolve without the need for acute surgical intervention.

The timing of any operative intervention requires clinical judgment. Rupture of the abscess with signs of generalized peritonitis requires urgent laparotomy to remove the infected organs, afford drainage, and lavage the peritoneal cavity. Traditionally, total (or subtotal) abdominal hysterectomy and bilateral salpingo-oophorectomy have been performed for ruptured tubo-ovarian abscess. Unilateral lesions do occur, however, particularly in women who have used IUDs. For such patients, unilateral salpingo-oophorectomy may be appropriate.

If the abscess is soft and fluctuant and is pointing into the cul-de-sac, as indicated by heat and edema of the posterior fornix, posterior colpotomy to allow drainage usually produces dramatic results. When the patient fails to respond to approximately 72 hours of multiagent broad-spectrum chemotherapy, with persistently spiking fever and pelvic and abdominal tenderness, laparotomy with extraperitoneal drainage is indicated if the abscess is not accessible to drainage through the vagina.

CHRONIC PELVIC INFLAMMATORY DISEASE

Clinical Features

Long-term sequelae of PID may include chronic pelvic pain, menometrorrhagia, dyspareunia, infertility, and ectopic pregnancy. Sterile hydrosalpinges or pyosalpinges, with multiple pelvic adhesions, may result, particularly if proper antibiotic therapy was not instituted early in the course of the acute episode of infection.

On physical examination, there is usually some lower abdominal tenderness. Pelvic examination may reveal tenderness in both adnexal regions, or there may be palpable masses and induration from hydrosalpinges or chronic abscesses. Hydrosalpinges may occasionally be quite large and mistaken for ovarian cysts. In long-standing cases, progressive adhesion formation may produce the so-called frozen pelvis, in which internal genital organs are fixed to the pelvic side walls by the indurated supporting ligaments. The uterus may be deviated from the midline or fixed in the cul-de-sac.

Differential Diagnosis

The most common problem clinically is to differentiate chronic PID from endometriosis, particularly if there is no well-documented history of acute infection. A normal sedimentation rate favors endometriosis. A number of conditions may be confused with chronic PID, however, including pelvic pain syndrome, pelvic tuberculosis, inflammatory bowel diseases, and pelvic malignancies. Often the diagnosis cannot be made without laparoscopy or laparotomy.

Treatment

In patients with less severe involvement who wish to become pregnant, various types of tuboplasties may be undertaken. For patients with more severe disease, medical management of large hydrosalpinges is disappointing, and, frequently, control of pelvic pain will necessitate total abdominal hysterectomy and bilateral salpingo-oophorectomy. Replacement hormonal therapy must then be administered to control hot flashes and prevent osteoporosis.

Prevention of Pelvic Inflammatory Disease

The sexually transmitted acquired immunodeficiency syndrome (AIDS) caused by the human immunodeficiency virus (HIV) should be considered the ultimate PID. AIDS, thus far, is always lethal. The "Safe Sexual Practices," as outlined by the Surgeon General of the United States, has in some sections of the population reduced the incidence of PID and decreased the spread of AIDS. The use of condoms as well as broad-spectrum polyantimicrobial vaginal suppositories (Inner Confidence) should decrease the spread of AIDS, PID, and vaginitis.

SUGGESTED READING

ACOG Technical Bulletin. Antimicrobial therapy for gynecologic infections. No 153, March 1991.

Centers for Disease Control. 1989 Sexually transmitted diseases treatment guidelines. MMWR 38:31, 1989.

Crombleholme WR, Ohm-Smith M, Robbie MO, et al: Ampicillin/sulbactam versus metronidazole-gentamicin in the treatment of soft tissue pelvic infections. Am J Obstet Gynecol 156:507, 1987.

Donowitz GR, Mandell GL: Beta-lactam antibiotics. N Engl J Med 318:419 & 490, 1988.

Hager WD, Pascuzzi M, and Vernon M: Efficacy of oral antibiotics following parenteral antibiotics for serious infections in obstetrics and gynecology. Obstet Gynecol 73:326, 1989.

Sweet RL: Imipenem/cilastatin in the treatment of obstetric and gynecologic infections: A review of worldwide experience. Rev Infect Dis 7(3 suppl):S522, 1985.

Styrt B, Gorbach SL: Recent developments in the understanding of the pathogenesis and treatment of anaerobic infections. N Engl J Med 321:240, 1989.

Toth A: Alternative causes of pelvic inflammatory disease. J Reprod Med 28:699, 1983.

Walters MD, Gibbs RS: A randomized comparison of gentamicin/clindamycin and cefoxitin-doxycycline in the treatment of acute pelvic inflammatory disease. Obstet Gynecol 75:867, 1990.

Thirty-seven

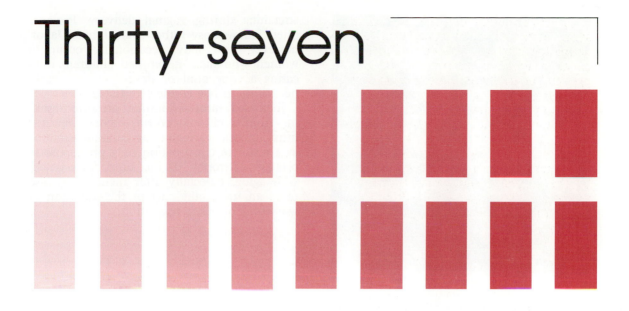

Pelvic Relaxation and Urinary Problems

NARENDER N. BHATIA

The pelvic organs, including the vagina, uterus, bladder, and rectum, are maintained in position by supporting ligaments, fascia, and pelvic floor muscles. The cardinal and uterosacral ligaments assist in maintaining the uterus in an anteflexed position and in preventing its descensus through the urogenital diaphragm. When these supports become damaged, one or more of the pelvic organs may prolapse within and, occasionally, protrude outside the vagina.

PROLAPSE

There are several types of genital prolapses. They may occur singly but are more commonly combined.

Uterine Prolapse

Although vaginal prolapse can occur without uterine prolapse, the uterus cannot descend without carrying the upper vagina with it. When the cervix remains within the vagina, it is called a first-degree prolapse. When the cervix protrudes beyond the introitus, it becomes a second-degree prolapse. A third-degree prolapse, or complete procidentia, implies descent of the entire uterus outside the vulva (Fig. 37–1).

Complete procidentia represents failure of all the genital supports. Hypertrophy, elongation, congestion, and edema of the cervix may sometimes cause a large protrusion of tissue beyond the introitus, which may be mistaken for a procidentia.

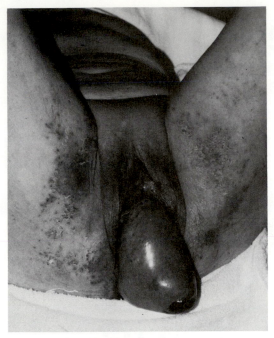

Figure 37–1. Complete procidentia. Note the ulceration of the cervix.

Vaginal Prolapse

The bulging or descent of the bladder into the upper anterior vaginal wall is called a cystocele (Fig. 37–2). It represents a weakness in the investing fascia of the vagina (pubocervical fascia). The bulging of the urethra into the lower anterior vaginal wall should be called urethral displacement. Older terminology would depict this as a urethrocele; however, there is no dilatation of the urethra in this condition.

Upper posterior vaginal wall prolapse is nearly always associated with herniation of the pouch of Douglas, and, since this is likely to contain loops of bowel, it is called an enterocele. Lower posterior vaginal wall prolapse is called a rectocele.

Vaginal vault prolapse or inversion of the vagina may be seen after vaginal or abdominal hysterectomy and represents failure of the supports around the upper vagina.

Etiology of Prolapse

The pelvic fascia, ligaments, and muscles may become attenuated from excessive stretching during vaginal delivery. Prolapse often follows easy rather than difficult labor, however, and may occasionally occur in women who have never had children, indicating a congenital or developmental weakness of the pelvic connective tissues.

Increased intra-abdominal pressure resulting from a chronic cough, ascites, repeated lifting of heavy weights, or habitual straining as a result of constipation may predispose to prolapse. Atrophy of the supporting tissues with aging, especially after menopause, also plays an important part in the initiation or worsening of pelvic relaxation.

Symptoms

The amount of discomfort and inconvenience experienced by a patient with prolapse is extremely variable. Often there is a feeling of heaviness or fullness in the pelvis. Patients may describe "something falling out" or a bearing down discomfort. Some patients may complain of backache at the level of the sacrum. The characteristic of nearly all symptoms is that they are worse after prolonged standing and immediately and completely relieved by lying down.

When the prolapse is extreme, the patient may experience difficulty in walking because of the exposed positions of the uterus, bladder, and rectum. Neglected cases of procidentia may be complicated by excessive purulent discharge, decubitus ulceration, bleeding, and, rarely, carcinoma of the cervix.

Symptoms of urinary frequency and urgency, urinary incontinence, and, occasionally, urinary retention may be seen in patients with anterior vaginal wall prolapse. Patients with a rectocele may have difficulty empting the rectum. Many of them learn to splint the posterior vaginal wall by placing two fingers along it to keep the rectocele from protruding during a bowel movement.

Diagnosis

Vaginal examination should be performed by using a Sim's speculum or by taking a standard Graves' speculum and removing the

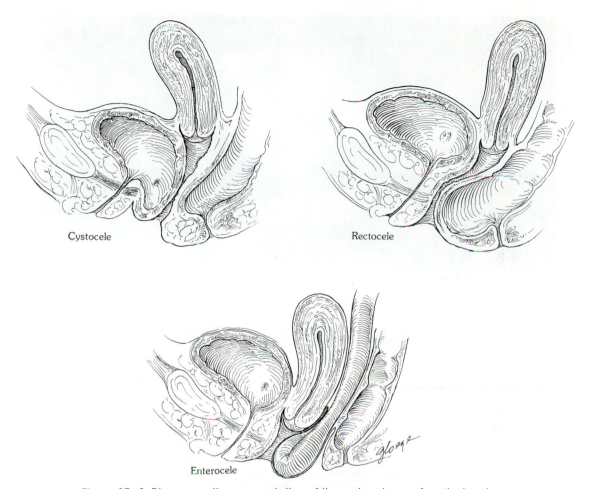

Figure 37–2. Diagrammatic representation of the various types of vaginal prolapse.

anterior blade. While depressing the posterior vaginal wall, the patient is asked to strain down. This will demonstrate the descent of the anterior vaginal wall consistent with cystocele and urethral displacement. Similarly, retraction of the anterior vaginal wall during straining demonstrates an enterocele and rectocele. Rectal examination is often useful to demonstrate a rectocele and to distinguish it from an enterocele.

Minor degrees of uterine prolapse may be recognized only by feeling descent of the cervix when the patient is straining. Occasionally, it is necessary to test for uterine prolapse by pulling on the cervix with a tenaculum. If there is doubt about the presence of prolapse, the patient may be asked to stand or walk for some time before the examination.

Treatment

Although treatment of pelvic relaxation is primarily surgical, nonoperative approaches may be used initially. The patient's age, marital status, desire for further childbearing, sexual activity, degree of prolapse, and presence or absence of associated pathologic conditions should be taken into consideration before institution of treatment. If it is difficult to be certain whether the prolapse is responsible for the symptoms, a trial of pessary may be undertaken.

Nonsurgical Treatment

When there is only a mild degree of pelvic relaxation, perineal exercises may improve

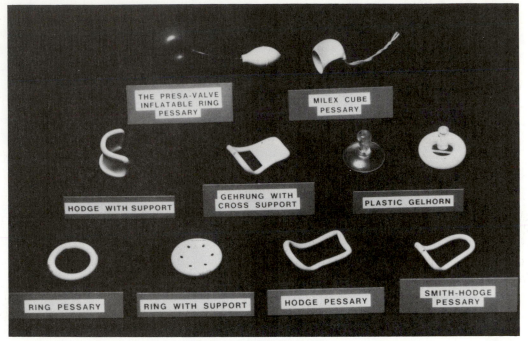

Figure 37–3. Vaginal pessaries.

the tone of the pelvic floor musculature. Their effect is limited, however, because they do not enhance support from the fascia and ligaments.

Pessaries may be used to correct prolapse in the following situations: (1) if the patient is medically unfit for surgery, (2) during pregnancy and the postpartum period, and (3) to promote healing of a decubitus ulcer before surgery. Pessaries require a great deal of care to avoid vaginal infection and leukorrhea. A variety of pessaries are shown in Figure 37–3.

Surgical Treatment

Surgical repair is the most satisfactory therapy, and the results are very good. Many surgical procedures have been proposed to correct the pelvic support defects.

Anterior Colporrhaphy. This is used to correct a cystocele and urethral displacement. It involves plication of the pubocervical fascia to support the bladder and urethra.

Posterior Colporrhaphy. This is the equivalent operation on the posterior vaginal wall. The endopelvic fascia and the perineal muscles are approximated in the midline to support the rectum and perineum.

Repair of Enterocele. The repair of an enterocele follows the general principles of hernia repair. The contents are reduced, the neck of the peritoneal sac is ligated, and the defect is repaired by approximating the uterosacral ligaments and levator ani muscles.

Manchester Operation. This operation combines anterior colporrhaphy, amputation of the cervix, posterior colpoperineorrhaphy, and suturing of the cardinal ligaments in front of the cervical stump to antevert the uterus. It is a low morbidity operation, and the uterus is preserved.

Vaginal Hysterectomy. This may be performed alone or in conjunction with anterior and posterior colporrhaphy. It may be used for any degree of uterine descent but is especially useful for procidentia.

LeFort's Partial Colpocleisis. This operation may be performed in elderly patients with substantial uterine prolapse. It involves suturing the partially denuded anterior and posterior vaginal walls together in such a way that the uterus is supported above the partially occluded vagina.

Vaginal Vault Suspension. When vaginal prolapse occurs following hysterectomy, it can be repaired by suspending the vaginal vault from the sacrum or sacrospinous ligaments. The procedure can be approached either vaginally or abdominally.

Complete Colpocleisis. This procedure may be performed for vaginal inversion after hysterectomy in older patients who are no longer sexually active. It involves total obliteration of the vagina.

URINARY INCONTINENCE

There are four common types of urinary incontinence: (1) stress incontinence, (2) total incontinence, (3) urge incontinence, and (4) overflow incontinence.

Anatomy and Physiology of the Lower Urinary Tract

The bladder detrusor is a smooth muscle appearing as a meshwork of fibers that are recognizable only at the bladder outlet as three distinct layers: the outer longitudinal, the middle circular, and the inner longitudinal

In the adult female, the urethra is a muscular tube, 3 to 4 cm in length, lined proximally with transitional epithelium and distally with stratified squamous epithelium. It is surrounded mainly by smooth muscle. The striated muscle urethral sphincter, which surrounds the middle one third of the urethra, contributes about 50 per cent of the total urethral resistance and serves as a secondary defense against incontinence. It is also responsible for the interruption of urine flow at the end of micturition.

The two posterior pubourethral ligaments provide a strong suspensory mechanism for the urethra and serve to hold it forward and in close proximity to the pubis under conditions of stress. They extend from the lower part of the pubic bone to the urethra at the junction of its middle and distal third.

Innervation

The lower urinary tract is under the control of both parasympathetic and sympathetic nerves. The parasympathetic fibers originate in the sacral spinal cord segments S2 through S4. Stimulation of the pelvic parasympathetic nerves and administration of cholinergic drugs cause the detrusor muscle to contract. Anticholinergic drugs reduce the vesicle pressure and increase the bladder capacity.

The sympathetic fibers originate from thoracolumbar segments (T10 through L2) of the spinal cord. The sympathetic system has α- and β-adrenergic components. The beta fibers terminate primarily in the detrusor muscle, whereas the alpha fibers terminate primarily in the urethra. α-Adrenergic stimulation contracts the bladder neck and urethra and relaxes the detrusor. β-Adrenergic stimulation relaxes the urethra and detrusor muscle. The pudendal nerve (S2 through S4) provides motor innervation to the striated urethral sphincter.

Factors Influencing Bladder Behavior

Sensory Innervation. Afferent impulses from the bladder, trigone, and proximal urethra pass to S2 through S4 levels of the spinal cord by means of the pelvic hypogastric nerves. The sensitivity of these nerve endings may be enhanced by acute infection, interstitial cystitis, radiation cystitis, and increased intravesical pressure. The latter may occur in the standing position; when bending forward; or in association with obesity, pregnancy, or pelvic tumors.

Inhibitory impulses, probably relayed by the pudendal nerve, also pass through S2 through S4 following mechanical stimulation of the perineum and anal canal. Their passage may explain why pain in this region can cause urinary retention.

Central Nervous System. In infancy, the storage and expulsion of urine is automatic and controlled at the level of the sacral reflex arc. Later, connections to the higher centers become established and, by training and conditioning, this spinal reflex becomes socially influenced so that voiding can be voluntarily accomplished. Although organic neurologic diseases may interrupt the influence of the higher centers on the spinal reflex arc, micturition patterns may also be profoundly altered by mental, environmental, and sociologic disturbances.

Continence Control

The normal bladder holds urine because the intraurethral pressure exceeds the intravesical pressure. The pubourethral ligaments and surrounding fascia support the urethra so that abrupt increases in intra-abdominal pressure are transmitted equally to the bladder and proximal one third of the urethra, thus maintaining a pressure gradient between the two. In addition, a reflex contraction of the levator ani compresses the midurethra.

Involuntary escape of urine is common. Approximately 50 per cent of young, healthy women occasionally experience some degree of urinary incontinence. The incidence of urinary incontinence increases with age and with increasing degrees of pelvic relaxation.

STRESS INCONTINENCE

Stress incontinence is the involuntary loss of urine through an intact urethra, secondary to a sudden increase in intra-abdominal pressure and in the absence of a bladder contraction. Based on the severity of the incontinence, the following gradation has been found to be of clinical value:

Grade I. Incontinence only with severe stress, such as coughing, sneezing, or jogging.

Grade II. Incontinence with moderate stress, such as rapid movement or walking up and down stairs.

Grade III. Incontinence with mild stress, such as standing. The patient is continent in the supine position.

Etiology

Most patients with clinically significant stress incontinence are multiparous. Pregnancy, labor, and delivery may damage the normal supports of the bladder neck and proximal urethra. In addition, continence deteriorates with increasing age, even in women who have not borne children, because intraurethral pressure decreases after the menopause.

The most commonly accepted theory for the pathogenesis of stress urinary incontinence is that the proximal urethra drops below the pelvic floor because of pelvic relaxation defects. Therefore, the increase in intra-abdominal pressure induced by coughing is not transmitted equally to the bladder and proximal urethra. The urethral resistance is overcome by the increased bladder pressure, and leakage of urine results.

Symptoms

When the sole complaint is of involuntary loss of urine on coughing or straining, urinary stress incontinence is the likely diagnosis. Frequently, the symptoms of stress and urge incontinence occur concurrently. The use of protective underwear is some guide to the severity of incontinence. Gradual onset of stress incontinence after bilateral oophorectomy or menopause may indicate estrogen deficiency. The history should include details of any neurologic diseases, vaginal repair, or bladder neck surgery.

Pelvic Examination

Inspection of the vaginal walls should be performed with a Sims' speculum, which allows optimal visualization of the anterior vaginal wall and urethrovesical junction. Scarring, tenderness, and rigidity of the urethra from previous vaginal surgeries or pelvic trauma may be reflected by a scarred anterior vaginal wall. Since the distal urethra is estrogen-dependent, the patient with atrophic vaginitis also has atrophic urethritis.

Diagnostic Tests

Stress Test

A stress test objectively demonstrates urinary incontinence. The patient is examined with a full bladder in the lithotomy position. While the physician observes the urethral meatus, the patient is asked to cough. Stress urinary incontinence is suggested if short spurts of urine escape simultaneously with each cough. A delayed leakage, or loss of large volumes of urine, suggests uninhibited bladder contractions. If loss of urine is not demonstrated in the lithotomy position, the test should be repeated with the patient in a standing position.

In patients with demonstrated stress urinary incontinence, elevation of the bladder neck with one finger on either side of the urethra (Bonney test) or a partially opened Allis clamp (Marshall-Marchetti test) should prevent leakage of urine on coughing. If urine loss stops, the test is considered positive and suggests that bladder neck suspension should control the incontinence. Both of these tests may occlude the urethra while elevating the bladder neck and, therefore, should not be relied on. A pessary test that does not cause urethral occlusion has been found to be reliable for the diagnosis of stress urinary incontinence.

Cotton-Tip Applicator Test

This test determines the mobility and descent of the urethrovesical junction on straining. With the patient in the lithotomy position, the examiner inserts a lubricated Q-tip into the urethra to the level of the urethrovesical junction and measures the angle between the Q-tip and the horizontal. The patient then strains maximally, which produces descent of the urethrovesical junction. Along with the descent, the Q-tip moves, producing a new angle with the horizontal. The normal change in angle is up to 30 degrees. In patients with pelvic relaxation and stress urinary incontinence, the change in Q-tip angle is in the range of 50 to 60 degrees or more (Fig. 37–4).

Urethrocystoscopy

Urethrocystoscopy allows the physician to examine the urethra, urethrovesical junction, bladder walls, and ureteral orifices. Either water or carbon dioxide may be employed as the filling medium. Ideally, urethrocystoscopy should be performed before any surgery on the urethra or bladder.

The following observations should be made:

1. The amount of residual urine.
2. The bladder capacity (normal capacity is 400 to 500 ml of water).
3. The appearance of the urethral and bladder urothelium, noting any inflammation, diverticula, or trabeculation.

4. The mobility of the urethrovesical junction in response to commands of rectal squeeze, urine hold, cough, and Valsalva. In a normal patient, the internal urethral orifice closes in response to these commands. Prior vaginal surgery may result in restricted urethral mobility (frozen urethra or drain-pipe urethra), which may also cause stress urinary incontinence.

Cystometrogram

Cystometry consists of distending the bladder with known volumes of water or carbon dioxide and observing pressure changes in the bladder during filling (Fig. 37–5). During the test, the patient is asked about the sensation of bladder fullness. The presence or absence of a detrusor reflex associated with a strong desire to void is noted. The most important observation is the presence of a detrusor reflex and the patient's ability to control or inhibit this reflex.

The ability of the patient to perceive the filling of the bladder indicates that sensory innervation of the bladder is intact. The first sensation of bladder filling should occur at volumes of 150 to 200 ml. The volume threshold for the detrusor reflex is a measure of the functional capacity of the bladder muscle. This critical volume (400 to 500 ml) is the capacity that the bladder musculature tolerates before the patient experiences a strong desire to urinate. At this point, if the patient is asked to void, a terminal contraction may appear and is seen as a sudden rise in intravesical pressure. At the peak of the contraction, the patient is instructed to inhibit this reflex (indicated by arrows in Fig. 37–5A and B). A normal person should be able to inhibit this detrusor reflex and bring down intravesical pressure (Fig. 37–5A). In a urologically or neurologically abnormal patient, the detrusor reflex may appear without the specific instruction to void, and the patient cannot inhibit it (Fig. 37–5B); this observation is referred to as an uninhibited detrusor contraction. Other terms for this disorder include detrusor dyssynergia, detrusor hyperreflexia, irritable bladder, hypertonic bladder, unstable bladder, and uninhibited neurogenic bladder.

These cystometric procedures allow differentiation between those patients who are in-

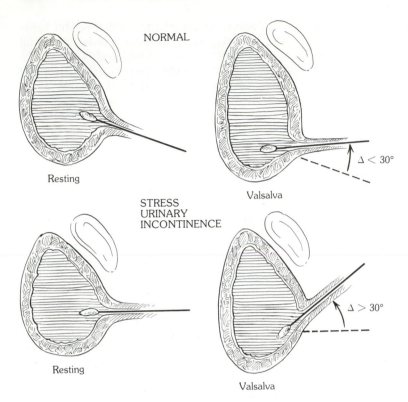

NORMAL

Resting

Valsalva

$\Delta < 30°$

STRESS
URINARY
INCONTINENCE

Resting

Valsalva

$\Delta > 30°$

Figure 37–4. Diagrammatic representation of the Q-tip test showing mobility of the urethrovesical junction in a continent patient and a patient with stress urinary incontinence.

continent as a result of uninhibited detrusor contraction and those who have stress urinary incontinence. Conversely, the hypotonic bladder accommodates excessive amounts of gas or water with little increase in intravesical pressure, and there is absence of the terminal detrusor contraction when the patient is asked to void (Fig. 37–5c).

Urethral Pressure Measurements

A low urethral pressure may be found in patients with stress urinary incontinence, whereas an abnormally high urethral closing pressure may be associated with voiding difficulties, hesitancy, and urinary retention.

The urethral closing pressure profile (UCPP) is a graphic record of pressure along the length of the urethra obtained by means of a pressure-sensitive recording catheter, which is slowly and progressively withdrawn through the urethra. The resulting bell-shaped curve provides a measurement of the urethral closing pressure (intraurethral minus intravesical pressure) and the functional length of the urethra (the length of the urethra along which urethral pressure exceeds bladder pres-

sure). The urethral closing pressure normally varies between 50 and 100 cm water and the functional length between 3 and 5 cm. A normal continent woman responds to the stress of bladder filling, postural change, coughing, sneezing, or jolting by increasing the urethral closing pressure and urethral length. Patients with stress urinary incontinence characteristically demonstrate decreases in urethral closing pressure.

Uroflowmetry

Uroflowmetry records rates of urine flow through the urethra when the patient is asked to void spontaneously while sitting on a uroflow chair. From the flow rate curve, the physician relates the voided volume to the maximum flow rate and the time for urine flow. The normal female voids by the "rule of twenties"—that is, the bladder is emptied in less than 20 seconds at a rate of 20 ml per second. For a flow rate to be significant, at least 200 ml of urine should be voided.

Uroflowmetry is indicated in patients complaining of difficulty or hesitancy in voiding, incomplete bladder emptying, poor stream,

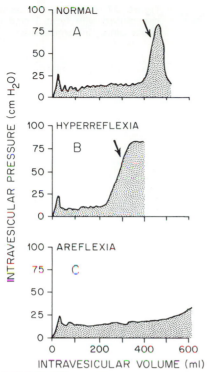

Figure 37-5. Water cystometrogram in (A) a normal patient, (B) a patient with detrusor hyperreflexia, and (C) a patient with detrusor areflexia (hypotonic bladder).

urinary retention, and in the assessment of patients for incontinence surgery.

Simultaneous Urethrocystometry

This technique employs simultaneous recording of the pressure in the urethra and bladder and allows the pressure changes during voiding to be recorded. Normally, urethral relaxation precedes bladder contraction. An observation of lack of bladder contraction and the use of abdominal straining during voiding may indicate a need for prolonged postoperative bladder drainage following incontinence surgery.

Voiding Cystourethrogram

In this radiologic investigation, fluoroscopy is used to observe bladder filling, the mobility of the urethra and bladder base, and the anatomic changes during voiding. The procedure provides valuable information regarding

bladder size and the competence of the bladder neck during coughing. It may detect any bladder trabeculation; vesicoureteral reflux during voiding; funnelling of the bladder neck, bladder, and urethral diverticula; and outflow obstruction.

Bead-Chain Cystourethrogram

This static cystourethrogram involves the introduction of a metallic bead-chain into the bladder transurethrally. A lateral x-ray film provides information regarding the location of the bladder and urethra in relation to the symphysis pubis and the urethrovesical anatomic configuration during rest and straining. On the basis of a static cystourethrogram, two basic types of anatomic disturbances have been described in patients with stress urinary incontinence (Fig. 37-6). Patients with a type 1 deformity have incomplete or complete loss of the posterior urethrovesical angle (normal 90 to 100 degrees). Patients with a type 2 deformity have an increased angle of urethral axis inclination to the vertical (normal is less than 30 degrees), in addition to loss of the posterior urethrovesical angle. Patients with a type 2 deformity have a more severe variety of stress urinary incontinence. This classification has been used to select the type of surgical approach—that is, anterior vaginal repair for patients with a type 1 deformity and an abdominal approach for patients with a type 2 deformity. With better understanding of the pathophysiology of urinary incontinence and increased utilization of urodynamic studies, the role of the static cystourethrogram has come under increasing criticism and is presently infrequently employed in the diagnostic work-up of stress urinary incontinence.

Ultrasonography

Employing real-time or sector ultrasonography, information can be obtained about the inclination of the urethra, flatness of the bladder base, and mobility and funnelling of the urethrovesical junction, both at rest and with a Valsalva's maneuver. In addition, any bladder or urethral diverticula may be identified.

STRESS INCONTINENCE

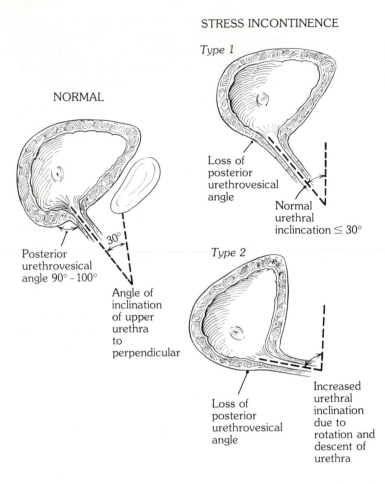

Figure 37-6. Anatomic deformities associated with type 1 and type 2 stress urinary incontinence.

Type 1

Loss of posterior urethrovesical angle

Normal urethral inclincation $\leq 30°$

NORMAL

Posterior urethrovesical angle 90°-100°

30°

Angle of inclination of upper urethra to perpendicular

Type 2

Loss of posterior urethrovesical angle

Increased urethral inclination due to rotation and descent of urethra

Summary

For about 90 per cent of patients with stress urinary incontinence, a good history and physical examination, uroflowmetry, cystourethroscopy, the Q-tip test, the stress test, the pessary test, and the cystometrogram are adequate investigations. Additional urodynamic, electromyographic, neurologic, and radiologic procedures may be necessary in patients with a history of multiple previous surgeries for urinary incontinence and for patients with associated neurologic disease.

Treatment

Medical Therapy

After the menopause, atrophic changes occur in the lower urinary tract. Estrogens improve urethral closing pressure, mucosal thickness and vascularity, and possible reflex urethral functions. α-Adrenergic stimulants, such as phenylpropanolamine (Propadrine) or pseudoephedrine, may enhance urethral closure and improve continence.

Physical Therapy

Pelvic diaphragm exercises (Kegel exercises) are known to improve or cure mild forms of stress incontinence. Because the entire pelvic floor exerts sphincteric action on the urethra, an increase in resting and active muscle tone will increase urethral closing pressure. To employ the exercises, the patient must be asked to learn to interrupt urine flow during voiding. Kegel exercises require diligence and willingness to practice at home and at work. Many women find them difficult, fatiguing, or time-consuming. Kegel exercises before and after delivery may help patients with postpartum urinary incontinence.

Intravaginal Devices

Large pelvic diaphragms, tampons, and various types of vaginal pessaries have been used to elevate and support the bladder neck and urethra. The pessary may provide an acceptable alternative for patients unfit for surgery. They must be regularly cleansed and replaced.

Surgical Therapy

Surgery is the most commonly employed treatment of stress urinary incontinence. The aim of all the surgical procedures is to correct the pelvic relaxation defect and to stabilize and restore the normal intra-abdominal position of the proximal urethra. The approach may be vaginal, abdominal, or combined abdominovaginal.

Vaginal Approach. Anterior vaginal repair (Kelly's operation) is an excellent procedure for correction of cystocele but less useful for correction of stress incontinence. It may be difficult to place the urethra high enough in the pelvis, thereby reducing the short-term and long-term success rate.

In patients with large cystoceles, overcorrection of the cystocele may result in postoperative stress incontinence in a previously continent patient. Such patients may require prophylactic retropubic urethropexy in addition to anterior colporrhaphy.

Abdominal Approach. The retropubic approach to urethrovesical elevation has a long-term success rate of approximately 85 per cent. The retropubic urethropexy is performed extraperitoneally (in the space of Retzius) by placing sutures in the fascia lateral to and on each side of the bladder neck and proximal urethra and elevating the vesicourethral junction by attaching the sutures to the symphysis pubis (Marshall-Marchetti-Kranz procedure) or to Cooper's ligament (Burch procedure). This restores the normal intra-abdominal position of the urethra. Care must be taken to correct any associated cystocele.

Postoperatively, a transurethral or suprapubic catheter is left in the bladder for continuous bladder drainage for 48 to 72 hours before instituting spontaneous voiding. Some patients (20 to 30 per cent) may need prolonged postoperative bladder drainage (more than 7 days). An occasional patient may develop osteitis pubis after the Marshall-Marchetti-Kranz procedure.

Combined Abdominovaginal Procedures. The modified Pereyra procedure is being increasingly employed because of its simplicity and short postoperative recovery period. The principle of the Pereyra technique is suspension of the vesical neck, as in the retropubic procedures, but the operation is primarily done via the vagina. Monofilament nylon sutures are placed in the endopelvic fascia on either side of the urethra, through a vaginal incision at the level of the bladder neck. The sutures are threaded through the space of Retzius with a special needle and are tied to the anterior rectus fascia through a small suprapubic incision.

In the Stamey procedure, a 1-cm sleeve of 5mm Dacron is threaded under the urethra at the bladder neck to provide additional support. Postoperative voiding difficulties and a need for prolonged postoperative bladder drainage or intermittent self-catheterization represent the main drawbacks of this procedure.

Comparison of Vaginal and Abdominal Procedures

Anterior colporrhaphy with plication of the vesical neck has been standard therapy for mild or moderate stress incontinence for decades. It is a convenient approach, especially when concomitant vaginal procedures are being performed, and avoids the necessity of an abdominal incision. Success rates are better in patients with mild incontinence, but not as good in the more severe forms. Long-term success rates are 55 to 65 per cent.

The Pereyra and Stamey procedures, with their several modifications, have about an 80 to 90 per cent success rate, which is comparable to open retropubic techniques. Some surgeons use these procedures routinely and achieve good results, even in cases of previous surgical failure. They require a relatively short amount of time to perform, and a wide abdominal incision is not required. An area of concern is the inability to control the amount of elevation of the bladder neck precisely. Avoidance of this problem comes only with experience with the technique.

Special Procedures

If conventional surgical procedures fail, special, more complicated operations may be performed. These include sling procedures, neourethra construction, implantation of an artificial urinary sphincter, and urinary diversion. The latter is the final solution for intractable incontinence.

It is important to recognize that the critical operation for urinary stress incontinence is the first one, and the cure rate declines more or less proportionately to the number of subsequent operations performed. Every effort should be made to use all necessary resources for a proper preoperative evaluation of patients before embarking on any kind of surgical procedure for incontinence.

TOTAL INCONTINENCE—
URINARY FISTULA

Pelvic surgery, irradiation, or both now account for 95 per cent of the vesicovaginal fistulas in the United States. More than 50 per cent occur following simple abdominal or vaginal hysterectomy. Obstetric injuries, once the leading cause for urinary fistulas, have almost disappeared in the United States, Canada, and Western Europe. They usually result from operative deliveries (e.g., forceps) rather than from neglected labor and pressure necrosis. One or 2 per cent of radical hysterectomies are followed in 10 to 21 days by a urinary fistula, usually ureterovaginal. These fistulas are usually due to devascularization of the ureter, rather than to direct injury.

Urethrovaginal fistulas generally occur as complications of surgery for urethral diverticula, anterior vaginal wall prolapse, or stress urinary incontinence.

Diagnosis of Fistulas

The usual history of painless and continuous vaginal leakage of urine soon after pelvic surgery is strongly suggestive of this problem. Installation of methylene blue dye into the bladder will discolor a vaginal pack if a vesicovaginal fistula is present. Intravenous indigo-carmine is excreted in the urine and will discolor a vaginal pack in the presence of a vesicovaginal or ureterovaginal fistula. In addition, cystourethroscopy should be performed to determine the site and number of fistulas. The majority of posthysterectomy vesicovaginal fistulas are located just anterior to the vaginal vault. An intravenous pyelogram and retrograde pyelogram should be undertaken to localize a ureterovaginal fistula.

Fistula Repair

Most of the obstetric fistulas can be repaired immediately on detection. For postsurgical fistulas, it is usual to wait 3 to 6 months to allow the inflammation to settle and the tissues to obtain good vascularity and pliability. During this waiting period, urinary tract infection should be treated and estrogen therapy instituted in postmenopausal women. Steroids have been advocated to hasten resolution of inflammatory changes and allow early surgical intervention. Their use in this circumstance is controversial.

In repairing urinary fistulas, the following principles must be observed:

1. All involved organs should be widely mobilized.
2. All scar tissue should be excised.
3. Nontraumatic instruments should be used.
4. Adequate hemostasis must be achieved.
5. A layer by layer closure should be used, without tension.
6. Minimal tissue necrosis should occur by nonstrangulating suture placement.
7. All dead space should be obliterated.
8. The bladder must be drained postoperatively.

Vesicovaginal Fistula. The vaginal approach (Latzko's operation) is suitable for most of these fistulas. After localization of the fistula, an area with a radius of 1.5 to 2 cm around the vaginal opening of the fistula is denuded of vaginal mucosa. Then, multiple layers of interrupted sutures are placed to bring together the denuded areas of anterior and posterior vaginal walls, Postoperatively, the bladder is drained suprapubically for a period of 7 to 14 days. Sexual intercourse is inadvisable for 2 months. A bulbocavernosus muscle flap (Martius graft) may be interposed between the bladder and vagina to provide support, vascularity, and strength to the suture line, especially in patients who have had multiple previous attempted repairs and in those with a postradiation fistula. Large radiation-induced fistulas may necessitate a continent urinary conduit for urinary diversion.

Ureterovaginal Fistula. Treatment of a ureterovaginal fistula depends on its location. If it is close to the ureterovesical junction, the ureter proximal to the fistula can be implanted into the bladder (ureteroneocystostomy). If the fistula is several centimeters from the bladder, a segment of ileum may be interposed between the proximal ureter and the bladder. Occasionally, it may be necessary to remove the kidney on the involved side.

URGE INCONTINENCE

Urge incontinence results from detrusor instability. It is characterized by the presence of involuntary and uninhibited detrusor contractions of 15 cm of water or more during cystometric evaluation.

The incidence of bladder instability in the general population varies from 10 to 15 per cent. In most patients, the exact etiology of bladder instability remains unknown. Clinical symptoms may include urinary urgency, frequency, urge incontinence, and nocturia.

Neurologic Examination

Because the innervation to the lower urinary tract is closely related to the innervation of the lower extremities and perineum, neurologic deficits of the bladder and rectum may be reflected in a systematic examination of the deep tendon reflexes and motor and sensory functions. For instance, the presence of hyperactive deep tendon reflexes and an extensor plantar response in a patient with a history of urinary frequency, urgency, or urge incontinence is likely to be associated with detrusor instability as a cause for the patient's symptoms. Similarly, in a patient with urinary retention or voiding difficulties, evidence of peripheral neuropathy, autonomic neuropathy, diminished tendon reflexes, or a

cauda equina lesion is more likely to be associated with a hypotonic or areflexic bladder.

Reflex contraction of the pelvic floor muscles indicates neuronal integrity of the sacral dermatomes S2, S3, and S4. Stroking the skin lateral to the anus elicits the anal reflex. The bulbocavernosus reflex involves contraction of the bulbo and ischiocavernosus muscles in response to gentle tapping or squeezing of the clitoris. Abnormalities of these reflexes are highly suggestive of peripheral or central nervous system disease as a cause for urinary tract problems.

Treatment

A number of therapeutic modalities are available, attesting to the unsatisfactory results with any kind of treatment. In treating urge incontinence, it is important to exclude significant outflow obstruction to avoid precipitating acute urinary retention.

Pharmacologic Treatment

It is reasonable to try several drugs, increasing the dose up to the maximum tolerated, until the most effective drug for a particular patient is found.

Anticholinergic Drugs. These are the most frequently employed agents. Propantheline (Pro-Banthine), 15 to 30 mg three times daily, and oxybutynin chloride (Ditropan), 5 mg three times daily, act by inhibiting the cholinergically innervated detrusor muscle.

Beta Sympathomimetic Agonists. The detrusor relaxing action of β-adrenergic receptors forms the basis for the use of drugs like metaproterenol (Alupent), 20 mg twice daily. They enhance the effect of propantheline.

Musculotropic Drugs. Flavoxate (Urispas), 200 mg three times daily, acts by causing direct relaxation of the detrusor muscle. Diazepam (Valium) acts by a combination of direct smooth muscle relaxation, anticholinergic effect, and central nervous system sedation.

Tricyclic Antidepressants. Imipramine (Tofranil), 25 to 50 mg two to three times a day, relaxes the detrusor muscle by virtue of its anticholinergic action, and it helps to enhance continence by its alpha-adrenergic stimulation of the urethra.

Dopamine Agonists. Bromocriptine (Parlodel), 2.5 mg three times daily, has been shown to be beneficial in detrusor instability, probably as a result of both central and peripheral actions.

Bladder Training

Bladder training represents a behavior modification designed to repeat the process of toilet training. The essential aim is to increase bladder capacity day by day and to prolong the intervals between voiding. Schedules are started at half-hour or 1-hour intervals and are changed weekly. No night-time schedule is kept. For some patients, hospital admission for a period of 7 to 10 days may be advisable. Supportive treatment may be provided by the use of various pharmacologic agents.

Biofeedback

Like bladder training, this is a technique in which an attempt is made to induce cortical control through recognition of physiologic changes using various instrumentation. Results seem to be similar to those from bladder retraining. With biofeedback, however, equipment cost, manpower, and inconvenience are significantly increased. This technique should, therefore, be reserved for resistant or complicated cases.

Bladder Denervation Procedures

Even total denervation may not paralyze the bladder. Therapeutic bladder denervation may be attempted at many levels from the bladder wall to the brain.

The vaginal approach is the most commonly employed approach for correction of detrusor instability. Through a U-shaped incision in the anterior vaginal wall, the vesical plexus can be identified on each side and resected unilaterally or bilaterally. This approach has the advantage of being close to the target organ and includes both parasympathetic and sympathetic nerves.

Bladder distention can provide useful rehabilitation of bladder function when other measures have failed. Results are uncertain, and repeated attempts may be required. When successful, it is not necessarily permanent; recurrence rates vary from 6 to 15 per cent.

OVERFLOW INCONTINENCE

Urinary retention and overflow incontinence may result from detrusor areflexia or hypotonic bladder, as is seen with lower motor neuron disease, spinal cord injuries, or autonomic neuropathy (diabetes mellitus). These patients are best managed by intermittent self-catheterization.

Overflow incontinence may also occur when there is an outflow obstruction. Straining to void, poor stream, retention of urine, and incomplete emptying may indicate an obstructive disorder. Overdistention of the bladder because of unrecognized urinary retention may occur in the postoperative period. This is a temporary problem related to postoperative pain and may be managed by continuous bladder drainage for 24 to 48 hours.

URETHRAL SYNDROME

The urethral syndrome occurs in a patient with various lower urinary tract symptoms, in the absence of obvious bladder or urethral abnormality, and with no evidence of urinary tract infection. Any combination of symptoms may be present, the most common being urinary frequency, urgency, dysuria, postvoid fullness, incontinence, and dyspareunia. The true incidence is unknown, although it is estimated to occur in 20 to 30 per cent of all adult females.

Possible causes include psychogenic factors, atrophic urethritis in perimenopausal or postmenopasual patients, bacterial infection, nonbacterial infection with organisms *Chlamydia* and *Mycoplasma,* urethral stenosis and spasm, allergy, neurogenic factors, and trauma during sexual intercourse.

Diagnosis is based on a detailed history and physical examination, negative urine cultures, dynamic cystourethroscopy, and urodynamic studies.

Treatment

Because of the diverse and indefinite etiologic factors, numerous forms of treatment are in current use. Serial urethral dilatation and urethral massage are the most commonly employed methods for treating chronic urethritis. The rationale is that stretching and massaging allow effective drainage of inspissated mucus from chronically infected periurethral glands and thereby lead to healing and relief of symptoms. Application of vaginal estrogen cream is effective in patients with atrophic urethritis. Some patients may improve with use of tetracyclines for 10 to 14 days. Internal urethrotomy and urethrolysis have also been employed with variable success. Supportive therapy is helpful in all patients with the urethral syndrome, regardless of cause.

URINARY TRACT INFECTIONS

It is estimated that 15 per cent of women will have at least one urinary tract infection (UTI) in their lifetime. Ninety-five per cent of UTI's are symptomatic, and of these symptomatic episodes, three quarters have positive urine cultures. Almost all asymptomatic patients have negative cultures.

Terminology

The terminology surrounding urinary tract infections is rather complex and requires some definition.

Bacteriuria. Bacteriuria literally means the presence of bacteria in the urine and may indicate contamination from the urethra, vaginal vestibule, or perineum if care is not exercised during collection of a urine specimen. Significant bacteriuria is generally accepted as indicating a bacterial colony count of 10^5 or more per milliliter of urine in a properly collected "clean catch" urine specimen. A colony count of 10^3 or more from a properly collected urine specimen, however, is an indication for treatment if the patient is symptomatic.

Asymptomatic Bacteriuria. Asymptomatic bacteriuria refers to the presence of a positive urine culture in a patient with no clinical symptoms.

Pyelonephritis. Pyelonephritis indicates bacterial infection of the renal parenchyma and the renal pelvicalyceal system. Acute pyelonephritis is commonly associated with fever, flank pain, costovertebral tenderness, urinary frequency, urgency, and dysuria. Chronic pyelonephritis denotes histologic changes of patchy interstitial nephritis, destruction of tubules, cellular infiltration, and inflammatory changes in the renal parenchyma. Chronic pyelonephritis is not synonymous with chronic urinary tract infection, which means only prolonged presence of bacteria.

Cystitis. Cystitis implies inflammation of the urinary bladder. Patients with cystitis usually have symptoms of lower urinary tract irritation, such as dysuria (burning on urination), urgency, frequency with small amounts of voided urine, nocturia, suprapubic discomfort, and, at times, urinary incontinence and hematuria.

Persistence of Bacteriuria. This indicates the presence of microorganisms that were isolated at the start of treatment and continue to be isolated while the patient is on therapy. Persistence may be caused by several factors, including the presence of resistant organisms, inadequate drug therapy, and poor patient compliance.

Superinfection. This implies appearance of a different organism while a patient is still on therapy. This new organism may be a different strain or a different serologic type.

Relapse. This implies recurrence of significant bacteriuria with the same species and serologic strain of organism. Relapse usually appears within 2 to 3 weeks of completion of therapy and most likely represents perineal colonization by the infecting organism.

Reinfection. This means infection occurring after cessation of therapy with a different strain of microorganism or a different serologic type of the original infecting strain. Typically, reinfection occurs 2 to 12 weeks after a previous episode of infection and indicates a recurrent bladder bacteriuria.

Incidence and Prevalence

After the age of 1 year and throughout adulthood, females are affected more frequently than males (10:1 ratio). Asymptomatic bacteriuria increases from an incidence in preschool children of 1 to 5 per cent to a peak of about 10 per cent in the postmenopausal female.

Pathogenesis

Bacteria may gain entry to the urinary tract by three pathways: the ascending route, the descending or hematogenous route, and the lymphatic route.

Ascending Infection. This route, which accounts for the majority of UTIs, is through the urethra into the bladder, and, on occasion, through the ureters into the kidneys. The female is more susceptible because of the short length of the urethra, urethral contamination by rectal pathogens, introital and vestibular colonization by pathogenic bacteria, and the decreased urethral resistance after menopause. Sexual activity is a related factor causing urethrovesical bacterial inoculation, especially in the presence of even minor degrees of hypospadias. Additional sources of infection include vulvovaginitis, urethral diverticula, poor hygiene, and indiscriminate urethral catheterization. Infrequent and incomplete voiding resulting in large bladder volumes increases the susceptibility to chronic urinary infection.

Hematogenous Infection. Urinary infection via the hematogenous route is very uncommon, but it is seen occasionally in elderly, debilitated, or immunosuppressed patients with overwhelming infections, in whom kidney infection is only part of the multisystemic involvement. Renal tuberculosis is almost always acquired via the hematogenous route.

Lymphatic Infection. Experimental evidence suggests the possibility of bacterial infection spreading along lymphatic channels connecting the bowel and the urinary tract.

Host Defense Mechanisms

Entrance of bacteria into the urinary tract does not necessarily result in infection. Natural barriers for invasion, such as the "washout" effect of normal periodic voiding, the antiseptic properties of the bladder's mucosa, and the high concentration of organic acids in normal urine prevent bacterial invasion. Other factors, such as the pH (below 5.5), urea ammonium, and organic acid content of the urine affect bacterial growth. If invasion takes place, the bacteria may remain in the bladder or may ascend to the kidney. Transient vesicoureteral reflux seen in association with severe lower urinary tract infections may allow the infected urine to reach the kidneys.

Perpetuating Factors

The following factors encourage and perpetuate urinary tract infections:

1. Mechanical urinary obstruction. Ureteropelvic junction obstruction, ureteral stricture, urethral stenosis, and caliculi are common to patients with recurrent or chronic urinary tract infections.
2. Functional urinary obstruction abnormalities. Incomplete bladder emptying and vesicoureteric reflux also encourage stasis of urine and bacterial growth. Pregnancy produces transient functional ureteral obstruction both mechanically and hormonally.
3. Systemic factors. Diabetes mellitus; gout; sickle cell trait; cystic renal disease; and metabolic disorders, such as nephrocalcinosis, chronic potassium deficiency, and renal tubular defects, increase susceptibility to pyelonephritis.

Clinical Classification

From the pathogenetic and management point of view, UTIs in nonpregnant females can be considered to be either uncomplicated or complicated. Uncomplicated UTIs account for 95 percent of urinary tract infections in women and seldom produce renal damage. They are either the first episode of infection or an episode far removed in time from a previous urinary infection. Ninety per cent of first infections are due to *Escherichia coli.* Seventy-five per cent of these infective episodes do not recur for at least 5 years. Complicated UTIs occur in patients with neurologic or obstructive abnormalities or in those with underlying parenchymal disease.

Investigations

Urinalysis

Microscopic examination of an uncentrifuged, unstained specimen (a drop of urine on the slide covered with a coverslip) provides better than 90 per cent accuracy in detecting significant bacteriuria when one or more bacteria are seen per high power field. A positive Gram's stain almost always correlates with a positive quantitative culture. A negative Gram's stain virtually eliminates significant bacteriuria.

Pyuria is arbitrarily defined as the presence of five or more white blood cells per high power field in the centrifuged specimen. The presence of white blood cells (pyuria) and red blood cells along with bacteriuria suggest infection. Pyuria without significant bacteria may indicate a nonbacterial inflammation or a urinary tract foreign body or tumor. It is a classic finding in urinary tuberculosis. Casts, when present, indicate renal parenchymal disease.

Urine Culture

A quantitative urine culture is the most important laboratory test in the diagnosis and management of complicated or uncomplicated UTIs. *Escherichia coli* is the predominant organism in 80 to 85 per cent of patients. The remaining less common organisms are *Klebsiella-Enterobacter, Proteus* species, *Enterococcus, Staphylococcus,* and group D *Streptococcus.* Anaerobic fecal bacteria do not grow well in urine and are rarely seen in urinary infections. Yeast, such as *Candida albicans,* may be seen in patients with diabetes mellitus or in individuals receiving immunosuppressive therapy, especially in the presence of foreign bodies or indwelling catheters.

There are three techniques for urine collection: (1) the midstream "clean-catch" method, (2) urethral catheterization, and (3) suprapubic aspiration. The midstream clean-catch method has an 80 per cent reliability, which increases to 95 per cent if two consecutive specimens show a colony count of 100,000 or more of the same organism. In routine cases of uncomplicated infections, the presence of two or more species of organisms in the same specimen normally suggests contamination. Urethral catheterization provides an optimal urine specimen. A positive culture has a 95 per cent accuracy, and false-positive cultures are rare. Suprapubic aspiration, although providing the most reliable specimen, is reserved for those in whom contamination is difficult to avoid (e.g., in young children and elderly people).

Radiologic Studies

An intravenous pyelogram is critical in the evaluation of patients whose recurrences are due to bacterial persistence (for example, due to stones or infected congenital anomalies), but almost of no value in the 99 per cent of patients with reinfections. Cystography and voiding urethrocystography may help to detect ureteric reflux, diverticuli, or fistulous tracts in patients with persistent bacteriuria.

Endoscopic Studies

Endoscopic studies such as urethroscopy and cystoscopy may be necessary to detect chronic trigonitis, urethritis, urethral or bladder diverticuli, fistulas, foreign bodies, or bladder wall trabeculation.

Renal Function Tests

Renal function tests are not required in a patient with an initial uncomplicated UTI. If recurrent episodes occur, blood urea nitrogen and serum creatinine levels should be obtained. If renal insufficiency is present, a creatinine clearance is helpful.

Urinary Tract Infection Localization Studies

The clinical presentation does not always allow differentiation between renal infections and lower UTIs. The clinical usefulness of localization lies in planning patient management, since the presence of renal infection usually necessitates a more vigorous and extended therapeutic approach than does the presence of lower UTI alone.

Indirect methods of localization include (1) special staining of urinary sediment to detect polymorphonuclear leukocytes originating in the kidney ("glitter cell" stain), (2) examination of urinary sediment after intravenous injection of bacterial pyrogen or adrenocorticosteroids, (3) measurement of the excretion of various urinary enzymes, (4) tests of maximal urinary concentrating ability, (5) determination of the immunologic response by estimating serum antibody titers against type-specific organisms in the urine, and (6) urine examination for bacteria that are antibody-coated. The latter test is based on the observation that, unlike bladder bacteriuria, renal infection produces a systemic antibody response.

Direct methods of localization, although invasive, are more accurate and include (1) selective ureteral catheterization via cystoscopy, (2) the bladder washout technique, and (3) examination of renal tissue for bacteria or bacterial antigen by the fluorescent antibody technique.

Management

Unless physical examination and urinalysis (bacteriuria) clearly indicate urinary infection, it is advisable to withhold definite antimicrobial therapy until culture and sensitivity reports are available. As a general rule, bacteriuria should be treated and not pyuria. General measures in the management of urinary tract infections involve the following:

1. Rest and hydration. Hydration promotes dilution of bacterial counts, frequent bladder emptying and reduction of medullary osmolality, which assists phagocytosis.

2. Acidification of the urine. Ascorbic acid (500 mg twice daily), ammonium chloride (12 gm per day in divided doses), or apricot, plum, prune, or cranberry juices have been employed to increase the antibacterial activity of urine and to inhibit bacterial multiplication. Grapefruit juice and carbonated drinks, particularly those containing citrates, turn the urine alkaline and should be avoided.

3. Urinary analgesics. Agents such as phenazopyridine hydrochloride (Pyridium), 100 mg twice daily for 2 to 3 days, are often helpful in relieving dysuria.

Basic Principles of Antimicrobial Therapy

The drug selected should be readily available, of low cost, rapidly absorbed from the upper gastrointestinal tract with minimal irritation, and selectively excreted in the urinary tract. A high serum level of antibiotic is undesirable in the treatment of acute cystitis, since it tends to alter normal bacterial flora. Nitrofurantoin (Macrodantin) produces low serum levels with a half-life of only 19 minutes, thereby minimizing the chances of alteration of intestinal and vaginal bacterial flora. Treatment with nitrofurantoin is effective against all uropathogens except *Proteus.*

On the other hand, for pyelonephritis, an antibiotic should be selected that will attain a significant serum level, since the badly infected renal tissue is poorly perfused. The cephalosporins are more effective and cause fewer side effects and relapses. Cephalosporins (Keflex, Duricef) are slowly and effectively excreted in urine, thereby reducing the frequency of daily drug administration (500 mg to 1000 mg twice daily). Antibiotics such as ampicillin, tetracyclines, and trimethoprim-sulfamethoxazole (Septra, Bactrim) alter the intestinal flora, destroy the normal vaginal and periurethral flora, and may result in a relapse of the UTI.

The high pH of urine associated with *Proteus* infection results from the splitting of urea with the subsequent liberation of ammonia. The urine has a characteristic "fishy" smell. If the urine is very alkaline (pH greater than 8.0), trimethoprim-sulfamethoxazole should be prescribed.

For patients with renal insufficiency, ampicillin, trimethoprim-sulfamethoxazole, and doxycycline have been shown to reach adequate levels in the urine without toxic levels in serum. Nitrofuratoin should be avoided, as high serum levels may lead to peripheral neuropathy. Similarly, tetracycline may lead to severe hepatic damage. Dosages of aminoglycosides should be adjusted in accordance

Table 37–1. ANTIMICROBIAL AGENTS USED IN THE MANAGEMENT OF URINARY TRACT INFECTIONS AND THEIR USUAL EFFECTIVENESS AGAINST COMMON PATHOGENS

AGENT	SERUM LEVELS	URINE LEVELS	ESCHERICHIA COLI	KLEBSIELLA	PSEUDO-MONAS	ENTERO-COCCUS	PROTEUS
Trimethoprim-sulfamethoxazole	±	+ +	+ +	+ +	−	−	+ +
Nitrofurantoin	−	+ +	+ +	±	−	±	−
Ampicillin	+	+ +	+ +	−	−	+ +	+ +
Cephalothin	+ +	+ +	+ +	+ +	−	±	+ +
Tetracycline	±	+	±	±	−	+ +	−
Kanamycin	+ +	+ +	+ +	+ +	−	−	+ +
Gentamicin	+ +	+ +	+ +	+ +	+ +	−	+ +
Carbenicillin	+ +	+ +	+ +	−	+ +	−	+ +

+ +, Good; +, adequate; ±, occasionally effective; −, not effective.

with creatinine clearance, and the serum levels should be monitored.

Antimicrobial agents commonly used in the management of urinary tract infections and their relative effectiveness against various organisms are shown in Table 37–1.

Symptoms Without Bacteria. Treatment should be symptomatic, such as increased fluid intake, the administration of Pyridium, and warm sitz baths.

Asymptomatic Bacteriuria. Although this condition may be ignored in many patients who have no evidence of mechanical obstruction or renal insufficiency, children and pregnant women should be given aggressive antimicrobial therapy. As many as 40 per cent of pregnant women with asymptomatic bacteriuria later develop symptomatic UTIs, usually pyelonephritis.

Acute Symptomatic Infections. Patients with evidence of bacteremia (e.g., shaking chills) or endotoxemia (e.g., hypotension or respiratory alkalosis) should be hospitalized. Almost always it is prudent to hospitalize the febrile diabetic. In the acutely ill patient with suspected bacteremia, aminoglycosides should be employed. The patient's temperature should be monitored. If the fever persists longer than 72 to 96 hours, a complication of infection, such as perinephric abscess, or of treatment, such as drug fever, should be contemplated and investigated.

For the patient without indications for hospitalization with the first episode of UTI, an inexpensive drug such as sulfonamide, nitrofuratoin, ampicillin, or tetracycline should be given for seven days.

Treatment with a single dose of an antimicrobial drug, e.g., trimethoprim, 320 mg, and sulfamethoxazole, 1600 mg, given as Bactrim or Septra in four single-strength or two double-strength tablets; kanamycin, 500 mg intramuscularly; or amoxicillin, 3 gm orally, is highly successful for bladder infections. Single-dose therapy fails in more than 50 per cent of patients with an upper tract infection, however, and as many as 40 per cent of women with only lower tract symptoms also have upper tract infections.

Recurrent Urinary Tract Infections

These patients demonstrate abnormal vaginal biologic factors. Colonization of vaginal and urethral mucosa usually precedes bacteriuria. Bacterial adherence to squamous cells and lack of vaginal antibody to *E. coli* probably lead to vaginal colonization. Women resistant to *E. coli* carry specific antibodies to their own *E. coli*.

The benefit of long-term (6 to 12 months) administration of antimicrobials in women with recurrent UTIs has been demonstrated. Trimethoprim-sulfamethoxazole has been found to be effective and is the only antibacterial agent known to be excreted in vaginal

Table 37–2. PRINCIPLES FOR BLADDER DRAINAGE

Avoid nonessential catheterization
Remove catheters promptly
Use correct sterile procedure for catheterization to avoid introducing bacteria
Maintain closed drainage
Disconnect the drainage system only when there is an obstruction
Avoid prophylactic antibiotics
Use suprapubic catheterization for prolonged bladder drainage

---

nary tract, particularly in association with catheterization. The principles shown in Table 37–2 should be employed in effecting drainage of the urinary bladder.

fluid. Sulfonamides, tetracycline, and ampicillin are not effective prophylactically because of the rapid emergence of resistant fecal strains. Recurrent infections tend to occur in clusters. There are often prolonged remissions between these clusters, and the timing of the clusters cannot be predicted. Prophylactic therapy should be initiated when the patient has had two infections within 6 months because she faces a 65 per cent chance of another infection within the next 6 months.

For women who are able to relate closely their frequently recurring infections to sexual activity, a single dose of an antimicrobial drug immediately after coitus has been shown to prevent bacteriuria and symptomatic infection.

Prevention of Hospital-Acquired Urinary Tract Infections in Gynecologic Patients

Sixty per cent of hospital-acquired infections in gynecologic patients involve the uri-

SUGGESTED READING

Bergman A, Koonings PP, Ballard CA: Primary stress urinary incontinence and pelvic relaxation: Prospective randomized comparison of three different operations. Am J Obstet Gynecol 161:637, 1989.

Bhatia NN: Neurophysiology of micturition. In Ostergard DR, Bent AE (eds): Urogynecology and Urodynamics: Theory and Practice. 3rd ed. Baltimore, Williams and Wilkins, 1991, pp 31–54.

Bhatia NN, Bergman A, Karram MM: Effects of estrogen on urethral function in women with urinary incontinence. Obstet Gynecol Surv 44:634, 1989.

Bhatia NN, Bradley WE: Neuroanatomy and neurophysiology of the lower urinary tract. Female incontinence. In Raz S (ed): Female Urology. Philadelphia, WB Saunders, 1983, pp 12–32.

Fantl JA, Wyman JF, McClish DK et al: Efficacy of bladder training in older women with urinary incontinence. Trans Am Gynecol Obstet Soc 9:43, 1991.

Karram MM, Bhatia NN: Management of co-existent stress and urge urinary incontinence. Obstet Gynecol 73:4, 1989.

Karram MM, Bhatia NN: Transvaginal needle bladder neck suspension for stress urinary incontinence: A comprehensive review. Obstet Gynecol 73:906, 1989.

Langer R, Neuman M, Ron-el R, et al: The effect of total abdominal hysterectomy on bladder function in asymptomatic women. Obstet Gynecol 74:205, 1989.

Pereyra AJ, Lebherz TB, Growdon WA, et al: Pubourethral support in perspective: Modified Pereyra procedure for urinary incontinence. Obstet Gynecol 59:643, 1982.

Rosenzweig BA, Bhatia NN, Nelson AL: Dynamic urethral pressure profilometry and pressure transmission ratio: What do the numbers mean? Obstet Gynecol 77:586, 1991.

Thomas S, Bhatia NN: New approaches in treatment of urinary tract infections. Obstet Gynecol Clin North Am 16:897–909, 1989.

Thirty-eight

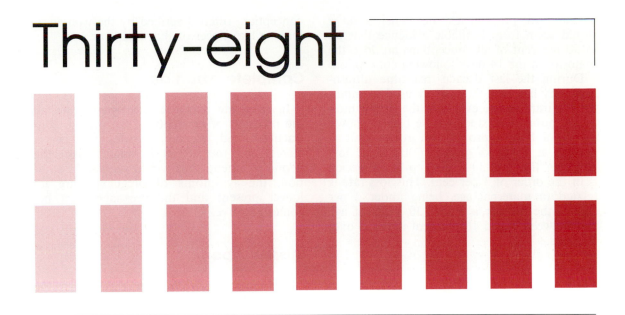

Abortion

MICHAEL J. BENNETT

In medical terminology, *abortion* is the unexpected, unplanned, spontaneous loss of a pregnancy before the fetus is sufficiently developed to survive outside its mother. In 1977, the World Health Organization defined abortion as "the expulsion or extraction from its mother of a fetus or an embryo weighing 500 gm or less," which approximated to 20 to 22 weeks of gestation. The lay public uses the word *miscarriage* to describe this spontaneous event. When a pregnancy is ended deliberately by any of a number of techniques, the lay public uses the term *abortion*, whereas medical persons use the phrase *termination of pregnancy*. In the United States and Australia, a spontaneous abortion can occur up to 20 weeks gestational age, after which such an event becomes a preterm birth until 37 completed gestational weeks.

INCIDENCE

The incidence of conception is unknown, and therefore the incidence of pregnancy loss cannot be derived with certainty. There have been studies of relatively small numbers of women attempting conception, and these suggest that spontaneous abortion occurs in 10 to 15 per cent of clinically recognizable pregnancies. The term *biochemical pregnancy* has evolved as a result of assisted reproductive technology such as in vitro fertilization. It refers to the presence of the beta subunit of human chorionic gonadotropin (β-hCG) in the blood of a woman 7 to 10 days after ovulation but in whom menstruation occurs when expected. In other words, conception has occurred, but spontaneous loss of the gestation takes place without prolongation of the menstrual cycle. When both clinical and

415

biochemical pregnancies are considered, it would seem from available evidence that up to 50 per cent of all conceptions are lost, the majority in the 14 days following conception.

During the last decade, real-time ultrasonography has been extensively used to monitor the intrauterine events of the first trimester. A number of studies have clearly shown that if a live, appropriately grown fetus is present at 8 weeks gestation, the fetal loss rate over the next 20 weeks (up to 28 weeks) is in the order of 3 per cent. This loss rate is related to maternal age, being under 2 per cent if the mother is under 30 years of age and between 5 and 10 per cent if she is over 40 years.

TYPES OF ABORTION

The remainder of this chapter deals with clinical pregnancies only.

Threatened Abortion

The term *threatened abortion* is used when a pregnancy is complicated by vaginal bleeding before the twentieth week. Pain is not a prominent feature of threatened abortion, although a lower abdominal dull ache sometimes accompanies the bleeding. Vaginal examination at this stage reveals a closed cervix. Approximately 25 per cent of pregnant women have some degree of vaginal bleeding during the first trimester. Fifty per cent of those who threaten eventually abort.

Inevitable Abortion

In a case of inevitable abortion, a clinical pregnancy is complicated by both vaginal bleeding and cramp-like lower abdominal pain. The cervix is frequently partially dilated, attesting to the inevitability of the process.

Incomplete Abortion

In addition to vaginal bleeding, cramp-like pain, and cervical dilatation, an incomplete abortion involves the passage of products of conception, often described by the woman as looking like pieces of skin and liver.

Complete Abortion

In complete abortion, after passage of all the products of conception, the uterine contractions and bleeding abate, the cervix closes, and the uterus is smaller than the period of amenorrhea would suggest. In addition, the symptoms of pregnancy are no longer present and the pregnancy test becomes negative.

Missed Abortion

The term *missed abortion* is used when the fetus has died but is retained in the uterus, usually for some weeks.

Recurrent Abortion

Convention dictates that three successive abortions label a patient a recurrent aborter. This convention was based on the concept proposed by Malpas in 1938 that when a single cause for abortion existed, the woman was likely to abort recurrently. On the basis of his calculations, three successive losses were likely to be associated with a single etiologic factor. Not only has this been subsequently shown to be false, but it also suggests that investigation of a couple should not be undertaken until three losses have occurred. In practical terms, this definition has little value except that it allows comparisons to be made between groups of couples. Two successive first-trimester losses or a single second trimester spontaneous abortion justifies investigation of a couple.

ETIOLOGY

There is at present much confusion about the etiology of spontaneous abortions. Although many factors may result in the loss of a single pregnancy, relatively few factors are present in couples who abort recurrently. Cause-effect relationships in individual patients are frequently difficult to ascertain.

General Maternal Factors

Infections

Despite the present recognition that microorganisms may cause spontaneous abortions, it is frequently difficult to identify unequivocally the infectious agent responsible for the loss of a specific pregnancy. Some microorganisms have a specific local effect on the conceptus (e.g., rubella, *Listeria monocytogenes,* cytomegalovirus, *Treponema pallidum*), whereas infection with others may cause general systemic effects and a fever that result in abortion. Very few microorganisms have been implicated in recurrent abortions. Infection with *Mycoplasma, Listeria,* or *Toxoplasma* should be specifically sought in women with recurrent abortions, since despite being infrequently found, they are all treatable with modern antibiotics.

Environmental Exposure

Epidemiologic evidence of a causal link between exposure to potentially mutagenic or teratogenic agents and subsequent abortion is sparse. Such exposures are likely to be uncommon and not an important cause of reproductive loss in the general population. Exceptions to this are maternal smoking and alcohol consumption, for which there is evidence of an increased incidence of chromosomally normal abortions. Women who smoke 20 cigarettes daily and consume more than seven standard alcoholic drinks per week have a fourfold increase in their risk of spontaneous abortion. It has also been reported that there is a doubling of the risk of spontaneous abortion with as little as two drinks a week.

Psychological Factors

There is very little evidence that a sudden physical or emotional shock can cause the subsequent loss of a pregnancy. Psychodynamic factors may contribute, however, to the etiology of recurrent abortion in a few cases and may even be the major factor on rare occasions. The importance of psychological support and inspiring confidence cannot be overemphasized in the management of patients with recurrent abortion.

Systemic Disorders

The three general medical disorders commonly related to spontaneous abortion are diabetes mellitus, hypothyroidism, and systemic lupus erythematosus (SLE). The evidence linking diabetes with spontaneous abortion is tenuous at best, with most studies unable to demonstrate a convincing difference in reproductive performance between patients with uncontrolled and controlled diabetes mellitus. Severe hypothyroidism is more often associated with disordered ovulation than spontaneous abortion but should be specifically tested for if other clinical features suggesting the condition are present. SLE is a widespread autoimmune disease with effects on a number of organs and systems. Various reports indicate that up to 40 per cent of clinical pregnancies are lost in women with this condition and that such patients have an increased risk of pregnancy loss prior to developing clinical stigmata of SLE.

The risk of abortion increases with maternal age, and studies linked to prenatal diagnostic procedures have revealed that if a live fetus is demonstrated by ultrasonography at 8 weeks gestational age, fewer than 2 per cent will abort spontaneously if the mother is under 30 years old. If, however, she is over 40 years of age, the risk exceeds 10 per cent and may be as high as 50 per cent at 45 years. The probable explanation is the increased incidence of chromosomally abnormal conceptuses in older women (Table 38–1).

Many modern texts still include chronic debilitating conditions such as cardiovascular and renal diseases as etiologic factors in spontaneous abortion, but these conditions, if severe, more often preclude conception. The question of essential hypertension is less clear cut, with one good study reporting a reduction in the incidence of spontaneous abortion in those women whose hypertension was treated. A randomized, controlled trial is needed to confirm or refute this suggestion.

Local Maternal Factors

Endocrine Factors. Despite a great deal of work worldwide, no prospective study has been able to demonstrate that a normal pregnancy can be lost as a result of abnormal

Table 38-1. NUMBER OF PREGNANCIES, SPONTANEOUS ABORTIONS, AND SPONTANEOUS ABORTION RATES BY MATERNAL AGE AT FIRST PREGNANCY

AGE AT LMP (YR)	PREGNANCIES	SPONTANEOUS ABORTIONS	SPONTANEOUS ABORTION RATE (%)
<30	1856	208	11.2
30-35	590	85	14.4
35-40	82	15	18.3
>40	25	14	56.0

Combined data from Alberman E: Maternal age and spontaneous abortion. In Bennett MJ, Edmonds DK (eds): Spontaneous and Recurrent Abortion. Oxford, Blackwell Scientific Publications, 1987.

hormone production by either the corpus luteum or the placenta. In addition to this, no controlled trial of exogenous hormones has been able to demonstrate any benefit, and there is good evidence that exogenous sex steroids may indeed be teratogenic. Until the existence of a "hormone deficiency" can be clearly demonstrated, it would be both scientifically and medicolegally sound to avoid prescribing progestogens or other such agents to women who are pregnant.

Uterine Abnormalities. Uterine abnormalities have been known to be associated with pregnancy loss since the turn of the century. The abnormalities may be cervical incompetence, congenital abnormalities of the uterine fundus, and acquired abnormalities of the uterine fundus.

Cervical Incompetence. Cervical incompetence occurs under a number of circumstances. The incompetence may be anatomic, and is usually the result of trauma in the form of rapid dilatation with tearing of fibers. This occurs most frequently as a result of mechanical dilatation at the time of termination of pregnancy by aspiration but may also occur at the time of curettage. The diagnosis of such incompetence is usually made when a mid-trimester pregnancy is lost with a clinical picture of sudden unexpected rupture of the membranes followed by painless expulsion of the products of conception. In addition, the cervix that is anatomically incompetent will accept a Hegar number 8 cervical dilator without any prior dilatation required and is seen to be much wider than usual on hysterography.

Functional incompetence of the cervix involves a cervix that is anatomically indistinguishable from a normal one and yet is associated with a pregnancy loss in the second trimester as previously described. Cervical incompetence is also frequently found in association with a congenital abnormality of the uterine fundus. It has been suggested that up to one third of these congenitally abnormal uteri have a cervix that exhibits a degree of incompetence.

Congenital Abnormalities. Fusion of the Müllerian ducts has been classified in a variety of ways, but it has only recently been recognized that both the internal and external contours of the uterus need to be evaluated. As a result, many former classifications have now been discarded. A congenitally abnormal uterus may be associated with pregnancy loss in both the first and the second trimester. Surgical correction of the abnormality can in many instances result in 80 per cent loss rates being turned into 80 per cent salvage rates. The diagnosis of these abnormalities is in the first instance suspected and then confirmed by either hysterography or hysteroscopy. Proper evaluation of the congenitally abnormal uterus requires laparoscopy, hysteroscopy, and hysterography before any proposals concerning therapy can be made.

Acquired Uterine Abnormalities. The most common acquired distorting influence on the uterus is the growth of submucous fibroids. Although these tend to occur more frequently in women in their late 30s and black women, they should always be sought by hysteroscopy or hysterography, since removal will frequently result in pregnancies continuing to term. Intrauterine adhesions result from trauma to the basal layer of the endometrium. This is almost always caused by overvigorous curettage at the time of either termination of pregnancy or evacuation of retained products of conception. When the entire uterine cavity has been obliterated (Asherman's syndrome), amenorrhea will result, but much more frequently there is no suggestion of intrauterine adhesions (synechiae) until a pregnancy is attempted and subsequently lost. Surgical correction of these intrauterine adhesions frequently results in subsequent pregnancies being successful.

Fetal Factors

The most common cause of spontaneous abortion is a significant genetic abnormality of the conceptus. In spontaneous first-trimester abortions, approximately two thirds have significant chromosomal anomalies, with approximately half of these being autosomal trisomies and the majority of the remainder being triploids, tetraploids, or 45X monosomies. Fortunately, the majority of these are not inherited from either mother or father and are single nonrecurring events. When seen on ultrasonography before spontaneous abortion occurs, many appear to be empty amniotic sacs and this condition is referred to as an *anembryonic pregnancy.* When a fetus is present in many late first-trimester and early second-trimester abortions, it is often significantly abnormal, either genetically or morphologically. It seems that nature has a way of identifying some of its major mistakes and causing them to be aborted.

Paternal Factors

The majority of chromosomal abnormalities occurring in the conceptus are, as already described, spontaneous events. Occasionally, however, they occur as a result of some form of chromosomal anomaly in either of the parents, and parental karyotyping is an important investigation in couples suffering from recurrent abortion.

There is increasing evidence that some pregnancies may be lost on the basis of disordered immunologic function in the female. A successful pregnancy depends on a number of immunologic factors that allow the host (mother) to retain an antigenetically foreign product (fetus) without rejection taking place. The precise mechanism of this immunologic anomaly is not yet fully understood, but it is recognized that some women, particularly those who abort recurrently, behave differently immunologically from those who carry pregnancies to term. The immunologic relationship between male and female in such a couple may therefore be regarded as abnormal, and current studies indicate that in some instances treatment of this condition may result in successful pregnancy.

MANAGEMENT

Threatened Abortion

A threatened abortion is best managed by an ultrasonic examination to determine whether the fetus is present and, if so, whether it is alive. Approximately 25 per cent of threatened abortions go on to pregnancy loss. Of those in whom a live fetus is present, 94 per cent will proceed to produce a live baby, although there is some evidence to suggest that the incidence of preterm delivery in these cases may be somewhat higher than in those who do not bleed in the first trimester. Once a live fetus has been demonstrated to the couple on ultrasonography, management consists essentially of reassurance. There is no need for admission to the hospital, nor is there any evidence that bed rest improves the prognosis. A repeat ultrasonic examination a week later will do more to elevate levels of confidence and provide reassurance to the couple than any other form of management.

Inevitable Abortion

Patients require admission to the hospital, analgesia for pain, and an ultrasonic examination to determine whether the process is inevitable or has gone further to become incomplete.

Incomplete Abortion

Patients require admission to the hospital, analgesia, and very possibly resuscitation. It is wise to insert an intravenous line into patients with an incomplete abortion and to take blood for cross-matching and blood grouping. These patients may suddenly become profoundly shocked as a result of hemorrhage, sepsis, or, rarely, products distending the cervical os. Once the patient's condition is stable, she should have the remaining products of conception evacuated from the uterus under appropriate anesthesia.

An incomplete abortion that has become septic is a condition fraught with danger and it must be managed vigorously. Overwhelming sepsis may lead to renal and hepatic failure, disseminated intravascular coagulation, and even death. Should the patient survive, the long-term sequelae of sepsis may be infertility or chronic pelvic inflammatory disease and its concomitant pain. Any physical signs suggesting sepsis in a woman with an incomplete abortion demand appropriate antibiotic therapy, which is best given intravenously in the first instance. The potential for disaster in these circumstances cannot be overemphasized.

Missed Abortion

The diagnosis is suggested by arrested increase in uterine size or inability to detect the fetal heart sounds. Missed abortion needs to be confirmed by ultrasonic examination. Once the diagnosis has been made, it is appropriate to evacuate the retained products of conception surgically to minimize the risk of sepsis and to reduce the extent of hemorrhage and the degree of pain that accompanies the spontaneous expulsive process.

General Management Considerations

Regardless of any of the above-mentioned diagnoses, if the patient is Rh negative and does not have Rh antibodies, prophylactic anti-D gamma globulin should be administered to prevent sensitization. All couples who have had a pregnancy loss should be seen and counseled some weeks after the event. At this time, questions that the couple may have can be answered and reassurance given about their chances of reproductive success in the future. In a typical couple who have suffered a reproductive loss, the woman has very marked guilt feelings and these need to be recognized. Further, the physician must explain to her that her recent loss was almost certainly not due to anything she did that she should not have done nor to anything she did not do that she should have done. Very often, a single counseling session for a couple who have lost one pregnancy is sufficient, but it must be recognized that there may be a need for further sessions, and indeed professional counseling help may be appropriate.

Recurrent Abortion

The investigation of a couple who present with more than one pregnancy loss can be determined from the previous discussion in this chapter. As far as the mother is concerned, it is appropriate to rule out the presence of systemic disorders such as diabetes mellitus, SLE, and thyroid disease, and it is also necessary to test for the presence of a lupus anticoagulant. Paternal and maternal chromosomes should be evaluated, and hysteroscopy or hysterography should be performed to evaluate the uterine anatomy.

Given the possibility of the pregnancy losses being caused by infectious agents, it is also appropriate to rule out the presence of *Mycoplasma, Listeria, Toxoplasma, Treponema,* cytomegalovirus, and *Brucella.*

In approximately half of the couples with recurrent losses, all of these tests will be normal, and this must be regarded both by the health care professional and the couple as being good news. The diagnosis of immunologic abnormalities requires complex investigations including assays for lymphocytotoxic antibodies and evaluation of cell-mediated immunity. There are a number of studies that indicate a significant success rate following the administration of purified paternal lymphocytes to the mother, but there are an equal number of well-conducted studies that fail to demonstrate any beneficial effect of such treatment. Studies from Scandinavia, North America, and Australia have demonstrated that a variety of disparate methods of raising patient confidence can produce success rates in the region of 85 to 90 per cent, and it would seem that many workers have underestimated the role played by reassurance and tender loving care in the management of patients with recurrent abortion.

In those couples in whom a specific etiologic factor(s) is found, appropriate management can be expected to be followed by reproductive success. Many of the congenital abnormalities of the uterus no longer require laparotomy for their correction and in expert hands are best dealt with through an operating hysteroscope. Cervical incompetence is managed by the placement of a cervical suture at the level of the internal os, and this suture is best placed in the first trimester, once a live fetus has been demonstrated on ultrasonography. The older texts suggest placement of a cervical cerclage at 12 to 14 weeks of gestation, but this was before the advent of ultrasonography, and it was believed that there was a significant risk of suturing a dead fetus into the uterus if the suture was placed before 14 weeks. We now know that if a live fetus is present in the uterus at 8 or 9 weeks, the likelihood of subsequent abortion is remote. The technical ease of placing a suture around the cervix while the uterus is still a pelvic organ far outweighs the very small risk of intrauterine death occurring.

There are some authorities who still believe that recurrent pregnancy loss is sometimes associated with the so-called luteal phase deficiency. The diagnosis of this condition is controversial at best, and the relationship between the two conditions is very tenuous. Moreover, studies aimed at giving hormones to correct the deficiency have been unable to show any improvement in pregnancy salvage.

TERMINATION OF PREGNANCY

Over the last 3 decades, many countries have moved to legalize termination of pregnancy. There is variation in the upper limit of gestational age beyond which termination is illegal, and the circumstances and conditions under which termination of pregnancy may be performed are similarly varied. Nevertheless, the loss of life, health, and fertility so commonplace when terminations were performed on desperate young women by untrained back-street criminals are, thankfully, rarely encountered today (Fig. 38–1).

Patient Assessment

Individual patient counseling should be an integral part of the service provided, since this is an emotionally difficult time for the patient and many women are plagued by guilt for many years after a termination of pregnancy. Physical assessment is as important as before any other surgical procedure, and special investigations are an integral adjunct. If there is any clinical discrepancy between dates and uterine size, an ultrasonic examination should be undertaken. The patient's blood group and Rhesus (Rh) type must be ascertained, since if she is Rh negative and has no anti-D antibodies, anti-D gamma globulin must be administered as prophylaxis against isoimmunization.

Techniques

In practical terms, the techniques used are determined by the duration of pregnancy. During the first trimester, the methods are either medical or surgical. Agents that have been called antiprogesterones (Ru 486) have been administered successfully in the first half of the first trimester. When given in conjunction with local prostaglandin, the success rate in causing expulsion of the uterine contents exceeds 90 per cent. This rate drops significantly if the pregnancy is more advanced than 7 weeks gestational age. One of the problems with these "abortion pills" is that countries like the United Kingdom have legislated that pregnancies can be terminated only in licensed premises, yet the tablets can be taken anywhere. As yet, few countries have licensed these products for use, but the very low rate of side effects and the high success rate suggest that the number of coun-

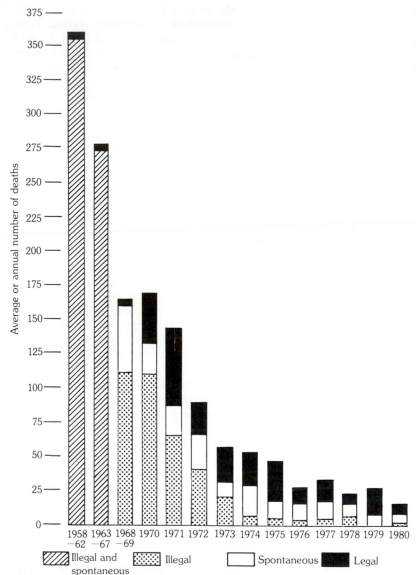

Figure 38–1. Number of deaths associated with abortion by type of abortion—United States, 1958–1980. (By permission of the Population Council from Tietze C: Induced Abortion: A World Review, 1983. 5th ed. New York, The Population Council Inc, 1983.)

tries permitting these compounds will increase in the future.

Dilatation and Aspiration

Dilatation of the cervix and aspiration curettage is the most common method used to terminate pregnancies in the first trimester. It can be performed under either local anesthesia (paracervical block) or general anesthesia and has a very low complication rate in trained hands. Dilatation of the cervix may be achieved surgically using graduated metal dilators or medically using either *Laminaria* or the local intravaginal placement of a prostaglandin E_1 analog. The medical methods have the advantage of dilating the cervix slowly and gently but take several hours to accomplish the task. The potential for physical damage to the cervix when it is surgically dilated is ever present, but there is no unequivocal evidence that cervical incompetence occurs more often as a result of first-trimester aspiration termination. Once the cervix is dilated, a hollow plastic curette is

Table 38–2. ABORTIFACIENT AGENTS

DRUG	DOSE AND ROUTE OF ADMINISTRATION	MEAN INSTILLATION TO ABORTION TIME	SUCCESS RATE (TIME)	SIDE EFFECTS
Prostaglandin $F_{2\alpha}$	40 mg in single Intra-amniotic dose	20 hr	80% (at 48 hr)	Diarrhea (15%) Vomiting (50%) Heavy uterine bleeding (5%) Bronchoconstriction (2%) Incomplete abortion (33%) Hypotension and hypertension Transverse rupture of posterior uterine wall at cervico-isthmic junction
Prostaglandin $F_{2\alpha}$ and urea	20 mg $PGF_{2\alpha}$ and 80 gm of urea dissolved in 130 to 150 ml of distilled water. Oxytocin infusion started 4 hr after rupture of membranes	13 hr	100% (at 24 hr)	Nausea and vomiting (60%) Incomplete abortion (45%) Hemorrhage (10%) Diarrhea (1%) Cervical laceration (3%)
Prostaglandin E_2	5 mg or 10 mg intra-amniotically. Oxytocin infusion started 6 hr later	15 hr	97% (at 36 hr)	Nausea (60%) Vomiting (45%) Diarrhea (17%) Pyrexia ($>38°C$) (15%) Blood loss >500 ml (1.7%)

Modified from Chaudhuri G: Abortion. In Hacker NF, Moore JG (eds): Essentials of Obstetrics and Gynecology. 1st ed. Philadelphia, WB Saunders, 1986, p 334.

inserted and the contents of the uterine cavity are aspirated under controlled negative pressure.

Second-Trimester Terminations

With an increasing number of women having prenatal diagnostic procedures, a significant number of second-trimester terminations are performed because of the diagnosis of serious genetic abnormalities. These terminations are all extremely distressing for the couple concerned, and careful, thoughtful, and knowledgeable counseling both before and after the termination is mandatory. The upper limit of gestational age after which termination can no longer be legally performed varies from country to country but does not influence the method used to achieve termination.

Since the introduction of prostaglandins, hysterotomy has become a very rarely performed operation and, in view of the increased risks of this procedure, should be avoided if at all possible. As for first-trimester terminations, the methods available are essentially medical or surgical.

The intrauterine instillation of prostaglandin E_2 or $F_{2\alpha}$ and hypertonic urea or the extra-amniotic placement of PGE_2 or $F_{2\alpha}$ will result in uterine contractions and expulsion of the fetus in the vast majority of cases (Table 38–2). The problem with this and related medical methods is that labor can take many hours and is painful unless conducted under epidural analgesia. The incidence of retention of the placenta is high, and there is the ever-present risk of hemorrhage, infection, or both. In addition, there are economic considerations of daily in-patient hospital costs.

Dilatation and evacuation of the fetus and

placenta piecemeal has become the most widely used method of termination of second-trimester pregnancies since the introduction of *Laminaria* in 1977. After gradual dilatation of the cervix, evacuation of the products of conception is the method of termination with the lowest complication rate.

The introduction of a new prostaglandin E_1 analog should undoubtedly replace *Laminaria* as the method of choice for cervical dilatation. If the evacuation is performed under ultrasonic control, the operator can be sure that no products are retained in the uterus at the end of the procedure and that undiagnosed uterine perforation will not occur. It is probably safe to suggest that the only indication for not doing a second-trimester termination by dilatation and evacuation under ultrasonic control is to obtain the fetus intact, to allow careful post-mortem evaluation for the diagnosis of a specific structural fetal abnormality. Dilatation and evacuation involves less emotional distress than the prolonged and painful process following the medical induction of termination at this stage of pregnancy.

CONCLUSION

Leaving aside the termination of pregnancy performed for genetic reasons, it must be remembered that in this, as in all other branches of medicine, prevention is better than cure. Adequate contraceptive methods will prevent all but the very rare unplanned pregnancy and should, therefore, be emphasized whenever and wherever the opportunity arises.

SUGGESTED READING

Bennett MJ, Edmonds DK: Recurrent and Spontaneous Abortion. Oxford, Blackwell Scientific Publications, 1987.

Bennett MJ, Horrowitz SDH, Wass DM, Hall R: The use of 16, 16-dimethyl-PGE-methyl ester (Cervagem*) vaginal pessaries for cervical dilatation prior to evacuation for second trimester termination. Aust NZ J Obstet Gynecol 31:44, 1990.

Byrne J, Warburton D, Kline J, et al: Morphology of early fetal deaths and their chromosomal characteristics. Teratology 32:297, 1985.

Harger JH: Early cerclage in habitual abortion. Fertil Steril 39(2):244, 1983.

Holzgreve W, Schonberg SA, Douglas RG, Golbus MS: X-chromosome hyperploidy in couples with multiple spontaneous abortions. Obstet Gynecol 63:237, 1984.

Quebbeman JF, Semprini AE, Beer AE: Clinical and immunological consequences of female immunization with paternal leukocytes in couples with recurrent abortion (abstr). Fertil Steril 41(suppl):2, 1984.

Quinn PA, Shewchuk AB, Schuber J, et al: Efficacy of antibiotic therapy in preventing spontaneous pregnancy loss among couples colonized with genital mycoplasmas. Am J Obstet Gynecol 145:239, 1983.

Simpson JL: Repetitive spontaneous abortion. In Porter IH (ed): Perinatal Genetics. New York, Academic Press, 1986.

Stray-Pedersen B, Stray-Pedersen S: Etiologic factors and subsequent reproductive performance in 195 couples with previous habitual abortion. Am J Obstet Gynecol 148:2, 1984.

Thirty-nine

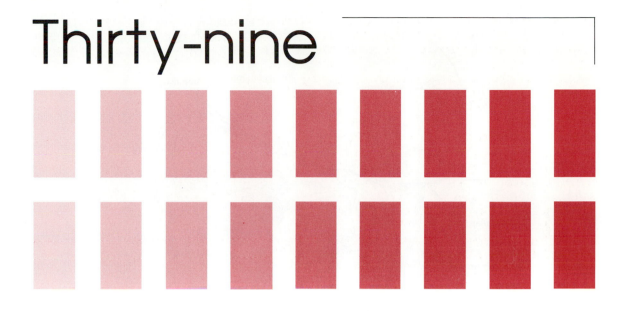

Ectopic Pregnancy

ALDO PALMIERI and J. GEORGE MOORE

An ectopic pregnancy is a gestation that implants outside of the endometrial cavity. It represents a serious hazard to a woman's health and reproductive potential, requiring prompt recognition and early aggressive intervention.

More than 95 per cent of ectopic pregnancies implant in various anatomic segments of the fallopian tube, including the interstitial (1 per cent), isthmic (5 per cent), ampullary (85 per cent), and infundibular portions (9 per cent). Other less common sites of ectopic implantation are the uterine cervix, ovary, and the peritoneal cavity (Fig. 39–1 and Table 39–1).

EPIDEMIOLOGY

Over the past 20 years, ectopic pregnancy and its related hospitalization have tripled, and currently this condition represents the fourth leading cause of maternal mortality overall and the most common cause of maternal mortality in the first trimester. Several factors have been implicated as contributing to this increased incidence:

1. Improved technology, which has allowed for earlier and more complete diagnosis of some patients who went undetected in the past.

2. The rising incidence of acute and chronic salpingitis, induced abortion, tubal ligation, tubal reconstructive surgery, and conservative management of tubal pregnancy, all of which result in histologic and structural damage to the tubes.

3. The use of intrauterine contraceptive devices (IUDs). Women with IUDs are four times more likely to suffer from an ectopic pregnancy. This effect is due to the better protection afforded by IUDs against intrauterine compared with extrauterine preg-

425

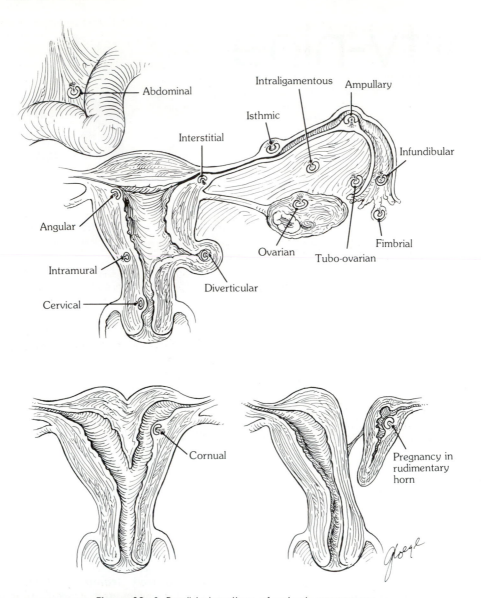

Figure 39–1. Possible locations of ectopic pregnancy.

nancy and the higher incidence of pelvic inflammatory disease among IUD users.

The overall incidence of ectopic pregnancy is estimated to be at least one in every 200 pregnancies.

ETIOLOGY

Several causative factors are known, but others remain unknown. Probably as many as 50 per cent of cases result from alteration of tubal transport mechanisms secondary to damage to the ciliated surface of the endosalpinx caused by infections such as chlamydia and gonorrhea. Others are the result of intrinsic abnormalities of the fertilized ovum and possibly transmigration of the oocyte to the contralateral tube, with resulting delays in passage.

EVOLUTION

Tubal pregnancies rapidly invade the mucosa, feeding from the tubal vessels, which

SITE	INCIDENCE
Abdominal	1:3372–1:7931
Ovarian	1:7000
Cervical	1:1000–1:18,000
Intraligamentous	1:49,765–1:183,900
Rudimentary horn	1:100,000

Table 39–1. INCIDENCE OF NONTUBAL ECTOPIC PREGNANCIES

(From Bayless RB: Nontubal ectopic pregnancy. Clin Obstet Gynecol 30:191, 1987.)

become enlarged and engorged. The segment of the affected tube is distended as the pregnancy grows. Possible outcomes of such abnormal gestations are as follows:

1. The pregnancy is unable to survive owing to its poor blood supply, thus resulting in a tubal abortion and resorption, or it is expelled from the fimbriated end into the abdominal cavity.

2. The pregnancy continues to grow until the overdistended tube ruptures, with resulting profuse intraperitoneal bleeding.

3. In rare instances, a tubal pregnancy will be expelled from the tube and seed onto sites in the abdominal cavity, for example, the omentum, the small or large bowel, or the parietal peritoneum, and give rise to a viable abdominal pregnancy.

SYMPTOMS AND CLINICAL DIAGNOSIS

Retrospective studies have shown that patients with an ectopic pregnancy may be seen several times by a physician before the correct diagnosis is made. The delayed diagnosis is related to a low index of suspicion by the clinician, often confused by a lack of typical symptoms. Pivotal to a prompt diagnosis of ectopic pregnancy is an awareness of the risk factors. High risk factors can be summarized as follows:

1. Previous history of pelvic inflammatory disease (ectopic rate of one in 24, as opposed to one in 200 in noninfected patients).

2. Previous ectopic pregnancy (15 to 50 per cent increase in incidence of ectopic gestation in subsequent pregnancies).

3. History of tubal sterilization within the past 1 to 2 years (higher incidence if cauterization was used).

4. Previous tubal reconstructive surgery (tuboplasty or end to end reanastomosis for sterilization reversal).

5. Pregnancy with an IUD in place or a patient with a history of IUD use.

6. Prolonged infertility.

7. More than one therapeutic abortion (controversial).

8. Diethylstilbestrol (DES) exposure (may have tubal abnormalities).

9. Pregnancy resulting from failed postcoital contraception (probably associated with abnormal tubal transport).

There are no pathognomonic symptoms of ectopic pregnancy, but the classic symptom triad consists of amenorrhea, vaginal bleeding, and abdominal pain.

Abdominal pain, usually in the lower abdomen in early cases, or generalized in ruptured ectopics with a hemoperitoneum, is present in more than 90 per cent of cases. Amenorrhea or a history of an abnormal last menstrual period is found in 75 to 90 per cent of ectopic pregnancies. Vaginal bleeding, from spotting to the equivalent of a menstrual period, results from a low human chorionic gonadotropin (hCG) production by the ectopic trophoblast and is seen in 50 to 80 per cent of patients.

Making the diagnosis of an acutely ruptured ectopic pregnancy is fairly straightforward. The patient presents with symptoms of increasing abdominal pain, abdominal distention, and hypovolemia (tachycardia, diaphoresis, orthostatic blood pressure changes). Sometimes shoulder pain, reflecting irritation of the phrenic nerve from intraperitoneal blood, is present. The entire abdomen is acutely tender with guarding and rebound tenderness.

Physical examination in patients with an unruptured ectopic pregnancy may be extremely variable. Most patients are afebrile, but 10 per cent of patients will have a temperature higher than 38°C. Ninety per cent have abdominal tenderness, but only 45 per cent have positive rebound tenderness, and only 50 per cent have an adnexal mass on pelvic examination. In half the cases, the mass is contralateral to the ectopic pregnancy and represents the corpus luteum. Twenty

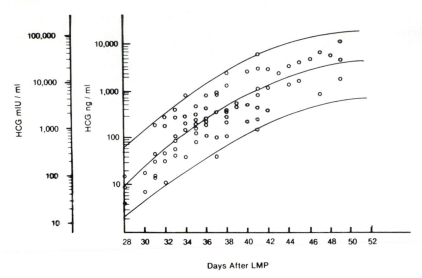

Figure 39–2. Distribution curve of hCG in normal pregnancies. (Modified from Pittaway DE, Reish RL, Wentz AC: Doubling times of human chorionic gonadotropin increase in early viable intrauterine pregnancies. Am J Obstet Gynecol 152:299, 1985.)

per cent present with bilateral adnexal masses owing to the presence of a contralateral corpus luteum cyst. The uterus is soft and either of normal size or slightly enlarged.

DIFFERENTIAL DIAGNOSIS

Many gynecologic and nongynecologic disorders have symptoms in common with ectopic pregnancy. Gynecologic disorders to be considered include:

1. Threatened or incomplete abortion (also presenting with pain, bleeding, and a positive pregnancy test).
2. A ruptured corpus luteum cyst (abdominal pain, moderate to severe, at times coexisting with a history of amenorrhea, vaginal spotting, and the presence or absence of pregnancy).
3. Acute pelvic inflammatory disease with fever, abdominal pain, leukocytosis, and, at times, adnexal masses.
4. Adnexal torsion or degenerating leiomyoma.

Among the nongynecologic problems, acute appendicitis, pyelonephritis, and pancreatitis must be considered.

The key to the successful management of ectopic pregnancy is early diagnosis. Although the number of new cases has increased threefold, fewer are arriving at the hospital ruptured, with the patient already in hemorrhagic shock. This decrease is evidence that a high index of suspicion and vigorous efforts at early diagnosis are effective. "Think ectopic!" is a sign frequently seen posted in emergency rooms.

Beta-hCG Testing

Human chorionic gonadotropin is a glycoprotein with a structure similar to luteinizing hormone (LH), consisting of two linked subunits, alpha and beta. The last 30 amino acids of the β subunit are different from the sequence of LH. Beta-hCG is secreted by the syncytiotrophoblast and has the sole function of supporting the corpus luteum. An accurate diagnosis of ectopic pregnancy requires knowledge of the dynamics of hCG in the first trimester of normal pregnancies. hCG increases exponentially following a nonlinear model (Fig. 39–2). The doubling time of beta-hCG in the serum will vary from 1.2 days shortly after implantation to 3.5 days 2 months after the last menstrual period.

Abnormal beta-hCG dynamics (prolonged doubling time, plateauing or decreasing levels) before the eighth week of gestation are indicative of a nonviable gestation but do not provide information on the location of the pregnancy (Fig. 39–3). When serial quantitative values of beta-hCG are obtained and they do not fall into the normal range, ultrasonography must be used to locate the gestation.

The rapidly dividing fertilized egg begins

Figure 39–3. Patterns of serial hCG concentrations from three surgically proved tubal pregnancies. The numbers indicate the doubling time for that interval of time (From Pittaway DE, Reisch RL, Wentz AC: Doubling time of human chorionic gonadotropin increase in early viable intrauterine pregnancies. Am J Obstet Gynecol 152:299, 1985.)

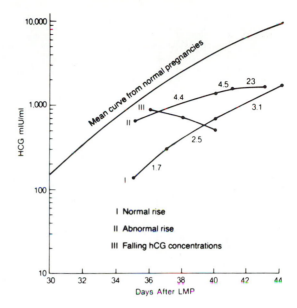

production of hCG even before implantation occurs. The sensitivity of the current methods for detection of beta-hCG in the maternal serum allows the confirmation of pregnancy even before a missed period (levels of > 10 mIU/ml). The commercially available urinary beta-hCG testing kits, based on monoclonal antibodies, are sensitive to 50 mIU/ml, corresponding to approximately 12 to 15 days from conception (Fig. 39–4).

Serum Progesterone

Serum progesterone levels of greater than 25 ng/ml virtually assure an intrauterine pregnancy. It is therefore helpful to obtain a progesterone level when suspecting an ectopic pregnancy. Should this level be below 15 ng/ml, additional testing with hCG and ultrasonography should be performed. Another limitation of progesterone testing is the relatively long waiting period for the result (approximately 24 hours in most situations), which further restricts its use.

Ultrasonography

This field has shown rapid technological improvements in recent years, and its application to the diagnosis of ectopic pregnancy, alone and in combination with hCG testing, is now the standard of care. Transvaginal

ultrasonography has allowed the detection of an intrauterine gestational sac as early as 5 weeks of amenorrhea (2 mm diameter), thus virtually ruling out an ectopic pregnancy, since the coexistence of an intrauterine pregnancy and an ectopic pregnancy occurs only once in 30,000 gestations.

When associated with beta-hCG determinations, it is important to recognize a "discriminatory zone." This can be defined as the level of beta-hCG at which an intrauterine sac must be seen with ultrasonography (Fig. 39–5). If the sac is not visualized at that discriminatory level of beta-hCG, the likelihood of an ectopic pregnancy is greater than 90 per cent (Fig. 39–6A). Special attention is needed to differentiate between a true sac and a pseudosac, which is a ring-like structure produced on ultrasound by a prominent decidual echo (Fig. 39–6B).

Discriminatory zones differ among institutions, depending on available technology and individual skills, but on average are equal to 1500 to 2000 mIU/ml of beta-hCG.

Culdocentesis

Culdocentesis is the technique by which a needle attached to a syringe is inserted transvaginally through the posterior vaginal fornix into the pouch of Douglas, detecting any fluid within the peritoneal cavity (Fig. 39–7). Although simple, inexpensive, and rapid, it is

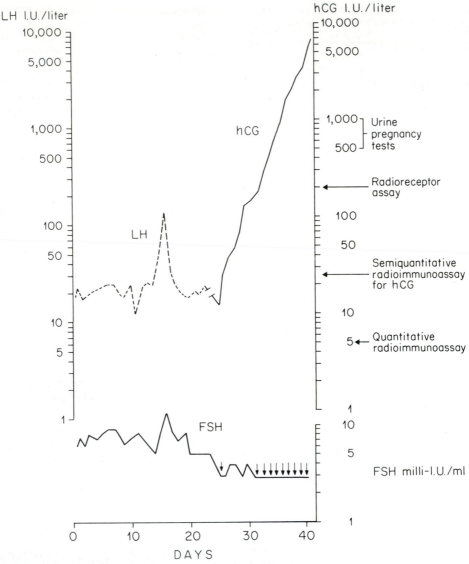

Figure 39–4. Graphic representation of serum chorionic gonadotropin titers in pregnancy and the sensitivity of the various pregnancy tests. Arrows indicate levels below the sensitivity of the assay. (From Dignam WJ: Ectopic pregnancy. In Hacker N, Moore JG (eds): Essentials of Obstetrics and Gynecology. 1st ed. Philadelphia, W. B. Saunders, 1986.)

quite uncomfortable for the patient and of limited use in an unruptured ectopic pregnancy. It is unnecessary when the diagnosis is obvious (i.e., hypovolemic patients) and has a high false-negative rate. Culdocentesis is progressively being replaced by transvaginal sonography and rapid beta-hCG assay.

Laparoscopy

Although extremely accurate for the diagnosis of ectopic pregnancy, laparoscopy is the last step to be entertained because it requires general anesthesia and there are infrequent, but serious risks associated with the procedure.

MANAGEMENT

The management of ectopic pregnancy has dramatically changed in recent years. The algorithm displayed in Figure 39–8 outlines a reasonably up-to-date approach to diagnosis and management. A condition that was in-

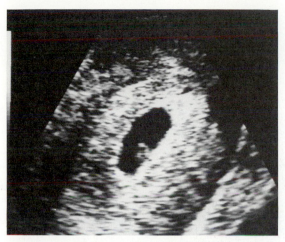

Figure 39–5. Transvaginal ultrasound view of intra-uterine gestational sac with embryo and placenta at 6½ weeks from last menstrual period (Courtesy of Dr. Gail Hanson, Department of Radiology, UCLA—Olive View Hospital, Sylmar, CA.)

Technique of Pelviscopic Removal of Ectopic Pregnancy

Under general anesthesia, the patient is placed in a steep Trendelenburg position to displace the bowels cephalad. A 10-mm laparoscope is placed intraumbilically, and lower quadrant 5-mm punctures are made on both sides to insert accessory probes, suction-irrigation cannulas, grasping forceps, and electrosurgical instruments (e.g., unipolar knife, laser probe, coagulating forceps).

The unruptured tube is incised longitudinally along the antimesenteric wall and the ectopic pregnancy removed with spoon forceps; bleeding is controlled with coagulating instruments, and the tube and pelvis are copiously irrigated with Ringer's lactate. The tubal incision is left open for spontaneous closure. All instruments are then removed and the three small cutaneous incisions closed (Fig. 39–9). If a partial or total salpingectomy is required, this is accomplished with the aid of endoscopic ligatures (Endoloops).

The laparoscopic approach offers several advantages over traditional exploratory laparotomy, as follows:

1. Decreased hospital stay. It can often be done on an outpatient basis.
2. Decreased disability and postoperative

variably treated by exploratory laparotomy and removal of the affected tube (salpingectomy) is now amenable to a variety of both surgical and nonsurgical treatments. Tubal gestations less than 3 cm in diameter and unruptured can be approached laparoscopically. If the patient is hemodynamically unstable with a substantial hemoperitoneum, the approach should be immediate laparotomy.

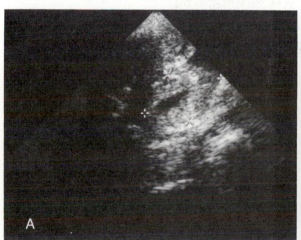
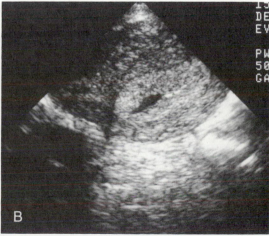

Figure 39–6. *A,* Tubal gestation in cul-de-sac. (Courtesy of Dr. Gail Hanson, Department of Radiology, UCLA—Olive View Hospital, Sylmar, CA.) *B,* Ultrasound view of pseudosac in uterus (same patient).

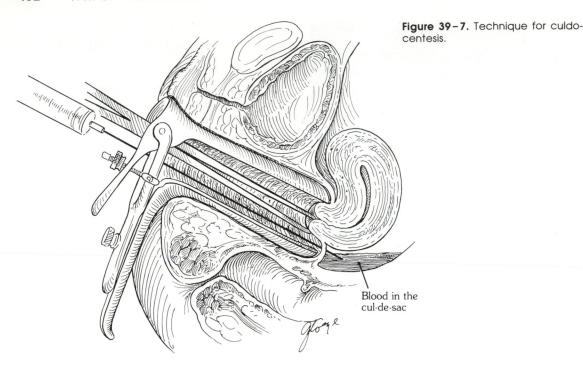

Figure 39–7. Technique for culdocentesis.

Blood in the cul-de-sac

pain. Time for recovery is often less than 1 week.

3. Decreased cost.

Sixty per cent of tubal pregnancies can be successfully managed with laparoscopy, and the subsequent pregnancy rates (60 per cent) are equal to those of laparotomy.

Laparotomy

Laparotomy is indicated in the following circumstances:

1. In all patients presenting with signs of hemodynamic compromise.
2. When the ectopic pregnancy is >3 cm in greatest dimension.
3. When extensive pelvic adhesions are suspected.
4. When there is failure or inadequacy of the laparoscopic equipment.
5. When the endoscopic skills of the operating surgeon are suboptimal.

As far as the surgeon's skill is concerned, it should be kept in mind that operative laparoscopy (or pelviscopy) is a recent acquisition in the armamentarium of the gynecologic surgeon, and exploratory laparotomy for the treatment of ectopic pregnancy is still the standard of care.

The type of procedure performed by either laparoscopy or laparotomy will be dictated by local findings at the time of surgery and the desire of the woman for future fertility. In patients who wish to conserve fertility, a linear salpingostomy is the treatment of choice in unruptured ampullary pregnancies. As an alternative, in ampullary pregnancies that have already ruptured, a segmental resection or partial salpingectomy can be offered, which implies the removal of only the affected segment of tube, leaving the rest intact for future reanastomosis, if desired.

All Rh-negative patients with an ectopic pregnancy should receive rhogam regardless of the mode of treatment.

Nonsurgical Management

A more recent approach to the medical management of ectopic pregnancy is the use of methotrexate, a folic acid inhibitor that blocks nucleic acid synthesis in the trophoblastic cells. The drug is administered intravenously for 8 days, alternating 1 mg/kg on

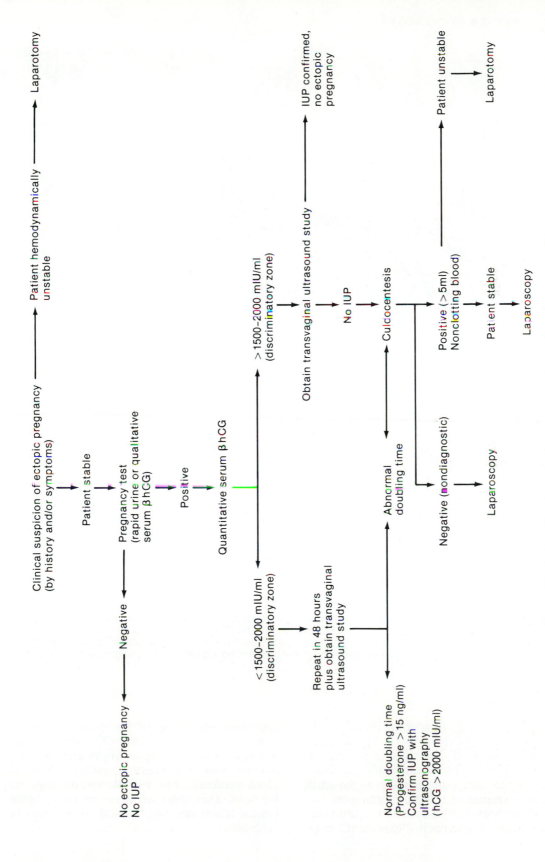

Figure 39-8. Algorithm for ectopic pregnancy diagnosis and management.

433

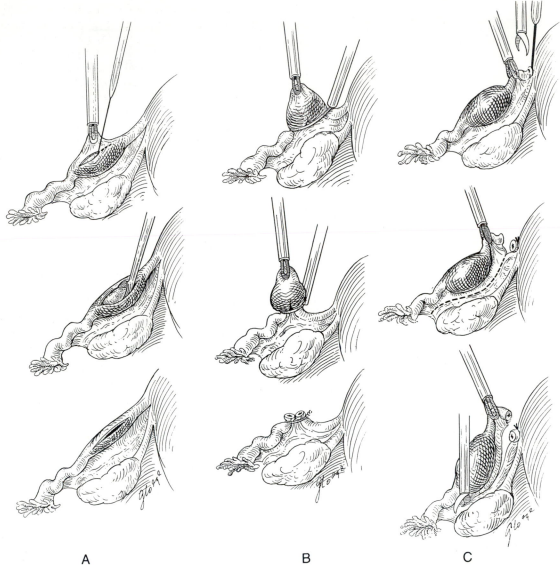

A   B   C

Figure 39-9. Methods of laparoscopic management of tubal pregnancy. *A,* Linear salpingostomy for an ampullary ectopic pregnancy. *B,* Partial salpingectomy with Endoloop. *C,* Salpingectomy using Endoloops and cautery scissors for isthmic tubal pregnancy. (From Reich H, et al: Laparoscopic treatment of 100 consecutive ectopic pregnancies. Proceedings of the Advanced Operative Laparoscopy Meeting, May 1990, Fort Worth, TX.)

days 1, 3, 5, 7 with citrovorum rescue on the intervening days (Table 39–2). Methotrexate can also be injected directly into the ectopic sac transvaginally under ultrasonic guidance. The use of methotrexate is reserved for small (<3 cm) unruptured ectopic pregnancies.

Some authors have advocated a nonsurgical, nonmedical approach ("expectant" management), consisting of hospitalizing the patient, with serial beta-hCG testing and monitoring of vital signs. Many ectopic pregnancies will not rupture spontaneously or bleed profusely but will slowly undergo resorption. This approach is not practical in the United States because hospital costs would be prohibitive.

Table 39-2. METHOTREXATE TREATMENT OF ECTOPIC PREGNANCY

DAY OF TREATMENT	THERAPY
1	Methotrexate, 1 mg/kg IV
2	Citrovorum factor, 0.1 mg/kg IM
3	Methotrexate, 1 mg/kg IV
4	Citrovorum factor, 0.1 mg/kg IM
5	Methotrexate, 1 mg/kg IV
6	Citrovorum factor, 0.1 mg/kg IM
7	Methotrexate, 1 mg/kg IV
8	Citrovorum factor, 0.1 mg/kg IM

IV = intravenous; IM = intramuscular.

Treatment of Uncommon Types of Ectopic Pregnancies

Ectopic pregnancy and *tubal pregnancy* are terms used interchangeably because other sites of ectopic implantation are rare. A pregnancy can implant on the surface of the ovary, however, producing identical symptoms to a tubal gestation. The treatment is aimed at removing the pregnancy and sacrificing as little as possible of the ovarian tissue. When this is deemed impossible, usually as a consequence of profuse bleeding, oophorectomy is indicated.

Cervical pregnancy usually presents with profuse vaginal bleeding, and attempts at removal of the pregnancy are often unsuccessful. Hysterectomy is frequently indicated and is usually quite difficult. In more recent years, methotrexate and arterial embolization have been used to manage cervical pregnancy.

Pregnancies can rarely implant in the abdominal cavity (e.g., example on the omentum, bowel, or the parietal peritoneum). At the time of laparotomy, a major technical difficulty is the removal of the placenta. Vital organs may be entirely or partially covered by the tenaciously attached placenta, and any attempt at removal may cause massive bleeding. Partial bowel resection may be required if the bowel is involved. In most cases, it is best to leave the placenta attached, especially if the pregnancy is in the second or third trimester.

SUGGESTED READING

Breen JL: A 21 year study of 645 ectopic pregnancies. Am J Obstet Gynecol 106:104, 1970.

Centers for Disease Control: Ectopic Pregnancy in the USA. MMWR 38:481, 1989.

Fritz MA, Guo S: Doubling time of human chorionic gonadotrophin (HCG) in early pregnancy: Relationship to HCG concentration and gestational age. Fertil Steril 47:584, 1987.

Henderson SR: Ectopic tubal pregnancy treated by operative laparoscopy. Am J Obstet Gynecol 160:1462, 1989.

Kadar N, De Vore G, Romer R: Discriminatory HCG zone: Its use in the sonographic evaluation for ectopic pregnancy. Obstet Gynecol 58:156, 1981.

Leach RE, Ory SJ: Modern management of ectopic pregnancy. J Reprod Med 34:324, 1989.

Pittaway DE, Reisch RL, Wentz AC: Doubling time of human chorionic gonadotropin increase in early viable intrauterine pregnancies. Am J Obstet Gynecol 152:299, 1985.

Stovall TG, Ling FW, Gray LA, et al: Methotrexate treatment of unruptured ectopic pregnancy: A report of 100 cases. Obstet Gynecol 77:749, 1991.

Vermesh M, Silva PD, Rosen GF, et al: Management of unruptured ectopic gestation by linear salpingostomy: A prospective, randomized clinical trial of laparoscopy vs. laparotomy. Obstet Gynecol 73:400, 1989.

Forty

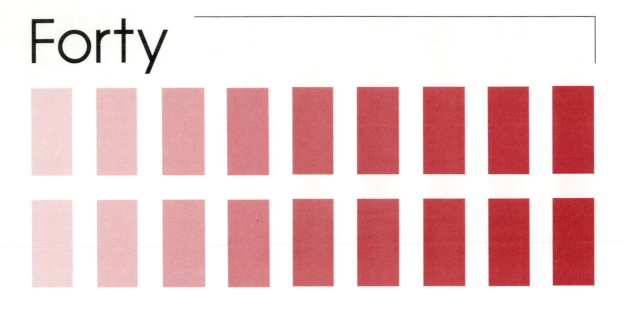

Chronic Pelvic Pain

ANDREA J. RAPKIN

Chronic pelvic pain refers to pain of greater than 6 months' duration. Although an enigmatic entity, it is one of the most common presenting complaints in a gynecologic practice. As a health problem, it incurs great cost to society in terms of hospital services, loss of productivity, and human misery.

Obviously, not all lower abdominal and low back pains are of gynecologic origin. Careful evaluation is needed to distinguish gynecologic pain from that of orthopedic, gastrointestinal, urologic, neurologic, and psychosomatic origin. The relationship between pelvic pain and the underlying gynecologic pathology is often inexplicable. For example, it is well known that women with severe endometriosis may experience no discomfort, whereas those with mild to moderate amounts of this disease may have disabling pain. Pelvic adhesions represent another puzzling entity. There is disagreement within the gynecologic community as

to whether adhesions can cause pelvic pain, and, if so, what types can be implicated. Finally, there are those situations in which no pathology can be found, but pain persists.

The discovery of the role of prostaglandins in primary dysmenorrhea, formerly believed to be a neurotic affectation, calls for caution in making a diagnosis of psychosomatic pelvic pain. There is still much to be learned about the mechanisms involved in the production and perception of pelvic pain.

ANATOMY AND PHYSIOLOGY

The pain fibers to pelvic organs are shown in Table 40–1. Painful impulses that originate in the skin, muscles, bones, joints, and parietal peritoneum travel in somatic nerve fibers, whereas those originating in the internal organs travel in visceral nerves. Visceral pain has a more diffuse localization than that

Table 40-1. NERVES CARRYING PAINFUL IMPULSES FROM THE PELVIC ORGANS

ORGAN	SPINAL SEGMENTS	NERVES
Perineum, vulva, lower vagina	S2-4	Pudendal Inguinal Genitofemoral Posterofemoral cutaneous
Upper vagina, cervix, lower uterine segment, posterior urethra, bladder trigone, utero-sacral and cardinal ligaments, rectosigmoid, lower ureters	S2-4	Pelvic parasympathetics
Uterine fundus, proximal fallopian tubes, broad ligament, upper bladder, cecum, appendix, terminal large bowel	T11-12, L1	Sympathetics via hypogastric plexus
Outer two thirds of fallopian tubes, upper ureter	T9-10	Sympathetics via aortic and superior mesenteric plexus
Ovaries	T9-10	Sympathetics via renal and aortic plexus and celiac and mesenteric ganglia

of somatic origin because there is no well-defined projection in the sensory cortex for its identification. Visceral pain is, therefore, usually referred to the skin, which is supplied by the corresponding spinal cord segment (referred pain). For example, the initial pain of appendicitis is referred to the epigastric area, since both structures are innervated by the thoracic cord segments 8, 9, and 10.

The structures of the female genital tract vary in their sensitivity to pain. The skin of the external genitalia is exquisitely sensitive. Pain sensation is variable in the vagina, since the upper segment is somewhat less sensitive than the lower. The cervix is relatively insensitive to small biopsies but is sensitive to deep incision or to dilatation. The uterus is quite sensitive. The ovaries are insensitive to many stimuli, but they are sensitive to rapid distention of the ovarian capsule or compression during physical examination.

PATIENT EVALUATION

History

The history should include a description of the localization, quality, radiation, intensity, and duration of the pain, together with any aggravating or alleviating factors. The rela-tionship of the pain to the menstrual cycle (including the presence of abnormal bleeding, menorrhagia, or metrorrhagia), bowel movements, urination, sexual intercourse, and physical activity should be noted. A history of similar painful episodes in the past should be sought, as should the presence of other somatic complaints, such as anorexia, weight loss, or gastrointestinal or urologic symptoms. One should establish whether there are solely musculoskeletal complaints, such as low or radicular back pain, or whether these accompany the patient's pelvic pain.

The degree to which the pain disrupts the patient's everyday activities should be ascertained, as should prominent events in the patient's life that may have occurred concurrently with the onset of pain. For example, the pain may have begun after the placement of an intrauterine device (IUD) (possible infectious etiology), rape (possible psychological trauma), or after lifting a heavy object (possible hernia). It should be established what pain medications the patient is taking and whether there are any compensation or litigation issues pending.

Symptoms of stress (e.g., palpitations, headaches) or depression (e.g., sleep disorders, loss of memory) should be elicited. Other psychological aspects to be investigated include the attitudes of both the patient and her significant others toward the pain, the illness, and her behavior resulting from the illness. The possibility of secondary gain or other psychological benefits should be explored, as should concurrent upheavals in the patient's life. Psychological evaluations should not preclude further diagnostic studies.

Gynecologic history should include inquiry regarding infertility, pelvic inflammation, usage of an IUD, gonococcal or chlamydial infection, endometriosis, and the time of the last pelvic examination. Details of abortion, childbirth, contraception, and sexual history should be sought. Surgical history should include all pelvic, orthopedic, urologic, and neurologic procedures. The medical history should focus on conditions that may impinge on the diagnosis of pelvic pain, such as irritable bowel syndrome, ulcerative colitis, Crohn's disease, and cystitis.

Physical Examination

The examination of the abdomen should be performed gently so as to prevent involuntary guarding, which may obstruct the findings. The patient should be asked to point to the exact location of the pain and its radiation, and an attempt should be made to duplicate the pain by palpation of each abdominal quadrant.

A gentle but thorough pelvic examination should be performed with an attempt to reproduce and localize the patient's pain. The examination may be suggestive of specific pelvic pathology. For example, patients with endometriosis may have a fixed retroverted uterus with tender uterosacral nodularity. Chronic salpingitis may be suggested by bilateral, tender, irregularly enlarged adnexal structures. A prolapsed uterus may account for pelvic pressure, pain, or low backache.

Further Investigations

Psychological evaluation should be requested if an obviously traumatic event has occurred with the onset of pain or if there is obvious neurosis, psychosis, or secondary gain.

Laboratory studies are of limited utility in the diagnosis of chronic pelvic pain, although

Table 40-2. GYNECOLOGIC CAUSES OF CHRONIC PELVIC PAIN

Endometriosis
Salpingo-oophoritis (PID)
Adhesions
Ovarian remnant syndrome
Pelvic congestion syndrome
Cyclic pelvic (uterine) pain
   Primary dysmenorrhea
    Secondary dysmenorrhea
     Myomata uteri
     Adenomyosis

a complete blood count, erythrocyte sedimentation rate (ESR), and urinalysis are indicated. The ESR is nonspecific and will be increased in any type of inflammatory condition, such as subacute salpingo-oophoritis, tuberculosis, or inflammatory bowel disease. If bowel or urinary signs and symptoms are present, a barium enema, upper gastrointestinal series, or intravenous pyelogram may be useful. Similarly, if there is clinical evidence of musculoskeletal disease, a lumbosacral x-ray film and orthopedic consultation may be in order.

If no obvious cause for the pain is uncovered, pelvic ultrasonography may be helpful, particularly in an obese or uncooperative patient. Diagnostic laparoscopy is the ultimate method of diagnosis for patients with chronic pelvic pain of undetermined etiology. Laparoscopic examination and bimanual examination may differ in 20 to 30 per cent of cases.

DIFFERENTIAL DIAGNOSIS

Organic Causes of Chronic Pelvic Pain

If women with chronic pelvic pain are subjected to diagnostic laparoscopy, approximately one third have no apparent pathology, one third have endometriosis, one quarter have adhesions or stigmata of chronic pelvic inflammatory disease (PID), and the remainder have various miscellaneous entities (Tables 40-2 and 40-3).

Endometriosis. Diagnostic laparoscopy is crucial for the diagnosis of endometriosis, since 30 per cent of women with this disease

Table 40-3. RESULTS OF LAPAROSCOPIC EXPLORATION FOR CHRONIC PELVIC PAIN

	NO. PATIENTS	NO PATHOLOGY (%)	ADHESIONS (%)	ENDOMETRIOSIS (%)
Liston, et al	134	77	16	5
Lundberg, et al	95	38	31	13
Renaer	108	28	23	22
Kresch	100	17	48	32
Rapkin	100	36	26	37

have normal pelvic findings. The size and location of the endometriotic implants do not appear to correlate with the presence of pain, and the reasons for the pain are not understood.

Chronic Pelvic Inflammatory Disease. Chronic PID may cause pain because of recurrent exacerbations that require active antibiotic therapy or because of hydrosalpinges and adhesions between the tubes, ovaries, and intestinal structures. Before ascribing symptoms to adhesions, one must have noted adhesions specifically in the area of pain localization, since some patients with extensive pelvic adhesions are asymptomatic.

Ovarian Pain. Ovarian cysts are usually asymptomatic, but pain may occur secondary to rapid distention of the ovarian capsule. An ovary or ovarian remnant may occasionally become retroperitoneal secondary to inflammation or previous surgery, and cyst formation in these circumstances may also be painful. Some women, for unknown reasons, may develop multiple recurrent hemorrhagic ovarian cysts that seem to cause pelvic pain and dyspareunia. Impaired blood supply to the ovaries has been implicated, especially when there has been previous pelvic surgery, such as a partial oophorectomy or hysterectomy.

Uterine Pain. Adenomyosis (or endometriosis interna) may cause dysmenorrhea and menorrhagia, but rarely does it cause chronic intermenstrual pain. Uterine myomata usually do not cause pelvic pain unless they are degenerating, torsing (twisting their pedicles), or compressing pelvic nerves. Occasionally, a submucous leiomyoma may attempt to deliver via the cervix, which may cause considerable pelvic pain akin to childbirth.

Pelvic pain is not likely to be due to variations in uterine position, but deep dyspareunia may occasionally be associated with retroversion. The pain has been ascribed to irritation of pelvic nerves by the stretching of the uterosacral ligaments as well as to congestion of pelvic veins secondary to retroversion. The dyspareunia is typically worse with the female in the missionary position and improved in the female superior position. If pressure in the posterior fornix reproduces the pain, ventral suspension of the uterus is very likely to be curative. A tender uterus that is in the fixed retroverted position is usually a sign of other intraperitoneal pathology, such as endometriosis or PID, and diagnosis rests on laparoscopic findings. Occasionally, pelvic heaviness and low back pain may be present with advanced degrees of uterine prolapse. Prior to electing hysterectomy, the resolution of these symptoms with uterine replacement may be evaluated with pessary placement.

Genitourinary Pelvic Pain. A variety of genitourinary problems result in pelvic pain as indicated in Chapter 37. Urinary retention, urethral syndrome, and trigonitis are prime examples. Such causes are often associated with gynecologic abnormalities such as uterine prolapse, vaginitis, and endometriosis. A thorough genitourinary evaluation is an important part of the work-up for chronic pelvic pain.

Gastrointestinal Pain. Chronic pelvic pain may be caused by various nongynecologic conditions. Gastrointestinal sources of chronic pelvic pain include penetrating neoplasms of the gastrointestinal tract, irritable bowel syndrome, partial bowel obstruction, inflammatory bowel disease, diverticulitis, and hernia formation. Because the innervation of the lower intestinal tract is the same as that of the uterus and fallopian tubes, the patient's complaint of pelvic pain may be confused with pain of gynecologic origin.

Neuromuscular Pain. Pain of neuromuscular origin, which is experienced as low back pain, usually increases with activity and stress. Chronic low back pain without lower abdominal pain is seldom of gynecologic etiology. Occasionally, neuromuscular symptoms are accompanied by a pelvic mass, and surgical exploration may reveal a neuroma or bony tumor.

Nonorganic Chronic Pelvic Pain

A pathologic diagnosis is unable to be made in approximately one third of patients with chronic pelvic pain, even after laparoscopy. Historically, various psychological and physiologic processes have been described to account for this enigmatic occurrence.

Pelvic Congestion Syndrome. The concept of a pelvic congestion syndrome still has many proponents. This entity has been described in multiparous women who have pelvic vein varicosities and congested pelvic organs. The pelvic pain is worse premenstrually and is increased by fatigue, standing, and sexual intercourse. Many women with this condition are noted to have a uterus that is mobile, retroverted, soft, boggy, and slightly enlarged. There may be associated menorrhagia and urinary frequency. Dilated veins may be seen on venographic studies. Factors other than venous congestion may be involved, however, since most women with pelvic varicosities have no pain, and surgery for this condition is not usually beneficial. There have been some noncontrolled observations of similar symptoms of pain and metrorrhagia occurring after tubal ligation, but no prospective studies have been performed.

Psychological Factors. The finding of chronic pelvic pain without pathology has led to the postulation that psychological factors may be etiologic. The patients have been assumed to be anxious, neurotic, anorgasmic, and insecure in their roles as women or as mothers. When subjected to the Minnesota Multiphasic Personality Inventory (MMPI), these patients have shown a greater degree of anxiety, hypochondriasis, and hysteria than control subjects. The profiles are similar, however, in patients who have chronic pain with organic pathology, suggesting that chronic pain per se engenders a complex, debilitating, psychological response. Chronic pain patients with and without pathology tend to feel depressed, helpless, and passive. They withdraw from social and sexual activity and are preoccupied with pain and suffering. There is no scientific evidence to support a pre-existing behavioral, personality, or sexual disorder, but no prospective studies have been undertaken.

Pain Perception Factors. More recent theories of the perception of chronic pain suggest that it is characterized by physiologic, emotional, and behavioral responses that are different from those of acute pain. Although both acute and chronic pain consist of a stimulus and a psychic response, for acute pain these may be adaptive and appropriate, whereas for chronic pain this may not be the case. In fact, the response to chronic pain may be greatly affected by learning. The patient's reaction to pain and the reaction of significant others to the patient and her pain may be so reinforcing that the behavior may persist even after the painful stimulus has resolved. Figure 40–1 illustrates the possible levels of agreement between sensory input, the pain sensation or perception, the patient's suffering, and the patient's pain behavior. In acute pain, the pain perception, suffering, and behavior are usually commensurate with the degree of sensory input. In chronic pain, the suffering and behavioral responses to a given sensory input may be quite exaggerated and may persist even after the stimulus has remitted.

Modulation of Sensation. It is now known that pain impulses are subjected to a large amount of modulation en route to the central nervous system. The first synapse in the dorsal horn is an important focus of enhancement, inhibition, or facilitation. Modulation of sensations may also occur within the spinothalamic system, the descending inhibitory neurosystems, and the frontal cortex. Within this context, anxiety and other psychological states may be considered to be facilitators or inhibitors for neurologic trans-

Figure 40–1. A model to illustrate the interplay between pain sensation and experience. (From Reading AE: Psychological Aspects of Pregnancy. New York, Longman Press, 1983, p 73.)

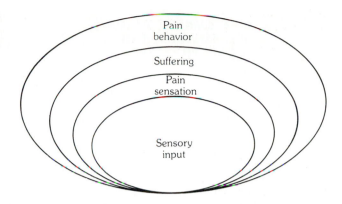

mission. It is possible that many forms of chronic pelvic pain, in particular those without pathology, may result from modulation of afferent impulses in the dorsal horn, spinal cord, or cerebral cortex.

MANAGEMENT

In dealing with patients with chronic pelvic pain, a therapeutic, supportive, and sympathetic, but structured, physician–patient relationship should be established. The patient should be given regular follow-up appointments and should not be told to call only if the pain persists. This reinforces pain behavior as a means of procuring sympathy and medical attention.

A negative evaluation and laparoscopy or the finding of pathology not amenable to therapy (for example, dense pelvic adhesions) does not mean that the patient should be discharged from care without therapy directed toward her symptoms. After initial reassurance that there is no serious underlying pathology, symptomatic therapy should be undertaken. The symptoms of pain should be approached with the seriousness and direction afforded to any other condition. The patient should not be placed in the position of "proving that she has pain," or she is apt to withdraw from the therapeutic situation and look for someone who will find out "what is wrong."

Team Management

The most productive strategy for the management of patients with chronic pelvic pain is referral to a multidisciplinary pain clinic. The personnel at such a facility should include a gynecologist, a psychologist who also has expertise in sexual and marital counseling, an anesthesiologist, and, occasionally, an acupuncturist. It is the role of the psychologist to provide marital and sexual counseling, assertiveness training, and adaptive coping strategies. This aspect of therapy is crucial, since many of these patients have become interpersonally, sexually, and sometimes even occupationally withdrawn. Relaxation, cognitive, and behavioral therapies are employed to replace the pain behavior and its secondary gain with effective behavioral responses.

Medical and Surgical Management

The gynecologist continues to assess progress, coordinate care, and provide periodic gynecologic examinations. In the initial stages of therapy, a trial of ovulation suppression with the birth control pill may be helpful, especially in patients who have midcycle, premenstrual, or menstrual exacerbation of pain, or in those who have ovarian pathology, such as periovarian adhesions or recurrent functional cyst formation. Nonsteroidal anti-inflammatory analgesics, such as ibuprofen (Motrin) or naproxen (Naprosyn), are also useful.

Surgical procedures that have *not* proved to be effective for chronic pelvic pain without pathology include unilateral adnexectomy for unilateral pain or total abdominal hysterectomy, presacral neurectomy, or uterine sus-

Table 40-4. SURGICAL MEASURES IN THE MANAGEMENT OF CHRONIC PELVIC PAIN

Diagnostic laparoscopy
Lysis of adhesions
Hysterectomy
Presacral neurectomy
Uterosacral nerve ablation

pension for generalized pelvic pain. Lysis of adhesions is usually also nonproductive, unless the site of adhesions visualized by the laparoscope specifically coincides with the localization of pain. It should be kept in mind that pelvic adhesions often recur following surgical lysis.

In contemplating surgical management, it must be realized that the scope of chronic pelvic pain is broad and has far-reaching implications. Stress, sexual dysfunction, interpersonal strife, and psychosocial problems may play important roles and are difficult to evaluate. Without proof of organic pathology or a reasonable functional explanation for the pelvic pain, a thorough psychosomatic evaluation should be carried out before a surgical corrective procedure is considered. Surgical measures that should be considered for management of chronic pelvic pain are listed in Table 40-4.

Anesthesia

Acupuncture, nerve blocks, and trigger-point injections of local anesthetics may provide prolonged pain relief. These therapeutic methods have only recently been directed toward chronic pelvic pain. Acupuncture has been used successfully for dysmenorrhea, and trigger-point injections of local anesthetics have been used successfully for pelvic pain. For pelvic pain, trigger points are either on the lower abdominal wall or in the vaginal and vulvar area. When these areas are subject to pressure, they give rise to pain, in the area depressed as well as at the site of possible noxious stimulation. Anesthesia of trigger points may abolish pain by lowering the impulses from the area of referred pain, thereby diminishing the afferent impulses reaching the dorsal horn to a level below the threshold for pain transmission.

SUGGESTED READING

Kumazawa T: Sensory innervation of reproductive organs: Visceral sensations. Progr Brain Res 67:115, 1986.

Lee RB, Stone K, Magelssen D, et al: Presacral neurectomy for chronic pelvic pain. Obstet Gynecol 68:517, 1986.

Malinek LR: Operative management of pelvic pain. Clin Obstet Gynecol 23:191, 1980.

Pettit PD, Lee RA: Ovarian remnant syndrome: Diagnostic dilemma and surgical challenges. Obstet Gynecol 71:580, 1988.

Rapkin AJ, Kames LD: The pain management approach to chronic pelvic pain. J Reprod Med 32:323, 1987.

Rapkin AJ, Reading AE: Chronic pelvic pain. Curr Probl Obstet Gynecol Fertil 14:99, 1991.

Reiter RC: A profile of women with chronic pelvic pain. Clin Obstet Gynecol 33:130, 1990.

Vereekin RL: Chronic pelvic pain of urologic origin. In Ranaer MR (ed): Chronic Pelvic Pain in Women. New York, Springer-Verlag, 1981, pp 155–161.

Wood DP, Weisner MG, Reiter RC: Psychogenic chronic pelvic pain, diagnosis and management. Clin Obstet Gynecol 33:179, 1990.

Forty-one

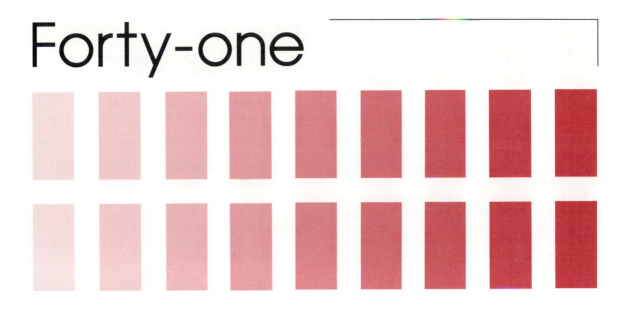

Breast Disease: A Gynecologic Perspective

NEVILLE F. HACKER

Because gynecologists are often regarded as the primary care physicians for most women, they are frequently the ones first to diagnose breast disease. Therefore, even though the treatment usually falls under the domain of the general surgeon, it is important that gynecologists be expert in breast examination, diligent about screening asymptomatic women for breast cancer, familiar with common benign and malignant disorders of the breast, and conversant with the various therapeutic options.

SCREENING OF THE BREAST IN ASYMPTOMATIC WOMEN

Self-Examination

Self-examination of the breast should be performed monthly by all women after the age of 20. Even though it is a simple and good screening technique for breast disease and is inexpensive, painless, harmless, and convenient, only about two thirds of women practice it at least once a year, and only one third practice it monthly as recommended. Of women performing the technique, only about half perform it correctly. When taught by physicians or nurses, however, more women practice regular breast self examination, and a greater proportion use the correct technique. Since it has been demonstrated that women who regularly practice the technique can discover breast disease at a significantly earlier stage, it behooves all gynecologists to promote self-examination among their patients.

Breast Self-Examination Technique. The patient should be taught to perform the examination after each menstrual period. She

443

should commence the technique in the upright position, carefully inspecting the breasts initially with her arms by her sides and then raised above her head. She should palpate the supraclavicular and axillary regions for the presence of nodes. The patient should then lie down and systematically palpate each quadrant of the breast against the chest wall, using the flat of the fingers. Finally, she should palpate the areolar areas and then compress the nipples for evidence of secretion.

Breast Examination by Physician. A complete breast examination should be performed by a physician at least annually. The breasts are first inspected with the patient in an upright position. The contour and symmetry are observed, and any skin changes or nipple retraction is noted. Skin retraction because of tethering to an underlying malignancy may be highlighted by having the patient extend her arms over her head.

Palpation of the breast, areola, and nipple is performed with the flat of the hand. If any mass is palpated, its fixation to deep tissues should be determined by asking the patient to place her hands over her hips and contract her pectoral muscles. Each axilla is then carefully examined while the patient's arm is supported. The supraclavicular fossae are also palpated for lymphadenopathy. Following palpation in the upright position, the examination is repeated in the supine position.

Mammography

Radiologic examination of the breast is an important component of the screening process carried out in asymptomatic women and should be performed in conjunction with a thorough physical examination. Densities and fine calcifications constitute suspicious findings, and clinically inapparent malignancies of less than 1 cm in diameter may be detected.

Studies of individuals who survived the atomic bomb, received frequent fluoroscopy for tuberculosis, or underwent breast irradiation for benign disease have indicated that radiation can induce breast cancer. In more recent years, there has been a marked improvement in the quality of mammography, with a concomitant decrease in the radiation

Table 41–1. AMERICAN CANCER SOCIETY GUIDELINES FOR MAMMOGRAPHIC SCREENING OF ASYMPTOMATIC WOMEN
Baseline mammogram for all women at age 35–40 yr
Mammography at 1- to 2-yr intervals from age 40–49 yr
Annual mammograms for women 50 yr or older

dose administered to the breasts. Mammograms of high quality can be made with about 0.3 cGy or less of radiation, so there is little, if any, risk of this technique causing breast cancer.

In the Breast Cancer Detection Demonstration Project carried out by the American Cancer Society and the National Cancer Institute, 89 per cent of 3557 cancers were correctly identified by mammography, 41.6 per cent of which were not clinically detectable. The optimal frequency for screening asymptomatic women has not been determined, but the current guidelines of the American Cancer Society are shown in Table 41–1.

Two techniques, film-screen mammography (which produces a regular x-ray film) and xeroradiography (which produces a blue image on paper), are currently available and are equally effective. Xeroradiography is especially good for finding the microcalcifications frequently associated with breast cancer.

Other Imaging Techniques

In addition to x-ray film, breast images may also be recorded using heat (thermography), sound (ultrasonography), light (diaphanography), and magnetism (nuclear magnetic resonance). The nonionizing properties of these modalities make them attractive, but there are no reported controlled studies that compare them favorably with the efficacy of x-ray mammography for widespread screening. Ultrasonography can differentiate cystic from solid masses and may demonstrate solid tissue that is potentially malignant within or adjacent to a cyst. It is also useful for imaging palpable focal masses in women under 30 years of age, reducing the need for x-ray studies in this population. Further research is needed to define the role that nuclear magnetic resonance may ultimately play in the evaluation of breast disease.

DIAGNOSIS OF BREAST LESIONS

Physiologic nodularity and cyclic tenderness caused by the changing hormonal milieu must be distinguished from benign or malignant pathologic changes. Definitive diagnosis of breast neoplasms has traditionally been made by open breast biopsy, although there has been a revival of interest in fine-needle (22-gauge) aspiration cytology.

Fine-Needle Biopsy

Fine-needle aspiration biopsy of the palpably suspicious lump in the breast can be performed in the outpatient clinic without anesthesia. Smears are prepared from the aspirate to allow cytologic evaluation. In experienced hands, the test is both sensitive and specific. A negative result should never be accepted as definitive, however, when there are clinical or mammographic indications that the lesion may be malignant. In the presence of a palpable lump, fine-needle aspiration cytology should make it possible to diagnose breast cancer without formal excisional biopsy in over 90 per cent of cases, allowing the subsequent management of the patient to be discussed prior to operation.

Open Breast Biopsy

Many factors should be considered prior to performing open biopsy, including the risk profile of the patient, the nature of the physical findings, the results of mammography, and the results of the aspiration cytology, if performed. Absolute indications for open breast biopsy are listed in Table 41–2.

Relative indications for breast biopsy include those women with a clinically benign mass but a positive family or personal history of breast cancer, a history of fibrocystic disease with atypia, or an equivocal finding on

Table 41–2. ABSOLUTE INDICATIONS FOR OPEN BREAST BIOPSY
Clinically suspicious (dominant) mass that persists through a menstrual cycle, regardless of mammographic findings. If fine-needle aspiration cytology is unequivocally positive, most surgeons proceed directly to definitive treatment
Cystic mass that does not completely collapse on aspiration (residual solid component) or contains bloody fluid
Spontaneous serous or serosanguineous nipple discharge. In the absence of a mass, a "trigger point" should be demonstrable
Suspicious mammographic abnormalities in the absence of a dominant nodule or discrete thickening

mammography or cytology. Patients suitable for observation would include those with a clinically benign mass or masses, no risk factors for breast cancer, and no evidence of malignancy on mammography.

Open breast biopsy may be performed as an outpatient procedure under local anesthesia or as an inpatient procedure under general anesthesia. Women with large breasts who have small deeply situated lesions are not good candidates for outpatient biopsies, nor are those who have a nonpalpable lesion detected by mammography.

COMMON BENIGN BREAST DISORDERS

Fibrocystic Disease

Fibrocystic disease is the most common breast disease and is clinically apparent in about 50 per cent of women. Histologically it is characterized by hyperplastic changes that may involve any or all of the breast tissues (lobular epithelium, ductal epithelium, and connective tissue). When the hyperplastic changes are associated with cellular atypia, there is an increased risk for subsequent malignant transformation.

It is postulated that the changes found associated with fibrocystic disease are due to a relative or absolute decrease in production

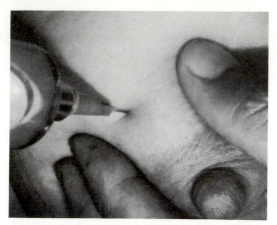

Figure 41–1. Aspiration of a breast cyst. The fluid is clear, and there are no other suspicious features in this breast. If the cytology is negative and the lump disappears, careful follow-up only is indicated.

of progesterone or an increase in the amount of estrogen. Estrogen promotes the growth of mammary ducts and the periductal stroma, whereas progesterone is responsible for the development of lobular and alveolar structures. Prolactin, insulin, corticotropin, thyroxine, and growth hormone are also required for complete functional development. Patients with fibrocystic disease improve dramatically during pregnancy and lactation because of the large amount of progesterone produced by the corpus luteum and placenta and the increased production of estriol, which blocks the hyperplastic changes produced by estradiol and estrone.

Clinically the lesions are usually multiple and bilateral and are characterized by pain and tenderness, particularly premenstrually. The disease usually occurs in the premenopausal years with a cessation of symptoms postmenopausally, unless exogenous estrogens are administered.

Treatment depends on the age of the patient, the severity of the symptoms, and the relative risk of the development of breast cancer. Women over 25 years of age should undergo baseline mammography to exclude carcinoma. Cysts may be aspirated to relieve pain (Fig. 41–1). If the fluid is clear and the lump disappears, careful follow-up only is indicated. Open biopsy is required if the fluid is bloody or if there is any residual mass

following aspiration. The only procedure offering complete protection against future breast cancer is bilateral total mastectomy. Although satisfactory breast reconstruction can be performed, no definitive surgery should be considered unless the patient is at high risk to develop breast cancer.

The medical management for fibrocystic disease has not been standardized. Progesterone, which can be administered orally as medroxyprogesterone acetate (Provera), 5 to 10 mg daily for 5 to 10 days at the end of each month, can be given to patients in whom there is a relative or absolute increase in estrogen. Tamoxifen, an antiestrogen that works by bonding to receptor sites, may be taken orally, 10 mg twice daily, and is usually tolerated without side effects. Bromocriptine (Parlodel), a potent dopamine receptor agonist that inhibits prolactin secretion, may relieve the mastalgia when taken orally in a dosage of 2.5 mg twice daily. Symptoms related to premenstrual breast edema may be relieved with the administration of diuretics for 7 to 10 days along with a low salt diet. Danazol (Danocrine), an orally active pituitary gonadotropin inhibitory agent, has been effective in ameliorating symptoms in about 80 per cent of patients when taken over a period of several months in a dosage of 100 to 400 mg daily. Further studies of the long-term effects of this drug are needed. Tamoxifen, Danocrine, and Parlodel are very expensive.

Fibroadenoma

Composed of both fibrous and glandular tissue, the fibroadenoma is the most common benign tumor found in the female breast. Clinically these tumors are sharply circumscribed, freely mobile nodules, which may occur at any age but are common before the age of 30. They usually are solitary and generally are removed when they reach 2 to 4 cm in diameter, although giant forms up to 15 cm in diameter occasionally occur. Pregnancy may stimulate their growth, and postmenopausally, regression and calcification usually eventuate. These tumors require surgical excision for definitive diagnosis and cure.

Intraductal Papilloma

Papillary neoplastic growths may develop within the ducts of the breast, most commonly just before or during the menopause. They are rarely palpable and usually present because of a bloody, serous, or turbid discharge from the nipple. If a trigger point from which palpation elicits a discharge is clearly identifiable, excisional biopsy of the involved duct should be performed whether or not a mass is palpable. Histologically there is a spectrum of lesions ranging from those that are clearly benign to those that are anaplastic and give evidence of invasive tendencies. These growths should be differentiated from other causes of benign nipple discharge that do not require surgery. Certain drugs, such as phenothiazines, may cause bilateral nipple discharge as a result of elevated prolactin levels. Mammography and cytologic examination of the fluid are helpful in investigating nipple discharges.

Mammary Duct Ectasia

Mammary duct ectasia (comedomastitis, plasma cell mastitis) is characterized by dilatation of ducts, inspissation of breast secretion, and chronic intraductal and periductal inflammation in which plasma cells predominate. It usually occurs in the fifth decade and is associated with nipple discharge, pain, and tenderness. The ducts, which are dilated and filled with thick, cheesy material, may be palpable through the skin, or the lesion may give the clinical impression of a homogeneous tumor mass. Nipple retraction from the inflammatory scarring and enlarged axillary glands may make the findings indistinguishable from breast cancer. Once the diagnosis is confirmed by breast biopsy, no further treatment is necessary.

Galactocele

A galactocele is a cystic dilatation of a duct that is filled with thick, inspissated, milky fluid. It presents during or shortly after lactation and implies some cause for ductal ob-

Table 41-3. RISK FACTORS FOR BREAST CANCER

TYPE	RISK FACTOR
Genetic	Positive family history
Hormonal	Nulliparity
	Late age at first pregnancy
	Early menarche
	Late menopause
	Age over 40 yr
	Prolonged unopposed estrogen usage
Nutritional	High dietary fat intake
Morphologic	Cancer of ovary or endometrium
	Cancer of the other breast
	Fibrocystic disease with cellular atypia
Irradiation	Breast irradiation

struction, such as inflammation, fibrocystic disease, or neoplasia. Often multiple cysts are present. Secondary infection may produce areas of acute mastitis or abscess formation. Needle aspiration is usually curative. If the fluid is bloody or the mass does not disappear completely, excisional biopsy is required.

BREAST CANCER

Breast cancer is the most common female malignancy, accounting for 29 per cent of malignancies in women. Approximately 150,000 new cases were diagnosed in the United States in 1990, and 44,000 of these women will die from the disease. There is a one in 12 chance (8.2 per cent) that a woman will develop breast cancer during her lifetime.

Etiology

Little is known about the actual cause of breast cancer. Several risk factors have been identified (Table 41–3), but there is still a substantial number of women who develop the disease in spite of having no apparent increased susceptibility.

The incidence and mortality rates for breast cancer are approximately five times higher in North America and northern Europe than they are in many Asian and African countries. Migrants to the United States from Asia (principally Chinese and Japanese) do not experience a substantial increase in risk, but their first-generation and second-generation descendants have rates approaching those of the white population in the United States. Since age-adjusted mortality rates for breast cancer exhibit a high correlation with per capita fat consumption, the difference may be related to dietary customs.

Unopposed estrogens may produce a small increase in the risk for breast cancer. The breast appears to be much less susceptible to the tumor-promoting effects of estrogens than the endometrium, however, and large amounts of estrogen are required to achieve any observable alteration in the risk of malignancy. Usage of combined oral contraceptives produces no significant alteration of risk. In contrast, oral contraceptive usage significantly decreases the risk for ovarian and endometrial cancer.

Tumor Types

The mammary epithelium gives rise to a wide variety of histologic tumor types. Approximately 90 per cent of cases arise in the ducts, and the remainder originate in the lobules. About 80 per cent of all breast cancers are nonspecific infiltrating duct carcinomas. These tumors usually induce a significant fibrotic response and are stony hard to clinical palpation. Less common types of ductal cancer include medullary, mucinous, tubular, and papillary types. In many tumors, several patterns coexist.

Paget's disease of the breast occurs in about 3 per cent of breast cancer patients. It represents a specialized form of intraductal carcinoma that arises in the main excretory ducts of the breasts and extends to involve the skin of the nipple and areola, producing an eczematoid appearance. The underlying carcinoma, although invariably present, can be palpated clinically in only about two thirds of patients.

Inflammatory breast cancer, often seen in pregnancy, is characterized clinically by warmth and redness of the overlying skin and induration of the surrounding breast tissues. Biopsies of the erythematous areas reveal malignant cells in subdermal lymphatics, causing an obstructive lymphangitis. Inflammatory cells are rarely present. Most patients have signs of advanced cancer at the time of diagnosis, including palpable regional lymph nodes and distant metastases.

Tumor Spread

Breast cancer spreads by local infiltration as well as by lymphatic or hematogenous routes. Locally, the tumor infiltrates directly into the breast parenchyma, eventually involving the overlying skin or the deep pectoral fascia.

Lymphatic spread is mainly to the axillary nodes, and 40 to 50 per cent of patients have involvement of these nodes at the time of diagnosis. Axillary node involvement is directly related to the size of the primary tumor, but not to the location of the tumor within the breast. The second major area for lymph node metastases is the internal mammary node chain. These nodes are most likely to be involved when the primary lesion is medially or centrally situated, but even in these circumstances, axillary node involvement is more common. The supraclavicular nodes are usually involved only after axillary node involvement.

Hematogenous spread occurs mainly to the lungs and liver, but other common sites of involvement include bone, pleura, adrenals, ovaries, and brain.

Staging

Several systems of staging for cancer of the breast have been recommended. The one recommended by the American Joint Committee on Cancer is shown in Table 41–4.

Clinical Features

Carcinoma of the breast is usually first discovered by the patient or physician as a breast lump. It is usually painless and may be freely mobile. A serous or bloody nipple discharge may be present. With progressive growth, the tumor may become fixed to the

Table 41-4. STAGING OF BREAST CANCER*

STAGE	DESCRIPTION
Stage Tis	In situ cancer (in situ lobular, pure intraductal, and Paget's disease of the nipple without palpable tumor)
Stage I	Tumor 2 cm or less in greatest diameter without evidence of regional or distant spread
Stage II	Tumor more than 2 cm but not more than 5 cm in greatest diameter with or without movable axillary nodes, but without distant spread
Stage IIIa	Tumor up to 5 cm in diameter, which may or may not be fixed, with homolateral clinically suspicious regional spread—or a tumor more than 5 cm in diameter, which may or may not be fixed, with or without clinically suspicious homolateral regional spread. No evidence of distant metastases
Stage IIIb	Tumor of any dimension with unequivocal homolateral metastatic supraclavicular or intraclavicular nodes or edema of the arm, but without distant metastases
Stage IV	Tumor of any size with or without regional spread, but with evidence of distant metastases

* As suggested by the American Joint Committee on Cancer.

deep fascia. Extension to the skin may cause retraction and dimpling, whereas ductal involvement may cause nipple retraction. Blockage of skin lymphatics may cause lymphedema and thickening of the skin, a change referred to as *peau d'orange* (Fig. 41-2).

Treatment

With increasing awareness of the likelihood of early hematogenous spread and an increasing number of early lesions being diagnosed, the present trend is toward a more conservative surgical approach to breast cancer in conjunction with adjuvant radiation and, if necessary, chemotherapy.

Surgery

Radical mastectomy, as first described in 1894 by Halsted and Meyer, was, until recently, the standard operation for operable breast cancer. The procedure consists of an en bloc dissection of the entire breast, together with the pectoralis major and minor muscles and the contents of the axilla. Presently, modified radical mastectomy, which leaves the pectoralis major intact, has supplanted radical mastectomy as the standard operation. It provides superior functional and cosmetic results, and survival data following both procedures appear to be comparable.

In 1971, a prospective study was initiated in the United States by the National Surgical Adjuvant Breast Project. Its purpose was to compare radical mastectomy with simple mastectomy plus local-regional radiation therapy with simple mastectomy alone for patients with clinically negative axillary nodes. The latter group underwent subsequent removal of axillary nodes only if they became positive. Ten years later, the survival statistics for all three groups were not significantly different, despite the fact that in those women believed to have clinically negative nodes, 40 per cent of the group undergoing radical mastectomy were found to have posi-

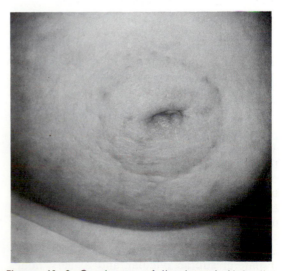

Figure 41-2. Carcinoma of the breast. Note the nipple retraction and the "peau d'orange." (Courtesy of Dr. Guy Juillard, Department of Radiation Oncology, UCLA School of Medicine, Los Angeles, CA.)

tive axillary nodes. Being a properly randomized trial, there is no reason to believe that patients in the other two groups did not have a similar incidence of positive nodes. The comparable survival statistics for the three groups indicate that by the time the patient reaches the physician, operable breast cancer is frequently already a systemic disease.

For small primary tumors, segmental mastectomy (also called partial mastectomy, quadrantectomy, or lumpectomy) has been advocated by some to improve the cosmetic outcome. This technique is combined with axillary node dissection and postoperative breast irradiation. With the short follow-up presently available, results appear to be comparable to the more radical approaches. To be suitable for conservative surgery, the primary tumor should be small relative to the breast, so that local excision with negative margins will result in an acceptable cosmetic appearance.

Breast reconstruction after mastectomy is an integral part of the treatment of breast cancer. It should be available to any woman who desires it, provided that her general condition allows for operation and her expectation for reconstruction is realistic. The procedure may be performed at the time of the mastectomy or may be delayed for at least 3 months.

Radiation Therapy

Radiation therapy was initially used postoperatively for patients with positive axillary nodes. Although it significantly decreased local recurrence, it did not improve survival. Currently, there is an increasing use of radiation as initial therapy for relatively small primary tumors, as mentioned previously. The radiation is given following excision of the primary lesion and axillary node sampling, the latter being undertaken to determine the need for adjuvant chemotherapy or axillary radiation. External beam therapy is used, with 4500 to 5000 cGy delivered to the entire breast and the anterior chest wall including the internal mammary chain. The ipsilateral supraclavicular and axillary nodes are treated if lymph node metastases are present. The primary tumor site may be boosted with external irradiation or with interstitial iridium-192. Functional and cos-

metic results are improved, and survival does not appear to be compromised, although longer follow-up studies are necessary. Major complications, such as arm edema, arm weakness, radiation pericarditis, and soft tissue necrosis are very uncommon, occurring in about 2 per cent of patients.

Chemotherapy

Although many drugs have some activity against breast cancer, the four most commonly used are cyclophosphamide (C), methotrexate (M), 5-fluorouracil (F) and doxorubicin (Adriamycin [A]). As single agents, each is capable of inducing responses in 25 to 45 per cent of patients. Combinations of drugs have been shown to be more effective than single agents. Various combinations have been used, the most popular being CMF and AC.

Because it is now clear that breast cancer is a systemic disease in many patients at the time of diagnosis, adjuvant systemic chemotherapy or hormonal therapy seems indicated if cure rates are to improve. Available data suggest that premenopausal women have improved survival (by about 15 per cent) and a longer disease-free interval with the use of adjuvant combination chemotherapy. Similarly, adjuvant hormonal therapy (tamoxifen) has been shown to have significant impact on disease-free survival and overall survival of postmenopausal patients with node-positive breast cancer. Whether adjuvant chemotherapy merely prolongs survival without actually increasing the cure rate will be determined by further follow-up studies.

In patients with established metastasis, symptoms may be palliated with combination chemotherapy. Partial responses are obtained in 50 to 75 per cent of patients, and complete clinical responses in 5 to 25 per cent. The median duration of response is about 12 months.

Endocrine Therapy

The response to hormonal manipulation of any type is correlated with the incidence of estrogen receptors (ER). Because the synthesis of progesterone receptors is estrogen-dependent, the presence of these receptors may be a better predictor of the response to endocrine treatment than that of estrogen receptors alone. The response rate to hormonal treatment in ER-positive tumors is 50 to 60 per cent, whereas it is less than 10 per cent in ER-negative tumors. The response is usually partial and temporary. Progesterone receptors (PR) have been found in about 40 per cent of ER-positive tumors. When both receptors are present, the response to hormonal therapy approaches 80 per cent. Premenopausal patients have a lower incidence of ER-positive tumors (30 per cent) than postmenopausal patients (60 per cent).

Antiestrogen therapy with tamoxifen has replaced additive hormones (e.g., diethylstilbestrol) as well as adrenalectomy and hypophysectomy as first-line hormonal treatment for postmenopausal women. Although fewer data are presently available, this treatment may replace oophorectomy in premenopausal women.

In addition to receptor positivity, there are clinical predictors for hormonal responsiveness and these include postmenopausal status, long disease-free survival, and the presence of soft tissue or bone metastases.

Prognosis

Although prognosis is related to the stage of the disease and the age of the patient (older patients have a better prognosis), the status of the axillary lymph nodes is the single most important prognosticator. More recently, evidence has indicated that estrogen-receptor status is also of independent prognostic significance, patients with ER-negative tumors having a poorer prognosis.

In the National Surgical Adjuvant Breast Project, patients with negative lymph nodes had an actuarial 5-year survival of 83 per cent, compared with 73 per cent for patients with one to three positive nodes, 45 per cent for those with four or more positive nodes, and 28 per cent for those with more than 13 positive nodes.

Breast Cancer in Pregnancy

About 3 per cent of breast cancers occur during pregnancy, complicating approximately one in every 3000 pregnancies. Diagnosis is usually delayed because small masses are more difficult to palpate in hypertrophied breasts. Needle aspiration or open biopsy, however, should be performed promptly on any suspicious mass.

The treatment is essentially that of the nonpregnant patient except that lumpectomy and removal of axillary nodes followed by postoperative irradiation would not be appropriate with a continuing pregnancy. For patients with nodal metastases, abortion is advisable in the first trimester of pregnancy because of the teratogenic risks of the adjuvant chemotherapy. In the third trimester, chemotherapy should be delayed until after delivery, although surgery should occur promptly after diagnosis.

Stage for stage prognosis is not much worse than for nonpregnant patients. There is no indication to advise against subsequent pregnancy for those who are without evidence of recurrence.

SUGGESTED READING

American Cancer Society: National Conference on Breast Cancer—1989. Cancer 66(supplt):1309, 1990.

Baket LH: Breast cancer detection demonstration project: Five year summary report. CA 32(4):194, 1982.

Black MM, Barclay THC, Cutler SJ, et al: Association of atypical characteristics of benign breast lesions with subsequent risk of breast cancer. Cancer 29:338, 1972.

Donegan WL: Cancer and pregnancy. CA 33:194, 1983.

Fisher B, Bauer M, Wickerham DL, et al: Relation of number of positive axillary nodes to the prognosis of patients with primary breast cancer. Cancer 52:1551, 1983.

Giuliano AE. Breast disease. In Berek JS, Hacker NF (eds): Practical Gynecologic Oncology. Baltimore, Williams & Wilkins, 1989, p 469.

Harris JR, Recht A, Connolly J et al: Conservative surgery and radiotherapy for early breast cancer. Cancer 66:1427, 1990.

Henderson JC: Adjuvant systemic therapy: State of the art, 1989. Breast Cancer Res Treat 14:3, 1989.

Huguley CM Jr, Brown RL: The value of breast self-examination. Cancer 47:989, 1981.

Kinne DW: Surgical management of stage I and stage II breast cancer. Cancer 66:1373, 1990.

UK Trial of Early Detection of Breast Cancer Group: First results on mortality reduction in the UK trial of early detection of breast cancer. Lancet 2:411, 1988.

Veronesi U, Saccozzi R, Del Vecchio M, et al: Comparing radical mastectomy with quadrantectomy, axillary dissection, and radiotherapy in patients with small cancers of the breast. N Engl J Med 305(1):6, 1981.

Winchester DP, Sener S, Immerman S, et al: A systematic approach to the evaluation and management of breast masses. Cancer 51:2535, 1983.

Forty-two

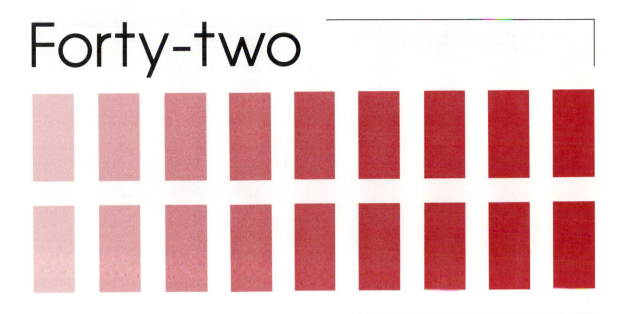

Contraception and Sterilization

J. GEORGE MOORE

Family planning generally refers to those birth control methods that allow patients to defer or prevent reproduction. These methods include deferral of pregnancy (contraception), permanent contraception (sterilization), and induced abortion. Abortion is discussed in Chapter 38. Family planning in a broader sense considers those factors that aid a couple in achieving pregnancy, treats the social and emotional factors associated with high parity, addresses the consequences of the world's burden of overpopulation, and weighs the advantages of allowing women to regulate their fertility in such a way that they can appropriately participate in societal and fiscal pursuits generally precluded by frequent and excessive pregnancies. This chapter primarily deals with contraception and sterilization.

CONTRACEPTION

Contraceptive methodologies may be divided into six general types: (1) hormonal, (2) intrauterine, (3) barrier, (4) chemical, (5) physiological, and (6) sterilization. None are 100 per cent effective and all are associated with some degree of risk. Consequently, the importance of appropriate and thorough counseling must be emphasized.

The preferred method of expressing contraceptive effectiveness depicts the percentage of women likely to become pregnant within the first year of applying the particular contraceptive method (Table 42–1). The effectiveness of a given method depends mainly on its biological method of action and its consistent and correct use (patient compliance). These

Table 42–1. FAILURE RATES FOR VARIOUS CONTRACEPTIVE METHODS

METHOD	ESTIMATED PREGNANCY RATES (%)*
Vasectomy	<1
Tubal sterilization	<1
Oral contraceptives	2–3
IUDs	5–6
Condoms	10–15
Spermicides alone	15–20
Diaphragm and spermicide	15–20
Natural family planning	20–25
Coitus interruptus	20–25
Postcoital douche	40
No method	25–90

* In the first year of use, assuming variations in consistency of use.

and other factors, such as combining methods, duration of use, and switching methods, account for a wide variation in reported effectiveness. Factors such as availability (cost, prescription requirement, governmental restrictions), acceptability (religious bias, personal responsibility, and "natural feeling"), coital dependence (e.g., the use of oral contraceptives, intrauterine devices [IUDs], and sterilization are most removed from the coital experience), and perceived safety have a great deal to do with patient compliance and hence the effectiveness of the method.

Hormonal Contraceptives

Although hormonal contraceptives are the most commonly used temporary contraceptive in the United States (20 to 30 per cent of sexually active women use oral contraceptives), there has been some decrease in use, attributable to reports of an association with an increased risk of breast cancer. Ovulatory escape resulting in an unintended pregnancy is rare in women using oral contraceptives consistently and correctly.

Drug interactions may reduce the effectiveness of oral contraceptives. Rifampin and phenantoin significantly reduce serum levels of oral contraceptive components and higher doses must be prescribed. Conversely, oral contraceptives may reduce the absorption of folates and block insulin receptor sites.

Monophasic or Fixed Combination Oral Contraceptives

Table 42–2 indicates the number of combination oral contraceptives that are commonly available for use in the United States. The estrogen used is ethinyl estradiol and the progestational agents are androgens in which the methyl group is absent at the 19 position.

Considering the relationship between dose, effectiveness, and adverse effects, a consensus suggests that appropriate agents and optimal doses for oral contraceptives are as follows:
Estrogen:
Ethinyl estradiol: 30 μg or 35 μg
Progestin:
Norethindrone: 1 μg
Norgestrol: 0.5 mg or 0.075 mg

The oral contraceptives are taken for 21 days out of the monthly (28-day) cycle, with either no pill or a placebo taken during days 22 to 28. The several progestins used in oral contraceptives have varying degrees of potency (Table 42–3). Lower doses of estrogen and progestins are associated with more breakthrough bleeding and higher failure rates. Higher doses, especially of estrogens, are associated with more untoward side effects and serious complications. Prudence would suggest using another method of contraception rather than prescribing a dose that might be hazardous.

Multiphasic or Varying Dose Pills

Multiphasic oral contraceptives generally maintain a low dose of estrogen throughout the cycle, combined with varying amounts of progestin in each of the 3 weeks of medication. Examples are cited in Table 42–2. Overall, the multiphasic oral contraceptives are highly effective and may provide a lower total amount of estrogen or progestin.

Both combined and multiphasic oral contraceptives are dispensed in color-coded, calendar-oriented packets to help maintain the

Table 42-2. STEROID CONTENT IN ORAL CONTRACEPTIVES COMMONLY AVAILABLE IN THE UNITED STATES

BRAND NAME	ESTROGEN	ESTROGEN μg/TABLET*	ESTROGEN μg/CYCLE	PROGESTOGEN	PROGESTOGEN μg/TABLET	PHARM. CO.
Monophasic						
Lo/Ovral	Ethinyl estradiol	30	630	Norgestrel	300	Wyeth
Ovcon 35	Ethinyl estradiol	35	735	Norethindrone	400	Mead Johnson
Brevicon	Ethinyl estradiol	35	735	Norethindrone	500	Syntex
Modicon	Ethinyl estradiol	35	735	Norethindrone	500	Ortho
Demulen 1/35	Ethinyl estradiol	35	735	Ethynodiol diacetate	1000	Searle
Norinyl 1 + 35	Ethinyl estradiol	35	735	Norethindrone	1000	Syntex
Ortho-Novum 1/35	Ethinyl estradiol	35	735	Norethindrone	1000	Ortho
Loestrin 1/20	Ethinyl estradiol	30	630	Norethindrone acetate	1500	Parke-Davis
Loestrin 1/20	Ethinyl estradiol	20	420	Norethindrone acetate	1000	Parke-Davis
Multiphasic						
Triphasil	Ethinyl estradiol	30 (6) 40 (5) 30 (10)	680	Levonorgestrol	50 75 125	Wyeth
Tri-Norinyl	Ethinyl estradiol	35 (7) 35 (9) 35 (5)	735	Norethindrone	500 1000 500	Syntex
Ortho-Novum 7/7/7	Ethinyl estradiol	35 (7) 35 (7) 35 (7)	735	Norethindrone	500 750 1000	Ortho
Progestin Only						
Micronor	—	—	—	Norethindrone	350	Ortho
Nor-Q.D.	—	—	—	Norethindrone	350	Syntex
Ovrette	—	—	—	d-1-Norgestrel	75	Wyeth

* Number of days the pill is used per 28-day cycle is given in parentheses.

correct schedule. During the fourth week (withdrawal period) of the 28-day cycle, the daily pill is eliminated or the packette provides a placebo pill for each of the last 7 days.

Progestin-Only Pills

As noted in Table 42-2, there are three progestin-only oral contraceptives. They are taken daily and may be associated with irregular, low-grade, breakthrough vaginal bleeding. They are generally not regarded as being as effective as combination or multiphasic pills but are prescribed for nursing mothers and those patients in whom estrogens are contraindicated.

Biological Action of Oral Contraceptives

The contraceptive effect stems from at least four actions:

1. Suppression of the follicle-stimulating hormone (FSH) and luteinizing hormone (LH) secretion from the anterior pituitary.
2. Suppression of the LH surge and the resulting ovulation.
3. Alteration of cervical mucus, making it less penetrable by spermatozoa.
4. Induction of an atrophic change in the endometrium that is probably not conducive to implantation.

Table 42–3. RELATIVE POTENCY OF PROGESTINS USED IN ORAL CONTRACEPTIVES

ANDROGENIC	ESTROGENIC	ENDOMETRIAL AND PROGESTATIONAL
1—Norgestrel	1—Ethynodiol diacetate	1—Norgestrel
2—Norethindrone acetate	2—Norethindrone acetate	2—Ethynodiol diacetate
3—Norethindrone	3—Norethindrone	3—Norethindrone acetate
4—Ethynodiol diacetate	4—Norgestrel	4—Norethindrone

1 = most active.
4 = least active

Remarkably low failure rates in spite of frequent ovulatory escapes suggest that all these factors are operative.

Patient compliance in the use of oral contraceptives relates to untoward side effects. Estrogens may cause nausea, edema, headaches, and weight gain. Progestogenic side effects include depression, mastodynia, acne, and hirsutism.

Complications of Oral Contraceptives

Complications of oral contraceptives include a number of serious and potentially lethal side effects (Table 42–4). When compared with other risks to which women are subjected (Figure 42–1), the relative risks of oral contraceptives are quite small.

Table 42–4. COMPLICATIONS OF ORAL CONTRACEPTIVES

Thromboembolism*
Cerebrovascular accidents*
Hypertension*
Post-pill amenorrhea
Increase in cholelithiasis
Benign hepatic tumors

* Mainly in smokers.

Cardiovascular complications include venous thrombosis, pulmonary embolism, cerebrovascular accident, and myocardial infarction. These complications can be attributed to changes in blood coagulability, thought to be due to an increase in coagulation factors VII and X and fibrinogen. This effect seems to be associated with estrogen doses in excess of 50 μg and is especially marked in older smokers. The progestin decreases the high-density lipoproteins and increases the low-density lipoproteins, which probably increases the tendency toward cerebrovascular accidents and myocardial infarction. Oral contraceptives increase the release of renin precursors from the liver and can result in hypertension in a small percentage of women.

Many of these complications are marginal, but the risks are greatly enhanced by smoking. In 1990, the Food and Drug Administration (FDA) authorized the labeling of oral contraceptives as follows: "The benefit of oral contraceptives use by healthy, nonsmoking women over 40 may outweigh the possible risks." Oral contraceptives do not increase the risk of myocardial infarction in nonsmokers (Fig. 42–2).

Neoplasia as a complication is rare. Benign hepatic tumors occur in approximately one in 10,000 users. The risk increases over time and seems to be related to pills containing mestranol. Serious intraperitoneal hemorrhage may result from these tumors.

Cervical dysplasia has been reported to occur with higher frequency among women using oral contraceptives, but this increase is

Figure 42–1. Risk of mortality associated with oral contraceptives compared with other associated risks to which women are subjected. (From Hatcher RA: Contraceptive Technology—International Edition. Atlanta, GA, Printed Matter, Inc., 1989.)

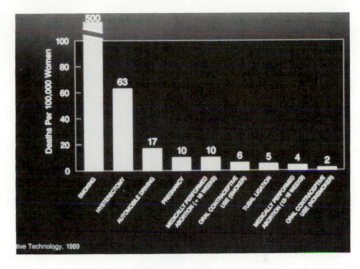

almost certainly related to other factors associated with the relative sexual freedom afforded by the pill.

In one study (British College of General Practitioners), an increased risk of breast cancer was correlated with long-term oral contraceptive use, but many other carefully controlled studies have shown no such increase (Fig. 42–3). There is possibly a relationship between the long-term use of oral contraceptives and breast cancer in young women (under the age of 35 years).

Gallbladder disease occurs with increased frequency in oral contraceptive users, especially during the first year of use and in those women who are at high risk for biliary tract disease (i.e., those who are fair, fat, and parous).

Amenorrhea is a disturbing complication. Women on oral contraceptives generally have a lighter withdrawal flow when compared with their prior menses, and some may even cease to have a withdrawal flow as a result of atrophic endometrial changes. In such cases, a serum prolactin level should be determined to rule out a prolactinoma, and a slightly more estrogenic pill should be substituted.

The vast majority of women who use oral contraceptives resume normal ovulatory menstruation promptly (1 to 3 months) after discontinuing the pill. A prepill history of oligo-ovulatory cycles may increase the risk

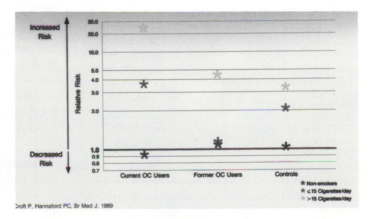

Figure 42–2. Relative risk of myocardial infarction in smokers using oral contraceptives (Royal College of General Practitioners Case-Control Study). (From Croft P, Hannaford PC: Br Med J, 1989.)

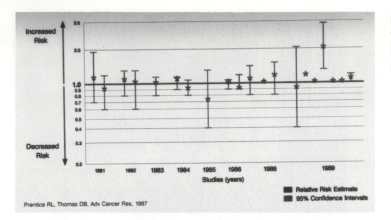

Figure 42–3. Risk of breast cancer associated with oral contraceptive use (20 case-control studies). (From Prentice L, Thomas DB: Adv Cancer Res 49:285, 1987.)

of "postpill" amenorrhea. There is some concern about a possible causal relationship between combination pills and pituitary microadenomas, especially if there is associated galactorrhea. If menstruation has not resumed after 6 months, a thorough endocrinologic appraisal must be made.

In contrast to the known complications that can occur, definite health benefits accrue from the use of oral contraceptives (Table 42–5). The incidence of ovarian cancer, endometrial cancer, and ectopic pregnancy, is significantly decreased. There is a protective effect against flareups of rheumatoid arthritis, and the progression of endometriosis is suppressed. It is estimated that although oral contraceptives are responsible for 9000 hospitalizations per year in the United States, their use prevents 57,000 hospitalizations (Fig. 42–4).

Contraindications to Oral Contraceptives

Contraindications to oral contraceptives vary from absolute to relative, as noted in Table 42–6.

Levonorgestrol Implants (Norplant System)

The Norplant kit contains a set of six flexible silastic capsules, each containing 36 mg of levonorgestrol. All six sealed capsules, each 34 mm in length, are surgically placed in the subcutaneous tissue of the inner surface of the upper arm. Initially, 85 μg is released daily, and the amount released daily declines to a level of 30 μg daily by 18 months. Levonorgestrol is highly progestational and has no estrogenic activity. Studies have shown the annual pregnancy rate to be less than one per 100 women through 5 years. Untoward effects relate to uterine bleeding and hyperlipidemia.

BARRIER AND CHEMICAL CONTRACEPTIVES

The objective of these methods is to prevent viable spermatozoa from gaining access to the endometrial cavity, fallopian tubes, and peritoneal cavity. They include condoms,

Table 42–5. NONCONTRACEPTIVE HEALTH BENEFITS OF ORAL CONTRACEPTIVES

DECREASES LIFE-THREATENING DISEASES	ALLEVIATES QUALITY-OF-LIFE PROBLEMS
Ovarian cancer	Anemia
Endometrial cancer	Dysmenorrhea
Ectopic pregnancy	Functional ovarian cysts
Anemia	Benign breast disease
Salpingitis	

After Grimes DA: Oral Contraceptives and Breast Cancer. Connforth, England, Parthenon Publishing, 1989.

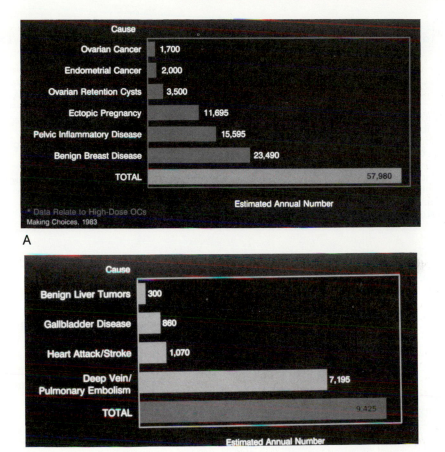

Figure 42–4. Hospitalizations prevented by oral contraceptive use *(A)* and hospitalizations attributed to oral contraceptives *(B)*, 1983. (From Ory HW, et al: Making Choices. Washington, D.C., The Alan Guttmacher Institute, 1983.)

cervical caps, vaginal diaphragms, chemically impregnated sponges, and chemical inserts (Fig. 42–5). Barrier methodologies extend far into the historical past, and presently those who use condoms and spermatocides enjoy the freedom of not requiring prescription by a physician.

Barrier methods and spermatocides have the drawback of varying degrees of coital dependence and must be used in close association with the precoital-coital sequence. Except for the risk of unintended pregnancy, they are free of serious complications.

Condoms

Condoms, in use since at least the sixteenth century, are rubberized sheaths applied over the erect penis prior to ejaculation. Many are packaged with contraceptive lubricants, and some are prepared with spermicidal agents added to their surface. It is important that a well be left at the end of the sheath for collection of the ejaculate and to avoid the inadvertent escape of semen as the penis is withdrawn from the vagina. Properly used, the condom is 98 per cent effective, but in couples reporting inconsistent use, the effectiveness drops to 90 per cent or lower.

Drawbacks of the condom include coital dependence, interruption of the coital sequence, and the occasional hypersensitivity to the rubber or lubricant. Some men associate erectile dysfunction with their use. Benefits include wide availability (pharmacies, markets, vending machines) and the possibility of preventing sexually transmitted diseases. The

Table 42-6. CONTRAINDICATIONS TO THE USE OF ORAL CONTRACEPTIVES

ABSOLUTE	RELATIVE CONTRAINDICATIONS TO ESTROGEN	OTHER RELATIVE CONTRAINDICATIONS
Venous thrombosis	Uterine fibroids	Anovulation/oligo-ovulation
Pulmonary embolism	Lactation	Depression
Coronary vascular disease	Diabetes mellitus	Severe headaches (especially
Cerebrovascular accident	Sickle cell disease	vascular)
Current pregnancy	Hypertension	Acne
Malignant tumor: breast, endo-	Age 35 + and cigarette smoking	Severe varicose veins
metrium, melanoma	Age 40 + and high risk for vas-	Hyperlipidemia
Hepatic tumor	cular disease	
Abnormal liver function		

threat of heterosexual and bisexual transmission of acquired immunodeficiency syndrome (AIDS) makes the condom a pressing contraceptive choice. The condom is well suited to couples who place a high value on male responsibility for contraception.

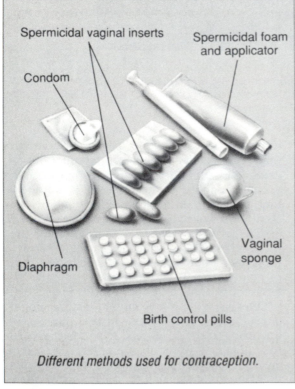

Spermicidal vaginal inserts
Spermicidal foam and applicator
Condom
Vaginal sponge
Diaphragm
Birth control pills

Different methods used for contraception.

Figure 42-5. Barrier and chemical contraceptives.

Spermicidal Agents

Various chemicals have been used for centuries to immobilize and destroy spermatozoa. Presently the most widely used spermicidal contraceptives contain nonoxynol-9 and octoxynol-9, which are surfactant agents that disrupt cell membranes. They are available as suppositories, creams, foams, and gels that are placed in the vagina up to 30 minutes before intercourse. Used properly and consistently, their effectiveness can be as high as 95 per cent. Sponges impregnated with spermicidal agents may be left in the vagina and used for up to 24 hours. If left in place for longer periods, they pose the risk of toxic shock syndrome. Postcoital douching with a weak solution of vinegar has a failure rate of approximately 40 per cent.

Vaginal Diaphragms

Vaginal diaphragms are a barrier of rubber or latex stretched across a circular rim that fits into the anterior vagina from the posterior fornix to a point just behind the hymenal rim, thus covering the cervix (Fig. 42-6). The barrier rings vary in diameter from 60 to 105 mm, increasing in increments of 5 mm. The size used should be the largest that fits comfortably. Nulliparous women generally take sizes 70 to 75 mm, and multipara generally require an 80 mm or larger size.

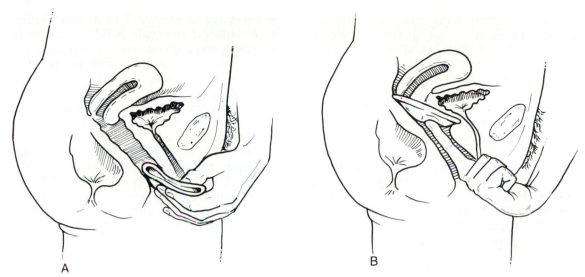

Figure 42–6. *A,* Insertion of a diaphragm into the vagina. *B,* Checking to ensure that the diaphragm covers the cervix.

Spermicidal jelly should be placed on either side of the diaphragm and it should be placed in the vagina before intercourse. It should be left in place for 6 to 8 hours thereafter, and if further intercourse occurs before removal, additional spermicide should be instilled without removing the diaphragm. The effectiveness, depending on proper and consistent use, can approach 98 per cent.

Untoward effects relate to bladder irritation, which occasionally leads to cystitis, and vaginal colonization with *Staphylococcus aureus* if the diaphragm is left in place for extended periods, thus raising concerns about toxic shock syndrome. Some women are unable to use the diaphragm because of hypersensitivity to the rubber or spermicide, and others cannot be properly fitted because of a cystocele, uterine prolapse, or perineal relaxation.

Cervical Caps

Cervical caps are soft rubber caps that fit over the cervix as a barrier and are held in place by suction and the flexible rim. They come in four sizes (in the United States) and must be carefully fitted to cervical size and used with a spermicidal jelly.

The technique of placement and removal is difficult for some women and the continuation rate is low (30 to 50 per cent). Although quite popular in Britain and Europe, the cervical cap is not widely available in the United States.

NATURAL FAMILY PLANNING AND FERTILITY AWARENESS

Physiologic contraception uses neither chemical nor mechanical barriers. The methods emphasize natural family planning, fertility awareness, and coitus interruptus. Natural family planning is generally meant to indicate abstinence shortly before and after ovulation, and fertility awareness refers to the use of various contraceptives (diaphragms, condoms, and spermicides) during periods of maximal fertility.

Natural family planning requires instruction in the physiology of menstruation and conception and more specifically in assessing the time ovulation occurs in the menstrual cycle. The time of ovulation is determined by the calendar method, the basal body temperature, and the character of the cervical mucus.

The basal body temperature uses the progesterone-induced thermogenic response, which indicates that ovulation has already occurred. The patient is instructed to record her temperature each morning before getting out of bed. The postovulatory rise is indicated by an increase of 0.5° to 1° F in temperature, which is maintained for 3 or more days. Occasionally ovulation is heralded by lower abdominal cramps (mittelschmerz) or by a show of vaginal bleeding (kleine regnung). For maximum effectiveness, intercourse should be avoided from the onset of menses until at least 2 days after ovulation has been suggested by the thermogenic shift.

The cervical mucus or spinnbarkeit method depends on differentiating between the scant, thick, opaque mucus of the preovulatory and postovulatory phases and the profuse, thin, clear mucus of the ovulatory phase. This thin, clear, stretchable (spinnbarkeit) mucus persists for 2 to 3 days, is readily apparent to most women, and represents the time of maximal fertility. Intercourse should be avoided until 48 to 72 hours after the last day of ovulatory mucus.

Most natural family planners depend on recording a menstrual calendar to avoid the periovulatory period. The beginning and end of each menstrual cycle is recorded for several months. Generally it is assumed that the onset of menses occurs 14 days after ovulation since the progestational phase of the cycle is fairly constant. If the length of the cycle is constant, the day of ovulation can be readily determined and the "unsafe" period is considered to be from 4 days before until 3 days after the day of ovulation. If the cycle length varies from month to month, the "unsafe" period can be determined by subtracting 18 days from the shortest cycle and 11 days from the longest cycle. Thus, if a patient's shortest cycle is 26 days and her longest is 32 days, her fertile period should be considered to be from the eighth to twenty-first day.

There is a great demand to increase the effectiveness of natural family planning, and for more accurate (and simpler) methods of determining the time of ovulation. Presently, poor reliability requires a prolonged period of abstinence—up to 17 days in some cases. Improvements could reduce the need for abstinence by more than 50 per cent. It would be necessary to provide 3 to 4 days warning of ovulation if the "safe period" were to be decreased, since spermatozoa can remain viable for this period in the female genital tract. The ovum, however, is relatively shortlived after ovulation (unless fertilized). The technology to assay the chemical determinants of the menstrual cycle is presently available and is being developed in industry. Highly accurate monoclonal antibody kits to determine the steady rise of estrogens in saliva or urine over a 48- to 168-hour period in the follicular phase would be one possible approach. The rising levels of LH leading to the surge occurs too close to ovulation (26 to 56 hours) to give sufficient warning to avoid intercourse, but the increasing levels of progesterone in the early postovulatory phase, and the concurrent secondary rise in estrogens, would give an accurate indication that the danger of conception had passed.

CONTRACEPTION DURING LACTATION

Lactational amenorrhea is in itself an inhibitor of ovulation, although its efficacy is questioned since 5 to 10 per cent of women become pregnant when exposed during the suckling period. Fifty per cent of nursing mothers will ovulate by 6 to 12 months even while nursing. Sterilization, barrier/spermicides, and IUDs have no effect on nursing. If combination oral contraceptives are used during lactation, there is concern about decreased milk production, the composition of the milk, and the passage of steroids into the milk. Progestin-only contraceptives offer no known adverse effects on the milk or the infant.

POSTCOITAL CONTRACEPTION

Rape, torn condoms, displaced diaphragms, expelled IUDs, and even second thoughts would seem to make postcoital contraception an urgent consideration, especially if termination of an eventual pregnancy is anticipated. Generally, two tablets of Ovral can be taken within 72 hours of intercourse and repeated in 12 hours. Premarin (10 mg)

Figure 42–7. Intrauterine devices presently available: *A*, Tatum-T, Paraguard-T; *B*, Progestasert.

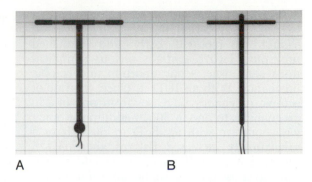

A   B

or stilbestrol (10 mg) may also be used. The patient must be followed to ensure that withdrawal bleeding occurs in 5 days. If a period does not ensue, termination of pregnancy should be advised because of possible teratogenic effects on the fetus. The postcoital pill is 99 per cent effective. In a broader sense, the antiprogestin RU 486 offers a similar approach to contraception by interrupting the established implantation. As of this writing, the drug is not available in the United States.

INTRAUTERINE DEVICES

IUDs have been used for decades. Modern devices are inserted into the endometrial cavity through a narrow plastic cannula and can be removed by traction on a string attached to the lower end of the device. Early devices without a string protruding from the cervix were the Graffenberg ring and the Birnbaum bow. The absence of the string, although theoretically preferable, makes removal difficult.

During the 1960s and 1970s, IUDs attained great popularity with the availability of the Lippes Loop, the Dalkon Shield, the Copper-7 and the Tatum-T. Because of serious pelvic infections associated with the method, however, only two IUDs are currently marketed in the United States: the copper Paraguard T380A and the Progestasert (Fig. 42–7).

The Progestasert releases progesterone from the vertical stem of the T. It reportedly results in less blood loss during menstruation and is associated with less dysmenorrhea. A disadvantage is that it must be replaced an-

nually. The Paraguard, shaped like the Tatum-T, has 380 mm of exposed copper and has somewhat better contraceptive effectiveness than previous copper-containing devices. It can be left in place for 4 to 6 years, and its effectiveness approaches that of oral contraceptives.

The precise mechanisms by which IUDs prevent pregnancy is not entirely clear. A number of mechanisms are postulated:

1. Inhibition of implantation.
2. Altered tubal motility.
3. Inflammatory changes in the endometrium.

During the first year of use, the failure rate for IUDs is approximately 5 per cent, probably because of unrecognized expulsions. After the first year, the failure rate drops to 1 to 2 per cent. Of women who do become pregnant with an IUD in place, the risk of ectopic pregnancy increases five fold.

Side effects and complications of IUDs can be severe and serious. IUDs generally increase the blood loss and duration of menses and increase the incidence of dysmenorrhea, especially in nulliparous women. Prostaglandin synthetase inhibitors may partially correct these problems, but in many instances the IUD must be removed. IUD expulsion is another problem occurring in 5 per cent of women, generally during the first year after insertion and in younger women of low parity. Symptoms of expulsion include lengthening of the string, ability to palpate the lower end of the device, and the sudden onset of uterine cramps or excessive bleeding. Partially expelled IUDs should be removed.

Pregnancy is a serious complication in a woman with an IUD. A delayed period should be reported early and evaluated promptly. Two potentially serious complications can ensue: septic abortion and ectopic pregnancy. With an IUD in place, the rate of ectopic pregnancy increases from one in 250 pregnancies to one in 50. In addition, women who conceive with an IUD in place have a substantially increased risk of abortion: 25 per cent if the IUD is removed and 50 per cent if it is not. A septic abortion in the presence of an IUD can have very serious consequences and the device should be removed promptly.

Insertion of an IUD can result in perforation of the uterine wall with protrusion through the serosa. The risk, although quite small overall (less than one per 5000), is increased with inexperience, uterine malposition, and myometrial softening as with the postabortal and puerperal state. Perforation should be suspected with a difficult or painful insertion, if the string is not visible, or if the patient becomes pregnant. A "misplaced" IUD can usually be detected by hysteroscopy, pelvic ultrasonography, hysterosalpingography, or by taking an abdominal x-ray film with a marker (uterine round) in the endometrial cavity. An intraperitoneal IUD should be removed by laparoscopy, colpotomy, or laparotomy. An IUD embedded in the myometrium can usually be removed by a long alligator-type forceps inserted through the cervical canal. It is sometimes necessary to dilate the cervical canal to facilitate this approach.

Women using IUDs are at higher risk to develop salpingo-oophoritis or a tubo-ovarian abscess, which may be unilateral. The risk of pelvic infection is greatest within the first few months after insertion and among younger, nulliparous women with more than one sexual partner. Because of the risk of infection and the consequent threat of infertility, many physicians advise against IUD use in nulliparous women.

Regular follow-up examinations are essential for women with IUDs to detect expulsion or infection. The IUD is less well tolerated by the nulliparous woman but is especially indicated for the multiparous woman for whom the oral contraceptive is contraindicated, that is, the smoker after her mid-thirties.

PERMANENT STERILIZATION

Permanent sterilizations on request have increased dramatically over the past 3 decades. The methods include vasectomy, postpartum tubal ligation, and interval tubal occlusion either by laparoscopy or minilaparotomy (Table 42–7). At the time of writing, 30 per cent of couples of reproductive age in the United States and Britain have opted for female sterilization. The procedure is increasing in popularity, and the age of those opting for it is declining.

Fatalities occur in four per 100,000 women being sterilized in the United States, and one ectopic pregnancy occurs per 15,000 women sterilized; however, 100,000 female sterilizations avert 1000 maternal deaths in the interval between sterilization and the end of the woman's fertile period. One per cent of women sterilized become pregnant, often because an early implantation is not detected at the time of the procedure. Clips have been somewhat less successful than rings, cautery, or the Pomeroy method. Cautery is most commonly used in the United States.

Counseling

The intended permanence and the surgical nature of permanent sterilization make patient evaluation and counseling critical. In the United States, if federal money is used to fund the sterilization, a 30-day interval is required between signing the consent and performing the procedure; however, the interval may be waived to 72 hours in the event of premature delivery or emergency abdominal surgery. Specific information concerning side effects and complications must be provided to the patient, and both men and women should understand that sterility cannot be guaranteed; that is, there are failures.

Vasectomy

Vasectomy would seem to be the simplest and safest option for permanent sterilization in a stable monogamous relationship. It causes no significant hormonal changes, and there is no change in spermatogenesis if re-

Table 42–7. METHODS OF TUBAL STERILIZATION

SURGICAL APPROACH	TECHNIQUE	SURGICAL PROCEDURE
Laparotomy	Pomeroy	Ligature around a "knuckle" (or loop) of tube; excision distally
	Madlener	Crushing and ligature of loop of tube
	Irving	Double ligation, excision between; proximal end buried in myometrium; distal end buried in broad ligament
	Uchida	Tubal serosa stripped from muscular coat; tubal segment excised; proximal end ligated and buried in broad ligament
	Fimbriectomy	Ligation of distal end of tube and mesosalpinx; excision of fimbriated end
Laparoscopy	Electrocoagulation	Electrical "burn" of two adjacent segments with/without transection
	Falope ring	Loop of tube drawn into applicator tube; plastic ring placed around both limbs of loop
	Hulka clip	Plastic crushing clip placed across tube (not a loop); kept closed by steel spring
"Mini-laparotomy"	Pomeroy ligation Electrocauterization	
Posterior colpotomy	Falope ring Pomeroy ligation Hulka clip	
Hysteroscopy	Insertion of tubal plug Electrocoagulation Chemical scarification	Cannulation of internal tubal ostia via a transcervical approach
Blind cannulation of tubes via transcervical approach	Chemical scarification	

versal is undertaken. Success of vasectomy reversal is in excess of 60 per cent.

Fallopian Tube Occlusion

Almost all tubal occlusions are carried out in hospital operating rooms or in surgicenters as outpatient procedures. They are done as an early puerperal tubal ligation, an interval laparoscopic tubal occlusion (after hospital discharge following obstetric delivery), or as a mini-laparotomy with tubal ligation (Table 42–7).

Types of Procedures

Laparoscopic tubal occlusion can be performed through a 1-cm incision in the inferior portion of the navel using bipolar electrocautery, the Hulka clip, or the Falope ring (Fig. 42–8). The occlusive devices should be applied to the mobile portion of the tubes at the junction of the isthmus and ampulla. This approach can be used concurrently with pregnancy interruption by dilatation and curettage (suction curettage).

The Falope ring applicator must be inserted through a 0.5-cm suprapubic incision just above the bladder reflection. Falope ring tubal occlusions are associated with a surprising amount of postoperative pain, probably because of the ischemic segment of tube within the constricting ring. Pelvic adhesions from prior pelvic infection may pose difficulties with this approach. Since a larger area of tube is destroyed with electrocautery, the method should not be used in younger women, in whom there is a somewhat greater likelihood that they may request reversal in later years, for example, following divorce and remarriage.

Laparotomy, using a small (3 to 4 cm) incision for open tubal ligation, is referred to as mini-laparotomy. A uterine elevator placed

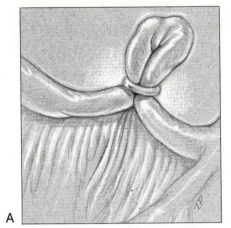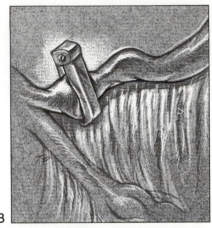

Figure 42–8. Tubal occlusion with (A) the Falope ring and (B) the Hulka clip. (Modified from McGonigle KF, Higgins GR: Tubal sterilization: Epidemiology of regret. Contemp Obstet Gyn 35(10):15, 1990.)

through the vagina into the cervix is used to raise the uterine fundus toward the incision where each tube can be occluded by the Pomeroy (Fig. 42–9) or other technique. An advantage of tubal resection at laparotomy is that tissue is obtained for histologic examination to confirm that the tubes have been interrupted.

Postpartum tubal occlusion is generally carried out 4 to 24 hours after vaginal deliv-

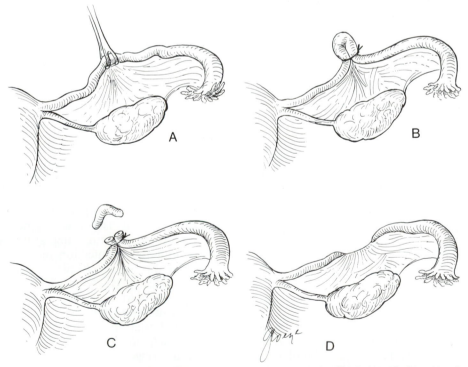

Figure 42–9. Pomeroy method of tubal ligation. A, Tube is grasped with Babcock forceps. B, A loop is ligated. C, The loop is excised. D, Several months later, the fibrosed ends of the tube separate.

ery through a small (2 to 3 cm) incision just below the navel. The large puerperal uterus extends almost to the navel just underneath the anterior abdominal wall, making the tubes easily accessible for the Pomeroy technique. There is a slightly higher failure rate when tubes are occluded puerperally or at the time of cesarean section.

Vaginal colpotomy by an incision through the posterior vaginal fornix into the pouch of Douglas provides access for tubal occlusion by either the Pomeroy technique or by the Kroener fimbriectomy. This approach is generally more difficult and is occasionally associated with postoperative infection; hence it is not commonly employed.

Hysteroscopic sterilization, by either cauterizing the internal tubal ostia or injecting a plug of an acrylate compound into them, has been the subject of large clinical trials. Although the method has minimal side effects, its clinical effectiveness is not yet established.

Sterilization reversal is requested in a substantial number of women previously sterilized (more than 1 per cent). The microsurgical techniques of tubal reanastomosis can achieve success rates up to 70 per cent. Success is more likely if the occluding technique has caused only minimal damage to the tube and has left the fimbriae intact. In vitro fertilization represents an alternative solution (see Chapter 51).

SUGGESTED READING

Centers for Disease Control, United States Public Health Service: Oral contraceptive use and the risk of breast cancer in young women. MMWR 33:353, 1984.

Chang RJ, Mackay HT: Current perspectives on low-dose oral contraceptives. Contemp Ob Gyn 35:13, 1990.

Djerassi C: Natural family planning. Science 248:1061, 1990.

Fazoli M, Parazzini F, Cecchetti G, et al: Postcoital contraception. Contraception 39:459, 1989.

Gosland IF, Crook D, Simpson R: The effects of oral contraceptives on lipid and carbohydrate metabolism. N Engl J Med 323:1375, 1990.

Gray RH: Contraceptive effects of lactation. Science 355:335, 1990.

Grimes DA: The Contraception Report, August 1990. Morris Plains, NJ, Emron Inc, 1990.

Hatcher RA: Contraceptive Technology—International Edition. Atlanta, GA, Printed Matter, Inc, 1989.

Kay CR: Oral contraceptives and diabetes mellitus, Br Med J 299:1315, 1989.

Kay CR, Hannaford PC: Breast cancer and the pill. Br J Cancer 58:675, 1988.

McGonigle KF, Higgins GR: Tubal sterilization: Epidemiology of regret. Contemp Ob Gyn 35(10):15, 1990.

Notelovitz M, Feldman EB, Gillespy M, Gudat J: Lipid and lipoprotein changes in women taking low-dose, triphasic oral contraceptives: A controlled, comparative, 12-month clinical trial. Am J Obstet Gynecol 160:1269, 1989.

Ory HW: Evaluating the health risks and benefits of birth control methods. Washington, D.C., The Alan Guttmacher Institute, 1983.

Romieu I: Prospective study of oral contraceptive use and risk of breast cancer in women. Journal of the National Cancer Institute 81:1313, 1989.

Seiler JS: The evaluation of tubal sterilization. Obstet Gynecol Surv 39:177, 1984.

Spellacy WN, Ellingson AB, Tsibris JCM, et al: The effects of triphasic oral contraceptives on carbohydrate metabolism. Fertil Steril 51:71, 1989.

Stadel BV, Lai S, Schlesselman JJ, et al: Oral contraceptives and premenopausal breast cancer. Contraception 38:287, 1988.

Stampfer MJ, Willet WC, Colditz GA, et al: Oral contraceptives and the risk of cardiovascular disease. N Engl J Med 319:131, 1988.

Forty-three

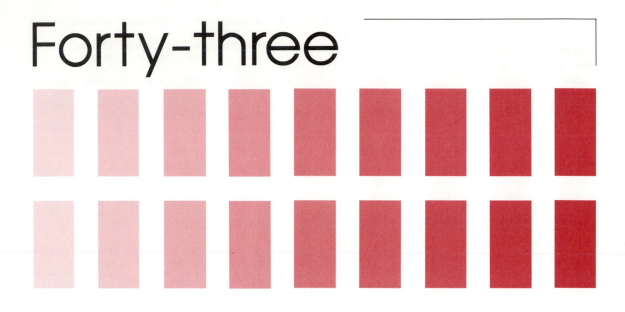

Human Sexuality

J. ROBERT BRAGONIER and ANTHONY E. READING

There is consensus that sexual functioning should be an integral part of a complete medical evaluation. A survey by Bachmann and coworkers in 1989 established the frequency of sexual problems in an outpatient gynecologic practice. A total of 887 women were interviewed. If a sexual complaint was not elicited as a reason for the visit, they were asked the following questions: "Are you sexually active?" and "Are you having any sexual difficulties or problems at this time?" Sexual complaints were the presenting problem in 3 per cent of the women, and the brief inquiry elicited a sexual concern from a further 16 per cent. Hence, 19 per cent of the total sample were experiencing sexual problems. The most common complaint was dyspareunia (48 per cent), with decreased sexual desire reported by 21 per cent, partner problems or dysfunction by 8 per cent, vaginismus by 6 per cent, anorgasmia by 4 per cent, and a variety of other problems including

sexual anxiety and decreased lubrication by the remaining 13 per cent. Problems were more common in women over 50, and difficulties were ascribable to physical factors (atrophic vaginitis, pelvic adhesions, endometriosis) in 32 per cent.

A comparable survey of gynecologic outpatients found the frequency of sexual problems to be 33 per cent. These studies confirm the high prevalence of problems and are reminders of the importance of direct inquiry because reliance on the patient to volunteer the information could mean many difficulties will be missed and therefore remain untreated.

Early research into uterine activity during orgasm was reported in 1896. Alfred Kinsey in the 1940s and 1950s observed and described sexual activity, but he was hesitant to publish his findings; he apparently considered his epidemiologic studies of sexual behavior that he did publish to be controversial enough for the times. It was not until the pioneering work of Masters and Johnson, published in 1966, that research into the physiology of sex was legitimized. Yet replication of even these studies has been slow.

ANATOMY AND PHYSIOLOGY OF THE FEMALE SEXUAL RESPONSE

Sexual response is mediated through three related, but neurophysiologically discrete, phases: (1) desire (libido), (2) excitement (arousal), and (3) orgasm (climax). Because each of these phases is mediated via different neuronal circuits, sexual dysfunction may affect one or another of them without affecting the others.

Desire Phase

Sexual desire appears to be an appetite similar to hunger, controlled by a dopamine-sensitive excitatory center, in balance with a serotonin (5-hydroxytryptamine)–sensitive inhibitory center. In both males and females, testosterone appears to be the hormone responsible for initially programming these centers in prenatal life and for maintaining their threshold of response. Stimulation and ablation experiments in cats and other mammalian species have located these centers within the limbic system, with significant nuclei in the hypothalamic and preoptic regions. These centers, therefore, are part of the archaic organizational system of the brain that is responsible for survival, reproduction, motivation, and emotion.

Desire is modulated by connections between these centers and other parts of the brain. For example, the activity of these centers can be markedly affected by neuro-electric and hormonal interactions with pleasure and pain centers. Connections with memory storage banks enable experience and learning to affect the frequency, direction, intensity, and mode of expression of sexual desire. The net effect of these positive and negative influences modulates genital sexual response via impulses passing down the spi-

nal cord to the spinal reflex centers that govern excitement and orgasm.

Excitement Phase

During the excitement phase, vascular engorgement occurs, mediated primarily by the parasympathetic nervous system. Genital changes include enlargement in the diameter and length of the clitoris; dilatation of perivaginal arterioles with seeping of vascular transudate across the vaginal membrane, resulting in lubrication; and expansion and "tenting" of the upper half of the vagina. Bartholin's glands may secrete several drops of mucoid fluid during the late excitement phase. The neuronal connections for the genital changes of excitement and orgasm are shown in Table 43–1.

Estrogen is the hormone responsible for maintaining the vaginal mucosa and allowing transudation and lubrication to occur. Its deficiency (postsurgically or postmenopausally) is by far the most common cause of excitement phase dysfunction in women.

Extragenital changes during the excitement phase include an increase in heart rate and blood pressure; enhanced muscle tension throughout the body; an increase in breast size, nipple erection, and engorgement of the surrounding areolae; and a sex flush. The latter is an erythematous rash over the chest, neck, and face that occurs to a noticeable degree in 75 per cent of women.

Orgasmic Phase

During the orgasmic phase, a series of reflex clonic contractions of the levator sling and related genital musculature occur, mediated primarily via the sympathetic nervous system.

Extragenital reactions during orgasm include contraction of muscle groups throughout the body; maximal intensity of the sex flush; and maximal elevations of heart rate, blood pressure, and respiratory rate.

Excitement and orgasm are reflexes. For the orgasmic reflex to be activated, the stimulus must be applied where the sensory nerve endings are located (primarily in the area of the clitoris), and the stimulation must be of

Table 43-1. NEUROANATOMY OF EXCITEMENT AND ORGASM

REFLEX	MEDIATION	AFFERENT (SENSORY) CONNECTIONS	SPINAL CORD CENTERS	EFFERENT (MOTOR) CONNECTIONS
Excitement	Parasympathetic	From clitoris via the dorsal nerve of clitoris to the pudendal nerve	S2–S4	Preganglionic fibers travel via the pelvic nerve (nervus erigentes) to the vesical and uterovaginal plexuses
		From anterior labia via ilioinguinal nerve and the perineal branch of the posterior femoral cutaneous nerve	T11–L2	Postganglionic fibers travel to the erectile tissue
Orgasm	Sympathetic	Same	T11–L2	Preganglionic fibers travel via the splanchnic nerve to the inferior mesenteric ganglion and ganglia in the hypogastric, vesical, and pelvic plexuses. Postganglionic fibers pass to genital smooth muscle
			S3–S4	Pudendal nerve to striated muscle (ischiocavernosus and bulbocavernosus)

sufficient intensity and duration to reach the threshold for the reflex. For many women, this involves more direct clitoral stimulation than can be achieved from male-superior, penile-vaginal thrusting alone. Many women have discovered that doing Kegel's exercises during sex or voluntarily tensing muscles in other parts of their body may lower the threshold for, or increase the intensity of, orgasm. Women generally experience an increased rate and intensity of orgasm with self-stimulation.

SEXUAL DYSFUNCTION

Classification

True sexual dysfunction is manifested by failure of one or more phases of the sexual response cycle: desire, excitement, and orgasm. It can be classified according to the earliest phase in which disruption is experienced. Disruption frequently begins with orgasmic disturbance, but if neglected, loss of excitement and, finally, loss of desire may follow.

Sexual dysfunction can also be subdivided into three different categories, depending on whether it is *primary* (realistic sexual expectations have never been met under any circumstances), *secondary* (all phases have functioned in the past, but one or more no longer do so), or *situational* (the response cycle functions under some circumstances, but not others).

Etiology

The etiology and classification of sexual dysfunction are summarized in Table 43-2. Most sexual problems are psychological (Table 43-3), but organic and pharmacologic causes must also be considered (Tables 43-4 and 43-5). Primary problems are predominantly psychogenic and tend to be of longer duration. Secondary problems are often associated with the onset of a disease process or the use of a pharmacologic agent. If such an association cannot be established, a deterioration in the patient's relationship or some other chronologically related change in the patient's life experience should be sought.

Table 43–2. CLASSIFICATION OF SEXUAL DYSFUNCTION*

Table 43–2. CLASSIFICATION OF SEXUAL DYSFUNCTION*

CATEGORY	CHARACTERISTICS	ETIOLOGY
Primary	Sexual expectations have never been met	Usually psychogenic
Secondary	All phases functioned in the past, but one or more no longer do so	May be organic or pharmacologic
Situational	Response cycle functions under some circumstances, but not others	May be psychogenic or relationship-related

* Any of the dysfunctions may involve desire, excitement, or orgasm.

The two situational problems of major clinical significance are represented by women who achieve climaxes with petting, oral sex, or self-stimulation, but not with penile thrusting alone (over one-half of all women complaining of orgasmic problems) and men who have erections in the morning, during sleep, or with masturbation, but not when needed for insertion and intercourse. Problems that are situational are noteworthy because they are almost invariably psychogenic or relational and not organic or pharmacologic in origin.

Factors initiating a problem may be different from those maintaining it. For example, drugs may precipitate a problem, but if anxiety and fear of failure sustain the difficulty, discontinuation of the drug may not rectify it.

SEXUAL ASSESSMENT

Sexual concerns may present as chief complaints or may become apparent during the review of systems. The likelihood of a woman expressing sexual concerns is a direct function of her perception of the clinician's level of comfort in discussing the subject.

Sexual Problem History

The sexual system can be reviewed by asking, "Is your sexual relationship meeting your expectations?" or "Are you experiencing any sexual difficulties?" If no concerns are expressed, no further assessment is warranted.

Table 43–3. PSYCHOLOGICAL CAUSES OF SEXUAL DYSFUNCTION IN WOMEN

INTRAPERSONAL
Inadequate self-esteem
Depression
Anxiety
  Performance
  Irrational fears
  Unresolved conflicts
  Developmental trauma
Diminished capacity for relationships
Psychosis

INTERPERSONAL
Distrust
Resentment
Disillusionment
Dissatisfaction
Poor communication

Table 43–4. ORGANIC CAUSES OF SEXUAL DYSFUNCTION IN WOMEN

DISORDERS	EXAMPLE
Neurogenic	Central, spinal, peripheral
Vascular	Local and systemic
Endocrine/metabolic	Diabetes mellitus, thyroid, pituitary
Systemic medical	Hepatic, renal, pulmonary
Musculoskeletal	Arthritis
Local pelvic	Genital infections, endometriosis, genital neoplasms, atrophic vaginitis

Table 43–5. DRUGS THAT CAN DIMINISH SEXUAL FUNCTION IN WOMEN

TYPE OF AGENT	EXAMPLES
Hypnotics	Alcohol, barbiturates
Tranquilizers	Chlordiazepoxide, diazepam
Narcotics	Heroin, methadone
Antipsychotics	Phenothiazines, butyrophenones
Antidepressants	Tricyclics, monoamine oxidase inhibitors
Stimulants	Cocaine, amphetamines
Anorectics	Fenfluramine
Hallucinogens	THC, LSD, PCP, mescaline
Hormones	Progestins, oral contraceptives
Antihypertensives	Reserpine, propranolol, methyldopa
Anticholinergics	Propantheline bromide
Diuretics	Acetazolamide

Once a concern has surfaced, a more detailed sexual history should be obtained by asking appropriate questions in specific problem areas. Questions listed under the following subheadings may be helpful.

Nature of the Problem. What do you perceive as the problem? Does it affect orgasm, excitement, or desire? How long has it been going on? Have things ever been better? Was its onset gradual or sudden? Is the problem intermittent? Is it getting worse, better, or staying about the same? If you have had more than one partner, did the problem occur with each of them? Were there any precipitating events? What does your partner think about the problem? How do you explain its occurrence to yourself? What seems to make the problem better? What makes it worse? What have you previously done to evaluate or treat the problem? What has your partner done to help? Does the problem decrease when you are by yourself (with self-stimulation)?

Earlier Sexual Experience. What were things like when they were the best they have ever been for you? How often were you having intercourse then? Who suggested it? How often did you want to have intercourse? Did you have the right to refuse? Compare and contrast your answers to your current situation.

Sexual Expectations. What do you expect to happen in a sexual encounter? Describe a current, typical sexual encounter. How are your expectations and actual experiences different? Who initiates sex? How much time elapses between initial caressing and entry? How is this decided? Would you ever like foreplay to last longer? Have you ever tried to let your partner know this? How long is the time from insertion until your partner ejaculates? Is this a problem for either of you?

Status of the Relationship. Are you and your partner good friends? What interests do you share? What changes have been occurring in other areas of your relationship?

General Coping Mechanisms. How are you coping with the problem and with life in general? Do you feel creative, successful, and competent in what you do? Do you like yourself? Are you frequently depressed, anxious, or fearful?

General Medical History

The sexual problem history should be accompanied by a general medical history and a physical examination with emphasis on the gynecologic examination. These routine procedures plus standard laboratory evaluation are adequate to rule out nearly all organic causes of sexual dysfunction in women.

MANAGEMENT

General Considerations

The challenge for the gynecologist or other primary care clinician is to (1) characterize the nature of the concern; (2) provide permission, reassurance, or limited information, as necessary; (3) recognize and manage problems caused by organic or pharmacologic factors; and (4) assess the need for referral of those patients with dysfunctions requiring more in-depth psychotherapeutic intervention.

For many patients, reassurance, information, and the opportunity to ventilate concerns and obtain permission and understanding can be extremely helpful. There may be a misfit between expectations and experience or between the expectations of the two partners; counseling might suggest more realistic expectations, more fulfilling practices, or appropriately negotiated compromises.

More serious sexual problems may require behavioral psychotherapy; for some patients, referral may be indicated. The approach is aimed at providing conditions conducive for sexual arousal by removing pejorative labels, extinguishing anxiety over performance, replacing avoidance behaviors, and facilitating communication about sexual issues.

Common Conditions

A detailed description of therapeutic techniques is beyond the scope of this chapter. Nonetheless, the principles of management for three common conditions are discussed.

Lack of Orgasm

Women who complain that they are not experiencing orgasm can be separated into four groups: (1) those who have erroneous expectations, (2) those who experience pressure from their partner, (3) those who have lost their orgasmic capacity, and (4) those lacking sufficient stimulation.

A large number of women experience orgasm only with manual or oral stimulation and not with penile thrusting alone. If they are capable of achieving orgasm with a partner by any means, their problem is primarily one of erroneous expectations. If they are willing to increase direct clitoral stimulation before, during, or after penile penetration, they may achieve a wholly satisfactory sexual adaptation.

Some women may enjoy intercourse but be under considerable pressure from partners to experience more intense orgasms. They may be uncertain as to whether they are currently experiencing orgasms at all. Exploring their feelings during resolution (euphoria versus frustration) may clarify this issue. Validation of a woman's current experience may relieve some of the pressure she is experiencing from her partner.

Women who have been orgasmic in the past but have lost that capacity should be carefully screened for organic or pharmacologic causes, and changes in their relationship(s) should be carefully explored.

Most women with primary anorgasmia have usually had minimal or no effective stimulation from self or partner. These patients should be encouraged to learn how to achieve orgasm through self-stimulation and then to share this new information with their partners. Increasing the intensity of stimulation should increase the intensity of response.

Vaginismus

With this condition, women experience severe pain on attempted penile penetration or are unable to allow any penetration at all. Examination reveals no organic pathology, but the pubococcygeal muscles are tight, and vaginal penetration by speculum or examining finger is painful and difficult, if not impossible.

Women with vaginismus may or may not remember episodes of sexual trauma, but the important issue is whether they are able and motivated to participate with their partners in a stepwise *desensitization* program. This involves the slow, gentle vaginal insertion of dilators of gradually increasing size, under the patient's own control. Once sufficient progress has been made, the partner's fingers and, ultimately, his penis may be substituted for the dilators. Alleviation of the problem is usually accomplished in 3 to 6 months. If anxiety precludes her participation, psychotherapeutic intervention may be required.

Secondary Lack of Desire

This complaint, once known as "frigidity," frequently surfaces in women under considerable psychological stress. It is nearly always due to loss of trust, resentment, or disillusionment with the relationship, although fatigue and boredom may play a role. When interpersonal strife is prominent, referral for therapy is generally necessary. For treatment to be effective, it must be focused on the relationship. If the partner is unwilling to participate in a serious renegotiation of the rules on which the relationship is based, desire is unlikely to return.

PROGNOSIS

The lack of controlled studies, standard definitions, uniform periods of follow-up, and standard criteria for improvement make more than a few general statements regarding prognosis impossible. As a group, orgasmic difficulties seem to respond to treatment most readily. For example, lack of orgasm in the female and premature ejaculation in the male can be resolved in 80 to 90 per cent of cases. Excitement phase dysfunctions do not have such positive outcomes. Although problems in females can nearly always be resolved satisfactorily, erectile difficulties in males respond only 60 to 70 per cent of the time. Lack of desire is the most resistant to treatment. Persons with little desire often have little internal motivation to seek more frequent sexual activity or to seek help. Fewer than 50 per cent of such patients show definite improvement. When the relationship is poor, behavioral approaches directed toward the sexual problem rarely are successful.

SUGGESTED READING

Annon JS: The Behavioral Treatment of Sexual Problems. Brief Therapy, Vol. I; Intensive Therapy, Vol. II. Honolulu, Enabling Systems, 1974, 1975.

Bachmann GA, Leiblum SR, Grill J: Brief sexual inquiry in gynecological practice. Obstet Gynecol 73:425, 1989.

Barnard M, Clancy B, Krantz K: Human Sexuality for Health Professionals. Philadelphia, WB Saunders, 1978.

Kaplan HS: The Evaluation of Sexual Disorders: Psychological and Medical Aspects. New York, Brunner/Mazel, 1983.

Kaplan HS: Disorders of Sexual Desire, and Other New Concepts and Techniques in Sex Therapy. New York, Simon & Schuster, 1979.

Kaplan HS: The New Sex Therapy. New York, Brunner/Mazel, 1974.

Kolodny RC, Masters WH, Johnson V: Textbook of Sexual Medicine. Boston, Little, Brown, 1979.

Lief HI (ed): Sexual Problems in Medical Practice. Monroe, WI, American Medical Association, 1981.

Munjack DJ, Oziel LJ: Sexual Medicine and Counseling in Office Practice. Boston, Little, Brown, 1980.

Plouffe L: Screening for sexual problems through a simple questionnaire. Am J Obstet Gynecol 151:166, 1985.

Forty-four

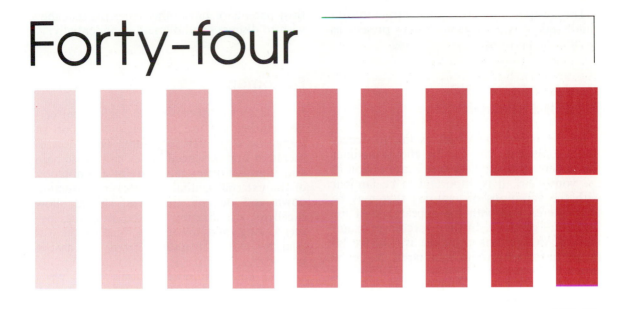

Pediatric Gynecology

JENNIFER BLAKE

Children experience fewer gynecologic problems than do adult women, but their concerns need to be met effectively and skillfully in a way that will allay anxiety and create a positive attitude toward their gynecologic health. Children's unique complaints fall generally into a handful of categories: congenital anomalies, genital injuries, inflammation of the unestrogenized genital tract, pubertal problems, and psychosexual concerns. Management of all of these conditions requires a good understanding of childhood and adolescent development.

ANATOMY

The child at birth typically exhibits evidence of exposure to maternal estrogen with prominent labia and a dull pink vaginal epithelium. As estrogen levels fall, the genitalia take on their juvenile appearance with small labial fat pads and labia minora. The healthy vaginal epithelium, only 1-cell thick, is bright red.

The hymen has a varied configuration. An imperforate hymen is evident in the newborn period as a thin bulging membrane. Most other anatomic configurations have no clinical significance. Much is made of the size of the hymenal opening, but there is a great deal of individual variation.

The uterus is also stimulated by maternal estrogens. It is larger in the newborn period than it will be for the next 5 or 6 years and therefore is easily palpated on rectal examination. Withdrawal bleeding in the newborn period is not uncommon. Involution takes place over the first 6 months of life. The fundus is relatively small in childhood, constituting approximately one third of the total volume of the uterus.

The ovaries are abdominal structures in childhood. Any enlargement may present as an abdominal mass.

EXAMINATION AND INSTRUMENTATION

Few examinations cause as much anxiety to the physician, the family, and sometimes the patient as the gynecologic examination of the young girl. It is important to be familiar with the variations of anatomy that may be encountered and with the appearance of the immature genitalia. In the gynecologic examination, the guiding principle is "Above all do no harm." Restraint may rarely be necessary with an infant but must *never* be used in a child, since they may recall the event as akin to a sexual assault, and it can give rise to long-term difficulties. Unless a child has had a painful examination in the past, a confident and unhurried approach will usually allow trust to develop, enabling the examiner to proceed.

The Setting

Privacy, quietness and comfort are essential to a successful examination. If there are personnel bustling in and out, other children popping up from behind privacy curtains, or the sounds of frightened or crying patients filling the air, it will be difficult to obtain a history, let alone a physical assessment.

Parents

A calm, confident parent can be a great help with some small children, but an anxious parent can ruin all the careful work of the most skilled of clinicians. The decision is a judgment call that can be best made after observing the interaction between parent and child during the interview. With teenagers, the parents should not be present, so the teen will have the opportunity to speak freely. It is important for children of any age to have some time when they are alone with the clinician. Children may disclose details of abuse that they could not discuss in front of their parents or have other concerns that they wish to discuss candidly and confidentially.

Equipment

Visualization of the upper vagina and cervix requires the use of a vaginoscope or, in teenagers, a slender speculum. These instruments in inexperienced hands can cause pain and injury. Fortunately, careful examination of the external genitalia, with gentle traction down and out on the labia, should allow excellent visualization of the introitus, hymenal ring, and lower one third of the vagina, so that instrumentation is not always needed.

Some basic equipment should be in place before the examination begins:

1. An excellent light source.
2. A hand lens or magnifying glasses.
3. A hand mirror (for the child to watch you or to distract herself).
4. Saline-moistened urethral swabs for vaginal samples.
5. Culture media.
6. A soft toy for the child to hold.

In the event that visualization is indicated, a vaginoscope, with or without a fiberoptic light source, is ideal. A nasal speculum or otoscope may be used if necessary.

In cases of genital injury, the following equipment is useful:

1. Lidocaine (Xylocaine) jelly.
2. Bags of chilled solution or compresses.
3. Warm saline for irrigation on an intravenous pole with tubing.
4. A sexual assault kit.

The physician using a sexual assault kit should be completely familiar with its contents and should know how to collect evidence that will stand up in court. The assessment for suspected child abuse is best left to a specialized team who have the skills to conduct the crucial initial history and examine a traumatized child. If such a team is not available, it is important to study the kit carefully beforehand, be gentle, and be painstakingly thorough.

The Examination

A better gynecologic assessment will be performed if it is included as part of a general examination. This allows time for the clinician to get to know the child and vice versa. Features to be noted include stage of pubertal development, endocrine status, presence of skin rashes or respiratory infections, evidence of infestations, presence of bruising, or signs of recent trauma to the kidneys or abdomen. Throughout the examination, it is important to explain what is about to be done clearly and simply.

The external genitalia can be examined most easily with the child in a "frog's leg" position. Teenagers and older girls can use lithotomy stirrups. The labia and perineum should be carefully inspected for foreign substances, trauma, or skin conditions. The vaginal orifice can be seen by gently pressing the labial pads downward and laterally or by using a light pulling motion. The child can often help, using her fingers to separate the labia. Most inexperienced observers are surprised by how bright red the tissues appear in childhood. The vaginal lining is extremely sensitive to any sort of insult and subject to minor infection and irritation. The hymen itself can be readily seen, and a hand lens or magnifying glass should help detect any breaks or trauma to this tissue. It is crucial to note even minor trauma to the hymen because it may be associated with a more significant lesion in the vagina or rectum and will necessitate further examination or, in the presence of acute trauma, examination under anesthesia. Finally, the anus should be inspected for evidence of scratching, suggesting pin worms or trauma. A patulous anus is suggestive of abuse. A careful rectal examination will enable the clinician to assess the uterus. The ovaries are abdominal structures in childhood and are not palpable under normal circumstances.

Obtaining Cultures

If cultures need to be obtained in a teenager, a speculum examination is essential to visualize the cervix and get a reliable sample. Because of the immature lining of the vagina, adequate samples can be obtained in a young girl either by collecting vaginal irrigant or by the careful use of a saline-moistened swab. A dry cotton swab should never be used on a young child because it will tear the fragile tissue.

Patient Confidentiality

There is an inevitable conflict between the patient's right to confidentiality and the parents' wish to be fully informed of all matters relevant to their child. Statutory guidelines vary as to the age at which parental consent is required and the settings in which it is mandatory. In general, when a child or minor is to be admitted to the hospital or is to undergo an operative procedure, parental consent must be obtained. The patient's right to confidentiality is also protected, and minors have an increasing right to make an informed choice and give or refuse consent according to their ability to understand the issues involved. The obligation of the physician is to ensure that the patient is fully informed and participates in the decision making to the extent of her ability. Issues of disclosure are more complex, but in general it is in the patient's best interest to protect her confidences, regardless of her age.

The circumstances of the case may have a bearing on these issues. For example, if a 15-year-old has freely chosen to become sexually active, her confidence should be protected; if she is being exploited or abused, she is in need of protection. These judgments require an extensive history. It may be necessary to involve the adolescent service or social worker with the patient to determine what will be in her best interests. The greatest obstacle to teenagers seeking medical care is their fear that their confidentiality will be violated.

In any case, you should discuss your policy with the patient at the outset and, in particular, the sort of information that you would feel obliged to report to her parents or to a child welfare agency. She then may decide whether or not to confide in you.

Genital Ambiguity

Genital ambiguity requires a coordinated and immediate response. Life-threatening illness may be missed in children with the salt-losing form of congenital adrenal hyperplasia. The family's psychological well-being must be addressed because they must feel confident in the gender identity of their child. Ambiguity can result from masculinization of a female child, exogenous hormone ingestion, or maternal or fetal overproduction of androgen. It may also result from incomplete virilization of a male infant, hormonal insensitivity, gonadal dysgenesis, or chromosomal anomalies. Some patients have associated major structural anomalies of the bladder or hindgut.

In assessing an infant with ambiguous genitals, electrolytes and fluid balance should be monitored and blood drawn for 17-hydroxyprogesterone and cortisol to rule out 21-hydroxylase deficiency. Rarer forms of adrenal hyperplasia should be considered. Buccal smears may be unreliable, so it is preferable to perform a karyotype. While awaiting results, the anatomy should be detailed, making careful identification of perineal structures and using ultrasonography to identify müllerian structures. It is also important to determine whether the genitalia are capable of responding to androgen.

The final gender assignment should take into account the function that the child may expect from his or her genitalia and the family's prior experience in the case of familial disorders, rather than the chromosomal makeup of the child. Any surgery that is required should be undertaken promptly so that the child looks congruent with the assigned gender. The exception to this is the creation of a neovagina, which is best delayed until adolescence because of the high probability of stenosis.

Trauma

Straddle injuries are the most common cause of trauma to the genitalia of a young girl and have a seasonal peak when bicycles come out in the spring. The majority of these injuries are to the labia. Penetrating vaginal injuries can cause major intra-abdominal damage, with minimal external findings. Sexual assault must always be considered.

The first step is a general assessment, including vital signs, a careful examination for evidence of trauma to other parts of the body, and an abdominal examination. If the child is frightened and in pain, it may be difficult to do a satisfactory gynecologic examination. An ice pack, chilled bag of intravenous solution, or cool compress may be applied and the child allowed to rest quietly for 20 minutes before being reassessed. To reduce the discomfort in the traumatized area, Xylocaine jelly can be applied and left in place for a few minutes to numb the perineal tissues. If the examination reveals old blood obscuring the view, a gentle stream of irrigant set up on an intravenous pole is helpful. Blood from a periurethral tear often accumulates in the vagina and may be easily confused with vaginal bleeding.

Small labial hematomas can generally be managed conservatively with ice packs and pressure dressings. Enlarging hematomas may require evacuation and ligation of bleeding vessels under general anesthesia.

Lacerations that are not deep and are not associated with any hymenal injury or vaginal bleeding can often be managed conservatively with sitz baths and simple dressings. More extensive injuries require examination under anesthesia and surgical repair.

In any case of trauma, concurrent damage to the rectum or urinary tract must be excluded. Abdominal examination and a digital rectal examination should detect gastrointestinal injury. After the genitalia have been cleansed and assessed, the child should be asked to void and kept in the emergency department until she is able to do so. An inability to void or gross hematuria are indications for further assessment. If there is any concern about disruption of the urethra, a catheter should not be passed because this may exacerbate the injury. Urologic consultation should be requested.

If there is any reason to suspect sexual abuse, the child protection authorities must be notified, and the examination should include the collection of medicolegal evidence. Collection of evidence is not, in itself, adequate justification to subject a child to the further risk of general anesthesia.

Vulvovaginitis

The most common complaint encountered among children is of irritation of the vulva, vagina, or both. They may present with discomfort or malodor or less frequently with a vaginal discharge. The prepubertal genital epithelium is vulnerable to nonspecific irritants and, with childhood hygiene being prone to lapses, is at risk from both gastrointestinal and skin organisms. The activities of childhood contribute, with sandboxes; tight, damp clothing; and touching or scratching playing a role. Once irritation is present, the complaint is perpetuated by the itch-scratch cycle. In some children, the touching may give rise to a pleasurable sensation, and in this way vulvitis may contribute to excessive self-stimulation.

Making a Diagnosis

During the examination, note should be made of any coexisting dermatologic conditions that may be manifest in the vulvar skin. Eczema, lichen planus, psoriasis, and lichen sclerosus may present with vulvar irritation.

During the genital examination, note should be made of the child's hygiene or of findings suggestive of sexual interference. Vaginal samples should be taken for culture for gonococci and *Chlamydia*. Samples for cytology may be taken from the lateral vaginal wall and submitted for a maturation index. The cytopathologist will not be able to interpret the smear if there is a marked inflammatory process present.

If there is a frank or bloody vaginal discharge present, vaginoscopy to search for a foreign body or local lesion is indicated. Most foreign bodies are not deliberately placed but enter the vagina during play or toileting. The child will likely be unaware of the presence of the foreign body, and the history is seldom helpful. The most likely foreign body is a fragment of toilet tissue, and this may be flushed from the vagina with a pediatric feeding tube and a gentle stream of saline. Metallic objects may "chink" against a metallic probe. Plastic objects can be more troublesome to identify. Attention should be paid to the fornices and to the suprapubic area, where a small foreign body may lodge.

Microbiology

The most frequent culture report is of nonspecific organisms or of coliform contaminants. Poor hygiene contributes to the incidence of enteric organisms that may be cultured in young girls, and many cases are asymptomatic. Urinary infections are frequently followed by contamination of the adjacent vagina. The pooling of small amounts of urine in the vagina (urinary vaginosis) can cause a malodor and mixed growth on culture. Respiratory pathogens may be found, particularly when vaginitis follows a cold or sore throat. Candidiasis is uncommon in the prepubertal child and, if not in response to antibiotic treatment, should prompt a screen for glycosuria.

Sexually transmitted organisms must be reported to child welfare authorities. Gonorrhea and *Chlamydia* infection are considered sexually transmitted. *Gardnerella* and *Trichomonas* infections are suspicious and require further assessment. Condylomata accuminata are increasingly reported in children and may present as genital warts or with bleeding. In infancy they have a lush, proliferative appearance rather than the dry, wart-like appearance seen in older patients. They may be transmitted perinatally, particularly if present in infancy, but sexual abuse must be excluded. Herpes genitalis may present with painful ulcers over the vulva. Sexual abuse must be considered and excluded. Typing the virus may be very helpful in cases in which the parent(s) suffers herpes type I to exclude the possibility of inadvertent contact during routine care.

Pinworm infestations are suggested by nocturnal itchiness and can be diagnosed by testing the anal margin with cellophane tape at night.

Management

Symptomatic and local measures to lessen the irritation and break the itch-scratch cycle are the starting point for vulvovaginitis. Correct wiping after toileting to avoid dragging contaminated paper across the vagina is basic advice. Urinary vaginosis is common in girls after toilet training. Their bottoms are not supported by the adult toilet seat so the vagina is dependent and susceptible to urine trickling in. A forward tilting posture on the toilet should correct this; fresh water rinses will also help.

Although many parents have been advised to go to great lengths to avoid contact irritants, these are probably only a factor in patients with sensitive skin or an atopic tendency. Excessive bathing or soaking, particularly in baking soda or vinegar, may exacerbate the problem by dehydrating the skin. Drying is also a problem in cold climates during the winter months, and skin hydration with bath emollients may be indicated. Sitz baths two to three times daily, night baths with colloidal oatmeal, and frequent changes of cotton underwear should be employed to reduce symptoms.

When the child is comfortable, routine bathing and adequate hygiene are all that is needed. Excessive attention to the genitals is not in anyone's best interest because it may give the child the feeling that she is "bad" or "dirty."

Approximately half the children who have vulvovaginitis will have it recurrently, and there are no good predictors of those who will experience recurrence. Parents need to be able to take a matter-of-fact helpful approach to the problem and should not be made to feel that they have neglected their daughter's hygiene.

Additional Measures

Topical estrogens have been advocated for nonspecific vulvovaginitis. Although a short course is unlikely to do harm, there is no sound evidence for or against this approach. Treatment with antibiotics should ideally be restricted to cases in which a specific pathogen has been identified. A short course of topical steroids may be useful to break the itch-scratch cycle.

Sexually Transmitted Infections

The treatment of sexually transmitted infections should follow public health guidelines. Because of the unestrogenized state of the genital tract, young children seem to be spared the risk of pelvic inflammatory disease and the complications that go with it.

Physiologic Leukorrhea

In peripubertal girls, a complaint of vaginal discharge is most likely physiologic. Unfortu-

nately, unopposed estrogen may cause a profuse leukorrhea that hardly seems benign to the patient. The use of impervious moisture shields, rather than pads to draw the moisture away from the body, may exacerbate the problem by causing local chafing or by setting up an environment conducive to secondary infection. Infection should be ruled out by culture, and cytology from the lateral vaginal wall should confirm the hormonal nature of the discharge.

Lichen Sclerosus

Lichen sclerosus may present with itchiness, discomfort, or even vulvar bleeding and fissuring. The vulva has a white, parchment-like appearance about the clitoral hood. The skin changes frequently occur in an hourglass configuration around the introitus and anal margin.

Symptomatic treatment is recommended, with good attention to hygiene and avoidance of dehydration of the skin through excessive bathing or harsh, defatting detergents. Topical steroids provide acute relief, but prolonged use may lead to atrophic changes. Topical progesterone has been used in this condition, although clinical data on its efficacy are lacking. Topical testosterone is to be avoided because of the potential for stimulation of the clitoris and masculinization.

Nonpatent Vagina

A variety of conditions may be referred because the parent or attending physician is unable to identify a vaginal opening. Fortunately, the majority are readily corrected, since vaginal agenesis is quite rare, occurring approximately once in every 5000 female births.

Labial Agglutination

Agglutination of the labia occurs frequently in the unestrogenized child. The etiology is presumed to be related to the presence of minor irritation, infection, or trauma to the skin, resulting in a fibrous tissue connection. Squamous epithelial cells in contiguity grow together, forming a thin bridge. The linear paper-thin junction between the two labia can be easily identified by gently shifting the labia from side to side. The process usually begins at the fourchette and may extend up to the clitoris. A pinpoint opening may be all that can be seen to allow for the escape of urine.

As long as the child is able to void, this condition is generally symptom free, and the presenting complaint is likely to be confusion with vaginal agenesis. If untreated, it usually resolves spontaneously with the rising hormone levels of puberty. Successful treatment can be very easily achieved with the application of estrogen cream to the line of agglutination nightly for 2 weeks. Medication should be applied in conjunction with a program of vulvar care. A nightly bath with an emollient is recommended for hygiene and skin hydration. After completing the course of estrogen cream, a barrier cream or petroleum jelly should be applied nightly for a further 2 weeks.

Recurrences may be expected in successfully treated patients. This is not an indication for a surgical separation but simply to repeat the medical course and re-emphasize the importance of hygiene and vulvar care. Forcible separation is not recommended because it may lead to the formation of scar tissue that will not be hormonally responsive.

Imperforate Hymen

There are a wide variety of configurations to the normal hymen. An imperforate hymen can be detected in the newborn infant on clinical examination or by the observation of a mucocolpos. If undetected in early infancy, the condition will remain unapparent until puberty, when it may present with hematocolpos and hematometros.

Diagnosis

It is important to distinguish between an imperforate hymen and other vaginal anomalies. The membrane should be thin and translucent and bulge with abdominal pressure. A mucocolpos will have a white appearance and a hematocolpos a dark color from the altered blood behind the hymen. If doubt remains, a rectal examination should define the upper margin. Vaginal cysts may be confused with a mucocolpos in infancy, but it is possible to introduce a fine urinary catheter into the vagina beside the cyst. To diagnose a *microperforate hymen,* a magnifying glass and a fine-gauge urinary catheter are extremely useful. It may be necessary to have an assistant place gentle traction on the labia to get adequate visualization. Pelvic ultrasonography can confirm the diagnosis. Needle aspiration should never be performed as a diagnostic maneuver on a hematocolpos except in the operating room immediately before the definitive procedure. Needle aspiration allows for the passage of bacteria, which will flourish in the entrapped blood and may cause severe pelvic infection.

Treatment

The optimal time to excise the membrane is when the tissues are estrogenized, either in the newborn period or at the time of thelarche. A general anesthetic is required, and treatment, once initiated, must be definitive. In the newborn, the central membrane is simply excised. In the peripubertal child, a wedge can be excised or a cruciate incision made and the four corners excised. If the tissues have been distended by a hematocolpos, it is important to excise widely, being careful of the urethra, because postoperative stenosis may otherwise be problematic.

Vaginal Septa

Vaginal septa occur in myriad forms. Transverse septa may be relatively thin or may be thick and involve the entire vagina including the cervix. It is imperative that the extent of the septum be well defined preoperatively; that the excision be done with care to avoid trauma to urethra, bladder, or bowel; and that it be wide enough to avoid a thick and unyielding vaginal ridge. The vaginal epithelium above and below the septum should be brought together to avoid postoperative stenosis and scarring.

Longitudinal septa are often found in conjunction with a duplex upper reproductive tract and may be entirely asymptomatic. If they are not causing difficulties with sexual function, they can be left alone. Problems occur if the septum is concealing a blind-ending vagina, creating a hemi-hematocolpos. Such a septum must be widely excised from below.

Vaginal Agenesis

Vaginal agenesis (Mayer-Rokitansky-Küster-Hauser syndrome) is not uncommon and presents in adolescence with amenorrhea in a young woman who has otherwise had normal pubertal growth and development. Pelvic ultrasonography will identify the ovaries, which may be lateral and superior to their usual location. A condensation of tissue may be seen in the region of the broad ligament and is sometimes described as a hypoplastic uterus. If the patient is well estrogenized, a functional uterus should be evident as a hematometros. Laparoscopy is not ordinarily indicated.

Complete androgen insensitivity can also present as vaginal agenesis and must be correctly diagnosed because of the risk of gonadoblastoma in the undescended gonad. Chromosomal analysis is the definitive investigation. Serum testosterone, luteinizing hormone, and follicle-stimulating hormone are elevated in these women.

Management

If the woman has an XY chromosome complement, gonadectomy must be carried out. There is considerable debate about the information that should be conveyed to the young woman and her family regarding her diagnosis. It has been the recommendation in the past that the chromosomal diagnosis be withheld because of the risk of psychic trauma. If this course is chosen, it is important not to give false information but to be selective in what is said. Direct questions should always be answered, and the parents should not be given information to conceal from the patient. Women with a well-established self-identity can often accept full knowledge of their diagnosis without threat, but this is much less likely to be true of a teenager. It is helpful to remember that the chromosomal definition of gender is a relatively recent development and has nothing to do with how we would otherwise attribute gender, that is, by appearance, behavior, and self-identity. The risk of withholding information is greater today, with the more ready access so many patients or their parents have to medical information.

Patients with vaginal agenesis will require gynecologic intervention to create a neovagina. Dilatation and surgical approaches are both in current practice. Referral to an experienced clinician is desirable.

Vaginal Bleeding in the Prepubertal Child

Vaginal bleeding is a frequent and distressing complaint in childhood. Although it will most often be of benign etiology, more serious pathology must always be ruled out.

Vaginal bleeding in the newborn is most often *physiologic* as a result of maternal estrogen withdrawal. In such cases, there should be supportive evidence of a hormonal effect such as the presence of breast tissue and pale engorged vaginal mucosa. *Bleeding disorders* are uncommon in this age group but should be considered. Vitamin K is routinely given to the newborn, but it is worth ensuring that the parents did not refuse the treatment.

Precocious puberty may present with vaginal bleeding, although most commonly other evidence of maturation will have preceded the bleeding and will be evident on examination. At the very least, a pale estrogenized vaginal mucosa will be seen, and cytology from the vagina will confirm the hormonal effect. Transient precocious puberty may occur in response to a functional ovarian cyst, and vaginal bleeding may be triggered by the spontaneous resolution of the cyst. Exogenous hormone exposure should be considered because children have been known to ingest birth control pills. Ovarian tumors causing pseudoprecocious puberty should be ruled out.

Vulvovaginitis is common but is a diagnosis of exclusion. When bleeding is present, it is necessary to assess the vagina and rule out a foreign body or vaginal tumor.

Vaginal tumors are the most serious possibility to be considered; sarcoma botryoides classically presents with vaginal bleeding and has an appearance of grape-like vesicles. Fortunately, this is a rare tumor.

It is important to ensure that the bleeding is originating in the vagina. *Cystitis* may cause bleeding but is usually associated with frequency and dysuria. *Urethral prolapse* is not uncommon in young girls aged 4 to 6. The bright red tender mass may be mistaken for a traumatized hymen or for a tumor. Many masses respond to sitz baths and topical estrogen, but others persist and require surgical management. Vulvar disturbances may cause bleeding. Particularly common is *lichen sclerosus,* which can cause fissures and bleeding in the genital skin. Finally, trauma or child abuse must always be considered.

Peripubertal Menstrual Disturbances

Menstrual disorders are common in adolescence, and excessive bleeding is a common presentation in emergency departments.

Menarche, the first menstrual flow, is almost always the shedding of an endometrium stimulated by rising levels of estrogen throughout puberty, without ovulation. The first several cycles may likewise be anovulatory. Until the feedback pathways are well established, teenagers are likely to fail to ovulate occasionally and return to an irregular pattern even after many apparently regular menses. Other causes of excessive, irregular, or acyclic bleeding that must always be considered are bleeding disorders, pregnancy, infections, metabolic conditions, and neoplastic conditions.

The initial history should include inquiry regarding age of menarche, menstrual pattern to date, faintness or syncopal episodes, abnormal bleeding or bruising, sexual activity, weight change, energy and activity level, and sleep patterns.

Investigations

The primary laboratory investigation is a complete blood count. A hemoglobin determination is not sufficient because both the white count and the platelet count are needed to rule out blood dyscrasias. Prothrombin time, partial thromboplastin time, and bleeding times are reasonable tests for any patient whose complaint is sufficiently severe to bring her to an emergency department.

Bleeding may occur in any early pregnancy but is a warning sign for either ectopic pregnancy or spontaneous abortion. A sensitive urinary pregnancy test or screening serum β human chorionic gonadotropin should be routinely ordered.

Acyclic bleeding may indicate an underlying malignancy. Leukemia and idiopathic thrombocytopenic purpura may present with dysfunctional bleeding. Cervical or endometrial cancer may rarely occur in young age groups; a prolonged history of menstrual irregularity, intermenstrual bleeding, or early age at first sexual exposure are risk factors that should lead to suspicion.

Metabolic causes of dysfunctional bleeding that may be encountered in adolescence include diabetes mellitus and hyperthyroidism or hypothyroidism. A urine dipstick for glucose and screening thyroid function studies are reasonable in an adolescent with a history of dysfunctional bleeding. Prolactinemia may be associated with oligomenorrhea or amenorrhea.

Management

Prolonged Bleeding. The typical presentation is for a young teen to come in with a history of bleeding of several weeks duration that is at times heavy and at other times just spotting but never stops completely. Her cycle up to that time may or may not have been regular. Because of the indolent course, she is usually hemodynamically stable, although she may be quite anemic. If investigation fails to reveal any specific cause, outpatient management may be recommended in a reliable patient using monophasic combination oral contraceptives such as Min-Ovral, Ovral, or Ovral 1/35 tablets, assuming there is no contraindication to their use. These should be given with instructions to take two every 6 hours until bleeding is controlled, then one daily until the packet is finished. Antinauseants may be needed, either in suppository or transdermal form. The patient should be warned to expect a heavy

Table 44–1. OBSTACLES AND STRATEGIES FOR CONTRACEPTION FOR TEENAGERS

OBSTACLE	STRATEGY
Acknowledgment of sexuality	Initiate frank discussion
Fear of reporting to parents	Assurance of confidentiality
Fear of side effects	Informative discussion, accessibility
Ambivalence toward sexuality	Stress non-contraceptive benefits
Cost	Consider in counseling
Use failure of birth control method	Have backup plans
Inappropriate discontinuation	Encourage dialogue before any changes or discontinuation

flow at the end of the pack and instructed to start a new package, one pill daily, after 1 week. A follow-up appointment should be made in 2 to 3 weeks for ongoing supervision.

Heavy Flow. The presentation in these cases is more dramatic, with the onset of heavy vaginal flow with the passage of clots and frequently accompanying syncope or faintness. It is particularly important to exclude bleeding disorders and pregnancy complications in these cases. Although some may be managed as outpatients, if there are any signs of hemodynamic instability, the hemoglobin is less than 90 gm/L, or she is saturating a pad in less than an hour, admission for control of blood loss is indicated. Management includes fluid replacement and hormonal control of bleeding, either with combination contraceptive tablets, two every 4 hours, or with intravenous Premarin, 25 mg every 4 hours. Bleeding should be controlled within 24 to 36 hours. If bleeding is persistent, an examination under anesthesia and dilatation and curettage may be necessary to rule out organic pathology.

BIRTH CONTROL COUNSELING IN ADOLESCENCE

Unplanned pregnancy remains one of the principal concerns for teenaged women, in spite of the availability of effective contraceptive technology (Table 44–1). Teens tend to delay contraceptive use for several months after the onset of sexual activity, and younger teens are likely to delay longer than older girls. Risk taking is commonplace in adolescence, in large part from a sense of invincibility.

Ambivalence toward their sexuality compounds the difficulty an adolescent may have in acknowledging that he or she is likely to be sexually active and ought to be using some form of birth control. The most commonly cited reason for not using birth control is that intercourse was not "planned." The fear that planning may take away the romance or cause a loss of reputation can have tragic consequences. It is worth ensuring that the patient has had a chance to consider whether she is choosing to become sexually active or whether she feels she has no choice. Young girls may feel that they have to have intercourse to hold onto a boyfriend, even though it goes against their wishes. Nonjudgmental counseling, emphasizing their right and power to say "no," is quite appropriate in these situations.

Fear that their parents may be informed causes many teens to take unnecessary chances. An assurance of confidentiality is essential. If the parents can be supportive of their teenager's decision to use birth control, it is a great aid to compliance. Few parents would want their young teens to be sexually active, but given the alternative of unprotected intercourse they may accept that their child should at least be safe. Physicians who do not think that they can provide birth control to an adolescent, whether because of their own beliefs or the conflict they might feel if the parent is a patient, should make an expedient referral to an appropriate source.

Any teenager starting to use a birth control method needs careful counseling to ensure that he or she can afford it, knows how to use it, knows how to deal with any errors in use, and has had his or her questions about mode of action and possible side effects answered. Teenagers should feel that the choices with respect to method have been theirs. They need an alternate method in the event of a slip-up and ideally should have both birth control and protection from sexually transmitted disease. More than anything else, a teenager needs support and ready access to the physician or nurse.

The objective for the physician should be to reduce, as much as possible, the incidence of unwanted pregnancy. Teenaged pregnancy per se is a more complex sociocultural phenomenon and beyond the scope of this chapter.

SUGGESTED READING

Berzonsky MD: Adolescent research, a life span developmental perspective. Human Devel 23:213, 1983.

Blake J: Gynecologic emergencies. In Fallis JC (ed): Pediatric Emergencies: Surgical Management. Philadelphia, BC Decker, 1991, p 162.

Blake J: Vulvovaginitis—a common but stressful complaint. Pediatr Med 2:101, 1987.

Emans SJH, Goldstein DP (eds): Pediatric and Adolescent Gynecology. 3rd ed. Boston, Little, Brown, 1990.

Jones HW, Rock JA: Reparative and Constructive Surgery of the Female Generative Tract. Baltimore, Williams & Wilkins, 1983.

Lavery JP, Sanfilippo JS: Pediatric and Adolescent Obstetrics and Gynecology. New York, Springer-Verlag, 1985.

1988 Canadian Guidelines for the Treatment of Sexually Transmitted Diseases in Neonates, Children, Adolescents and Adults. Canada Diseases Weekly Report, Health and Welfare Canada, vol 14S2, 1988.

Rapp CE: The adolescent patient. Ann Intern Med 99:52, 1983.

Redmond CA, Cowell CA, Krafchik BR: Genital lichen sclerosus in prepubertal girls. Adolesc Pediatr Gynecol 1:177, 1988.

Sanfilippo JS, Wakim NG: Bleeding and vulvovaginitis in the pediatric age group. Clin Obstet Gynecol 30(3):653, 1987.

Zelnik M, Shah FK: First intercourse among young Americans. Fam Plan Perspect 15:64, 1983.

Forty-five

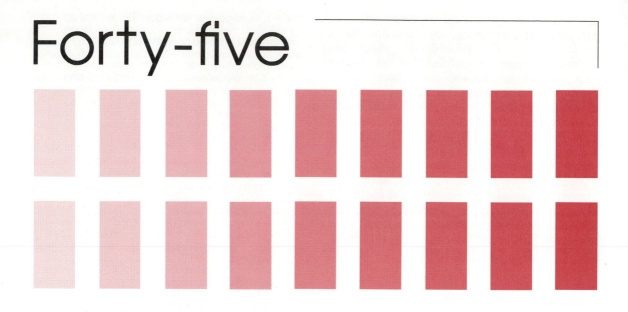

Sexual Assault

ANTHONY E. READING and J. ROBERT BRAGONIER

Rape is the fastest-growing violent crime in the United States, with one woman in six likely to be raped in her lifetime. A large random sample of women living in San Francisco found 24 per cent had experienced rape, whereas a national survey of female university students reported 54 per cent had experienced some form of unwanted sexual contact and 27 per cent rape or attempted rape. Such figures are undoubtedly underestimates, since many women fail to report their experience. In this chapter, the gynecologic management of cases of sexual assault is discussed.

The medical management of sexual assault cannot be discussed without recognizing the broader social and moral context. In the past, rape was considered to be a sexual experience, and a stigma was attached to the victim. Modern society is increasingly recognizing rape as a violent attack that may or may not stem from the perpetrator's sexual drive

or arousal. Research has shown many rapists to be sexually incompetent in the rape setting. Whatever the male intent, rape is definitely not a sexual experience for the victim. During the assault, the victim's predominant feeling is a fear of death or mutilation.

PSYCHOLOGICAL SEQUELAE OF SEXUAL ASSAULT

Sexual assault is associated with both immediate and long-term effects on all victims. These effects have been termed the *rape trauma syndrome.* Immediately after the experience, victims frequently appear outwardly calm, although preoccupied and inattentive. As they become more comfortable with the medical personnel, they commonly express shock, disbelief, fear, guilt, and shame. The long-term sequelae include changes in life-

Table 45-1. DIAGNOSTIC CRITERIA FOR POST-TRAUMATIC STRESS DISORDER

Existence of a recognizable stressor that would evoke symptoms of distress in almost everyone

Re-experiencing the trauma, as evidenced by at least one of the following:
  Recurrent and intrusive recollections of the event
  Recurrent dreams of the event
  Suddenly acting or feeling as if the traumatic event were recurring because of an association with an environmental or ideational stimulus

Numbing of responsiveness to or reduced involvement with the external world, beginning some time after the trauma, as shown by at least one of the following:
  Markedly diminished interest in one or more significant activities
  Feeling of detachment or estrangement from others
  Constricted affect

At least two of the following symptoms that were not present before the trauma:
  Hyperalertness or exaggerated startle response
  Sleep disturbance
  Guilt about surviving when others have not or about behavior required for survival
  Memory impairment or trouble concentrating
  Avoidance of activities that arouse recollection of the traumatic event
  Intensification of symptoms by exposure to events that symbolize or resemble the traumatic event

Reprinted with permission from the American Psychiatric Association Committee on Nomenclature and Statistics, Diagnostic and Statistical Manual of Mental Disorders. 3rd ed. Washington, DC, American Psychiatric Association, 1980.

style, the occurrence of disturbing dreams and nightmares, and the persistence of phobic reactions. Fear persists as the predominant feeling. These reactions often make it difficult for the victim to concentrate effectively on everyday activities and relationships.

The management of the rape victim in the acute phase influences longer term adjustment. Many rape victims may manifest a *post-traumatic stress disorder,* the diagnostic criteria for which are shown in Table 45-1. The likelihood of this disorder developing is high, owing to the abrupt nature of the crime, its violence, the passivity and helplessness imposed on the victim, and the high probability of physical as well as psychological trauma ensuing.

THE MEDICAL CARE PROCESS

The medical consultation should proceed only after a supportive, caring relationship has been established. Some victims have a need to ventilate their feelings, and it is important to provide sufficient opportunity for them to do this. The woman should be actively involved in the consultation so she may regain a feeling of control over what is happening to her. The purposes of the consultation should be explained, and she should be allowed to dictate the pace of the questioning and the order of the examination.

Medical History

In taking the victim's history, questions regarding the assault should be confined to those necessary to determine the need for any acute medical care and to direct the examination toward the appropriate collection of evidence. Prefacing questions with remarks that certain acts are not uncommon may avoid embarrassment and humiliation. Facts to be determined in the medical history of a rape victim are listed in Table 45-2.

Physical Examination

Separate informed consents must be obtained for examination and collection of evidence. During these procedures, it is important to be gentle and to explain the purpose of everything that is being performed. Steps to be observed in the examination are listed in Table 45-3.

TREATMENT

Medical Treatment

All injuries should be appropriately treated. Tetanus toxoid should be given if injuries are present and no toxoid has been received in the past 10 years. Prophylactic treatment for sexually transmitted diseases should be of-

Table 45-2. HISTORY REQUIRED OF A RAPE VICTIM

Date and time of the assault; date and time of the present examination
Physical surroundings and circumstances in which the assault occurred
Nature of the assault and any associated pain experienced
Weapons or foreign objects used and where they were used
The number of assailants
Any acts that were committed, such as coitus, fellatio, cunnilingus, sodomy
Whether or not ejaculation occurred and where; whether or not a condom was used
Whether or not there was vomiting or loss of consciousness
Whether or not the patient washed, wiped, bathed, douched, defecated, brushed her teeth or changed her clothes after the assault
Use of drugs, alcohol, or medications in proximity to the time of the assault; current medication history
Allergies
Date of last tetanus immunization
Date and time of last consensual intercourse
Gravity, parity, and menstrual history
Contraceptive history
General past medical history, as indicated

fered; many facilities provide this routinely. Current recommendations are that 4.8 million units of procaine penicillin be administered intramuscularly, following 1 gm of probenecid orally. If the oral route is preferred, ampicillin, 3.5 gm immediately (given with 1 gm of probenecid), followed by tetracycline, 0.5 gm four times a day for 7 days, is effective treatment for incubating syphilis, gonorrhea, and *Chlamydia* infection. For penicillin-allergic patients, tetracycline, 0.5 gm four times a day for 7 days, may be prescribed orally.

If the possibility of pregnancy is likely, alternatives should be discussed, including continuation, first-trimester induced abortion if pregnancy ensues, or postcoital drug contraception.

Psychological Management at the Initial Evaluation

In addition to attending to immediate physical and emotional needs, the initial evaluation provides an opportunity to pre-

pare the victim for the longer term psychological impact of the experience. This preparation is intended to diminish the long-term consequences and to enable the woman to recognize the common psychosocial sequelae when they occur, thus enabling her to seek professional help at an early stage.

The psychological problems that may result are varied and may mimic those seen in the aftermath of other kinds of traumatic experiences. Among those expected in the acute phase of adjustment are irritability, tension, anxiety, depression, fatigue, and persistent ruminations. Somatic symptoms of a general nature may occur, such as headaches or irritable bowel syndrome, or symptoms may be more specific to the reproductive system, such as vaginal irritation or discharge. Behavioral problems may also surface, particularly when these have been evident in the past, such as overeating and alcohol or substance abuse.

Stimuli associated with the rape, such as a similar-looking man or similar surroundings,

Table 45-3. PHYSICAL EXAMINATION OF A RAPE VICTIM AND COLLECTION OF EVIDENCE

Note and record vital signs
Examine clothing and skin for loose hair, stains, or other debris, and collect as evidence
Inspect fingernails and preserve cleanings
Collect clothing
Comb pubic hair for loose strands and save
Clip and label samples of head and pubic hair for comparison with any loose strands found
Perform and record general physical examination, as indicated, with special attention to evidence of trauma
Carefully inspect the external genitalia for lacerations, abrasions, ecchymoses, or hematomas; give special attention to the posterior fourchette
Gently insert a warmed speculum and carefully inspect for evidence of trauma
Prepare a gonococcal culture and appropriate smears for the detection of spermatozoa
Obtain similar cultures and smears from the throat and anus, as indicated
Collect baseline blood specimens for grouping, syphilis serology, pregnancy testing, and drug or alcohol levels; a reference saliva specimen should be obtained to determine ABO secretor status of the victim
Handle all specimens so as to insure preservation and maintenance of the chain of custody

may be associated with *flashbacks*. These are common reactions and relate to the process of classic conditioning, whereby peripheral stimuli associated with an event eliciting a strong emotional response can subsequently elicit an attenuated form of that response. Research on the etiology and maintenance of fears and phobias indicates that avoidance of potentially frightening situations will only strengthen the conditioned emotional reaction and may, in some cases, lead to full-blown phobic avoidance. If the woman continues to engage in normal life experiences rather than trying to avoid such stimuli, the emotional reaction to such innocuous stimuli will extinguish over time. By introducing this principle, the gynecologist may suggest to the woman the most appropriate course of action.

Reactions to the sexual assault may result in problems with sexual behavior and functioning. Loss of libido is a common response to stressful or traumatic circumstances of any kind. Other complaints include vaginismus, impaired vaginal lubrication, and loss of orgasmic capacity. These problems may be even more likely if the assault occurred at home while asleep. Preparing the woman for these eventualities can be extremely helpful in preventing sexual dysfunctions from developing. Giving permission for a lower-than-usual sexual drive during the postassault period may remove some performance anxiety. Explaining how anxiety and stress can inhibit sexual responsiveness and providing ways in which this can be overcome are also important.

After-Care Planning

Whether or not the patient elects to have prophylaxis against sexually transmitted dis-eases or pregnancy, careful follow-up must be arranged. Tests for gonorrhea should be performed in 2 weeks and for syphilis in 6 weeks; if pregnancy is suspected, it should be confirmed or refuted. If any of these tests are positive, appropriate management should be instituted immediately.

Before discharging the patient, it is important to ensure that she has a safe place to go and a suitable means of transportation. She should also be given the names, addresses, and phone numbers in writing of resources available in the community to meet medical, legal, and psychosocial needs related to the assault.

SUGGESTED READING

American Psychiatric Association Committee on Nomenclature and Statistics: Diagnostic and Statistical Manual of Mental Disorders. 3rd ed. Washington, DC, American Psychiatric Association, 1980.

Bragonier JR, Nadelson CC: Caring for the rape victim. Interact 1:1, 1977.

Burgess AW, Holstrom LL: Rape trauma syndrome. Am J Psychiatry 131:981, 1974.

Burgess AW, Holstrom LL: Crisis and counselling requests of rape victims. Nurs Res 23:196, 1974.

Ellis L, Beattie C: The feminist explanation for rape: An empirical test. J Sex Res 19:74, 1983.

Koss MP, Gidycz CA, Wisniewski N: The scope of rape: Incidence and prevalence of sexual aggression and victimization. J Consult Clin Psychol 50:455, 1987.

Martin CA, Warfield MC, Braen ER: Physician's management of the psychological aspects of rape. JAMA 249:501, 1983.

Reading AE: The management of anxiety related to vaginal examination. J Psychosom Obstet Gynecol 1:99, 1982.

Russell DEH: Sexual exploitation. Rape, Child Sexual Abuse, and Workplace Harassment. Beverly Hills, CA, Sage, 1984.

State of California Department of Health Services: Guidelines for Treatment of Victims of Sexual Assault, 1976.

Forty-six

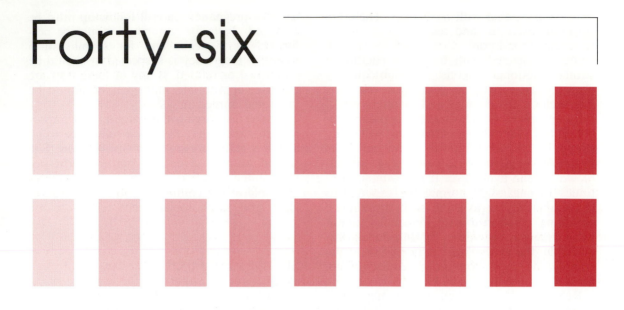

Gynecologic Operative Techniques

RONALD S. LEUCHTER, JOSEPH GAMBONE, and PHILIP G. BROOKS

It is not the purpose of this chapter to qualify the reader as a gynecologic surgeon. It is, however, essential that students and residents become familiar with the basic principles of common gynecologic surgical procedures so that they can properly assist in the operating room.

APPROPRIATENESS OF ELECTIVE GYNECOLOGIC SURGICAL PROCEDURES

At least 80 per cent of gynecologic surgical procedures are considered to be elective, that is, there are other alternative treatments to be considered. The appropriateness of performing these procedures should be evaluated by physician and patient on an individual basis.

A useful mnemonic to assess preoperatively the appropriateness of health care procedures, including elective gynecologic surgery, is *PREPARED*, where:

P   is the procedure
R   is the reason or indication
E   is the expectation
P   is the probability that the expectation will occur
A   is the alternative(s)
R   is the risk(s)
E   is the expense (hospital costs and surgeon's fees)
D   is the decision to perform or not perform the procedure

An analysis of each gynecologic procedure can be carried out and the patient counseled using this format.

DILATATION AND CURETTAGE

The most common gynecologic surgical procedure is dilatation of the cervix and curettage of the endometrium. If cancer of the cervix or endometrium is suspected, a fractional curettage should be performed. In this procedure, the endocervix is initially curetted, even before sounding the uterine depth. The cervix is then dilated and the endometrium curetted. The curettings from the endocervix and endometrium are submitted separately.

Indications

Dilatation and curettage may be a diagnostic or a therapeutic procedure. A diagnostic dilatation and curettage is performed for irregular menstrual bleeding, heavy menstrual bleeding, or postmenopausal bleeding, unless an endometrial biopsy has already revealed a diagnosis of malignancy. In patients younger than 35 years with irregular bleeding, hormone manipulation frequently obviates the need for curettage. Irregularities in the contour of the endometrial cavity, either congenital (e.g., uterine septum) or acquired (e.g., submucous myomata), are frequently determined during the operation.

The dilatation and curettage may have a therapeutic effect in patients with heavy or irregular bleeding from endometrial hyperplasia; endometrial polyps; or small, pedunculated submucous myomas. Unwanted first-trimester pregnancies are usually evacuated by dilatation and suction curettage.

Technique

The operation is performed with the patient in the dorsal lithotomy position. In the past, dilatation and curettage was considered an inpatient procedure because of the need for general anesthesia. Most curettages are now performed on an outpatient basis. Paracervical blocks and local anesthesia are frequently employed.

A repeat pelvic examination is done under anesthesia, and, after sterile preparation, a weighted speculum is placed in the posterior vagina. The cervix is grasped with a single-toothed or double-toothed tenaculum. A Kevorkian curette is used to curette the endocervical canal. The depth of the uterine cavity is determined with a uterine sound, and the cervix is then dilated with a set of graduated dilators. Dilatation to a no. 8 Hegar dilator is sufficient for a diagnostic curettage in a premenopausal patient. In postmenopausal women with increasing stenosis of the cervix, extreme caution must be exercised in the dilatation to avoid lacerating the cervix or perforating the uterus. In such patients, *Laminaria* tents or prostaglandin E_2 suppositories or gel may be inserted some hours preoperatively to enhance cervical dilatation.

A small polyp or ovum forceps is introduced through the dilated cervix and gently rotated to remove any endometrial polyps. A thorough curettage is done with a sharp curette, proceeding with each stroke in either a clockwise or counterclockwise manner to ensure that the entire uterine cavity has been covered. Particular attention must be directed to each cornu. The surgical instruments required for this procedure are shown in Fig. 46–1.

Complications

The most common surgical complications of dilatation and curettage are hemorrhage, infection, perforation of the uterus, and laceration of the cervix. Perforation of the uterus, even in experienced hands, is a common complication. As long as no bowel or large blood vessels are injured, careful observation and antibiotics may be all the therapy required. Except in an acute emergency, such as an infected incomplete abortion, no dilatation and curettage should be done in the presence of infection. Any suspicion of infection postoperatively should be vigorously treated with antibiotics. Lacerations of the cervix occurring during the operation must be repaired at the conclusion of the surgery.

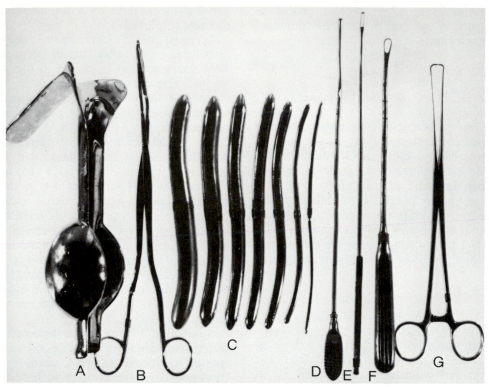

Figure 46–1. Instruments used for dilatation and curettage: *A*, weighted (Auvard) speculum; *B*, polyp forceps; *C*, Hegar dilators; *D*, uterine sound; *E*, Kevorkian curette for endocervical curettage; *F*, sharp uterine curette; and *G*, tenaculum.

CONIZATION OF THE CERVIX

Conization of the cervix is a procedure in which a cone-shaped portion of the cervix is removed for diagnostic or therapeutic purposes. The section of the tissue surrounding the external os represents the base of the removed specimen. The apex is either near or at the internal os.

Indications

Although the use of the colposcope has significantly reduced the need for cone biopsy in the evaluation of an abnormal Papanicolaou smear, diagnostic conization (Fig. 46–2A) is still required under the following circumstances: (1) if the squamocolumnar junction cannot be visualized colposcopically, (2) if the endocervical curettage is positive, (3) if there is a significant discrepancy between the Papanicolaou smear and the colposcopically directed cervical biopsy, (4) if the

cervical biopsy reveals microinvasive squamous cell carcinoma, and (5) if the cervical biopsy reveals adenocarcinoma in situ.

A therapeutic conization may be performed for extensive carcinoma in situ of the cervix, particularly in women who have completed childbearing (Fig. 46–2B). Provided that the surgical margins are free of disease, a diagnostic cone frequently becomes a therapeutic cone once lack of invasion has been established. The amount of tissue excised depends on the indications for the procedure and the extent of the disease as determined by colposcopy. On rare occasions, the surgery may be employed to eradicate an intractable chronic cervicitis.

Technique

The patient is placed in the dorsal lithotomy position, and a weighted speculum is placed in the vagina. Whenever possible, a colposcopic examination should be per-

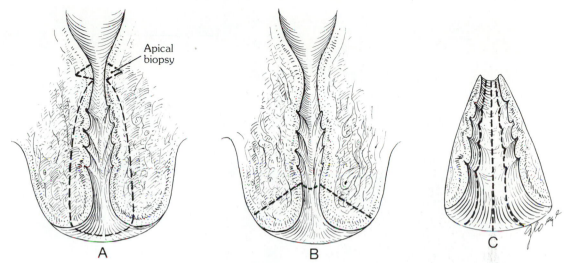

Figure 46-2. Cone biopsy of the cervix. *A*, Diagnostic conization performed when transformation zone is not fully visualized colposcopically; *B*, therapeutic conization performed for disease involving ectocervix and distal endocervical canal; and *C*, specimen opened for serial sectioning.

formed in the operating room to determine the extent of the dysplastic epithelium on the ectocervix. If colposcopy is not available in the operating room, the cervix is stained with Lugol's solution (Schiller's test). Dysplastic epithelium, which lacks glycogen, will not stain with iodine and will appear pale (Schiller-positive).

To help control bleeding from the descending branch of the uterine artery, hemostatic sutures are placed at the 3 and 9 o'clock positions. Some surgeons also inject a saline and epinephrine solution into the cervix to aid hemostasis. A circular incision is made around the external os to incorporate all of the Schiller-positive or colposcopically abnormal areas. The incision is continued into the stroma, angulating toward the canal. The apex is reached just below or at the level of the internal os. After removing the cone, biopsies are taken at the retained apex, and the procedure is completed with a dilatation and curettage. It is usually necessary to place hemostatic sutures in the anterior and posterior lips of the cervix to control bleeding.

The excised cone should be sent fresh to the pathologist. The cone is opened at 12 o'clock, pinned to a cork board, then fixed in formalin (Fig. 46-2*C*). Serial blocks are made, and several sections from each block are examined in a serial manner.

The CO_2 laser is now commonly used to perform conization of the cervix. If the cervix is adequately infiltrated with a hemostatic solution, bleeding is usually minimal. Following a laser cone biopsy, there is less risk of cervical stenosis developing, which makes it easier to evaluate the endocervical canal cytologically in the future.

Complications

The most common complication of conization of the cervix is immediate or delayed bleeding. Secondary hemorrhage, which is due to infection, occurs in about 10 per cent of patients. It usually requires antibiotics and vaginal packing but may necessitate resuturing.

HYSTEROSCOPY

With the increasing refinement of fiberoptics and instrumentation, endoscopy has become a valuable adjunct to the practice of gynecology. The hysteroscope, an instrument for viewing the endocervix and endometrial cavity, may be used for diagnosis or therapy.

Instrumentation

The telescope used for diagnostic and operative hysteroscopic procedures is the same. It

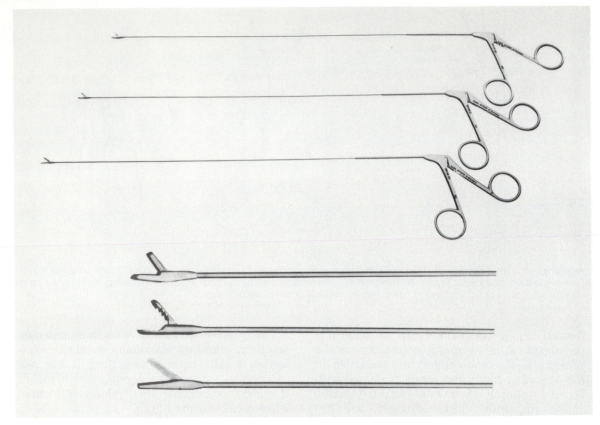

Figure 46–3. Accessory instruments for the flexible hysteroscope. *Top to bottom:* Scissors, grasping forceps, biopsy forceps. (Courtesy of Karl Storz Endoscopy America, Inc.)

has a 4-mm outer diameter and a viewing angle anywhere from 0 degrees (i.e., straight ahead) to 30 degrees (oblique angle). Angled telescopes are particularly useful because they enhance visualization of the cornual areas and the lateral walls of the lower uterine segment.

Although the outer sheaths of diagnostic hysteroscopic systems are narrower (usually 5 mm), allowing only the telescope and a small channel for the flow of a gas or fluid medium, operative sheaths must be wider to allow channels for operating instruments or laser beams. All operating hysteroscope sets include flexible or semirigid instruments such as scissors, grasping forceps, and biopsy punches (Fig. 46–3), which are inserted into a separate channel and are manipulated independently from the locked-together telescope and sheath. Some sheaths have a mechanical deflector (albarans bridge) (Fig. 46–4) to assist in directing the accessory instrument toward an off-center target.

When a stronger accessory instrument (scissors, biopsy punch) (Fig. 46–5) is needed, an outer sheath with the instrument welded to it is available. This rigid instrument has the main advantage of allowing the operator to exert more force, as when incising a thick intrauterine septum. Disadvantages include a reduction in the field of vision and the need to move the telescope, sheath, and operating instrument in unison.

The newest of operative hysteroscopy systems is the gynecologic resectoscope (Fig. 46–6). Adapted from the time-proved urologic resectoscope, this instrument uses wire loop or roller-ball electrodes and electrical energy to excise, shave, or coagulate intrauterine lesions. It should be noted that the gynecologic resectoscope is a continuous-flow device, designed to use low-viscosity liquid distention media that continually rinse blood and debris while allowing constant uterine distention.

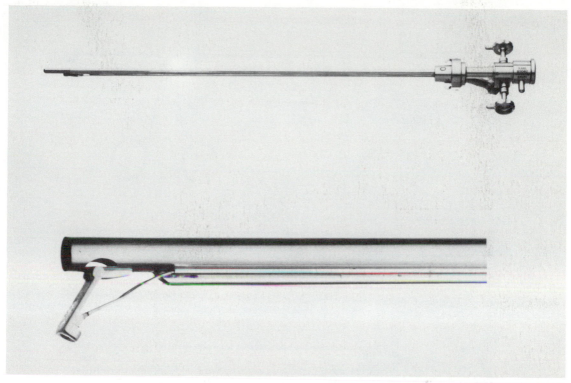

Figure 46–4. *Top:* Hysteroscopy instrument deflector (Albarans Bridge). *Bottom:* Close-up of tip with deflector extended. (Courtesy of Karl Storz Endoscopy America, Inc.)

Distention Medium

Most diagnostic hysteroscopy is performed using carbon dioxide for uterine distention. Some simple operative procedures can also be performed with CO_2 as the distention medium, but bleeding that may result during longer procedures markedly limits the use of CO_2. Intrauterine electrosurgical procedures similarly are unsuccessful because of the excessive smoke produced if used in the presence of gas.

Dextran-70 (Hyskon) is the most frequently used distention medium for operative procedures because it provides good distention and is not miscible with blood. Disadvantages of dextran-70 are its viscosity and stickiness, requiring immediate rinsing of the instruments to prevent deterioration, and its potential for serious allergic reactions including ascites and anaphylactic-like events.

Low-viscosity, nonelectrolytic liquids, such as sorbitol or glycine, are becoming favorites as distention media for continuous-flow procedures, such as resectoscopic ablations and resections. Their miscibility with blood requires continual rinsing for adequate visualization.

Diagnostic Hysteroscopy

Diagnostic indications for hysteroscopy may include primary and secondary infertility, habitual spontaneous abortion, abnormal uterine bleeding, lost intrauterine device, or suspected intrauterine abnormalities. The hysteroscope has also been used to determine the extent of cervical or endometrial malignancies. Biopsies may be obtained by the hysteroscope, and hysteroscopic biopsy is more accurate than random biopsy or blind curettage.

Operative Hysteroscopy

The most significant success for operative hysteroscopy has been in the treatment of infertility or reproductive wastage due to intrauterine abnormalities. The lysis of intra-

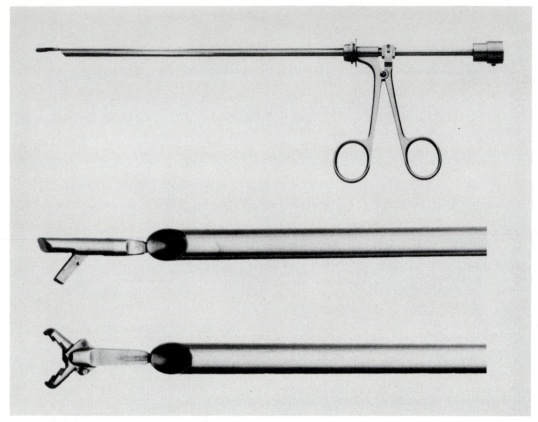

Figure 46–5. *Top:* Rigid hysteroscopy instrument. *Bottom:* Close-ups of tips of rigid scissors and grasping forceps. (Courtesy of Karl Storz Endoscopy America, Inc.)

uterine adhesions, from the thin filmy ones on up to thick, dense, and extensive synechiae, as in Asherman's syndrome, results in improvement in term pregnancy rates from less than 20 per cent before surgery to greater than 75 per cent after treatment. In most cases, these adhesions are readily incised with flexible scissors under simple outpatient conditions. When dense synechiae make the procedure more difficult and increase the risk of uterine perforation, concomitant laparoscopy is useful to help avoid this hazard.

Another highly successful hysteroscopic procedure is the incision of congenital uterine septae, known as transcervical metroplasty. This condition is usually associated with repeated mid-trimester abortion. What used to be performed transabdominally as a very traumatic and bloody procedure, inevitably requiring cesarean section for subsequent delivery, can now be successfully done with hysteroscopic scissors, either flexible or rigid.

This is a relatively short, bloodless outpatient procedure, and vaginal delivery is satisfactory for subsequent pregnancies. Because of the need to ensure that the anomaly is a septate and not a bicornuate uterus and also to prevent perforation, hysteroscopic metroplasty is always performed with laparoscopic guidance. Up to 80 per cent of patients will have a successful pregnancy following this procedure.

When large or small polyps or small pedunculated submucous myomata are associated with either infertility or abnormal uterine bleeding, hysteroscopic removal is indicated. In most cases, this can be achieved with scissors and grasping forceps. When the myoma or polyp virtually fills the endometrial cavity, however, the gynecologic resectoscope allows the neoplasm to be resected. Using a nonconductive distention medium (sorbitol, glycine, dextran-70) in a continuous-flow system and with an electric genera-

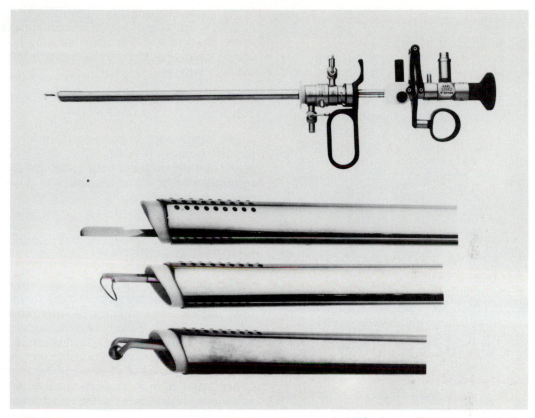

Figure 46–6. *Top:* Gynecologic resectoscope. *Bottom:* Close-up of electrodes available (electric knife, wire loop, roller-ball). (Courtesy of Karl Storz Endoscopy America, Inc.)

tor providing 60 to 120 watts of energy, the resectoscope can morcellate large myomas (up to 7 to 8 cm) or giant polyps. When no visible lesion is found for the patient with uncontrollable uterine bleeding, the endometrium can be ablated.

Abnormal bleeding is reduced in up to 95 per cent of patients following resection of myomata. Up to 65 per cent of patients will have amenorrhea and over 90 per cent amenorrhea or hypomenorrhea after an ablative procedure. These are short, low-risk, minor outpatient procedures that almost always reduce the need for hysterectomy for this benign but debilitating problem.

The Neodymium Yttrium Aluminum Garnet (Nd:YAG) laser has also been used for destruction of submucous myomata or endometrial ablation. There may be a slightly increased margin of safety with the laser, but the disadvantages are the greater expense of the procedure and the instrumentation, the

more extensive training required, and the much longer time needed to perform the procedures.

Complications

Complications of operative hysteroscopy are infrequent and can be divided into hemorrhagic (traumatic), infective, distention medium hazards, and electrical/laser tissue damage.

Traumatic-hemorrhagic problems occur from laceration of the cervix as a result of vigorous dilatation or use of the tenaculum and are usually managed by suturing the tear. Uncontrollable bleeding from uterine sinuses or raw surfaces after resections or ablations are best controlled with intrauterine tamponade using one of several kinds of balloon catheters. Perforation of the uterus is a rare occurrence during operative hysteroscopy and usually requires diagnostic laparoscopy to detect excessive intra-abdominal bleeding or trauma to adjacent organs.

Postoperative infection resulting from hysteroscopic procedures is uncommon and readily managed by oral antibiotics. It is recommended that prophylactic antibiotic coverage be provided for procedures done for infertility or when prolonged instrumentation may increase the chances of contamination.

To avoid gas embolism during CO_2 hysteroscopy, it is mandatory to use low-pressure, low-flow insufflation. Hysteroscopic insufflation is usually adequate at flow rates of 40 to 70 ml per minute (as contrasted to laparoscopic insufflation flow rates of 1 to 3 L per minute).

The use of dextran-70 for uterine distention has been associated with rare but serious problems of fluid overload (owing to its osmotic attraction for fluid when intravascular intravasation occurs) and allergic reactions. It is essential to use small amounts of this liquid medium and to monitor patients well.

Low-viscosity fluid overload also occurs but can be predicted and more easily managed if the inflow and outflow of the medium are closely monitored. When there exists a large discrepancy between the amount of fluid infused and that collected from the outflow port, prompt postoperative assessment of the patient's serum electrolytes will detect early significant changes.

The tissue effects of both electrical and laser energies are relatively similar and depend on the watts of power, the size and configuration of the electrode tip or laser spot (defined as current density or power density, respectively), and the duration of exposure in the same location. The thickness of the myometrium in most areas of the uterus affords a cushion to protect against perforation or thermal damage to adjacent organs. Caution is advised, however, when applying energy to the thinner parts (e.g., cornual areas) or where the large vessels are fairly superficial (e.g., the lateral lower uterine segment).

In 1990, an unusual complication of intrauterine laser surgery was reported and prompted a warning from the Food and Drug Administration. Laser fibers, when used with special tips (sapphire or ceramic) require the cooling of the tips with either gas (CO_2) or liquid to reduce the risk of fracturing the tips.

When gas is chosen, flow rates must be high, and CO_2 embolism has occurred in several cases, prompting a warning that only liquid-cooled fibers should be used during intrauterine laser surgery.

LAPAROSCOPY

The laparoscope is an instrument for viewing the peritoneal cavity (Fig. 46–7). Both pelvic and upper abdominal structures can be inspected. Most laparoscopies are done as outpatient procedures.

Indications and Contraindications

The indications for laparoscopy are both diagnostic and therapeutic. *Diagnostic indications* include the evaluation of infertility, pelvic pain, small pelvic masses, congenital anomalies, and a small hemoperitoneum. The most common indication for *therapeutic laparoscopy* (pelviscopy) is tubal sterilization. Other therapeutic indications include lysis of adhesions, fulguration of endometriotic implants, aspiration of small cysts, and retrieval of lost intrauterine devices. Laser technology can now be applied to operative laparoscopic procedures both to cut and to vaporize areas of pathology.

Absolute contraindications to laparoscopy include bowel obstruction and large hemoperitoneum. A relative contraindication is obesity. In patients who have had multiple previous laparotomies, a history of peritonitis, previous bowel surgery, or a lower midline abdominal incision, open laparoscopy is preferable. In this procedure, the peritoneal cavity is opened through a small subumbilical incision under direct vision prior to introduction of the trocar and sheath.

Technique

The procedure is performed in a modified dorsal lithotomy position, usually under general anesthesia. An intrauterine manipulator is inserted to help in the visualization of the pelvic organs. A pneumoperitoneum is created by inserting a spring-loaded needle, such as a Veress needle, into the peritoneal cavity

Figure 46–7. Instruments required for single puncture laparoscopy: *A*, trocar and cannula; *B*, Veress needle; and *C*, Wolf laparoscope (10 mm).

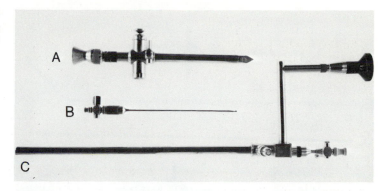

via the subumbilical fold. Proper placement of the needle is checked by disappearance of a hanging drop from the needle hub with elevation of the diaphragm or injection of 10 ml of saline and observation of its passage without resistance. The gas line is then connected, and insufflation with either carbon dioxide or nitrous oxide is begun. Between 2 and 4 L of gas are required. The trocar and surrounding sheath are then inserted through a small subumbilical incision, the trocar is withdrawn, and the valve is opened manually. A hiss of escaping gas ensures that the instrument is in the peritoneal cavity.

The lighted telescope is inserted into the sheath and advanced slowly. Visualization of pelvic organs confirms that the peritoneal cavity has been entered. Gas may be added intermittently to maintain a good pneumoperitoneum. To perform a second puncture, which is sometimes necessary, especially in laparoscopic surgical procedures, the abdominal wall is transilluminated, and a 4- or 6-mm trocar and sheath are inserted under laparoscopic guidance through a small incision at the pubic hairline. A probe or other surgical instrument (e.g., Falope ring applicator) is passed through the second sheath (Fig. 46–8).

Upon completion of the procedure, hemostasis is checked, the gas is released from the peritoneal cavity, and the instruments are withdrawn. The small skin incisions are closed with a clip or single suture.

Complications

Insufflation of the abdominal wall may occur from failure to enter the peritoneal cavity with the Veress needle. Perforation of a viscus, especially bowel, may occur at the time of insertion of the trocar and sheath. Once the instruments have been successfully introduced into the peritoneal cavity, lack of proper intraperitoneal hemostasis and coagulation burns of a viscus may occur. A poor pneumoperitoneum increases the risk of these complications.

Bowel burns during fulguration are the most serious complications of laparoscopy, although the most common complications are related to the anesthesia. Bowel burns result either from direct contact with the bowel or from a spark and are usually not detected at the time of the procedure. Several days later bowel perforation with peritonitis may occur. The increased use of bipolar instruments has diminished the occurrence of this serious complication.

In addition to the surgical complications, there is an increased risk of anesthetic complications in a patient with a pneumoperitoneum. Both surgical and anesthetic complications are frequently the result of lack of adequate experience with laparoscopy by the relevant physician.

HYSTERECTOMY

Hysterectomy, the most common major gynecologic operation and the second most common major surgical procedure, can be performed abdominally or vaginally. Before performing any hysterectomy, cervical cytology must be evaluated and, if necessary, colposcopy performed to exclude occult cervical cancer.

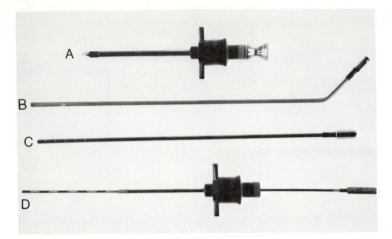

Figure 46-8. Instruments used for second puncture: *A*, 6-mm trocar; *B*, suction catheter; *C*, 6-mm probe; and *D*, 4-mm trocar with secondary probe.

There are more indications listed for hysterectomy than any other operation. A useful list of indications for abdominal or vaginal hysterectomy with criteria-sets is shown in Table 46-1.

Abdominal Hysterectomy

Total hysterectomy or panhysterectomy implies removal of both the corpus and the cervix. Subtotal hysterectomy implies preservation of the cervix. Extrafascial hysterectomy implies removal of the uterus with its outer fascial layer in toto. Intrafascial hysterectomy implies that the cervix is cored out, and the outer (endopelvic) fascial layer is left attached to the bladder. Radical hysterectomy implies removal of the parametrial tissue and uterosacral ligaments in conjunction with the corpus and cervix after dissecting each ureter from its tunnel beneath the uterine artery. Figure 46-9 demonstrates diagrammatically the differences between the various types of hysterectomy.

Indications

The indications for abdominal hysterectomy include benign diseases, such as fibroids, endometriosis, chronic pelvic inflammatory disease, and recurrent uterine bleeding that is unresponsive to conservative medical measures, or malignant diseases, such as stage I carcinoma of the endometrium, microinvasive carcinoma of the cervix,

or ovarian cancer. A total extrafascial hysterectomy should normally be performed. A subtotal hysterectomy is sometimes performed for disseminated ovarian cancer to prevent tumor growth at the vaginal vault. Intrafascial hysterectomy may occasionally be used when it is difficult to dissect the bladder from the front of the cervix, as may occur in patients who have had multiple lower segment cesarean sections. Radical hysterectomy is performed for stage Ib or IIa carcinoma of the cervix and sometimes for stage II carcinoma of the endometrium.

The question of whether to remove the ovaries depends on the individual case. Bilateral salpingo-oophorectomy is routinely performed, along with abdominal hysterectomy, in postmenopausal women. Prior to the menopause, the merits of removing normal ovaries to prevent subsequent neoplastic disease versus leaving them so that hormonal function can be maintained must be thoroughly discussed with the patient. Prior to age 45 years, the ovaries are generally preserved, unless there is a family history of ovarian cancer.

Technique

The operation is performed in the supine position, usually under general anesthesia. The type of skin incision chosen depends on the nature of the disease. In most patients with benign disease, a low transverse (Pfannenstiel's) incision can be used. In the presence of proved or suspected malignant dis-

Table 46–1. HYSTERECTOMY INDICATION LIST WITH CRITERIA

ACUTE CONDITION
A-1*   Pregnancy catastrophe (e.g., severe hemorrhage)
A-2   Severe infection (e.g., ruptured tubo-ovarian abscess)
A-3*   Operative complication (e.g., uterine perforation)

BENIGN DISEASE
B-1   Leiomyomata
       Symptomatic (e.g., bleeding, pressure)
       Asymptomatic (≥ 12 week size, confuses adnexal evaluation)
B-2   Endometriosis (distinct endometriosis, unresponsive to hormonal suppression or conservative surgery)
B-3   Adenomyosis
B-4   Chronic infection (e.g., recurrent pelvic inflammatory disease)
B-5   Adnexal mass (e.g., ovarian neoplasm)
B-6   Other (operator defined, criteria specified)

CANCER OR SIGNIFICANT PREMALIGNANT DISEASE
C-1   Invasive disease of reproductive organs
C-2   Significant preinvasive disease of the uterus (CIN-3† or adenomatous hyperplasia of the endometrium with cellular atypia)
C-3   Cancer of adjacent or distant organ (gastrointestinal, genitourinary, or breast cancer)

DISCOMFORT (NO TISSUE PATHOLOGY EXPECTED)
D-1*   Chronic pelvic pain (negative laparoscopy and nonsurgical treatment attempted)
D-2*   Pelvic relaxation (symptomatic)
D-3*   Recurrent uterine bleeding (unresponsive to hormone regulation and curettage—normal size uterus)
D-4*   Other (operator defined, criteria specified)

EXTENUATING CIRCUMSTANCES
(not specifically indicated but possibly justified—requires preoperative peer review)
E-1*   Sterilization (extenuating circumstances)
E-2*   Cancer prophylaxis (e.g., recurrent CIN-2 after cone biopsy or persistent adenomatous hyperplasia of the endometrium without atypia)
E-3*   Other—listing extenuating circumstances

* Denotes indications where tissue pathology is not expected to confirm the preoperative diagnosis.
† CIN = cervical intraepithelial neoplasia.
Modified from Gambone JC, Lench JB, Slesinski MJ, et al: Obstet Gynecol 73:1045, 1989. By permission of The American College of Obstetricians and Gynecologists.

ease of the uterus or ovaries, however, or in cases in which potential complications are anticipated, such as in very obese patients or in those who have had previous surgeries or pelvic inflammatory disease, a vertical lower abdominal incision provides better exposure. The various lower abdominal incisions are discussed in Chapter 1.

After evaluating the upper abdomen, the abdominal contents are packed out of the pelvis, and the patient is placed in a modified Trendelenburg position. The round ligaments are clamped, cut, and tied (Fig. 46–10*A*). This allows entrance between the leaves of the broad ligament, exposing the retroperitoneal space so that the ureter and pelvic vessels can be identified (Fig. 46–10*B*). The vesicouterine fold of peritoneum is incised, and the bladder is dissected from the front of the uterus and cervix. If the ovaries are to be removed, each infundibulopelvic ligament is clamped and doubly tied once the ureters have been identified. If the ovaries are to be left behind, each utero-ovarian pedicle, as it attaches to the uterus, is clamped, cut, and tied. The posterior peritoneum between the rectum and the cervix is incised, thereby moving the ureters further down into the pelvis. The uterine vessels are isolated as they come up the side of the uterus at the level of the internal os; they are clamped and doubly tied. The cardinal and uterosacral ligaments are taken down sequentially as they attach to the lateral and posterolateral aspect of the

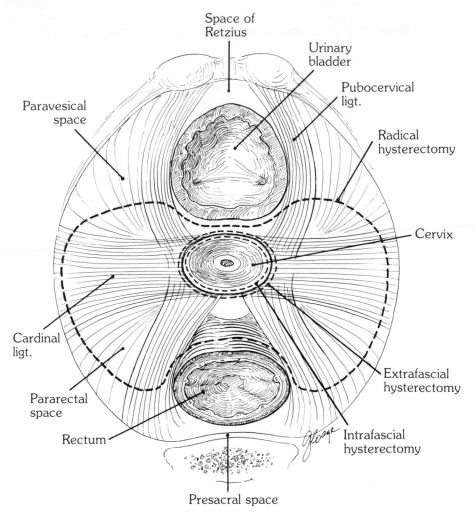

Figure 46-9. Types of hysterectomy: extrafascial, intrafascial, and radical. Note the extensive amount of parametrial tissue that is removed in a radical hysterectomy.

uterus (Fig. 46–10C). This is continued until the cervicovaginal junction is reached, at which point the clamps are placed underneath the cervix across the upper vagina and the specimen is removed (Fig. 46–10D).

The vagina is normally closed, and the cardinal and uterosacral ligaments are incorporated into each angle to prevent vaginal vault prolapse (Fig. 46–10E). The pelvic peritoneum is closed with a running suture after hemostasis has been secured. The uterus, once removed, should be opened in the operating room to exclude unsuspected malignancy, which may necessitate more extensive evaluation and dissection.

Vaginal Hysterectomy

This approach avoids an abdominal scar and is associated with minimal postoperative discomfort.

Indications

Vaginal hysterectomy may be performed provided that the uterus is mobile and not larger than 10 weeks gestational size; there are no adhesions from pelvic inflammatory disease, endometriosis, or multiple laparotomies; and ovarian disease is not suspected. The most common indication for this ap-

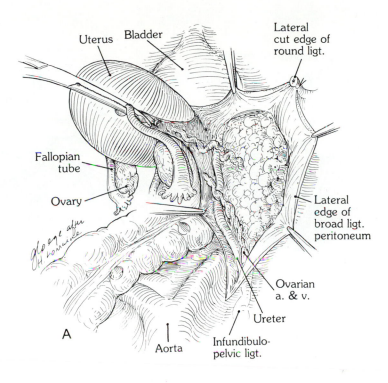

Figure 46-10. Technique for abdominal hysterectomy. *A*, The round ligament has been clamped, cut, and tied and the broad ligament opened. *B*, The retroperitoneal space has been opened, revealing the ureter and pelvic vessels.

Illustration continued on following page

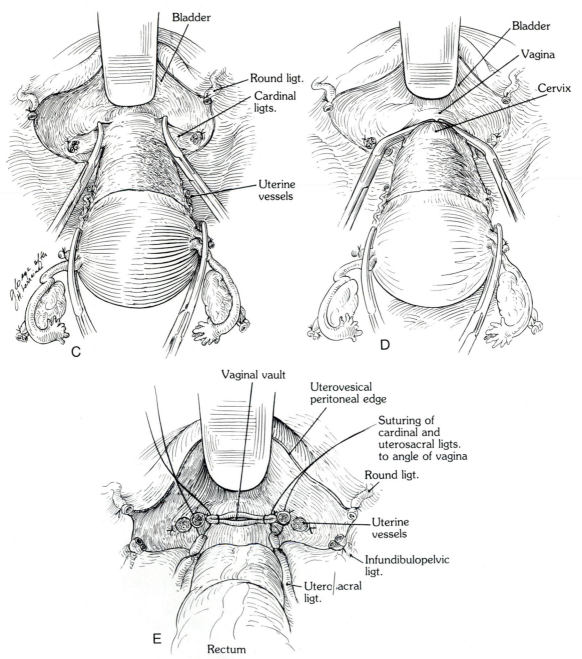

Figure 46–10. *Continued C,* The infundibulopelvic ligaments and uterine arteries have been secured, the bladder dissected off the cervix, and the cardinal ligaments clamped. *D,* Clamps have been placed across the upper vagina. *E,* The uterus has been removed. The vaginal vault is being closed.

proach is uterine prolapse, with or without associated cystocele, enterocele, or rectocele. Other indications include carcinoma in situ with positive margins on cone biopsy and sterilization in the presence of other gynecologic conditions that are amenable to vaginal surgery. The ovaries are not routinely removed through the vaginal approach, since this is technically more difficult and occasionally not technically feasible.

Technique

The principles of this operation are similar to those for abdominal hysterectomy except the ligaments and vessels are clamped and tied in reverse order. The patient is placed in the lithotomy position, and a weighted speculum is placed in the vagina. A tenaculum is placed on the cervix to pull the uterus down into the vagina. A circumferential incision is made at the cervicovaginal junction, and the posterior cul-de-sac is entered (Fig. 46–11A). A finger is placed in the cul-de-sac to make sure there are no unsuspected adhesions that would contraindicate proceeding with the surgery vaginally.

The uterosacral ligaments are isolated, clamped, cut, and tied. The cardinal ligaments are isolated, clamped, cut, and tied (Fig. 46–11B). Then the bladder is separated from the cervix to expose the anterior peritoneal reflection. The peritoneal cavity is entered anteriorly, and a retractor is placed beneath the bladder. The uterine vessels are secured (Fig. 46–11C), and, once this is achieved, the uterus can be brought further down into the vagina, exposing the utero-ovarian pedicles and round ligaments, which are clamped, cut, and tied (Fig. 46–11D). The ovaries are inspected, hemostasis is secured, and the peritoneum is then closed in a purse-string fashion (Fig. 46–11E).

All pedicles are left extraperitoneally to prevent a hemoperitoneum should secondary bleeding occur. Each cardinal ligament is sutured to the superior angle of the vagina on either side to protect against vaginal vault prolapse, and the uterosacral ligaments are tied in the midline to prevent a subsequent enterocele (Fig. 46–11F). The vaginal cuff is closed with interrupted absorbable sutures (Fig. 46–11G).

Complications of Hysterectomy

General complications associated with any abdominal or pelvic surgery include atelectasis, wound infection, urinary tract infection, thrombophlebitis, and pulmonary embolism. Atelectasis occurs most commonly in the first 24 to 48 hours and can be prevented and treated with aggressive pulmonary toilet. Wound infection usually occurs about 5 days postoperatively and is associated with redness, tenderness, swelling, and increased warmth around the wound. Treatment may require systemic antibiotics, opening the incision, draining the discharge, local debridement, and wound care. Urinary tract infection can occur at any time in the postoperative period, and urine for microscopy and culture should be obtained on any patient with a postoperative fever. Thrombophlebitis (with possible subsequent pulmonary embolism) is manifested by fever and leg swelling or pain; it usually occurs 7 to 10 days postoperatively. Pulmonary embolism may occur, even in the absence of signs of thrombophlebitis. Wound disruption, with evisceration of intestine, is generally heralded by a profuse serous discharge from the wound (peritoneal fluid) 4 to 8 days postoperatively. When evisceration is suspected, the wound should be explored in the operating room.

The most common intraoperative complication of abdominal or vaginal hysterectomy is bleeding, from the infundibulopelvic or utero-ovarian pedicle, the uterine pedicle, or the vaginal angle. When postoperative hemorrhage occurs, bleeding from the vaginal angle can sometimes be identified and controlled vaginally. If bleeding is sufficient to cause hypotension, however, laparotomy may be required to tie off the bleeding vascular pedicle.

Infection is common to both procedures and is manifested by fever and lower abdominal pain. Examination often reveals tenderness and induration of the vaginal cuff, indicative of a pelvic cellulitis. This can usually be treated with antibiotic therapy. When there has been seroma or hematoma formation, a pelvic abscess or infected pelvic hematoma can develop. This will be manifested by a hot, tender mass on rectovaginal examination. Such patients require the appropriate

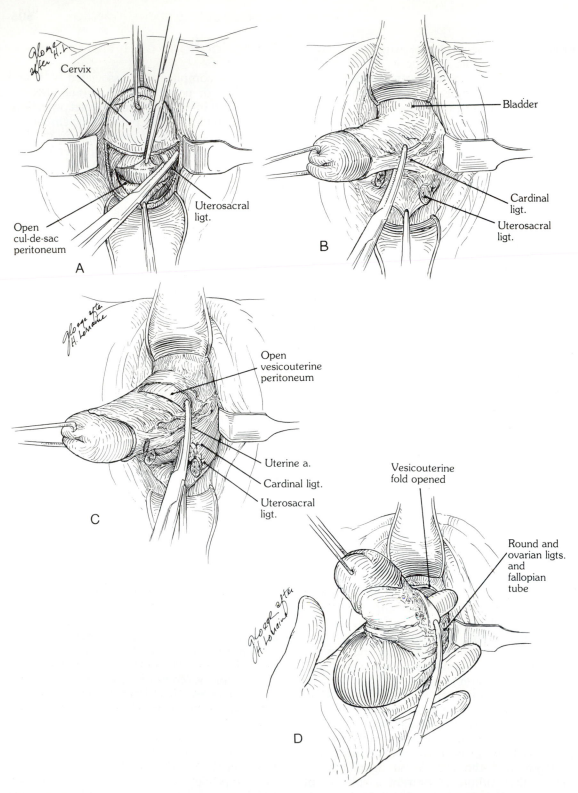

Figure 46–11. Technique for vaginal hysterectomy. *A,* A circumferential incision has been made at the cervicovaginal junction and the posterior cul-de-sac entered. *B,* The uterosacral ligaments have been secured and the cardinal ligaments clamped. *C,* The peritoneal cavity has been entered anteriorly, and the uterine vessels have been clamped. *D,* The final pedicle, containing the round and ovarian ligaments and the fallopian tube, has been clamped.

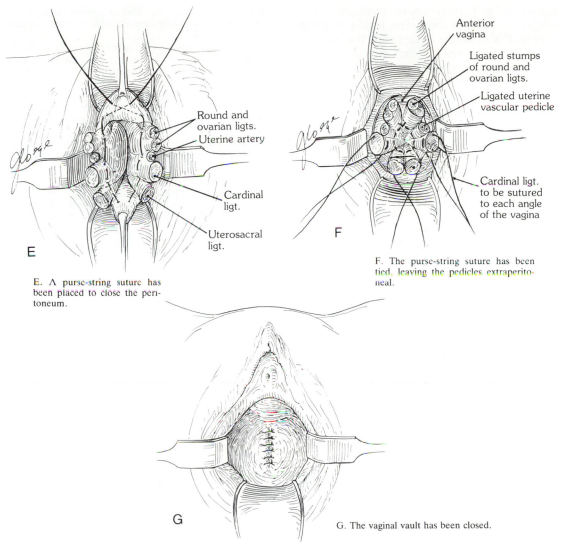

E. A purse-string suture has been placed to close the peritoneum.

F. The purse-string suture has been tied, leaving the pedicles extraperitoneal.

G. The vaginal vault has been closed.

Figure 46–11. *Continued E,* A purse-string suture has been placed to close the peritoneum. *F,* The purse-string suture has been tied, leaving the pedicles extraperitoneal. *G,* The vaginal vault has been closed.

drainage of the infected material through the vaginal cuff, in addition to the administration of parenteral antibiotics. Prophylactic cephalosporin intraoperatively and for 24 hours postoperatively has proved beneficial in controlling infection in vaginal hysterectomies done on premenopausal patients.

Injury to the ureter is the most serious complication of hysterectomy and usually occurs during the abdominal procedure, particularly during a difficult dissection for pelvic inflammatory disease, endometriosis, or pelvic cancer. The most common site of injury is just lateral to the cervix; the second most common site is beneath the infundibulopelvic ligament. A suture can be placed through the ureter, or it may be clamped and cut. It is important to identify the ureter before ligating and incising the infundibulopelvic ligament. Postoperatively, the patient will develop a fever and flank pain, and a ureterovaginal fistula or urinoma may occur 5 to 21 days postoperatively. If fluid begins to leak from the vagina, a work-up, including cystoscopy and intravenous pyelography, is necessary. A ureterovaginal fistula requires reimplantation of the ureter into the bladder, but it is usual to wait several months to allow the inflammatory reaction to settle.

Intraoperative injury to the bladder or intestine can occur and, if recognized, should be repaired immediately. If a bladder repair is necessary, 7 days of postoperative drainage with a Foley catheter is necessary to allow optimal healing.

SUGGESTED READING

Brooks PG, Serden SP: Hysteroscopic findings after unsuccessful dilatation and curettage for abnormal uterine bleeding. Am J Obstet Gynecol 158:1354, 1988.

Brooks PG, Loffer FD, Serden SP: Resectoscopic removal of symptomatic lesions. J Reprod Med 34:435, 1989.

Daly DC, Maier D, Soto-Albors C: Hysteroscopic metroplasty: Six years' experience. Obstet Gynecol 73:201, 1989.

Gambone JC, Reiter RC, Lench JB, Moore JG: The impact of a quality assurance process on the frequency and confirmation rate of hysterectomy. Am J Obstet Gynecol 163:545, 1990.

Gimpelson RJ, Rappold HO: A comparative study between panoramic hysteroscopy with directed biopsies and dilatation and curettage. Am J Obstet Gynecol 158:489, 1988.

Goldrath MH, Fuller T, Segal S: Laser photovaporization of endometrium for the treatment of menorrhagia. Am J Obstet Gynecol 140:14, 1981.

Gray LA: Techniques of abdominal total hysterectomy. Am J Obstet Gynecol 75:334, 1958.

Pratt JH: Operative and postoperative difficulties of vaginal hysterectomy. Obstet Gynecol 21:220, 1963.

Reiter RC, Lench JB, Gambone JC: Consumer advocacy, elective surgery, and the "golden era of medicine." Obstet Gynecol 4:815, 1989.

Vancaillie TG: Electrocoagulation of the endometrium with the ball-end resectoscope ("rollerball"). Obstet Gynecol 74:425, 1989.

Part 4

Reproductive Endocrinology

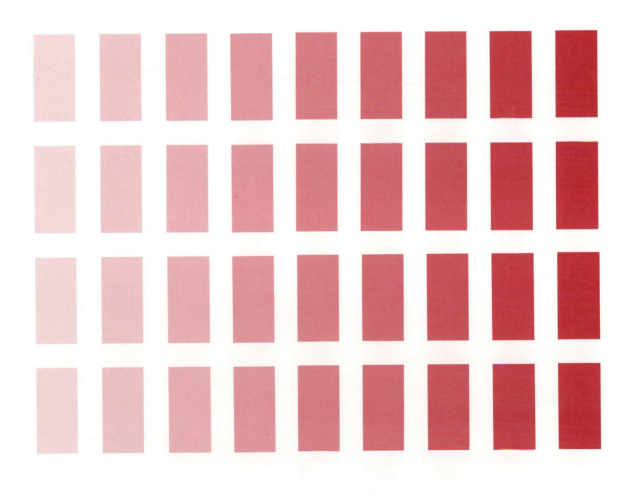

Forty-seven

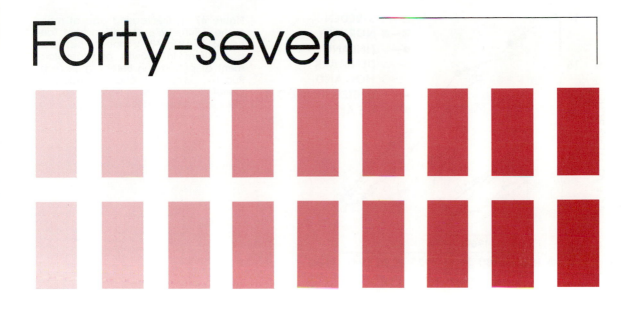

Puberty and Precocious Puberty

RICHARD P. BUYALOS, Jr.

Puberty is the sequence of events in the transformation of a child into a young adult, with the development of secondary sexual characteristics and reproductive capability. During this transition, a variety of physical, endocrinologic, and psychological changes occur, accompanying the increasing levels of sex steroids. These changes usually occur between the ages of 10 and 16 years.

The onset of pubertal changes is determined primarily by genetic factors. Geographic location, nutritional status, and psychological factors also influence the age at which puberty is initiated. For example, children with mild to moderate obesity, who reside in metropolitan areas, at altitudes near sea level, or latitudes close to the equator tend to begin puberty at an earlier age than children of normal weight or those residing in rural areas, at higher altitudes or at latitudes further from the equator.

In the United States and Western Europe, a decrease in the age of *menarche* (age at first menses) was noted between 1840 and 1970. This trend has slowed in the last 20 years (Fig. 47–1). Presently, the mean age of menarche is approximately 12.8 years in the United States.

ENDOCRINOLOGIC CHANGES OF PUBERTY

Evidence suggests that the fetal hypothalamic-pituitary-gonadal axis is capable of producing adult levels of gonadotropins and sex steroids. In this context, the endocrine

511

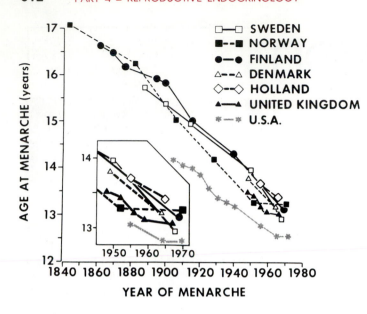

Figure 47–1. Decreasing age at menarche, 1840–1978. (Modified from Tanner M, Eveleth PB: Variability between populations in growth and development at puberty. In Bereberg SR (ed): Puberty, Biologic and Physiological Correlations. Leiden, Netherlands, HF Stenfert Kroese Publishers, 1976, p 256.)

changes involved in the pubertal transition and the development of sexual maturation are more clearly understood.

Fetal and Newborn Period

By 20 weeks gestation, serum levels of the gonadotropins, follicle-stimulating hormone (FSH) and luteinizing hormone (LH), rise dramatically in both male and female fetuses (Fig. 47–2). The female fetus has significantly higher concentrations of both FSH and LH than the male fetus. Autopsy studies have demonstrated that the female fetus has a maximal number of oocytes by midgestation and experiences a brief period of follicular maturation and sex steroid production in response to elevated gonadotropin levels in utero. The transient increase in serum estradiol acts on the fetal hypothalamic-pituitary unit, resulting in a reduction of gonadotropin secretion (negative feedback effect). This suggests that the inhibitory effect of sex steroids on gonadotropin release is operative before delivery.

In both male and female fetuses, serum estradiol is primarily of maternal and placental origin. With birth and the acute loss of maternal and placental sex steroids, the nega-

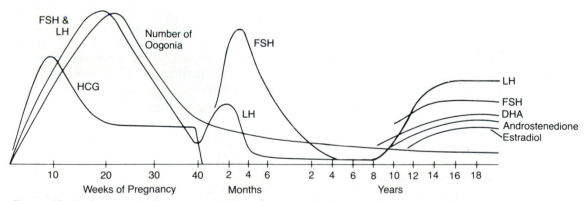

Figure 47–2. Changes in the concentration of gonadotropins, sex steroids, and the number of oogonia throughout fetal life and puberty. (Adapted from Speroff L, Glass RH, Kase NG: Neuroendocrinology. In Clinical Gynecologic Endocrinology and Infertility. Baltimore, Williams & Wilkins, 1989, p 83 © 1989, the Williams & Wilkins Co., Baltimore.)

tive feedback action on the hypothalamic-pituitary axis is lost and gonadotropins are once again released from the pituitary gland, reaching adult or near adult concentrations in the early neonatal period. In the female infant, peak levels of gonadotropins are generally seen by 3 months of age and then slowly decrease until a nadir is reached by the age of 4 years. In contrast to gonadotropin levels, sex steroid concentrations decrease rapidly to prepubertal values within 1 week following delivery and remain low until the onset of puberty.

Childhood

Between the ages of 4 and 10 years, the hypothalamic-pituitary-gonadal axis in the young child is suppressed. The hypothalamic-pituitary system regulating gonadotropin release has been termed the "gonadostat." Low levels of gonadotropins and sex steroids during this prepubertal period are a function of two mechanisms: (1) maximal sensitivity of the gonadostat to the negative feedback effect of the low circulating levels of estradiol present in prepubertal children and (2) intrinsic central nervous system inhibition of hypothalamic gonadotropin-releasing hormone (GnRH) secretion. These mechanisms occur independently of the presence of functional gonadal tissue, because the pattern of gonadotropin secretion in early childhood is similar in both normal and agonadal children. Children display elevated gonadotropin concentrations during the first 2 to 4 years of life, followed by a decline in circulating FSH and LH levels by 6 to 8 years of age. By 10 to 12 years of age, gonadotropin concentrations spontaneously rise once again, eventually achieving castrate levels. This pattern of gonadotropin secretion in children with gonadal dysgenesis is similar to that of children with normal gonadal function. This suggests that intrinsic central nervous system inhibition of GnRH release is the principal inhibitor of gonadotropin secretion, from 4 years of age until the peripubertal period.

Late Prepubertal Period

Generally, androgen production and differentiation by the zona reticularis of the adrenal cortex are the initial endocrine changes associated with puberty. Serum concentrations of dehydroepiandrosterone (DHEA), dehydroepiandrosterone-sulfate (DHEAS), and androstenedione (A_4) rise between the ages of 6 and 9 years. This rise in adrenal androgens induces the growth of both axillary and pubic hair and is known as *adrenarche* or *pubarche*. This increase in adrenal androgen production occurs independently of gonadotropin secretion or gonadal steroid levels.

Pubertal Onset

By approximately the eleventh year of life, there is a gradual loss of sensitivity of the gonadostat to the negative feedback of sex steroids (Fig. 47–3). The factor(s) that causes the derepression of the gonadostat is unknown. A further decrease in sensitivity of the gonadostat combined with the loss of intrinsic central nervous system inhibition of hypothalamic GnRH release is heralded by prominent sleep-associated increases in GnRH secretion. This nocturnal-dominant pattern gradually evolves into an adult-type secretory pattern, with GnRH pulses occurring every 90 to 120 minutes throughout the 24-hour day. The secretion of FSH and LH by the pituitary gland mirrors the pattern of GnRH pulses. This increase in gonadotropin release promotes ovarian follicular maturation and sex steroid production, which induces the development of secondary sexual characteristics. By mid to late puberty, maturation of the positive feedback mechanism of estradiol on LH release from the anterior pituitary gland is complete, and ovulatory cycles are established.

CRITICAL WEIGHT HYPOTHESIS

Events involved in the initiation of puberty are poorly understood. It has been proposed that an "invariant mean weight" of 48 kg (106 lb) is essential for the initiation of menarche in healthy girls. The proposed relationship between a critical body weight and the onset of puberty is speculative and has not been confirmed by prospective analyses. Menarche does tend to occur earlier in moderately obese females (20 to 30 per cent above ideal body weight), however, and is

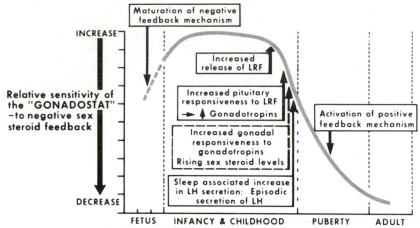

Figure 47–3. Changes in setpoint of the hypothalamic-pituitary unit (gonadostat) *(denoted by solid lines)* and the maturation of the negative and positive feedback mechanism from fetal life to adulthood in relation to the normal changes of puberty. This figure does not illustrate the change in the sex steroid–independent intrinsic central nervous system inhibitory mechanism that is observed from late infancy to puberty. (From Grumbach MM, Roth JC, Kaplan SL, Kelch RP: Hypothalamic pituitary regulation of puberty in man: evidence and concepts derived from clinical research. In Grumbach MM, Grave GD, Mayer FE (eds): Control of the Onset of Puberty. New York, John Wiley & Sons, 1974, p 115.)

delayed in children who are malnourished or those with chronic illnesses associated with weight loss.

The loss of a critical percentage of body fat provoking an aberration in gonadotropin secretion has also been postulated as the mechanism for amenorrhea observed in females with anorexia nervosa or excessive weight loss or following strenuous physical conditioning regimens.

SOMATIC CHANGES OF PUBERTY

Physical changes of puberty involve the development of secondary sexual characteristics and the acceleration of linear growth (gain in height). The somatic changes of puberty were first standardized by Marshall and Tanner on a population of Anglo-Saxon adolescents. Their classification of breast and pubic hair development is generally employed for descriptive and diagnostic purposes (Figs. 47–4 and 47–5).

Stages of Pubertal Development

The first physical sign of puberty is usually breast budding *(thelarche),* followed by the appearance of pubic or axillary hair *(pubarche or adrenarche).* Maximal growth or *peak height velocity* is usually the next stage, followed by *menarche* (the onset of menstrual periods). The final somatic changes are the appearance of adult pubic hair distribution and adult-type breasts. The sequence of pubertal changes generally occurs over a period of 4.5 years, with a normal range of 1.5 to 6 years (Fig. 47–6).

Adolescent Growth Spurt

Generally, the pubertal female's growth spurt is seen 2 years earlier than that of a male. Growth hormone, estradiol, and insulin-like growth factor-I (IGF-I or somatomedin-C) are involved in the adolescent growth spurt. Peak height velocity occurs approximately 1 year before the onset of menarche. Therefore, there is limited linear growth after menarche, since gonadal steroid production accelerates fusion of the long bone epiphyses.

Body Composition and Bone Age

Changes in body composition occur as a result of the sex steroid release accompanying

Figure 47-4. Stages of breast development as defined by Marshall and Tanner. *Stage 1:* Preadolescent; elevation of papilla only. *Stage 2:* Breast bud stage; elevation of breast and papilla as a small mound with enlargement of the areolar region. *Stage 3:* Further enlargement of breast and areola without separation of their contours. *Stage 4:* Projection of areola and papilla to form a secondary mound above the level of the breast. *Stage 5:* Mature stage; projection of papilla only, resulting from recession of the areola to the general contour of the breast.

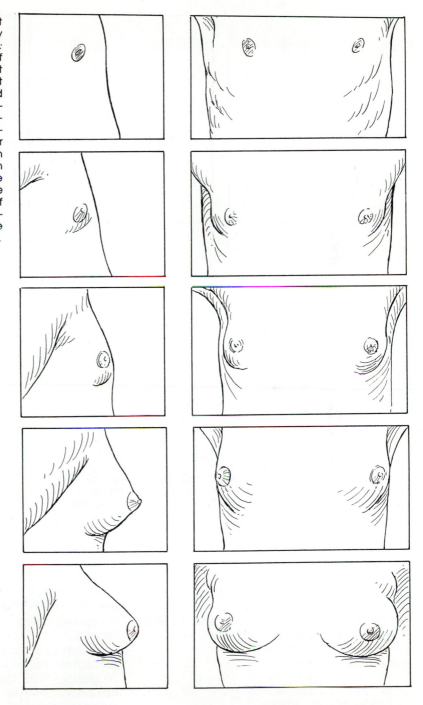

puberty, which induces the development of secondary sexual characteristics. There are no significant differences in skeletal mass, lean body mass, or the percentage of body fat between prepubertal males and females. Upon attaining sexual maturity, females generally have less skeletal and lean body mass and a greater percentage of body fat than males.

Bone age correlates well with the onset of secondary sexual characteristics and menarche. Bone age is determined by utilizing radiographs of the hand-wrist, elbow, or knee and comparing them with an index popula-

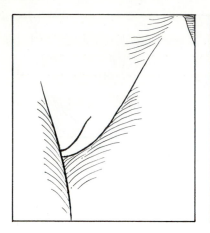
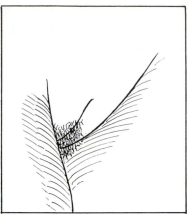
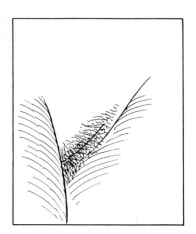

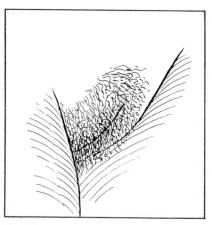
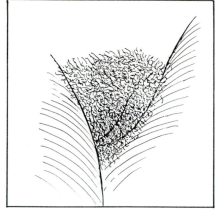

Figure 47–5. Stage of female pubic hair development according to Marshall and Tanner. *Stage 1:* Preadolescent; absence of pubic hair. *Stage 2:* Sparse hair along the labia. Hair downy with slight pigment. *Stage 3:* Hair spreads sparsely over the junction of the pubes. Hair is darker and coarser. *Stage 4:* Adult type hair. There is no spread to the medial surface of the thighs. *Stage 5:* Adult type hair with spread to the medial thighs assuming an inverse triangle pattern.

tion. Osseous maturation is particularly useful in the evaluation of adolescents with the delayed onset of puberty. Bone maturation, chronologic age, and height can also be used to predict the final adult stature from standardized nomograms such as the Bayley-Pinneau table.

PRECOCIOUS PUBERTY

Precocious puberty refers to the development of any sign of secondary sexual maturation at an age earlier than 2.5 standard deviations below the expected age of pubertal onset. In North America, these ages are 8 years for females and 9 years for males. Sexual precocity has an overall incidence of one in 10,000 children in North America and is approximately five times more common in females.

In approximately 75 per cent of cases of precocious puberty in females, the cause is *idiopathic.* With the apparent onset of sexual precocity, however, a thorough evaluation to eliminate a serious disease process and to arrest potential premature osseous maturation is mandatory.

The early development of secondary sexual characteristics may promote psychosocial problems for the child and should be carefully addressed. Typically, these girls are

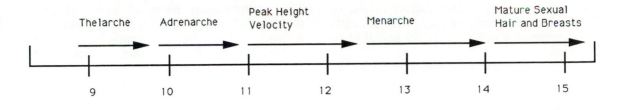

Figure 47–6. Sequence of physical changes in pubertal development.

taller than their peers as children but ultimately are shorter as adults owing to the premature fusion of the long bone epiphyses. A classification system for female precocious puberty is shown in Table 47–1.

Heterosexual Precocity

Precocious puberty may be divided into two major subgroups. The first, *heterosexual*

<table>
<tr><td colspan="2" align="center">**Table 47–1. CLASSIFICATION OF FEMALE PRECOCIOUS PUBERTY**</td></tr>
</table>

HETEROSEXUAL PRECOCIOUS PUBERTY
Virilizing neoplasm
  Ovarian
  Adrenal
Congenital adrenal hyperplasia
Exogenous androgen exposure

ISOSEXUAL PRECOCIOUS PUBERTY
Incomplete isosexual precocious puberty
  Premature thelarche
  Premature adrenarche
  Premature pubarche
Complete isosexual precocious puberty
  True isosexual precocious puberty
    Constitutional (idiopathic)
    Organic brain disease
  Pseudoisosexual precocious puberty
    Ovarian neoplasm
    Adrenal neoplasm
    Exogenous estrogen exposure
    Advanced hypothyroidism
    McCune-Albright syndrome
    Peutz-Jeghers syndrome

Adapted from Brenner PF: Precocious puberty in the female. In Mishell DR Jr, Davajan V (eds): Infertility, Contraception and Reproductive Endocrinology. 2nd ed. New Jersey, Medical Economics Books, 1986.

precocious puberty, refers to the development of secondary sexual characteristics opposite from the anticipated phenotypic sex; for example, virilization in females or feminization in males. In females, heterosexual precocity results from virilizing neoplasms, congenital adrenal hyperplasia, or exposure to exogenous androgens.

Androgen-secreting neoplasms in females are either ovarian (most commonly an arrhenoblastoma) or adrenal in origin and are exceedingly rare in childhood.

Virilization at birth in females is most frequently observed in congenital adrenal hyperplasia (CAH). The majority of cases of CAH result from an adrenal enzyme deficiency of 21-hydroxylase. Other causes of CAH include 11-β-hydroxylase and 3-β-hydroxysteroid dehydrogenase deficiencies (see Chapter 49). In utero exposure to high adrenal androgen concentrations results in the development of a female fetus with ambiguous genitalia. If untreated, progressive virilization during childhood and short adult stature will ensue.

Chronic exposure to anabolic steroids or androgenic agents can also induce heterosexual precocity in females.

Isosexual Precocious Puberty

Isosexual precocious puberty refers to premature sexual maturation that is appropriate for the phenotype of the affected individual; for example, precocious feminization in females and virilization in males. Isosexual precocious puberty may be subdivided into *complete isosexual precocious puberty*, referring to the development of the full complement of secondary sexual characteristics, or *incomplete isosexual precocity,* with the early appearance of a single secondary sexual characteristic.

Incomplete Isosexual Precocity. The incomplete forms of isosexual precocity are *premature thelarche* (the isolated appearance of breast development), *premature adrenarche* (the isolated appearance of axillary hair), and *premature pubarche* (the isolated appearance of pubic hair), occurring in females before 8 years of age.

Premature thelarche usually occurs before the age of 4 years and may be unilateral or bilateral. It resolves spontaneously within months and is probably secondary to transient estradiol secretion by the ovary. Premature adrenarche usually occurs after the age of 6 and is the result of premature adrenal gland androgen secretion. Generally, premature thelarche and premature adrenarche are of little clinical significance and are associated with appropriate sexual maturation. They do not require therapy. Both conditions are more common in females than males. Premature pubarche is associated with central nervous system disorders in approximately 50 per cent of cases and requires thorough evaluation. Premature pubarche is more common in boys.

It is usually not possible to diagnose an incomplete form of sexual precocity on a single evaluation and interval examinations are necessary. In any form of incomplete precocity, advancing bone age requires immediate treatment.

Complete Isosexual Precocity. Complete isosexual precocious puberty is the development of premature sexual maturation in association with increased levels of sex steroids. Complete isosexual precocity may be subdivided into *true isosexual precocity,* in which there is a premature activation of the hypothalamic-pituitary-gonadal axis, and *pseudoisosexual precocity,* in which the development of sexual maturation occurs without activation of the hypothalamic-pituitary axis. Thus, in pseudoisosexual precocious puberty, sex steroid levels are independent of pituitary gonadotropin release.

True Precocious Puberty. Approximately 90 per cent of cases of true isosexual precocity in females are constitutional or idiopathic. The constitutional form of isosexual precocious puberty results from the premature activation of the hypothalamic-pituitary axis and is associated with the normal sequence of pubertal changes. Constitutional precocious puberty is a diagnosis of exclusion. The diagnostic administration of exogenous GnRH (GnRH stimulation test) induces a rise in gonadotropin levels, as normally seen in older girls undergoing puberty.

In approximately 10 per cent of girls with the true form of precocious puberty, a central nervous system disorder is the underlying etiology. Tumors (including gliomas, astrocytomas, and hamartomas), obstructive lesions (hydrocephalus), granulomatous diseases (sarcoidosis, tuberculosis), infective processes (meningitis, encephalitis, or brain abscess), neurofibromatosis (von Recklinghausen's disease), and head trauma may cause sexual precocity. It is postulated that these conditions interfere with the normal inhibition of hypothalamic GnRH release. Children with precocious puberty secondary to organic brain disease generally exhibit neurologic symptoms before the appearance of premature sexual maturation. The majority of organic central nervous system lesions associated with precocity have an unfavorable prognosis.

Pseudoisosexual Precocious Puberty. Individuals with pseudoisosexual precocious puberty develop secondary sexual characteristics without activation of the hypothalamic-pituitary apparatus. Therefore, folliculogenesis and ovulatory cycles are not established. Females with pseudoisosexual precocity have elevated estrogen levels, which induce physical sexual maturational changes. The categories of pseudoisosexual precocious puberty are listed in Table 47–1.

Estrogen-secreting neoplasms of the ovary are most commonly granulosa-theca cell tumors. Only 5 per cent of granulosa cell tumors and 1 per cent of theca cell tumors occur in prepubertal girls and they are usually unilateral. The majority of these tumors are detectable on pelvic or abdominal examination and require surgical extirpation.

Functional follicular cysts may secrete estrogens and induce the development of secondary sexual characteristics. Other benign ovarian tumors (cystadenomas, gonadoblastomas, or teratomas) and rarely ovarian malignancies have been reported with sexual precocity.

Rare adrenal tumors have been reported to induce pseudoisosexual precocious puberty in females but are much more commonly associated with masculinization (heterosexual precocity).

Ectopic human chorionic gonadotropin (hCG) production from hepatoblastomas, teratomas, and choriocarcinomas has been reported to cause sexual precocity but almost exclusively in males.

Agents containing *exogenous estrogenic compounds* can induce sexual precocity in children. A careful history is mandatory to identify lotions, creams, cosmetics, or medications to which the child may have been exposed. Meat from hormonally treated livestock has been implicated in provoking pseudoisosexual precocity.

The *McCune-Albright syndrome* (polyostotic fibrous dysplasia) is a rare syndrome consisting of sexual precocity, multiple cystic bone defects that fracture easily, and café au lait spots with irregular borders most frequently on the face, neck, shoulders, and back. Skeletal deformities frequently occur after pubertal changes. This condition is now thought to occur from autonomous gonadal estrogen production and is much more common in females than males.

Prolonged severe *hypothyroidism* in childhood can cause pseudoisosexual precocity, occurring almost exclusively in girls. It is hypothesized that pituitary gonadotropin release occurs in response to the persistently elevated secretion of thyroid-releasing hormone (TRH). Concomitant elevated prolactin levels may also occur with the development of galactorrhea. Ovarian cysts may occasionally develop, and bone age may be retarded. This is the only form of precocious puberty associated with *delayed bone age*. Upon achieving a euthyroid state, gonadotropin, prolactin, and sex steroid levels return to prepubertal concentrations with regression of precocious physical changes, cessation of galactorrhea, and appropriate osseous maturation.

The *Peutz-Jeghers syndrome* has been associated with a rare sex-cord tumor with annular tubules, which may be estrogen-secreting, and has been reported to induce sexual precocity in females. This syndrome of gastrointestinal tract polyposis and mucocutaneous pigmentation has also been reported in a female with a granulosa-theca cell tumor. Therefore, children with Peutz-Jeghers syndrome should be screened for the development of gonadal neoplasms.

Diagnosis of Precocious Puberty

History. The sequence and velocity of sexual maturational changes should be carefully outlined. A familial history of premature pubertal development should be excluded. Parents should be questioned about potential ingestion of or exposure to medications, tonics, lotions, and powders containing hormones. A careful history regarding a previous central nervous system infection, head trauma, or chronic illness should be obtained. Of particular importance is a detailed history of behavioral changes, seizure-like activity, or persistent headaches.

Physical and Laboratory Diagnosis. Physical examination, including records of serial heights and weights, and a detailed evaluation of secondary sexual characteristics, including Tanner stages, is obligatory. Careful abdominal and pelvic examination must be performed. A thorough neurologic examination is necessary to identify potential focal deficits. Cutaneous examination for café au lait lesions, neurofibromas, and acne should be performed. Breast examination should also evaluate the presence of expressible galactorrhea. Diagnostic studies indicated in the evaluation of female precocious puberty are outlined in Table 47–2. A GnRH stimulation test may prove useful in distinguishing between true versus pseudoisosexual precocious puberty.

The clinical history and physical examination may dictate a particular diagnostic sequence. For example, females with masculinizing signs or symptoms (heterosexual precocity) and elevated adrenal androgens should have a magnetic resonance imaging (MRI) or computed tomographic (CT) scan of the adrenal glands.

Table 47–2. RADIOLOGIC AND LABORATORY EVALUATION OF FEMALE PRECOCIOUS PUBERTY

RADIOLOGIC
Skull film
Serial bone age
MRI or CT scan of brain with optimal visualization of hypothalamic region and sella turcica
MRI, CT scan, or ultrasonography of abdomen, pelvis, or adrenal gland

LABORATORY
LH, FSH, hCG
DHEAS, androstenedione, testosterone, estradiol, progesterone
17-OH progesterone, 11-deoxycortisol
Thyroid function tests (TSH, free T_4 or free T_4 index)
Prolactin (if galactorrhea present)
GnRH stimulation test
EEG
Visual field testing

Treatment of Precocious Puberty

Approximately 75 per cent of females with precocious puberty will prove to have constitutional or idiopathic etiology. These girls require treatment to prevent further sex steroid release and accelerated epiphyseal fusion. If untreated, fewer than 50 per cent of girls with idiopathic precocity will attain an adult height of 5 feet.

GnRH analogs presently are the most effective therapy for idiopathic precocity. They are available in long-acting formulations administered as intramuscular injections. These preparations are also available for daily administration as subcutaneous injections and intranasal sprays. Long-term GnRH analog treatment will suppress pituitary release of LH and FSH, resulting in the decline of gonadotropin levels to prepubertal concentrations and arrest of gonadal steroid secretion. Clinically normal gonadotropin release, sex steroid production, and pubertal maturation will resume following discontinuation of GnRH analog therapy. GnRH analog treatment is generally not indicated in precocity that is independent of gonadotropin release (e.g., estrogen-secreting neoplasms), unless the chronic elevation of sex steroids has acti-

vated the hypothalamic-pituitary axis. Long-term follow-up is needed to confirm the predicted improvement in final adult stature.

Medroxyprogesterone acetate (MPA) had been widely used for idiopathic precocious puberty, in oral and intramuscular regimens. MPA is effective in retarding breast and genital development but does not consistently slow peak height velocity or osseous maturation. Long-term therapy has been reported to cause signs of glucocorticoid excess.

Other formulations that have previously been employed in the treatment of sexual precocity include the potent progestin and antiandrogen *cyproterone acetate*, not currently available in the United States, and danazol, a weak androgenic compound that may induce virilization. Neither compound is more efficacious than MPA, and they generally have more adverse side effects.

Individuals with tumors, infections, or other central nervous system disorders require neurosurgical consultation. Pelvic, abdominal, or adrenal neoplasms generally require surgical exploration.

Exposure to exogenous steroid compounds requires identification and removal of offending agents. Precocity from advanced hypothyroidism necessitates thyroid hormone replacement. Adrenal hyperplasia requires careful glucocorticoid and mineralocorticoid replacement.

The majority of children with sexual precocity have few significant behavioral problems. Emotional support is important in these children, however. Expectations by family members and teachers must be based on the child's chronologic age, which determines psychosocial development, and not on the presence of secondary sexual characteristics.

SUGGESTED READING

Bayley N, Pinneau SR: Tables for predicting adult height from skeletal age: Revised for use with the Greulich-Pyle hand standards. J Pediatr 40:423, 1952.
Brenner PF: Precocious puberty in the female. In Mishell D, Davajan V (eds): Infertility, Contraception, and Reproductive Endocrinology. Cambridge, MA, Medical Economics Books, 1986, p 223.

Crowley WF Jr, Comite F, Vale W, et al: Therapeutic use of pituitary desensitization with a long-acting LHRH agonist: A potential new treatment for idiopathic precocious puberty. J Clin Endocrinol Metab 52:370, 1981.

Frisch RE, Revelle R: Height and weight at menarche and a hypothesis of critical body weights and adolescent events. Science 169:397, 1970.

Kaplan S, Grumbach MM: Pathogenesis of sexual precocity. In Grumbach MM, Sizonenko P, Aubert M (eds): Control of the Onset of Puberty. Baltimore, Williams & Wilkins, 1990, p 620.

Marshall WA, Tanner JM: Variations in pattern of pubertal changes in girls. Arch Dis Child 44:291, 1969.

Roy S, Brenner PF: Puberty. In Mishell D, Davajan V (eds): Infertility, Contraception, and Reproductive Endocrinology. Cambridge, MA, Medical Economics Books, 1986, p 163.

Speroff L, Glass RH, Kase NG: Abnormal puberty and growth problems. In Clinical Gynecologic Endocrinology and Infertility. Baltimore, Williams & Wilkins, 1989, p 409.

Styne DM, Grumbach MM: Puberty in the male and female: Its physiology and disorders. In Yen SSC, Jaffe RB (eds): Reproductive Endocrinology. Physiology, Pathophysiology and Clinical Management. Philadelphia, WB Saunders, 1991, p 511.

Styne DM, Harris D, Egli CA et al: Treatment of true precocious puberty with a potent luteinizing hormone-releasing factor agonist: Effect on growth, sexual maturation, pelvic sonography, and the hypothalamic-pituitary-gonadal axis. J Clin Endocrinol Metab 61:142, 1985.

Forty-eight

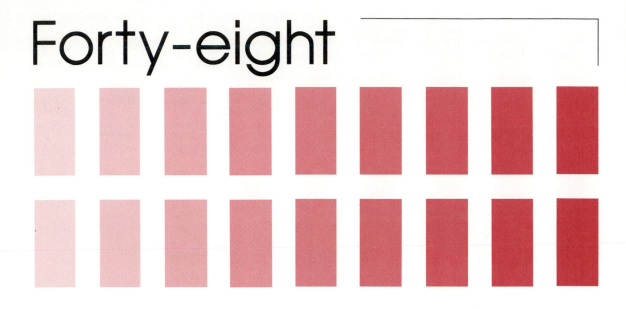

Amenorrhea and Abnormal Uterine Bleeding

OSCAR A. KLETZKY

Amenorrhea (*A* [Greek for negative], *men* [month or moon], *rhoia* [flow]) is a common symptom of a variety of pathophysiologic states. Amenorrhea usually occurs when the dynamic and rhythmic changes occurring in the reproductive endocrine system are not initiated or are interrupted by anatomic, genetic, or functional alterations. It is usually divided into primary and secondary amenorrhea. Before the evaluation of amenorrhea is initiated, chronic diseases, such as anemia, diabetes mellitus, and thyroid abnormalities, as well as pregnancy should be ruled out.

PRIMARY AMENORRHEA

The diagnosis of primary amenorrhea is usually made when no spontaneous uterine bleeding has occurred by the age of 16½ years. Thus, a woman who menstruates only in response to exogenous hormones should be classified as having primary amenorrhea. The work-up should be initiated sooner if the patient presents with no breast development by the age of 15 or has failed to menstruate spontaneously within 2 years of the onset of breast development (thelarche) and pubic or axillary hair development (adrenarche).

Depending on the presence or absence of the uterus and the presence or absence of breast development, patients with primary amenorrhea and normal female external genitalia can be subdivided into four categories (Fig. 48–1):

1. Patients with no breast development and uterus present.
2. Patients with breast development and uterus absent.

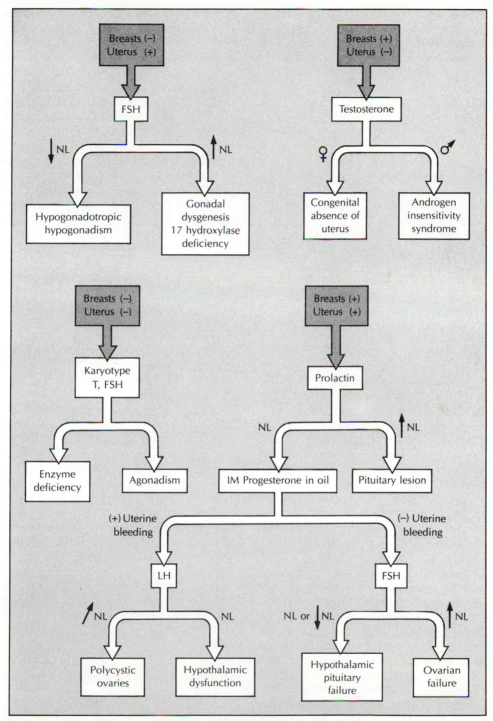

Figure 48–1. Systematic approach to the diagnostic evaluation of patients with primary amenorrhea based on presence or absence of breast development and uterus. IM = intramuscular; NL = normal level. Arrow pointing up indicates level above normal; arrow pointing down indicates level below normal; slanted arrow indicates moderate elevation. (From Mashchak CA, Kletzky OA, Davajan V, Mishell DR Jr: Clinical and laboratory evaluation of patients with primary amenorrhea. Obstet Gynecol 57:715–721, 1981.)

3. Patients with no breast development and uterus absent.

4. Patients with breast development and uterus present.

Primary Amenorrhea with No Breast Development and Uterus Present

The differential diagnosis of these patients includes *hypogonadotropic hypogonadism* caused by either hypothalamic or pituitary failure and *gonadal dysgenesis.*

The differential diagnosis is easily made by the measurement of a single serum follicle-stimulating hormone (FSH) sample. Patients with hypogonadotropic hypogonadism have low or low normal serum FSH levels, whereas patients with gonadal dysgenesis have elevated FSH levels in the menopausal range. The measurement of serum luteinizing hormone (LH) is of no additional diagnostic value. The absence of breast development is indicative of inadequate secretion of estradiol, and thus its measurement adds nothing further to the differential diagnosis.

Hypogonadotropic hypogonadism is the most common cause of amenorrhea in this group of patients. It may be due to an intrinsic hypothalamic derangement or to abnormalities of the neural regulatory mechanism that controls the qualitative or quantitative adequacy of gonadotropin-releasing hormone (GnRH) synthesis and release. Some patients with amenorrhea also have anosmia (Kallmann's syndrome). Substances such as coffee, tobacco, orange, and cocoa can be used to determine the integrity of the olfactory system. Although a pituitary tumor is rarely seen in patients with hypogonadotropic hypogonadism, a patient with a craniopharyngioma may present with amenorrhea, and therefore a computed tomographic (CT) scan or magnetic resonance imaging (MRI) of the hypothalamic-pituitary area is recommended.

The differentiation between a hypothalamic and a pituitary origin of the hypogonadotropic hypogonadism can be established by performing a GnRH test. If there is an appropriate LH response following the administration of exogenous GnRH, the diagnosis is hypothalamic failure to produce or secrete adequate endogenous GnRH. If the pituitary has not been previously primed with endogenous or exogenous GnRH, lack of response to a bolus of GnRH may not necessarily indicate primary pituitary gonadotropin deficiency. Therefore, such patients should be treated with daily doses of GnRH for up to 10 days and retested. Absence of LH response to a subsequent GnRH test usually indicates pituitary failure.

Patients with *gonadal dysgenesis* have hypergonadotropic hypogonadism caused by a genetic or enzymatic abnormality that results in the failure of gonadal development or abnormal functioning of the ovary. The differential diagnosis includes patients with 45,X (Turner's syndrome), structurally abnormal X chromosome, mosaicism with or without a Y chromosome, pure gonadal dysgenesis (46,XX and 46,XY), and 17 hydroxylase deficiency with 46,XX. Patients with hydroxylase deficiency have hypertension and hypokalemia. Only patients with primary amenorrhea and an elevated serum FSH level need a karyotype to confirm the diagnosis of ovarian failure or to establish the presence of a Y chromosome.

Patients with gonadal dysgenesis are sterile and can carry a pregnancy only if a donor egg is fertilized in vitro and transferred into the uterus. Although most of these patients show no signs of secondary sexual characteristics, occasionally an individual with mosaicism or Turner's syndrome can synthesize enough estrogen to cause breast development, menstruation, ovulation, and even pregnancy. If pregnancy is not an issue, all patients with primary amenorrhea should be treated with estrogen-progestin replacement to induce breast development and cyclic menstrual bleeding. This therapy is also important in preventing osteoporosis and coronary heart disease.

Primary Amenorrhea with Breast Development and Absent Uterus

The differential diagnosis is between patients with androgen insensitivity *(testicular feminization syndrome)* and *congenital absence of the uterus.* Patients with androgen insensitivity syndrome have testicles, and patients with absence of the uterus have ovaries. Therefore, any method that will detect ovulation could be sufficient to establish the differential diagnosis. Alternatively, measurement of serum testosterone clearly establishes the differential diagnosis. Those with congenital absence of the uterus will have a serum testosterone level in the normal female range and those with androgen insensitivity syndrome will have a serum testosterone level in the normal male range. Only those patients with serum testosterone level in the male range should have a karyotype to confirm the diagnosis.

In patients with androgen insensitivity, the gonads (testicles) should be removed to prevent malignant transformation (25 per cent chance) and the patient should be treated with estrogen. In counseling these patients, it is desirable to use the word *gonad* and not *testicle* because it is very difficult for these phenotypical females to accept the fact that there are functioning testicles present.

Patients with congenital absence of the uterus usually do not require any endocrine replacement treatment. Patients in either group cannot conceive or carry a pregnancy, unless the patient with an absent uterus undergoes in vitro fertilization with embryo transfer to a surrogate mother.

Primary Amenorrhea with Neither Breast Development Nor Uterus

These patients are extremely rare. Often they have a male karyotype (46,XY), elevated gonadotropins, and serum testosterone level within the normal female range. They differ from patients with gonadal failure in that they do not have a uterus and from patients with androgen insensitivity syndrome in that they do not have breast development or normal male testosterone levels. The differential diagnosis includes 17,20 demolase deficiency, agonadism (also known as vanishing testicles syndrome), or 17-hydroxylate deficiency with 46,XY karyotype. The diagnosis of 17,20 demolase deficiency can be made only by incubation studies with a portion of gonadal tissue. The presence of agonadism can be suspected by the lack of testosterone response following the daily administration of hCG and confirmed by laparotomy. Patients with 17-hydroxylate deficiency and 46,XY karyotype have elevated blood pressure and hypokalemia. If gonadal tissue is present, it should be removed to prevent malignant transformation. They should be treated with estrogen replacement to induce breast development and to prevent osteoporosis and cardiovascular disease.

Primary Amenorrhea with Breast Development and Uterus Present

About 25 per cent of these patients have an elevated serum prolactin level, no galactorrhea, and radiographic abnormalities of the sella turcica compatible with the presence of a pituitary adenoma. Therefore, in such patients, a prolactinoma needs to be ruled out. If the serum prolactin is normal, the differential diagnosis includes *polycystic ovary disease* (PCO), *hypothalamic dysfunction, hypothalamic-pituitary failure,* and *ovarian failure.* Because patients with secondary amenorrhea have the same differential diagnosis, both groups of patients undergo a similar systematic evaluation.

SECONDARY AMENORRHEA

Only patients with amenorrhea and no evidence of galactorrhea or excess cortisol or androgen are discussed here. Secondary amenorrhea is usually defined as the absence of menses for 6 months or more in a woman who previously had regular menses or the absence of menses for 12 months if the patient has a history of oligomenorrhea.

After pregnancy has been ruled out, a careful history should be taken to identify the use of drug(s) or medication(s), any unusual degree of stress or exercise, or any significant weight reduction or weight gain. Special consideration should be given to a history of intrauterine instrumentation, particularly if associated with pregnancy termination. In these circumstances, the presence of intrauterine synechiae should be suspected and the uterine cavity investigated with hyster-

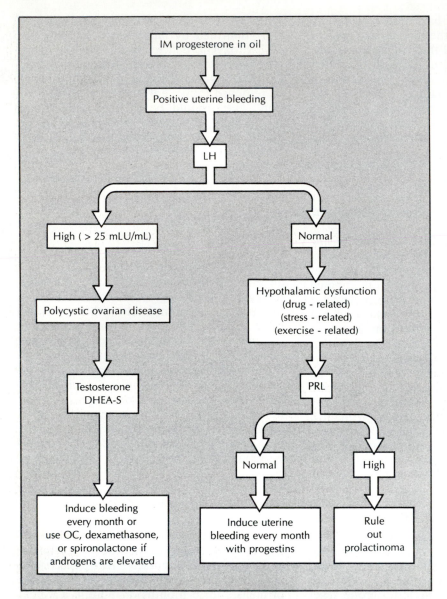

Figure 48–2. Systematic approach to the diagnostic evaluation of patients with secondary amenorrhea. OC = oral contraceptives; PRL = prolactin. (From Kletzky OA, Davajan V, Nakamura RM, Mishell DR Jr: Clinical categorization of patients with secondary amenorrhea using progesterone induced uterine bleeding and measurement of serum gonadotropin levels. Am. J Obstet Gynecol 121:695–703, 1975.)

ography, hysteroscopy, or both. Once intrauterine synechiae have been ruled out, the next step is to determine the patient's estrogen status. This can be done by giving 100 mg of progesterone in oil intramuscularly or 30 mg of oral progestin for 3 days. Patients with low levels of estrogen (<40 pg/ml) will not have uterine bleeding. Even a minimal amount of bleeding occurring 2 to 14 days later is sufficient to be considered a positive response.

The major differential diagnosis in patients bleeding following the administration of progesterone is between *PCO* and *hypothalamic dysfunction* (Fig. 48–2). A serum LH value

of 25 mIU/ml or greater is diagnostic of PCO in about 70 per cent of patients. The determination of the serum LH to FSH ratio does not add additional diagnostic value. If clinically indicated, patients with PCO should also have androgen studies performed.

Patients with a normal serum LH level are diagnosed as having hypothalamic dysfunction. This includes those with idiopathic amenorrhea and those with amenorrhea induced by medication, stress, or simple weight loss.

Regardless of the etiologic diagnosis, clomiphene citrate is the treatment of choice for patients wishing to conceive. For the patient not desiring to conceive, monthly administration of an oral progestin for 12 days is recommended to induce periodic bleeding and sloughing of the endometrium. Owing to the small likelihood of ovulation, a barrier method of contraception is appropriate for these patients. Because sufficient levels of endogenous estrogen are secreted by these patients, oral steroid contraceptives are not necessary. Steroid contraceptives may be indicated, however, in patients with PCO, hirsutism, acne, in whom it is important to reduce the level of serum testosterone.

If the amenorrhea is associated with the use of medication(s) or secondary to stress, the treatment should be directed toward correction of the etiologic factor.

The differential diagnosis for patients with amenorrhea who do not bleed following the administration of progesterone is between *hypothalamic failure* and *premature ovarian failure* (Fig. 48–3). A single serum FSH level identifies two distinct populations: Patients with a low serum FSH level have hypothalamic-pituitary failure, and patients with an elevated serum FSH level have premature ovarian failure (POF).

The *hypothalamic-pituitary failure* group includes patients with severe weight loss (which may be associated with anorexia nervosa), hypothalamic lesions, Sheehan's syndrome, and nonsecreting pituitary adenomas. Patients with a pituitary adenoma or Sheehan's syndrome should have an insulin-induced hypoglycemia test for the evaluation of growth hormone, prolactin, and adrenocorticotropic hormone (ACTH) reserve secretion. Patients with hypothalamic-pituitary failure who wish to conceive require human menopausal gonadotropins. Otherwise, they should be given estrogen-progestin replacement therapy. Patients with a nonsecreting pituitary adenoma may require adenomectomy.

Patients with POF may present with either primary or secondary amenorrhea. If the patient is younger than 25 years, a karyotype should be ordered to exclude the presence of a Y chromosome, which would necessitate gonadectomy to prevent malignant transformation. An autoimmune disorder is probably the most common cause of POF. Autoantibodies may be produced against ovaries, oocytes, or gonadotropin receptors and in some instances against other endocrine glands as well (e.g., adrenal glands, thyroid, and parathyroid glands). Since the measurements of antithyroid antibodies and antimicrosomal antibodies are the only tests available to the clinician, these should be ordered in all patients with POF who are younger than 35 years. It is not infrequent for patients with POF to fluctuate between normal and abnormal secretion of estrogen and gonadotropins, so spontaneous menses, ovulation, and pregnancy may occasionally occur. A few pregnancies have been reported in patients with POF following treatment with estrogen alone or with human gonadotropins. Patients with persistent ovarian failure secrete very low levels of estrogen and require estrogen-progestogen replacement therapy.

AMENORRHEA WITH HYPERPROLACTINEMIA

Symptoms and Signs Related to Hyperprolactinemia

Galactorrhea is the most frequently observed abnormality associated with hyperprolactinemia. Galactorrhea is defined as a nonpuerperal watery or milky breast secretion that contains neither pus nor blood. The secretion may be manifested spontaneously or obtained only by breast examination. It is usually bilateral but has the same significance if it is present in only one breast. The important factor is the presence or absence of milk, not the amount of secretion. Both breasts should be gently examined by expressing the gland from the periphery to the nipple. To ascertain the quality of the secretion and to determine the presence of true galactorrhea (milk), a smear is prepared and examined microscopically. If multiple fat droplets are present, the secretion contains milk.

Besides galactorrhea, hyperprolactinemia frequently also causes oligomenorrhea or amenorrhea. The mechanism of the menstrual irregularity varies with the etiology of hyperprolactinemia. Drugs affecting the normal pathways for dopamine and norepinephrine secretion can produce amenorrhea-galactorrhea. Hyperprolactinemia may affect the synthesis and secretion of GnRH or the secretion (but not the synthesis) of gonadotropins.

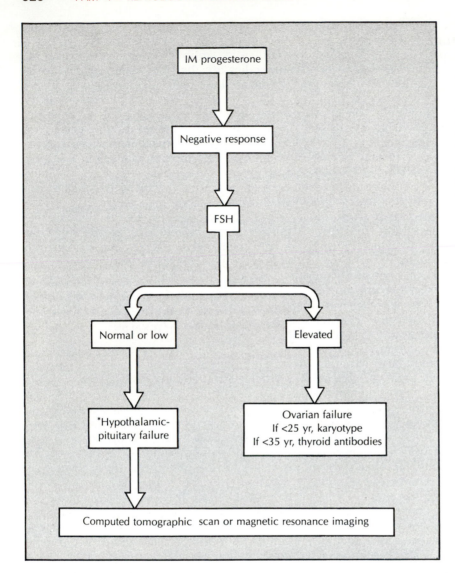

Figure 48–3. Systematic approach to diagnostic evaluation of patients with secondary amenorrhea. Patients with simple weight loss; a history of drug intake, stress, or exercise; or those who do not have hyperprolactinemia do not need a computed tomographic scan. (From Kletzky OA, Davajan V, Nakamura RM, Mishell DR Jr: Clinical categorization of patients with secondary amenorrhea using progesterone induced uterine bleeding and measurement of serum gonadotropin levels. Am J Obstet Gynecol 121:695–703, 1975.)

Pharmacologic Agents Affecting the Secretion of Prolactin

Drug-induced hyperprolactinemia appears to be the most common cause of nonphysiologic galactorrhea or hyperprolactinemia. Responsible drugs include tranquilizers, tricyclic antidepressants, antihypertensive agents, narcotics, and oral contraceptive steroids. Tranquilizers induce hyperprolactinemia by depleting the hypothalamus of catecholamines or by blocking binding sites. This lowers the levels of dopamine or interferes with its action, which in turn deprives the pitui-

tary of its natural inhibitor and results in the increased prolactin. Tricyclic antidepressants block catecholamine reuptake, reserpine causes depletion of catecholamines, and methyldopa blocks the conversion of tyrosine to dihydroxyphenylalanine and dopamine.

If clinically indicated, patients with galactorrhea caused by medications should be encouraged to discontinue the medication for at least 1 month. If galactorrhea persists or if the patient cannot interrupt the medication, a complete evaluation is indicated if the serum prolactin is greater than 50 ng/ml. Bromocriptine is a semisynthetic ergot alkaloid with potent dopamine agonist effects that inhibits prolactin secretion by acting directly on the pituitary. Presently, this is the only medication available to treat hyperprolactinemia.

Pathologic Factors Affecting Prolactin Secretion

Hypothyroidism. In about 3 to 5 per cent of patients with galactorrhea and hyperprolactinemia, the underlying etiology is primary hypothyroidism. These patients have a low serum thyroxine (T_4) level, so consequently they lack negative feedback on the hypothalamic-pituitary axis. They also have a decreased positive feedback on dopamine. Thus, diminished dopamine secretion results in elevated levels of serum thyroid-stimulating hormone (TSH) and prolactin. Patients with primary hypothyroidism should be given T_4 replacement therapy without further evaluation.

Hypothalamic Causes. A craniopharyngioma is the nonpituitary tumor most commonly associated with hyperprolactinemia. These tumors arise from epithelial remnants of Rathke's pouch, which are distributed along the pituitary stalk from the pars distalis to the floor of the third ventricle. Approximately 250 cases of craniopharyngioma are diagnosed in the United States annually. A craniopharyngioma is most frequently diagnosed during the second and third decades of life. Classically, a plain skull x-ray film or CT scan during childhood reveals calcifications. The incidence of calcifications diminishes during the third decade of life.

A craniopharyngioma either damages the hypothalamus or extends into the sella turcica, where it interferes with the transport of hypothalamic hormones and neurotransmitters, resulting in pituitary dysfunction. Although some degree of impairment of pituitary function is almost universally found, the extent of impairment depends on whether the hypothalamus or the pituitary stalk is more involved. In either case, gonadotropin deficiency is always present, resulting in amenorrhea. Galactorrhea is present in those patients with hyperprolactinemia. Diminished levels of growth hormone (GH), TSH, ACTH, and antidiuretic hormone (ADH) are also present.

As a craniopharyngioma expands, it produces local compression, especially of the optic chiasm. Therefore, surgical decompression is necessary.

Pituitary Causes. Although a tenfold increase in the incidence of all types of pituitary adenomas has been reported since 1970, the exact incidence of prolactin-secreting pituitary adenomas is still unknown. Patients with prolactin-secreting pituitary adenomas have galactorrhea, hyperprolactinemia, or both. The etiology of these adenomas is unknown. About 50 per cent of patients with hyperprolactinemia will have radiographic changes in the sella turcica compatible with an adenoma. Most patients have normal baseline levels of FSH and LH.

Hyperplasia of the Lactotrophs. Patients with hyperplasia of the lactotrophs cannot be distinguished from those having a microadenoma by any clinical, laboratory, or radiologic method. It is a histologic diagnosis made only at the time of surgical exploration of the pituitary gland.

Empty Sella Syndrome. Empty sella is characterized by herniation of the subarachnoid membrane into the sella turcica through a defective or incompetent sella diaphragm. Primary empty sella may result from alterations in the circulatory dynamics of the cerebrospinal fluid or coexist with prolactin-secreting, GH-secreting, or ACTH-secreting pituitary adenomas. Secondary empty sella is seen after radiation therapy or surgical intervention in the sellar region. The subarachnoid herniation results in compression of the pituitary gland and remodeling of the sella contour. Radiographically, the sella is symmetrically enlarged, with or without bone erosion. A definitive diagnosis can accurately be made by MRI. Patients with this diagnosis require a less stringent follow-up than those with a prolactinoma. Although most patients with empty sella have no endocrine abnormalities, some may have pituitary dysfunction and even panhypopituitarism.

Acromegaly. About 30 per cent of patients with acromegaly can have galactorrhea and an elevated serum prolactin level. Galactorrhea in patients with acromegaly is most likely due to the secretion of both prolactin and growth hormone.

Sheehan's Syndrome. Sheehan's syndrome is the only entity with lower than normal levels of serum prolactin ($<$5ng/ml) that is of clinical significance. Typically, these patients fail to lactate postpartum. If the insult to the pituitary results in complete damage to the anterior pituitary, these women will also have a blunted LH, FSH, prolactin, and TSH response following the administration of GnRH and TRH.

Other Causes of Hyperprolactinemia

Renal Disease. Patients with acute or chronic renal failure have hyperprolactinemia because of delayed clearance of the hormone. These patients rarely require treatment other than that for acute or chronic renal failure.

Chest Surgery. Patients with previous chest surgery, including breast implants, may have galactorrhea with normal serum prolactin levels. This is probably due to peripheral nerve stimulation.

Diagnostic Evaluation

The use of drugs or medications that stimulate prolactin production can be ruled out by history.

The most consistently abnormal hormone response in patients with a pituitary tumor is the failure of TRH to induce a rise in serum prolactin. If the increase of serum prolactin following an intravenous bolus of 500 mg of TRH is blunted or does not triple over the baseline level, an MRI to rule out a prolactinoma should be ordered. The TRH test is clinically useful only in patients with hyperprolactinemia of 20 to 60 ng/ml. Patients with serum prolactin levels above 60 ng/ml need to have an MRI of the sella turcica.

Hyperprolactinemia, Pituitary Adenomas, and the Menstrual Cycle. Patients with galactorrhea, regular menses, and a normal serum prolactin (<20 ng/ml) are at low risk to have a prolactin-secreting pituitary adenoma. These patients should be followed annually with measurement of serum prolactin. If it becomes elevated, further work-up is necessary, even in the presence of normal menses.

Patients with oligomenorrhea, galactorrhea, and normal prolactin levels should have an anteroposterior and lateral cone view x-ray study of the sella turcica. If necessary, a skull MRI will confirm the diagnosis of empty sella. Patients with secondary amenorrhea and low levels of serum estrogen (<40 pg/ml) have a significantly greater risk of having a pituitary adenoma. Regardless of the menstrual pattern, if the serum prolactin level is between 20 and 60 ng/ml, a TRH test is indicated. If the test result is normal, the patient should be followed annually with a TRH test. If the test result becomes abnormal (less than three times the baseline), a skull MRI is indicated. If the initial serum prolactin level is greater than 60 ng/ml, a skull MRI should be performed without a TRH test.

Treatment of Galactorrhea and Hyperprolactinemia

The objectives of therapy for patients with galactorrhea or hyperprolactinemia include (1) the elimination of lactation, (2) the establishment of normal estrogen secretion, (3) the induction of ovulation, and (4) the treatment of prolactin-secreting pituitary adenomas. The recommended forms of management are periodic observation, drug therapy, surgery, and radiation.

Periodic Observation

This form of management is indicated in menstruating women with galactorrhea who either have normal serum prolactin levels or have idiopathic elevations of prolactin. As long as the galactorrhea is not socially embarrassing and the patient has regular or irregular menses, there is no need to institute any treatment. Patients with oligomenorrhea can be treated with progestins to induce regular uterine bleeding. Long-term treatment with bromocriptine is unnecessary since no risk is known to occur in euestrogenic patients with idiopathic hyperprolactinemia.

Observation can be extended to some women with radiologic evidence of a microadenoma (<1 cm in diameter). Because the growth rate of microadenomas is slow, an annual measurement of serum prolactin and a skull MRI every 2 to 3 years is appropriate in selected patients. Only a small percentage of women with a microadenoma who do not receive any treatment have an increase in size of the tumor.

Drug Therapy

Patients with primary hypothyroidism should be treated with T_4. Patients with hyperprolactinemia and low estrogen levels are at increased risk to develop osteoporosis and cardiovascular disease. Bromocriptine induces a cyclic and physiologic estrogen secretion. Ninety-five per cent of women without radiographic evidence of an adenoma require 5 mg/day. About 50 per cent of those with an adenoma require higher doses of bromocriptine to resume regular menses. Menses resume and galactorrhea resolves after about 6 weeks of bromocriptine therapy in women without an adenoma. If an adenoma is present, bromocriptine takes another 3 or 4 weeks to become effective. Discontinuation of therapy usually results in the return of hyperprolactinemia, leading to galactorrhea and amenorrhea. Fewer than 10 per cent of patients will remain euprolactinemic following 2 or more years of uninterrupted therapy.

Patients with a pituitary macroadenoma should have a repeat MRI 6 months after reaching the full therapeutic dose of bromocriptine. As long as shrinkage of the adenoma is demonstrated, bromocriptine therapy is continued. After obtaining maximal shrinkage of the adenoma, adenomectomy may be considered for some patients. Surgery should also be performed in patients who do not respond to bromocriptine therapy.

The induction of ovulation in patients with hyperprolactinemia can be accomplished with bromocriptine. Approximately 50 per cent of women will require only 5 mg/day; the remaining patients will require larger doses. The length of treatment necessary to induce ovulation in women with a pituitary adenoma (16 weeks) is significantly longer than that in patients without an adenoma (10 weeks). Restoration of normal menstrual cycles and pregnancy may occur without complete normalization of the serum prolactin level. Bromocriptine therapy is discontinued as soon as the pregnancy is confirmed, unless the patient has a macroadenoma, in which case the treatment is maintained throughout pregnancy.

Several studies have shown that most patients do not have a significant enlargement of the adenoma during pregnancy. The patient's visual fields should be examined, however, at 20, 28, and 38 weeks. If abnormal visual fields develop, a limited MRI is indicated. If suprasellar extension is demonstrated, bromocriptine treatment should be instituted or increased and maintained for the rest of the pregnancy. There is no increase in fetal malformations as a result of bromocriptine treatment, and the drug can be discontinued after the completion of pregnancy to allow for unrestricted breast feeding. Radiographic studies of the pituitary should be repeated 10 to 12 weeks after completion of pregnancy. In patients not responding to bromocriptine, adenomectomy can be performed during the pregnancy since no increased surgical morbidity has been reported.

In 50 to 70 per cent of women, the oral administration of bromocriptine is associated with nausea, vomiting, headaches, and dizziness. Most of these side effects are mild and tend to be short-lived if the medication is taken with food. In up to 10 per cent of patients, however, bromocriptine needs to be discontinued because of severe side effects. For women with severe nausea or vomiting, vaginal bromocriptine administration is a viable alternative.

Surgery

The transsphenoidal route for the microsurgical exploration of the sella turcica permits the removal of the pituitary adenoma (adenomectomy) while preserving the functional capacity of the remaining gland. Cure rates of 50 to 80 per cent have been reported for patients with microadenomas and 10 to 30 per cent for patients with macroadenomas. Transient or definitive diabetes insipidus, hemorrhage, meningitis, cerebrospinal fluid leak, and panhypopituitarism have been reported following adenomectomy. Fifty per cent of patients followed for 5 to 10 years after successful adenomectomy will develop recurrence of hyperprolactinemia without radiologic evidence of tumor. Considering the good results obtained with bromocriptine, the low rate of side effects, and the possibility of reducing the adenoma size, surgery should be instituted only in patients with complete or partial failure of medical therapy or poor compliance. Patients with extrasellar extension of the adenoma may be treated surgically after maximum reduction of the tumor size has been obtained with bromocriptine. Surgery should be performed without discontinuing bromocriptine because a rapid regrowth of the adenoma can occur.

Radiation Therapy

Cobalt radiation (4500 cGy) may arrest the growth of a pituitary adenoma. Following this treatment, however, regular menses usually do not return and it takes up to 1 year for the galactorrhea to be corrected. Because the adenoma tissue may be more resistant than the surrounding organs, secondary hypothalamic or pituitary damage can occur. Alternatively, heavy-particle irradiation has been used, but visual field defects or oculomotor palsies have been reported. Neither form of radiation therapy is recommended.

ABNORMAL UTERINE BLEEDING

Menstruation is considered normal when bleeding occurs every 21 to 35 days and lasts for 1 to 5 days. Abnormal uterine bleeding occurs when the frequency or intensity of uterine bleeding changes. The following types of abnormal uterine bleeding can occur:

1. *Hypermenorrhea* or *menorrhagia,* which is defined as cyclic or regular menstrual bleeding that is excessive in either amount or duration.

2. *Hypomenorrhea,* which is defined as a diminished menstrual flow. Sometimes there is only vaginal spotting.

3. *Polymenorrhea,* which is defined as episodes of vaginal bleeding occurring more frequently than every 21 days.

4. *Oligomenorrhea,* which is defined as episodic vaginal bleeding occurring at intervals greater than 35 days.

5. *Metrorrhagia,* which is defined as uterine bleeding occurring between menstrual periods.

6. *Menometrorrhagia,* which is defined as uterine bleeding that is irregular in frequency and also excessive in amount.

7. *Postmenopausal bleeding,* which is any vaginal bleeding that occurs at least 1 year following the cessation of spontaneous menstruation.

8. *Estrogen withdrawal bleeding,* which occurs following the acute cessation of estrogen after constant exposure to estrogen.

9. *Breakthrough bleeding,* which occurs during chronic estrogen stimulation without any decline in estrogen levels.

10. *Progesterone withdrawal bleeding,* which occurs after the administration and sudden discontinuation of progesterone or a gestagen. Bleeding can occur only if the endometrium has been previously stimulated with estrogen.

11. *Progesterone breakthrough bleeding,* which occurs only when there is a high ratio of progesterone to estrogen or when there is insufficient estrogen.

Some types of abnormal uterine bleeding are seen in specific circumstances, such as hypomenorrhea that is frequently seen during oral contraceptive use. Oligomenorrhea is frequently seen in anovulatory cycles, and menometrorrhagia is seen when organic pathology is present. This loose association is not sufficient, however, to make a diagnosis.

Gynecologic cases of abnormal bleeding include alterations of the hypothalamic pituitary-ovarian axis resulting in anovulation and pathologic abnormalities of the uterus such as uterine myomas and endometrial or cervical polyps or carcinomas. Therefore, a complete history, physical examination, and appropriate laboratory evaluation should be performed in most cases before instituting any therapeutic modalities. Abnormal uterine bleeding can also occur in association with nongynecologic diseases. Examples include blood clotting disorders, like thrombocytopenia and von Willebrand's disease, or leukemia.

DYSFUNCTIONAL UTERINE BLEEDING

Dysfunctional uterine bleeding is defined as bleeding occurring from a proliferative endometrium as a result of anovulation in the absence of any organic disease. It is a diagnosis of exclusion in which local and systemic diseases must be ruled out. About 50 per cent of these patients are at least 40 years of age and another 20 per cent are adolescents, as these are the times when anovulatory cycles are more commonly seen.

The mechanism of chronic anovulation may be different in adolescents than in older women. In adolescents, blood concentrations of both estrone and estradiol are in the normal range, but the positive estrogen feedback effect that induces the midcycle LH surge is absent, thereby resulting in anovulation. On the other hand, studies performed in patients with perimenopausal dysfunctional uterine bleeding demonstrate that the hypothalamic-pituitary axis is intact, but the ovarian response to gonadotropin is diminished. Therefore, abnormal ovarian function seems to be the primary cause of abnormal bleeding in these patients.

Dysfunctional uterine bleeding occurring during the reproductive age could be due to various causes such as failure of the positive feedback effect of estrogen, abnormal peripheral conversion of androgen to estrogen, or an endometrial defect that could be either at the receptor level or in the secretion or release of prostaglandins.

In the absence of progesterone secretion (anovulation) and under persistent estrogen stimulation, the endometrium proliferates, reaching an abnormal height. There is intense vascularity and glandular growth without stromal support. The endometrium finally outgrows the stimulation produced by estrogen and bleeding occurs, with irregular endometrial shedding.

Investigation of Dysfunctional Uterine Bleeding

A careful history and pelvic examination should be performed on all patients. The extent of laboratory evaluation should be individualized depending on the patient's age and the severity of the bleeding. In general, all patients should have a Papanicolaou smear, a pregnancy test, and a complete blood count. With the exception of the very young patient, an endometrial biopsy for tissue diagnosis should be obtained in most patients. Usually it can be performed in the office using the Pipelle curette.

Management of Dysfunctional Uterine Bleeding

Some patients may require supportive therapy with iron or blood transfusions. Those with a normal pelvic examination and with proliferative endometrium confirmed at endometrial biopsy are best treated with hormonal therapy. Patients who fail to respond to hormonal therapy rapidly or those older than 35 years of age should have a curettage to rule out endometrial carcinoma. Patients failing to respond to hormonal therapy also may have a submucosal myoma or endometrial polyp and may require a hysterosalpingogram or hysteroscopy for diagnosis and treatment.

Hormonal therapy includes progestins alone, oral contraceptives, or sequential estrogen-progestin therapy. If the initial endometrial biopsy demonstrates proliferative endometrium, the treatment of choice is 5 mg of medroxyprogesterone acetate daily, either for the first 13 days of every month or for 13 consecutive days starting on day 14 of the cycle. This treatment will convert the proliferative endometrium into a secretory-like type and prevent recurrent bleeding. Progestin therapy should be continued for as long as necessary. If the patient wishes to conceive, clomiphene citrate is the treatment of choice.

If the initial endometrial biopsy demonstrates secretory endometrium and the abnormal bleeding persists or recurs, a pathologic defect within the uterine cavity should be suspected and hysterosalpingography or hysteroscopy performed. Treatment of the acute episode of bleeding can be accomplished using either oral contraceptives alone or a sequential estrogen-progestin combination. Both methods are equally effective in arresting the bleeding episode. If oral contraceptives are prescribed, 4 tablets a day should be used for 7 days. Usually bleeding will cease within 24 to 48 hours. The patient should be informed that at the end of this treatment heavier than usual vaginal bleeding may ensue. The patient should be continued on a daily dose of oral contraceptives as prescribed for contraception and maintained for at least 6 months.

If a decision is made to use the sequential estrogen-progestin therapy, treatment should commence with 2.5 mg of oral conjugated estrogen four times a day for 21 consecutive days. Five mg of medroxyprogesterone acetate daily is added during the last 10 days of treatment and then both steroids are discontinued. Usually vaginal bleeding occurs a few days later. Monthly administration of oral medroxyprogesterone acetate will prevent future abnormal uterine bleeding. The administration of intravenous estrogen offers no advantage over its oral administration.

Several reports have established that the use of prostaglandin synthetase inhibitors are useful in reducing blood loss in women with menorrhagia. Women presenting with abnormal uterine bleeding associated with submucous myomata, blood clotting disorders, or leukemia may be best treated with monthly intramuscular injections with GnRH agonists. This treatment is reversible and produces a medical oophorectomy.

SUGGESTED READING

Burrow GN, Wortzman G, Rewcastle NB, et al: Microadenomas of the pituitary and abnormal sellar tomograms in an unselected autopsy series. N Engl J Med 304:156, 1981.

Drinkwater BL, Nilson K, Chesnut C, et al: Bone mineral content of amenorrheic and eumenorrheic athletes. N Engl J Med 311:277, 1984.

Fraser IS, Michie EA, Wide L, Baird DT: Pituitary gonadotropins and ovarian function in adolescent dysfunctional bleeding. J Clin Endocrinol Metab 37:407, 1973.

Kletzky OA, Davajan V, Nakamura RM, Mishell DR Jr: Clinical categorization of patients with secondary amenorrhea using progesterone induced uterine bleeding and measurement of serum gonadotropin levels. Am J Obstet Gynecol 121:695, 1975.

Kletzky OA, Marrs RP, Davajan V: Management of patients with hyperprolactinemia and normal or abnormal tomograms. Am J Obstet Gynecol 147:528, 1983.

Kletzky OA, Vermesh M: Effectiveness of vaginal bromocriptine in treating women with hyperprolactinemia. Fertil Steril 51:269, 1989.

March CM, Mishell DR Jr, Kletzky OA, et al: Galactorrhea and pituitary tumors in postpill and nonpostpill amenorrhea. Am J Obstet Gynecol 134:45, 1979.

Martin TL, Kim M, Malarkey WB: The natural history of idiopathic hyperprolactinemia. J Clin Endocrinol Metab 60:855, 1985.

Mashchak CA, Kletzky OA, Davajan V, Mishell DR Jr: Clinical and laboratory evaluation of patients with primary amenorrhea. Obstet Gynecol 57:715, 1981.

Forty-nine

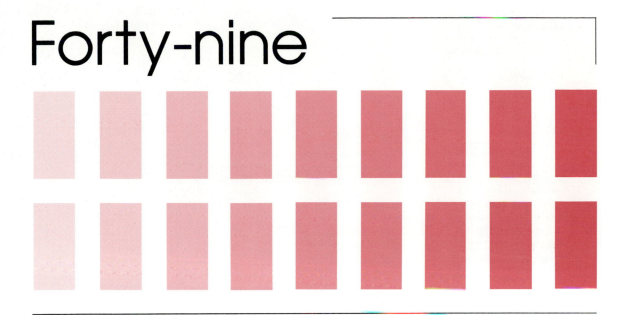

Virilism and Hirsutism

R. JEFFREY CHANG

Virilism and hirsutism are clinical manifestations of increased androgen effect. Androgens are produced by the ovaries and adrenal glands in women. The effects of these hormones are related to their production rates, their transportation in the circulation, and the target organ response. The most common abnormality is an increased production rate, which may arise from a functional or neoplastic process. Thus, the evaluation of virilism and hirsutism is directed toward exclusion of an androgen-secreting tumor and identification of the site of hormone production.

NORMAL ANDROGEN METABOLISM

Androgens represent a class of steroid hormones that are structurally related to estrogens and progestins. The formation of an-drogens results from the metabolism of cholesterol via the Δ^5 or Δ^4 pathway (Fig. 49–1). Glucocorticoids (cortisol), mineralocorticoids (aldosterone), estrogens, and progestins are also derived from the metabolic breakdown of cholesterol. The most commonly studied androgens are testosterone, androstenedione, dehydroepiandrosterone (DHEA), and dehydroepiandrosterone sulfate (DHEA-S). Other androgens exist that may possess greater or lesser biological potency. The stimulus for ovarian androgen production is pituitary luteinizing hormone (LH); that for the adrenal gland is pituitary adrenocorticotropic hormone (ACTH).

Approximately one half of serum testosterone and androstenedione originates from the ovary, whereas the other half arises from the adrenal gland. DHEA and DHEA-S are chiefly products of adrenal androgen production and, as such, serve as markers for this tissue. The circulating levels, rates of produc-

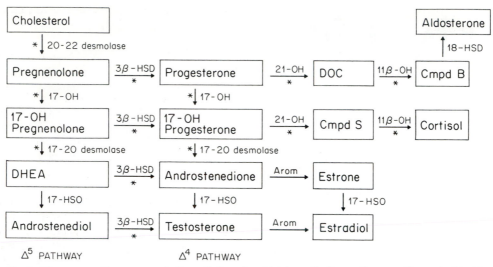

Figure 49–1. Diagrammatic representation of the steroid biosynthetic pathways. The asterisk (*) refers to specific enzyme defects that result in congenital adrenal hyperplasia. OH = hydroxylase; HSD = hydroxysteroid dehydrogenase; HSO = hydroxysteroid oxidoreductase; Arom = aromatase.

tion, and metabolic clearance rates of the common androgens are shown in Table 49–1. After secretion by the ovaries or adrenals, most androgens are bound to specific protein hormones in the circulation. In the bound form, androgens are biologically inactive. For example, in normal women, approximately 99 per cent of serum testosterone is protein-bound and, thus, inactive. The active nonprotein-bound or free fraction represents only about 1 per cent of the total circulating testosterone.

When androgens reach the target tissue, they are further metabolized, which may result in more potent intracellular hormones. Testosterone is converted within the cell to dihydrotestosterone, which possesses greater biological potency than its precursor. The skin is capable of this conversion. The pilosebaceous unit in the skin consists of the sebaceous gland and hair follicle, both of which are sensitive to androgens. The development, growth, and activity of these units appear to be regulated by hormonal as well as genetic

Table 49–1. MEAN VALUES FOR THE PLASMA CONCENTRATION, PRODUCTION RATE, AND METABOLIC CLEARANCE RATE (MCR) OF VARIOUS ANDROGENS IN NORMAL PREMENOPAUSAL WOMEN*

ANDROGEN	PLASMA CONCENTRATION (ng/ml)	PRODUCTION RATE (mg/day)	MCR (L/day)
Testosterone	0.31	0.27	830
Androstenedione	1.90	3.44	1900
DHEA	4.20	6.34	1500
DHEA-S	1700.00	28.90	17

* Modified with permission from Abraham GE: Adrenal androgens in hirsutism. In Genazzani AR, Thijssen JHH, Siiteri PK (eds): Adrenal Androgens. New York, Raven Press, 1980, p 268.

factors. The sebaceous component is more sensitive to androgen stimulation than is the hair follicle.

ABNORMAL ANDROGEN METABOLISM

Hirsutism and virilism are the principal clinical signs of excess androgen production. Hirsutism, defined as excessive body hair, is most commonly manifested by excessive facial hair on the sideburns, chin, and upper lip. Increased body hair occurs as an extension of pubic hair toward the umbilicus, on the chest, or in the periareolar area of the breast. Frequently, hirsutism is accompanied by oily skin and acne. If the hyperandrogenism is severe, virilizing signs may be present. These include temporal balding, deepening of the voice, a male body habitus, and clitoromegaly.

Functional Adrenal Disorders

Two major conditions comprise functional disorders of the adrenal gland resulting in hirsutism or virilism: congenital adrenal hyperplasia and Cushing's syndrome.

Congenital Adrenal Hyperplasia

Congenital adrenal hyperplasia is a general term used to describe an assortment of clinical entities that arise from inborn errors of steroid synthesis. Symptomatology associated with each entity is due to steroid overproduction, underproduction, or both, secondary to an enzyme deficiency. Although there have been six enzyme-deficiency states associated with congenital adrenal hyperplasia, only three lead to androgen overproduction and hirsutism or virilism.

The most common condition is 21-hydroxylase deficiency. In 20 per cent of cases, the defect is complete, whereas in 80 per cent it is incomplete or partial. The most severe form of the disease usually occurs in the neonate and is manifest by ambiguous genitalia in female newborns and life-threatening salt-wasting. Fortunately, in the majority of cases, the enzyme deficiency is only partial, which accounts for lack of salt-wasting in 50 per cent of patients.

This disorder has been recognized in young women soon after puberty (late onset 21-hydroxylase deficiency). In these patients, the diagnosis is discovered after an evaluation of hirsutism or virilization. The diagnosis is suggested by an adolescent onset of severe hirsutism or virilism, particularly in the presence of regular menstrual function.

Because 21-hydroxylase is responsible for the conversion of 17-hydroxyprogesterone to desoxycortisol (compound S), a deficiency of this enzyme results in an accumulation of the precursor hormone, which is detectable in the circulation (see Fig. 49–1). As a result, this specific enzyme disorder is marked by an elevated serum 17-hydroxyprogesterone level as well as increases in its Δ^4 metabolites androstenedione and testosterone. This disease is inherited as an autosomal recessive trait, and there is a familial tendency of occurrence. Thus far, only 21-hydroxylase deficiency has been found to exhibit this familial tendency.

The second most common condition is 11-β hydroxylase deficiency, which is associated with hirsutism or virilism and hypertension as a result of excessive production of androgens and mineralocorticoids. In contrast to 21-hydroxylase deficiency, salt-retention may exist because of an accumulation of desoxycorticosterone (DOC). Testosterone and androstenedione are usually elevated, whereas DHEA-S is uncommonly increased.

A rare cause of congenital adrenal hyperplasia resulting in androgen excess is 3-β hydroxysteroid dehydrogenase deficiency. This condition is marked by a decrease of testosterone, mineralocorticoid, and glucocorticoid. DHEA-S, however, is elevated. Affected genetic males fail to develop normal external genitalia secondary to a lack of testosterone, whereas females are slightly masculinized by the overproduction of DHEA-S.

Cushing's Syndrome

The second major adrenal disease leading to excess androgen production is Cushing's syndrome, in which a constellation of clinical features occurs as a result of hy-

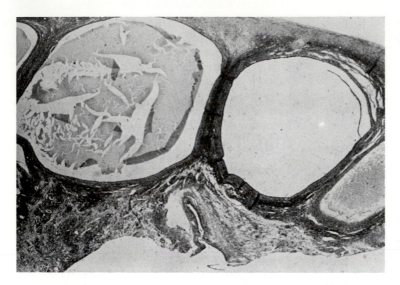

Figure 49–2. Low-power magnification of a polycystic ovary showing multiple cystic follicles with dense overlying cortical stroma.

percortisolism. Characteristic manifestations include truncal obesity, moon-like facies, hypertension, impaired glucose tolerance, muscle wasting, osteoporosis, abdominal striae, and easy bruisability. Other symptoms include hirsutism, acne, and irregular menstrual function. Emotional lability is common in Cushing's syndrome. This disorder may arise from a cortisol-producing tumor or from excessive ACTH production, which serves to overstimulate the adrenal glands.

Adrenal Neoplasms

Adrenal tumors resulting in androgenization without symptoms and signs of glucocorticoid excess are rare. Glucocorticoid-producing adenomas are usually associated with minimal, if any, elevation of androgens. Adenomas, which produce androgens only, generally secrete large amounts of DHEA-S. Adrenal carcinomas may produce large amounts of both glucocorticoids and androgens.

Functional Ovarian Disorders

Polycystic Ovarian Syndrome

In general, 1 to 4 per cent of women of reproductive age suffer from polycystic ovarian syndrome (PCO) (Fig. 49–2). The hallmark features of this disorder are (1) andro-

gen excess, (2) chronic anovulation, and (3) anabolic effect. Clinically, the most common symptoms are hirsutism (90 per cent), menstrual irregularity (90 per cent), and infertility (75 per cent). Obesity is found in approximately one half of patients, and 15 per cent of patients are virilized. In most patients, the ovaries contain multiple follicle cysts that are inactive and arrested in the midantral stage of development. The ovarian stroma consists of luteinized thecal cells that produce androgens.

In PCO, hyperandrogenism commonly results from an overproduction of androgen by both the ovary and the adrenal gland. These hormonal abnormalities may represent a vicious cycle of events that perpetuate the syndrome. Pituitary LH levels are increased and stimulate excess ovarian androgen production leading to hirsutism and acne. The excessive amounts of androgen are peripherally converted to estrogen. Since patients with PCO fail to ovulate, their estrogen secretion is acyclic and unopposed by progesterone. The unopposed estrogens may cause adenomatous hyperplasia of the endometrium or even endometrial carcinoma. Other important effects of the increased estrogen secretion are the stimulation of pituitary LH release and the inhibition of follicle-stimulating hormone (FSH) release. Increased LH results in the continued androgen production, whereas decreased FSH is largely responsible for the chronic anovulation.

PCO is unique in that excessive androgen production originates from both the adrenal glands and the ovaries. The mechanism of excess adrenal androgen production is unknown. Basal ACTH concentrations in PCO are similar to those of normal ovulating women. The secretion pattern of ACTH over 24 hours in this disease has not been reported, although normal circadian rhythms of cortisol have been observed, which suggest that corresponding ACTH release is normal. These findings imply that in PCO, factors other than ACTH stimulate adrenal androgen production, adrenal androgen responsiveness to ACTH is altered, or both.

A pituitary factor other than ACTH may contribute to stimulation of adrenal steroidogenesis, in particular adrenal androgens. This putative adrenal androgen-stimulating factor (CASH) has not been identified as yet. Moreover, the precise relationship of CASH to ACTH is not clear.

Hyperthecosis and Hilus Cell Hyperplasia

Hyperthecosis and hilus cell hyperplasia are also examples of chronic stimulation of the ovarian stroma caused by disruption of feedback signals to the hypothalamus and pituitary. In hyperthecosis, nests of luteinized stroma are seen. The appearance of the remainder of the ovary is similar to PCO. Hyperthecosis may be simply one part of the spectrum of the ovarian response to overstimulation.

Hilus cell hyperplasia is seen most often when estrogen feedback from ovarian follicles is minimal or absent as a result of gonadal dysgenesis, menopause, or, occasionally, gonadotropin-resistant ovary syndrome. The resulting elevation of gonadotropin leads to hilus cell hyperplasia, which is functionally significant in only a minority of patients with the above-mentioned disturbances.

Ovarian Neoplasms

Androgen-producing ovarian tumors are extremely uncommon. An arrhenoblastoma or Sertoli-Leydig cell tumor usually gives rise to a palpable mass, a large overproduction of testosterone, and a lesser increase of androstenedione. Hilus cell tumors are often nonpalpable and similarly give rise mainly to an increase in testosterone. Lipoid cell tumors, probably stromal in origin, are also frequently nonpalpable and produce androstenedione and testosterone in large amounts. Finally, there are virilizing conditions associated with hyperplasia of the stroma surrounding neoplasms, which themselves generally do not produce androgens. These tumors include cystic teratomas, Brenner tumors, serous cystadenomas, and Krukenberg's tumors, all of which are frequently associated with increased androstenedione production.

Idiopathic Hirsutism

Occasionally, some patients exhibit mild to moderate hirsutism without an elevation in circulating levels of androgens. This condition has been referred to as "familial," "constitutional," or "idiopathic" hirsutism. Serum 3-α-androstanediol glucuronide levels are increased in these individuals compared with those of normal women. Because 3-α-androstanediol glucuronide is derived from intracellular testosterone metabolism, the excess hair growth may occur as a result of increased tissue utilization of testosterone.

EVALUATION

Hirsutism and virilism are elevated by history, physical examination, and laboratory assessment.

History

Functional disorders often first appear in the pubertal period and tend to progress slowly, with the signs of androgen excess developing over several years. In contrast, neoplastic disorders can occur at any time. They most often arise several years after puberty, however, and their manifestations appear abruptly. Progression is rapid, and these patients frequently present with frank virilism. There is some overlap with functional disorders; 15 per cent of PCO patients can also exhibit signs of virilization, particularly temporal balding or clitoromegaly.

Evaluation of a Tumor

Physical Examination

A bimanual pelvic examination may identify ovarian enlargement. Asymmetrical ovarian enlargement associated with the rapid onset of virilizing signs usually indicates an androgen-producing tumor. Adrenal neoplasms are usually nonpalpable, and laboratory techniques are required for their diagnosis.

Laboratory Evaluation

The laboratory evaluation of patients with virilism, hirsutism, or both is aimed primarily at identification of a neoplastic disorder. The most appropriate screening tests are measurement of serum total testosterone and DHEA-S. DHEA-S serves as a marker of adrenal androgen production and is extremely useful in the detection of an adrenal neoplasm. Values of DHEA-S in excess of 8000 ng/ml should be viewed as highly suspicious for an adrenal tumor.

Marked elevations of testosterone may indicate the presence of an ovarian or adrenal androgen-producing tumor. About 80 per cent of patients with an androgen-producing ovarian tumor have peripheral testosterone concentrations over 200 ng/dl. Because only rare patients with functional disorders have levels above 200 ng/dl, such a finding demands that a neoplasm be ruled out.

Almost 20 per cent of patients with tumors have levels under 200 ng/dl, and there is a broad overlap with functional disease. In this group of patients, clinical features, such as the sudden onset and rapid progression of signs, are important in raising sufficient suspicion to go on to more definitive evaluation. Virilism is present in 98 per cent of tumors, regardless of the peripheral level of testosterone.

A pelvic sonogram should be done whenever any high-risk features are present and the ovaries cannot be adequately delineated clinically. Androgen-secreting tumors of the adrenal gland may occasionally be detected by CT scan. Magnetic resonance imaging of the adrenal glands may prove very helpful.

If any of these factors suggests the presence of an androgen-secreting tumor and it cannot be located by pelvic examination, sonogram, or adrenal computed tomographic scan, selective venous catheterization should be carried out and androgens measured in the venous blood from each adrenal gland and ovary. Selective venous catheterization is well suited to the localization of an ovarian neoplasm, particularly one measuring 5 cm or less in diameter.

Evaluation of a Functional Disorder

Once an androgen-producing tumor has been excluded, attention is focused on possible functional disorders. With respect to the ovary, the presence of hirsutism and oligomenorrhea indicates PCO in the vast majority of cases.

Physical Examination

Approximately half of the patients are obese and many exhibit evidence of acne. On physical examination, the ovaries are usually bilaterally cystic and enlarged, although in some women ovarian enlargement does not occur. The diagnosis is based primarily on the history and physical examination, with an assessment of circulating androgens to rule out a neoplasm.

Laboratory Tests

Serum 17-Hydroxyprogesterone. In the presence of regular menstrual cycles, congenital adrenal hyperplasia due to 21-hydroxylase deficiency should be considered. The appropriate screening test for this condition is a serum 17-hydroxyprogesterone obtained at 8:00 AM. The time of day is important. Steroid levels are greatest in the early morning owing to the normal diurnal adrenal secretion pattern. Concentrations above 3 ng/ml warrant an ACTH stimulation test as the definitive method of diagnosis. Since ACTH regulates steroid production by the adrenal gland, subtle enzyme deficiencies are exaggerated by its administration.

Adrenocorticotropic Hormone Stimulation Test. One milligram of dexamethasone is given at bedtime on the night before testing. This suppresses endogenous ACTH secretion, which may interfere with the steroid response. The following morning, after an overnight fast, ACTH (Cortrosyn), 0.25 mg, is injected intravenously. Blood samples are obtained before and 1 hour after injection. In normal individuals, baseline 17-hydroxyprogesterone levels are less than 3 ng/ml and rise twofold to threefold in response to ACTH. In most instances, maximal stimulation does not exceed 5 ng/ml. In patients with 21-hydroxylase deficiency, the 17-hydroxyprogesterone response to ACTH is greater than that of normal individuals and may achieve peak levels in excess of 100 ng/ml.

Dexamethasone Suppression Test. If Cushing's syndrome is suspected, an overnight dexamethasone suppression test should be done. Dexamethasone, 1 mg, is given orally at bedtime, and blood is drawn at 8:00 AM after an overnight fast. This dose of dexamethasone suppresses serum cortisol concentrations to less than 5 μg/100 ml in the normal person. Occasionally, false-positive (> 5 μg/100 ml) results are found, which can be due to obesity or a poor night of sleep. If cortisol levels are nonsuppressible, a formal low-dose, high-dose dexamethasone suppression test should be done.

TREATMENT

Treatment of hirsutism or virilism is determined by the nature of the underlying disease, the clinical symptoms and signs, and the ultimate desires of the patient. If an ovarian or adrenal neoplasm exists, surgical removal of the tumor is indicated. In premenopausal women, unilateral salpingo-oophorectomy is usually sufficient for an ovarian tumor and preserves future childbearing potential. In postmenopausal women, the treatment of choice is a total abdominal hysterectomy and bilateral salpingo-oophorectomy.

PCO is by far the most common functional ovarian disorder causing hirsutism. If necessary, therapy for the hirsutism is ovarian suppression, which is best achieved by administration of an estrogen-progestin oral contraceptive. Estrogen-progestin treatment suppresses gonadotropins, which allows regression of the testosterone and androstenedione overproduction by the ovary. The estrogen component also stimulates sex hormone–binding globulin, which decreases free testosterone. Estrogen-progestin also causes regular cyclic bleeding and progestin opposition to the estrogenic stimulation of the endometrium. The use of an estrogen-progestin combination is not without risk, particularly in women who are smokers and over the age of 35.

Treatment of functional adrenal androgen excess is determined by the type of disorder. Congenital adrenal hyperplasia is treated by the administration of glucocorticoid, which replaces any deficient cortisol and provides sufficient negative pituitary feedback to restore normal ACTH secretion. Cushing's syndrome should be treated by surgical removal of the source of excess cortisol or ACTH.

Corticosteroid administration is not without risk. Significant long-term complications include osteoporosis and adrenal atrophy. Bothersome side effects, such as weight gain, fluid retention, and emotional disturbances, may also occur.

Antiandrogenic Agents

Antiandrogenic agents have been advocated for the treatment of hirsutism, particularly when ovarian or adrenal suppression has failed or is contraindicated. The most commonly used drug in the United States is spironolactone. This aldosterone antagonist competes for testosterone-binding sites, thereby exerting a direct antiandrogenic effect at the target organ. In addition, spironolactone interferes with steroid enzymes and decreases testosterone production. Because this medication opposes the action of aldosterone, serum potassium levels may rise and, therefore, should be monitored.

Cyproterone acetate, a potent antiandrogen that has received wide acceptance, particularly in Europe, has demonstrated a beneficial effect in the vast majority of patients treated. This drug is not available for clinical use in the United States. Another antiandrogen is cimetidine. Its utility in the treatment of hirsutism, however, has not been fully substantiated.

Cosmetic Treatment

Suppression of abnormal androgen production generally halts hair growth but does not immediately cause the hirsutism to disappear. Improvement of the hirsutism may not be observed for up to 1 year, at which time most old hairs have degenerated and fallen out. To obtain good cosmetic results, some local hair removal is usually required in addition to the biochemical manipulation. Local methods include shaving, depilatory creams, and electrolysis. Plucking of individual hairs should be discouraged because growth of surrounding hair follicles is stimulated by this technique.

Treatment of Infertility

Because most women suffering from androgen excess also exhibit infrequent or absent menses, infertility is a common problem. In this group of women, it is often necessary to induce ovulation with clomiphene citrate or human menopausal gonadotropin, sometimes coupled with corticosteroid suppression (see Chapter 51). Overall, these methods of ovulation induction have proved extremely successful.

SUGGESTED READING

Abraham GE: Adrenal androgens in hirsutism. In Genazzani AR, Thijssen JHH, Siiteri PK (eds): Adrenal Androgens. New York, Raven Press, 1980, p 267.

Abraham GE: Ovarian and adrenal contribution to peripheral androgens during the menstrual cycle. J Clin Endocrinol Metab 39:340, 1974.

Adreyko JL, Monroe SE, Jaffe RB: Treatment of hirsutism with a gonadotropin-releasing hormone agonist (Nafarelin). J Clin Endocrinol Metab 63:854, 1986.

Chang RJ, Mandel FP, Wolfsen AR, Judd HL: Circulating levels of plasma adrenocorticotropin in polycystic ovarian disease. J Clin Endocrinol Metab 54:1265, 1982.

Chapman MG, Dowsett M, Dewhurst CT, Jeffcoate SL: Spironolactone in combination with an oral contraceptive: An alternative treatment for hirsutism. Br J Obstet Gynaecol 92:983, 1985.

Goldzieher JW: Polycystic ovarian disease. Fertil Steril 35:371, 1981.

Greep N, Hoopes M, Horton R: Androstenediol glucuronide plasma clearance and production rates in normal and hirsute women. J Clin Endocrinol Metab 62:22, 1986.

Lobo RA, Shoupe D, Serafini P, et al: The effects of two doses of spironolactone on serum androgens and anagen hair in hirsute women. Fertil Steril 43:200, 1985.

Meldrum DR, Abraham GE: Peripheral and ovarian venous concentrations of various steroid hormones in virilizing ovarian tumors. Obstet Gynecol 53:36, 1979.

Parker LN, Odell WD: Control of adrenal androgen secretion. Endocr Rev 1:392, 1980.

Yen SSC: The polycystic ovary syndrome. Clin Endocrinol 12:177, 1980.

Fifty

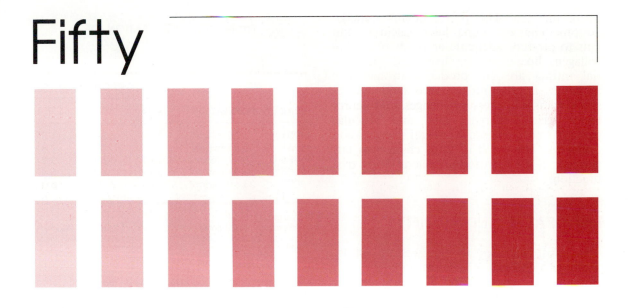

The Menopause

BARRY G. WREN

The menopause, as its name implies, is that time in a woman's life when she has her last menstrual period. It occurs because she no longer produces sufficient estrogen to maintain responsive tissue in an active physiologic mode. In most women, the menopause occurs between 50 and 55 years with an average of 51 years, but some women reach their menopause as early as the fourth decade, whereas a few may menstruate until they are in their sixties.

Women are born with about 1.5 million ova and reach their menarche with about 400,000. Most women menstruate about 400 times between the menarche and the menopause, but during this time they use all their responsive ova. When all these ova become atretic, the ovary is no longer capable of responding to pituitary gonadotropins, and the production of estrogen, progesterone, and other ovarian hormones is reduced. The result of these low levels of hormones is often

manifest by deleterious physical, psychological, and sexual changes in postmenopausal women. This postmenopausal phase is now being recognized as a time of decreased hormonal production with associated problems that reduce the quality and quantity of life for a large number of women.

Hormones are chemical messengers generated in one part of the body to produce a specific cellular response in another group of cells. Target or responsive tissue requires receptors to be present within the cell for the hormonal messenger to act and produce the appropriate response. It has now been established that receptors for estrogen are found in tissues as far distant from each other as the vagina, cervix, uterus, ovary, pelvic fascia, bladder, skin, bone, heart, arteries, liver, brain, muscle, breasts, and other endocrine glands. Although all may not be causally related, when estrogen levels are low or absent, cells within these tissues become relatively inactive. The pelvic organs undergo atrophic changes, bone loses calcium, skin fails to produce adequate amounts of quality collagen, lipases in the liver and the arterial intima are not produced in adequate amounts, arterial musculature tends to respond poorly to pressure changes, and neurologic tissue undergoes glial and reticular changes that may lead to neural transmission problems. The result of these changes in target cells is an increase in general body dysfunction.

MENOPAUSE AND SOCIETY

In most societies in the western world, about 13 to 14 per cent of the population are women over the age of 50 years. In the United States, this would suggest that about 33 million women are postmenopausal. If a woman lives to the age of 50 years, she can expect to live about another 30 years of her life in an estrogen-deficient state, during which time she will have an increasing number of sex hormone–related problems. These problems not only cause the individual woman considerable distress and disability but also place a strain on the scarce resources of the health care system. It has been stated that in Scandinavia, 70 per cent of the health care budget is being spent on those members of the community who will die within the following 8 months. Women over the age of 60 years occupy 40 per cent of all the health care beds available in Australia, and they consume about 28 per cent of the total health care "cake." Therefore, any reduction in the incidence of diseases in these older women will have a considerable impact on reducing total health costs. It is clear also that prophylactic medicine must play the greatest role in lowering health care costs in our aging population. In this regard, estrogen replacement therapy is likely to have a significant impact.

In 1986, Australia had about 10.5 per cent of its population over the age of 65 years and 23 per cent under the age of 15 years, but these figures are projected to change dramatically over the next 30 years (Table 50–1). By 2025, it is expected the population will include 16 to 17 per cent of elderly people and only 19 to 20 per cent of the young. The

Table 50–1. POPULATION OF AUSTRALIA, 1901–2025				
		PROPORTION AGED (%)		
YEAR	**POPULATION**	**<14**	**65–74**	**75+**
1901	3.79 million	35.2	3.0	1.0
1961	10.51 million	30.2	5.7	2.8
1986	15.97 million	23.2	6.6	3.9
2005	20.21 million*	20.9	6.9	5.4
2025	23.86 million*	19.1	9.5	6.6

* Estimated.
Information obtained from Economic Planning Advisory Council, Council Paper 29. Commonwealth of Australia, 1988.

burden of looking after the rapidly increasing older generation is likely to become difficult for the workforce to support unless every effort is made to keep the older members of society fit and independent of health care institutions.

HORMONAL CHANGES

The menopause rarely occurs as a sudden loss of ovarian function. For some years prior to the menopause, the ovary begins to show signs of impending failure. Anovulation becomes common, there is unopposed estrogen production, menstrual cycles become irregular, occasionally there are heavy menses or evidence of endometrial hyperplasia, and there are increasing mood and emotional changes with premenstrual syndrome symptoms becoming more marked. In some women, hot flashes (flushes) and sweats occur well before they reach their menopause. These *perimenopausal* symptoms usually last for 3 to 5 years before there is complete loss of menses or postmenopausal levels of hormones are reached.

Some women suffer a dramatic loss of estrogen. This usually occurs following a hysterectomy or other surgical intervention that removes or damages the ovaries or their blood supply. Occasionally women suffer an early ("artificial") menopause following surgery, chemotherapy, or radiotherapy for on-

Figure 50–1. Skin temperature of the finger and serum gonadotropin, estrone (E₁), and estradiol (E₂) levels in a woman with frequent hot flushes. Note the close correlation of skin temperature elevations and pulsatile LH release with occurrence of subjectively experienced hot flushes *(arrows)*. (From Meldrum DR, et al: Gonadotropins, estrogens, and adrenal steroids during menopausal hot flash. J Clin Endocrinol Metab 50:687, 1980.)

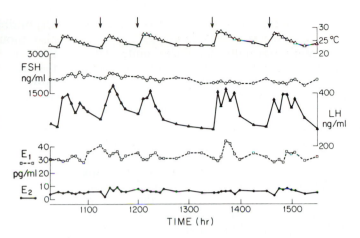

cologic diseases or endometriosis. Women who reach their menopause before the age of 40 years are said to have a *premature menopause.*

Some women continue to produce estrogen in quite adequate amounts for many years following their menopause. Androstenedione from the ovary or the adrenal gland is converted in peripheral fat to estrone, which is then capable of maintaining the vagina, skin, and bone in reasonable cellular tone and reducing the incidence of flushes and sweats. Although this unopposed estrogen is beneficial to women, it may be responsible for the increased incidence of endometrial cancer among obese women. For this reason, it is important that obese, postmenopausal women, who have no signs or symptoms of estrogen deficiency, have a regular check-up to monitor their endometrial and breast tissue.

OVARIAN DYSFUNCTION

The ovary produces a sequence of hormones during a normal menstrual cycle, each sequence being induced by gonadotropic hormones from the pituitary. Under the influence of luteinizing hormone (LH), cholesterol from the liver is converted in theca cells to pregnenolone. Pregnenolone then becomes the substrate for all further ovarian sex steroid genesis, and under the influence of enzymes within the granulosa and luteal cells, progesterone, androgen, and estrogen are produced (Fig. 50–1). The induction of these

sex hormones depends on the presence of viable ova and normal ovarian stroma and the production of follicle-stimulating hormone (FSH) and LH in adequate amounts. When the ovary becomes depleted of ova, the ability to ovulate and produce sex hormones is diminished. As women approach their menopause, ovulation becomes more infrequent, progesterone is often not produced or the levels are insufficient to induce endometrial changes, menses may become irregular (dysfunctional uterine bleeding), and premenstrual symptoms may become more prominent. Some women develop long episodes of amenorrhea during which estrogen levels are low and the first symptoms of the menopause occur. Hot flushes, sweats, and formication (feeling of ants in the skin) may be present, and mood changes, agitation, panic attacks, and depression are common complaints. This perimenopausal phase may last for 3 to 5 years before menses cease altogether; if no menses have occurred for 12 months or longer, the menopause can be said to have occurred.

Estrogen

Following the menopause, ovarian estradiol values decline to subfunctional levels (10 to 50 pgm/ml of estradiol are usual), but estrone levels may be higher. Estrone can be produced by peripheral conversion of androstenedione from the adrenal gland. In some women, the amount of postmenopausal estrogen can be quite considerable.

Androgens

Women normally produce quite large quantities of androgens during the metabolic conversion of cholesterol to estradiol. In this process, both androstenedione and testosterone are formed, and although the majority is aromatized to estradiol, some androgens circulate. It is claimed that androgens, particularly testosterone, are responsible for a sense of well-being and libido as well as influencing the clitoris and labia. Following the menopause, there is a decrease in the level of circulating androgens, with androstenedione falling to less than half that found in normal young women, while testosterone gradually diminishes over about 3 to 4 years. Dehydroepiandrosterone (DHEA) and DHEA-S (sulfate) are produced by the adrenal gland. Although levels are unaffected by ovarian failure, the values gradually decline after the age of 40.

Progesterone

With anovulation before, and ovarian failure during, the menopause, the production of progesterone declines to very low levels that are insufficient to induce those cytoplasmic enzymes (estradiol dehydrogenase and estrone sulfurtransferase) that convert estradiol to the relatively inactive estrone sulfate. Not only is there insufficient progesterone to prevent the mitotic activity of estrogen, there is also insufficient progesterone to induce secretory activity in the endometrium. As a consequence, the perimenopause is often associated with irregular vaginal bleeding, endometrial hyperplasia and atypia, and an increased incidence of endometrial cancer.

Gonadotropins

The two gonadotropins, LH and FSH, are produced in the anterior pituitary. When levels of estrogen are low, the arcuate nucleus and paraventricular nucleus in the hypothalamus are induced to secrete increasing amounts of gonadotropic-releasing hormone (GnRH) into the portal circulation. This in turn stimulates an increased release of FSH and LH into the circulation. The mechanism responsible for pulsatile release of GnRH is also thought to be responsible for inducing the hot flush, which so much characterizes the menopause. One hypothesis for the hot flush involves episodic pulses of dopamine and GnRH together with a "down-setting" of the thermoregulatory center in the midbrain (see Fig. 50–1).

CLINICAL MANIFESTATIONS

Loss of estrogen is associated with an increased risk of adverse changes such as osteoporosis, atherosclerosis, myocardial infarction, stroke, and cancer.

General Symptoms

About 85 per cent of women experience hot flushes as they pass through the menopause, but about half of these women are not seriously disturbed by them. For about 40 per cent of postmenopausal women, however, the hot flush is a most distressing experience. Flushes may occur as frequently as every 30 to 40 minutes but more often occur about eight to 15 times daily. There may be associated sweating, dizziness, formication, and palpitations. Often, the flush is preceded by an aura, which may awaken the patient and disturb her sleep. As a consequence of frequent night flushes, insomnia, tiredness, and irritability are common accompanying symptoms. Women are often given sedatives, hypnotics, or psychotropic drugs in an attempt to relieve symptoms that are caused by estrogen deficiency. Some complain of confusion, loss of memory, lethargy, and inability to cope as well as depression and loss of interest. It is uncertain whether these symptoms are directly due to estrogen deficiency affecting the neurotransmission processes or whether they are secondary to the disturbing vasovagal symptoms. Whatever the etiology, women improve considerably when an appropriate hormonal replacement therapy is initiated.

Urogenital Symptoms

The vagina is the organ most sensitive to estrogen, and it responds to this hormone by producing a thick moist epithelium with an acid secretion (pH 4.0). Absence of estrogen results in a thin dry epithelium with an alkaline secretion (pH 7.0). The postmenopausal vagina shrinks in diameter, splits and tears easily, and causes severe dyspareunia. A loving couple often avoid sexual intercourse because of this extreme discomfort, excusing their deprivation as being "because we're too old for that sort of thing."

The bladder and vagina are derived from the same embryologic tissue, so it is not surprising that some postmenopausal women also complain of urinary frequency and dysuria. The elastic capacity of the bladder is decreased even though the urinary output remains constant. As a result, frequency, urgency, and nocturia occur.

Collagen and Cell Response

Skin, bone, and joints all contain cells that respond to estrogen by producing better quality collagen. There is an improvement in the thickness and elasticity of skin, joints become less stiff, and osteoid is laid down in bone under the influence of estrogen. Estrogen appears to control the function of both osteoclasts and osteoblasts in bone and thus influences the rate of absorption and deposition of calcium. Remodeling of bone continues throughout life, but after estrogen deprivation, the osteoclastic activity far exceeds the osteoblasts' ability to lay down calcium. Under these conditions, osteopenia and finally osteoporosis occur. Ten to 15 years following the menopause, women begin to fracture their bones at a rate that exceeds that occurring among men by a factor of threefold to fivefold (Fig. 50–2). This increased fracture rate can be seen in the community, being manifest by women with a dowager's hump (crush fracture of thoracic vertebrae) or women struggling to rehabilitate themselves with a walking frame for a hip fracture.

About 200,000 women break a hip each year in the United States and the cost in 1990 was estimated in excess of $10 billion. The earlier women are deprived of estrogen in their lives, the earlier osteoporosis occurs. Most calcium is lost from trabecular bone, and as a consequence, the spinal column and femoral neck are the bones most commonly fractured. The amount of calcium in these sites can be calculated using specific bone mineral analysis machines. These machines pass two beams of energy (using either x-ray or gamma irradiation) through the affected bone site, and using sophisticated equipment and computer-assisted calculations (dual photon densitometry), a very accurate measure of bone mineral content can be achieved.

Appropriate estrogen replacement following the menopause results in maintenance of bone mineral content. The amount of estrogen necessary to inhibit osteoporosis has been calculated to be 0.625 mg for equine estrogens (Premarin), 1.25 mg piperazine estrone sulfate (Ogen), or 2 mg estradiol valerate (Progynova). There is some evidence that higher doses of estrogen may result in a gain in bone calcium, but caution must be exercised that increasing oral estrogen does not result in abnormal blood coagulation activity.

Not every woman loses calcium to the extent of developing osteoporosis, and it would be advantageous if the at-risk patient could be identified. Women at greatest risk are those who have a family history of osteoporosis, are slender, of Caucasian or Chinese origin, lead a sedentary lifestyle, drink alcohol, smoke cigarettes, or take corticosteroids. Those at risk of developing osteoporosis should have their progress monitored by a bone mineral analysis. They should be encouraged to take appropriate hormonal replacement therapy, partake of adequate weight-bearing exercise, (walking for 30 minutes daily), and ingest about 1000 mg of calcium each day (about 0.5 L milk). Calcium is deposited in bone during the formative years of a woman's life, so educational strategies should be devised to persuade young women to consume over 1000 mg of calcium daily between the ages of 10 and 25 years. By so doing, they are more likely to have a higher bone mass when they reach the menopause.

For women who have developed osteoporosis following the menopause, etidronate and calcitonin can be administered as well as hormone replacement therapy (HRT) and calcium. Education, physiotherapy, and exercise are also important in helping prevent falls and fractures in the elderly, but it is important to remember that no woman is too old to receive some benefit from HRT. It has

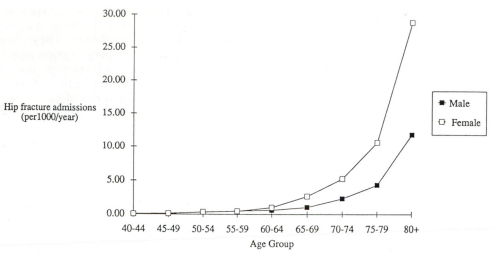

Figure 50–2. Age-specific admission rates of hip fractures (per 1000/year) in New South Wales, Australia (in-hospital morbidity data, 1986).

been shown that estrogen helps to improve muscle tone and balance in older individuals and thus reduces the incidence of traumatic falls.

Cardiovascular Changes

Over the last decade, it has also become evident that estrogen plays a highly significant role in preventing cardiovascular disease in women. Following the menopause, women appear to have a rapidly increasing incidence of atherosclerotic changes, myocardial infarction, ischemic heart disease, hypertension, and stroke. Administration of estrogen from the time of the menopause reduces the risk of death from myocardial infarction by 50 to 70 per cent, and from stroke by 50 per cent. Not only is there a reduction in these cardiovascular accidents, there is also an associated fall in blood pressure as a result of estrogen therapy.

These positive changes are thought to be mediated through two major pathways: First, estrogen by mouth influences lipase activity within the liver. This results in a reduced total cholesterol level and an increased level of high-density lipoproteins. Second, estrogen is also thought to influence the production of lipase enzymes within the intimal cells of arteries so that cholesterol esters do not accumulate to produce "foam cells" or athero-

sclerotic plaques. Cardiac and arterial musculature contains large quantities of estrogen receptors and thus responds positively to circulating estrogen. Vessels tend to dilate, cardiac palpitations and arrhythmias are reduced, and peripheral blood flow is improved under the influence of estrogen.

General Systemic Response

Not only do vasovagal symptoms cease with estrogen administration, but body tone is improved. There is an increased sense of well-being and less cardiovascular and locomotor disease processes, and epidemiologic evidence suggests a significant reduction in the incidence of nongenital cancer. Women given estrogen from the time of the menopause live, on average, 4 years longer than women not given HRT.

Progestogens may have a counteractive effect to estrogen, in which case the benefit gained from estrogen in protecting the cardiovascular system might be lost.

THERAPY REGIMENS

Estrogen may be administered as equine estrogen (Premarin) or as conjugated estrone or estradiol in dosage regimens sufficient to prevent osteoporosis and to inhibit hot flushes. Unless the patient has had a hysterectomy, it is advisable to add a progestogen such as medroxyprogesterone acetate (Provera, 5 to 10 mg) or norethisterone (Primolut-N, 1.25 to 5.0 mg) for 10 to 14 days in each cycle. If withdrawal bleeding becomes intolerable, the concurrent daily use of estrogen (Premarin, 0.625 mg) and progestogen (Provera, 2.5 mg) will often prevent endometrial growth and thus inhibit withdrawal bleeding. Following a hysterectomy, estrogen can be taken every day without the need for added progestogen.

Routes of Administration

Estrogens are generally administered orally, passing through the gut and the liver. If there is a history of thrombosis or liver disease, however, it is advisable not to administer the estrogen by mouth, at least until there is evidence that no adverse hepatic activity exists. Women with thrombosis may have some increased production of coagulation proteins as a result of oral estrogen therapy, and until it is certain that coagulation factors have not been increased by this route of administration, it is wise to cease the oral estrogen.

To bypass the gut and liver, estrogens can be administered vaginally, dermally, or subdermally. All routes have excellent absorption, and each has an advantage under certain conditions for individual women. Progestogens are currently available as oral preparations, but new delivery techniques will allow a choice of oral, vaginal, or dermal preparations in the future.

Side Effects of Therapy

Breakthrough bleeding is common when using combined continuous therapy but is less likely to occur in sequential regimens. Bleeding can be controlled by manipulating the dosage and regimen of estrogen and progestogens.

Weight gain and fluid retention are common symptoms of therapy regimens. Progestogens tend to slow bowel activity and induce a bloated sensation, whereas weight gain and fluid retention are probably a result of both estrogen and progestogen. Changing the dosage or type of hormone may help reduce these somatic symptoms, but diet must be disciplined if weight gain is a problem.

Adverse Effects

Women given unopposed estrogen replacement therapy (ERT) have an increased incidence of endometrial hyperplasia, endometrial cancer, and abnormal bleeding patterns, and for these reasons women who still have a uterus are often advised not to take ERT. There is now clear evidence, however, that progestogens given for 10 to 14 days in a cycle reduce the risk of abnormal bleeding, endometrial hyperplasia, and cancer to negligible proportions. For that reason, a number of regimens of HRT have been developed to reduce endometrial cellular activity. Less endometrial proliferation and withdrawal bleeding occur if higher doses of progestogen are given for longer periods in each cycle. Some regimens now use progestogen concurrently with estrogen every day for months on end. The problem with these regimens is the untoward effect that continuous progestogens have on blood lipids and lipase activity.

Breast cancer is probably not induced by hormonal replacement therapy, and there is no clear evidence to support either a positive or a negative influence. Once a breast malignancy has occurred, however, HRT should be ceased. It has been found that ovarian cancer is reduced and nongenital cancer is significantly reduced among women taking HRT.

In the past, when potent stable estrogens, such as ethinyl estradiol, stilbestrol, and mestranol, were used to treat postmenopausal women, there was a risk that coagulation proteins from the liver might be increased. Under these conditions, there was a theoretical risk that thrombosis might increase among women on HRT. With use of low-dose "natural" estrogens, however, there has been no demonstrable increase in coagulation factors or thrombosis among postmenopausal women.

Hypertension has been associated with medium-dose to high-dose oral contraceptive pills, and for this reason, some medical practitioners have suggested that postmenopausal women using HRT may also be at risk of developing high blood pressure. Investigation has shown that estrogens are more likely to produce a small fall in blood pressure as well as increasing blood flow to tissues.

Contraindications

There are very few contraindications to hormonal replacement therapy, but hormonally dependent genital tract cancer is certainly an indication to cease treatment. Women who have developed a thrombosis should cease treatment until evidence of organization of the thrombosis is available, whereas women who have hepatitis or liver disease should not take oral estrogen.

SUGGESTED READING

Antunes CM, Stolley PD, Rosenshein NB: Endometrial cancer and estrogen use: Report of a large case-control study. N Engl J Med 300:9, 1979.

Bergkvist L, Adami HO, Persson I, et al: The risk of breast cancer after estrogen and estrogen-progestin replacement. N Engl J Med 321:293, 1989.

Bush T: The Lipid Research Clinics Program. In Peck WA, Lobo RA (eds): Long-term Effects of Estrogen Deprivation. Minneapolis, McGraw-Hill Healthcare Publications, 1989, p 45.

Christiansen C, Riis BJ: Five years with continuous combined estrogen/progestogen therapy. Effects on calcium, metabolism, lipoproteins and bleeding patterns. Br J Obstet Gynaecol 97:1087, 1990.

Hammond CB, Jelovsek FR, Lee KL, et al: Effects of long-term estrogen replacement therapy. I. Metabolic effects. Am J Obstet Gynecol 133:525, 1979.

Henderson BE, Paganini-Hill A, Ross RK: Decreased mortality in users of estrogen replacement therapy. Arch Intern Med 151:75, 1991.

Hirvonen E, Malkonen M, Manninen V: Effects of different progestogens on lipoproteins during postmenopausal replacement therapy. N Engl J Med 304:560, 1981.

Judd HL, Meldrum DR, Deftos LJ, et al: Estrogen replacement therapy: Indications and complications. Ann Intern Med 98:195, 1983.

Lindsay R, Hart DM, Aitken JM, et al: Long-term prevention of postmenopausal osteoporosis by oestrogen: Evidence of an increased bone mass after delayed onset of oestrogen treatment. Lancet 1:1038, 1976.

Paganini-Hill A, Ross RK, Henderson BE: Postmenopausal oestrogen treatment and stroke: A prospective study. Br Med J 297:519, 1988.

Sullivan JM, Vander Zwaag R, Lemp GF, et al: Postmenopausal estrogen use and coronary atherosclerosis. Ann Intern Med 108:358, 1988.

Studd JWW, Whitehead MI (eds): The Menopause. Oxford, Blackwell, 1988.

Wren BG: Oestrogen replacement therapy: The management of an endocrine deficiency disease. Med J Aust 142 (Suppl 1):(II, Spec Suppl S1–15), 1985.

Wren BG, Routledge AD: The effect of type and dose of oestrogen on the blood pressure of postmenopausal women. Maturitas 5:134, 1983.

Fifty-one

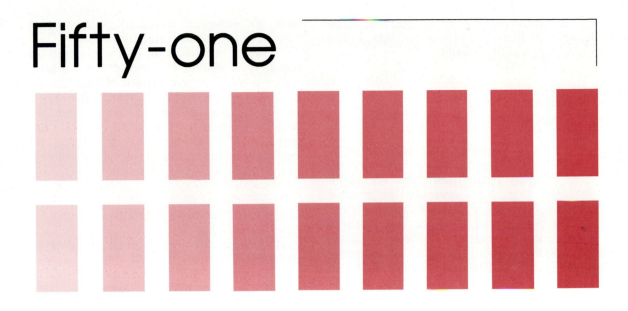

Infertility

DAVID R. MELDRUM

A couple is considered infertile after unsuccessfully attempting pregnancy for 1 year. Infertility is termed *primary* when it occurs without any prior pregnancy and *secondary* when it follows a previous conception. Some conditions, such as azoospermia, endometriosis, and tubal occlusion, are more common in women with primary infertility, but virtually all conditions occur in both settings, making the distinction of little clinical benefit.

Conception requires the juxtaposition of the male and female gametes at the optimal stage of their maturation, followed by transportation of the conceptus to the uterine cavity at a time when the endometrium is supportive to its continued development and implantation. For these events to occur, the male and female reproductive systems must be both anatomically and physiologically intact, and coitus must occur with sufficient frequency for the semen to be deposited in close temporal relationship to the release of the oocyte from the follicle. Even when fertilization occurs, it is estimated that over 70 per cent of resulting embryos are abnormal and fail to develop or become nonviable shortly after implantation. Therefore, it is not surprising that 10 to 15 per cent of couples experience infertility. The physiology of conception is fully discussed in Chapter 4.

Considering the vast complexity of the reproductive process, it is remarkable that 80 per cent of couples achieve conception within 1 year. More precisely, 25 per cent conceive within the first month, 60 per cent within 6 months, 75 per cent by 9 months, and 90 per cent by 18 months. The steadily decreasing rate of monthly conception demonstrated by these figures most likely reflects a spectrum of fertility extending from highly fertile couples through to those with relative infertility. After 18 months of unprotected sexual intercourse, the remaining couples have a very low monthly conception rate without treatment, and many may have absolute defects preventing fertility (sterility).

GENERAL PRINCIPLES OF EVALUATION

Conception requires adequate function of multiple physiologic systems in both partners. Infertility may result from either one major deficiency (e.g., tubal occlusion) or multiple minor deficiencies. Failure to realize this important dictum may lead the inexperienced practitioner to overlook additional factors that might be more amenable to treatment than the one that has been identified. About 40 per cent of infertile couples have multiple causes. Therefore, with rare exceptions, a complete infertility evaluation should be performed on each couple.

Age substantially decreases the rate of conception because of decreased coital frequency and other poorly defined effects on fertility. From a large study of donor insemination, the strictly age-related reduction appears to be about one third in women aged 35 to 45. The tendency to embark on investigations and therapy at an earlier point in these older couples should be tempered by the expected delay and the consequence that unnecessary risks and expenses may be induced. A reasonable compromise is to telescope somewhat the testing and treatments during the second year of infertility in women over 35.

Basic Evaluations

Evaluation and therapy may be started at an earlier point when obvious defects are identified, or they may be delayed, for instance, when a correctable coital factor, such as infrequent intercourse, is identified. Generally, the first 6 to 8 months of evaluation involve relatively simple and noninvasive tests and the performance of a radiologic evaluation of tubal patency (hysterosalpingogram [HSG]), which can sometimes have a therapeutic effect. Operative evaluation by laparoscopy is thus reserved for the small proportion of couples (5 to 10 per cent) who

have not conceived by 18 to 24 months or who have specific abnormalities.

To keep the status of the evaluation in mind, it is helpful to arrange the work-up under a series of five categories that can be mentally reviewed at each visit. Table 51–1 shows the approximate incidence and the tests involved in the evaluation of each category. In 5 to 10 per cent of couples, no explanation can be found (idiopathic infertility).

Effects of Social Trends

Modern social trends, such as delayed childbirth, use of the intrauterine device (IUD), and the "sexual revolution," with its accompanying epidemic of salpingitis, have made infertility more common. According to the National Center for Health Statistics, infertility increased 177 per cent among married women aged 20 to 24 between 1965 and 1982. In addition, the legalization of abortion and the increased acceptance of single motherhood have largely removed the principal alternative of adoption. The infertile couple, therefore, has little choice but to go through a complex, expensive, and often lengthy series of evaluations and treatments.

Psychological Effects

The infertility specialist must be aware of and sensitive to the psychological stresses associated with infertility. The expectations of friends and family, the loss of self-esteem associated with the inability to fulfill this basic function, the associated stresses to the marital and sexual relationship, and the inability of the couple to plan their personal lives and careers all contribute to the emotional impact of the condition. At the same time, the couple can be reassured that with the exception of effects on libido and occasional transient anovulation, there is no evidence of any significant effect of these psychological stresses on fertility. A supportive relationship with the physician, frank discussion on the sometimes lengthy nature of various treatments, realistic expectations as to their prognosis, and participation in support

Table 51-1. COMMON INFERTILITY FACTORS

FACTOR	INCIDENCE (%)	BASIC INVESTIGATIONS
Male-coital	40	Semen analysis, postcoital test
Ovulatory	15-20	Basal body temperature, serum progesterone, endometrial biopsy*
Cervical	5-10	Postcoital test
Uterine-tubal	30	Hysterosalpingogram, laparoscopy
Peritoneal	40	Laparoscopy

* Investigations when menses are regular (every 22 to 35 days); oligoamenorrhea requires additional testing (see Chapter 48).

groups such as Resolve all help these couples to adjust successfully to their condition.

Prognosis

Without therapy, spontaneous conception occurs at a decreased rate in infertile couples. Treatments are thus aimed at increasing the rate as well as the likelihood of conception. Unfortunately, most therapeutic regimens are based on collective clinical experience rather than controlled clinical trials. With a thorough evaluation and application of current treatments short of in vitro fertilization (IVF) or ovum transfer, 50 to 60 per cent of infertile couples will conceive. With the full utilization of the latter techniques, it is anticipated that most couples who pursue all available treatment methods will eventually be successful.

ETIOLOGIC FACTORS

Male Coital Factor

History

The history from the male partner should cover any pregnancies previously sired; any history of genital tract infections, such as prostatitis or mumps orchitis; surgery or trauma to the male genitals or inguinal region (e.g., hernia repair); and any exposure to lead, cadmium, radiation, or chemotherapeutic agents. Excessive consumption of alcohol or cigarettes or unusual exposure to environmental heat should be elicited.

Physical Examination

Lack of either sexual hair or masculine build may indicate insufficient testosterone production. The normal location of the urethral meatus should be ensured. Testicular size is estimated by comparison to a set of standard ovoids. The presence of a varicocele is elicited by asking the patient to perform Valsalva's maneuver in the standing position. Rectal massage of the prostate and seminal vesicles brings forth sufficient secretions at the urethral meatus to allow microscopic examination for white blood cells.

Investigations

A semen analysis should be performed following a 2- to 3-day period of abstinence. The entire ejaculate should be collected in a clean glass container. Until relatively recently, the full range of normal variation has not been appreciated. Characteristics of a normal semen analysis are shown in Table 51-2.

An excessive number of leukocytes (more than 10 per high power field) may indicate infection, but special stains are required to differentiate polymorphonuclear leukocytes from immature germ cells. Semen quality varies markedly with repeated samples. A conclusion of normality should be based on at least two specimens, and an accurate ap-

Table 51-2. CHARACTERISTICS OF NORMAL SEMEN ANALYSIS

CHARACTERISTIC	QUANTITY
Semen volume	2–5 ml
Sperm count	Greater than 20 million/ml
Sperm motility	Greater than 50%
Normal forms	Greater than 60%
White blood cells	Fewer than 10 per high power field or 1×10^6/ml

praisal of abnormal semen requires at least three analyses. Periodic reassessment is necessary. A few weeks should pass between each sample to reflect fluctuations in spermatogenesis. Although infertility does not occur until semen quality is below the above-mentioned levels, fecundability continues to increase as the count, percentage, quality of motility, and percentage of morphologically normal sperm increase.

Endocrine evaluation of the male with subnormal semen quality may uncover a specific cause. Hypothyroidism can cause infertility, but there is no place for the empiric use of thyroxine. Low levels of gonadotropins and testosterone may indicate hypothalamic-pituitary failure. An elevated prolactin concentration suggests the presence of a prolactin-producing pituitary tumor. An elevated level of follicle-stimulating hormone (FSH) generally indicates substantial parenchymal damage to the testes, since inhibin, produced by the Sertoli cells of the seminiferous tubules, provides the principal feedback control of FSH secretion. A response to any treatment is unlikely in the presence of an elevated level of FSH.

Treatment

The couple should be advised to have intercourse approximately every 2 days during the periovulatory period (e.g., days 10 through 18 and particularly days 12 through 16 of a 28-day cycle). Because infrequent coitus is a common contributing factor, firm advice in this regard can be very beneficial. This "scheduled intercourse" can be very disruptive and stressful, however, and insemi-

nation may relieve considerable pressure on a couple whose biological drives do not match the physiologic necessity.

Lubricants and postcoital douching should be avoided, and the woman should be advised to lie on her back for at least 15 minutes following coitus with her knees bent and even a pillow under the buttocks to prevent rapid loss of semen from the vagina.

Smoking should be reduced or stopped, as should alcohol intake. Use of saunas, hot tubs, or tight underwear should be discouraged, as should exposure to other environments that raise scrotal temperature, because these factors may affect spermatogenesis.

Low semen volume may provide insufficient contact with the cervical mucus for adequate sperm migration to occur. This may be remedied by artificial insemination with the husband's semen. Following liquefaction (20 to 30 minutes), 0.1 ml of the semen is placed in the endocervical canal and the remainder in a cup over the cervix. When a high semen volume coexists with a low count, the sperm can be concentrated by collecting the specimen as a "split ejaculate." In most instances, the first small portion of the ejaculate contains most of the sperm and can be used for insemination. Currently these abnormalities of volume are most commonly treated with sperm washing and intrauterine insemination.

If low sperm density (oligospermia) or low motility (asthenospermia) is due to hypothalamic-pituitary failure, injections of human menopausal gonadotropins (hMGs) are effective. The suppressive effects of hyperprolactinemia on hypothalamic function can be reversed by the administration of bromocriptine, a dopamine agonist. When low semen quality coexists with a varicocele (dilatation and incompetence of the spermatic veins), improved semen quality, particularly motility, may occur with ligation of this venous plexus. Various medications (clomiphene, human chorionic gonadotropin [hCG], testosterone, and hMG) have been tried when no cause is apparent (idiopathic oligoasthenospermia). Although still inconclusive, the bulk of information does suggest a therapeutic role for clomiphene, but it is not yet approved for this purpose. Since approximately 3 months are required for spermatogenesis and transportation, frequent semen checks during treatment are unnecessary and serve only to discourage the patient.

If semen quality cannot be improved, intrauterine insemination with close timing of the insemination to the precise point of ovulation is effective. By washing and concentrating the sperm into a small volume by slow centrifugation, large numbers of sperm can be placed into the uterus. Without washing, intrauterine insemination must be limited to very small amounts of semen, owing to marked cramping. Accurate timing may be accomplished either by measurement of daily luteinizing hormone (LH) concentrations or by controlled stimulation of the cycle with clomiphene or hMG, followed by administration of hCG when follicular diameter by ultrasonography indicates maturity. Insemination may then be carried out within a few hours of ovulation, which occurs 36 to 44 hours following the LH surge or hCG injection. When urinary LH testing is used, there is a delay of several hours between the onset of the surge and the positive urine test. It is advisable to test in the afternoon or evening, with insemination the following morning.

In vitro fertilization is also used to treat the male factor because a relatively small number of sperm is required to inseminate each oocyte. Finally, artificial insemination with donor sperm is very effective when the male factor is refractory to treatment.

Ovulatory Factor

History

Most women with regular cycles (every 22 to 35 days) are ovulating, particularly if they have premenstrual molimina (e.g., breast changes, bloating, and mood change).

Investigations

The simplest screening tests to confirm reasonably normal ovulation are the basal body temperature (BBT), which assesses the duration of luteal function, and the midluteal level of serum progesterone, which assesses the level of luteal function. The interval from the urinary LH surge to the onset of menses may also be used to detect a short luteal phase.

The BBT is the temperature on awakening before any activity. It rises about 0.4°F at ovulation owing to the thermogenic effect of progesterone and should remain elevated for at least 11 days (Fig. 51–1). The point of rise does not have a precise relationship to ovulation, and the BBT should not be used to predict the best time for the couple to attempt pregnancy. A progesterone level of greater than 5 ng/ml indicates ovulatory activity, but midluteal concentrations usually exceed 10 ng/ml in cycles capable of conception.

In spite of ovulation, an inadequate luteal phase may be responsible for infertility. If there are suggestions that a luteal phase defect may be present (abnormal BBT, history of spontaneous abortion or endometriosis, poor cervical mucus), an endometrial biopsy should be taken from the upper anterior aspect of the uterine fundus and the histologic development carefully dated. If the day of the biopsy, retrospectively determined by its relationship to the onset of the next menses, lags by more than 2 days in at least two cycles, a luteal phase defect is present. It has been shown that prospective timing from the LH surge helps to reduce false-positive results.

Treatment

Correction of a luteal phase defect is generally possible by the use of vaginal progesterone suppositories, 25 mg twice daily, beginning on the second or third day of the temperature rise. Response should be documented in a subsequent cycle by repeat biopsy. Clomiphene citrate or hMG may be used if simple progesterone supplementation does not result in correction of the defect or pregnancy. By resulting in higher levels of FSH, these latter treatments more directly correct the underlying pathophysiology (insufficient FSH stimulation of the follicle) and may correct accompanying defects of oocyte maturation or extrusion. They are accompanied by an increased risk of multiple pregnancy, however, and clomiphene citrate may itself cause a luteal phase defect.

In women whose menses are less frequent than every 35 days (oligoamenorrhea), it is helpful to induce more frequent ovulation, thus increasing the opportunity for pregnancy

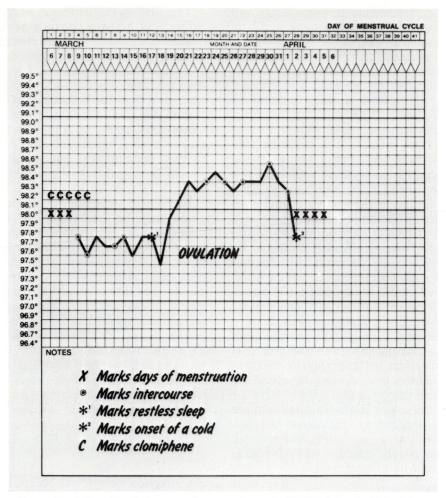

Figure 51-1. Basal body temperature graph used at UCLA School of Medicine.

and improving the ability to time coitus. Luteal activity associated with infrequent ovulation is often abnormal. Ovulation induction should always be preceded by a thorough work-up, as discussed in Chapter 48, because conditions causing anovulation may be worsened by pregnancy or may complicate it. In addition, ovarian failure seldom responds to attempts to induce ovulation.

Choice of the most appropriate technique for ovulation induction is determined by the patient's specific diagnosis. With this approach, regular ovulation can be restored in over 90 per cent of anovulatory women. Provided that these patients persist with treatment for an adequate period of time and no other infertility factors are present, their fertility should approximate that of normal women.

Pituitary insufficiency requires the intramuscular administration of purified FSH and LH, which are extracted from menopausal urine and, therefore, are called hMGs. Hypothalamic amenorrhea is due to infrequent or absent pulsatile release of gonadotropin-releasing hormone (GnRH). The latter is highly effective when administered in small pulses subcutaneously or intravenously in these patients every 90 to 120 minutes by a small portable infusion pump. Hyperprolactinemia and its suppressive effect on the hypothalamus are specifically treated by use of the dopamine agonist bromocriptine (Parlodel).

Most of the remaining patients with anovulation have some form of polycystic ovarian syndrome and generally respond to clomiphene, an orally active antiestrogen. Anovulation occurs in patients with polycystic ovaries because of chronic, mild suppression of FSH release and the antagonistic effect of androgens on the response of the follicle to FSH. These women often have both increased ovarian and increased adrenal androgen production. Clomiphene, by inhibiting the negative feedback effect of endogenous estrogen, causes a rise of FSH and stimulation of follicular maturation.

Two other treatments have been used to decrease the inhibitory effect of androgens. First, surgical excision of androgen-producing ovarian stroma (wedge resection) induces ovulation, but it is not as effective as clomiphene treatment and may cause infertility by inducing periadnexal adhesions. Laparoscopic procedures to create multiple craters in the ovary with cautery or laser have been used to achieve similar effects. Second, dexamethasone, which suppresses adrenal androgens, may be helpful in selected cases. In those anovulatory women with levels of dehydroepiandrosterone sulfate above the mean for normal women, clomiphene treatment is more effective in inducing ovulation and pregnancy at lower dose levels when dexamethasone is given concomitantly, since dehydroepiandrosterone sulfate has been shown to act as a circulating precursor for the production of ovarian androgens. If ovulation does not occur at a maximal clomiphene dose, follicular development may be occurring, but the normal LH surge may fail to occur. This results in lack of follicular rupture. Assessment by serial pelvic ultrasonography and carefully timed hCG may lead to normal ovulation. If follicular maturation is not occurring, ovulation induction will require hMG/hCG with or without clomiphene pretreatment.

Complications of Ovulation Induction. The main complications are related to excessive stimulation of the ovaries. Substantial enlargement of the ovary with clomiphene citrate can generally be avoided by examining the adnexae before each treatment course and by using the lowest effective dose. Cystic ovarian enlargement is not an uncommon complication of hMG treatment. The hyperstimulation syndrome is a critical illness associated with marked ovarian enlargement and exudation of fluid and protein into the peritoneal and pleural cavities. The use of serum estradiol measurements and transva-ginal ultrasonic scanning with hMG treatment has markedly reduced the incidence of hyperstimulation syndrome, provided that hCG is withheld if the estradiol concentration is excessive or there are more than 10 intermediate-sized follicles present.

Multiple pregnancy occurs in 6 to 8 per cent of clomiphene citrate conceptions, but more than twins is unusual (fewer than 1 per cent). Multiple gestation occurs in 20 to 30 per cent of hMG conceptions, and 5 per cent are more than twins. Ultrasonic monitoring appears to reduce this risk if the hCG is withheld in the presence of an excessive number of mature follicles. Current trends toward use of a low-dose regimen of hMG or pure FSH may further reduce the risks of excessive stimulation.

Cervical Factor

During the few days before ovulation, the cervix produces a profuse watery mucus that exudes out of the cervix to contact the seminal ejaculate. To assess its quality, the patient must be seen during the immediate preovulatory phase (days 12 to 14 of a 28-day cycle).

Investigations

The amount and clarity of the mucus are recorded. The spinnbarkeit may be tested by contacting the mucus with a piece of pH paper and lifting vertically. The mucus should thread out to at least 6 cm. The pH should be 6.5 or greater. A postcoital (Sims-Huhner) test is done 2 to 4 hours after intercourse to assess the number and motility of spermatozoa that have entered the cervical canal. The number of sperm, however, does not correlate well with semen quality, recovery of sperm from the cul-de-sac, or subsequent fertility. If the number of sperm is greater than 20 per high power field, it is probable that the semen analysis is normal and that there is a better prognosis for fertility. When 0 to 20 sperm are seen, which is the case in most infertile couples, limited information is gained. For this reason, and because psychosexual stress can result when coitus must occur at a prescribed time, it is important to emphasize to the couple that they should not be concerned if problems arise, since mucus quality can still be evaluated.

Treatment

Any cervical infection is treated by prescribing a 10-day course of doxycycline, 100 mg twice daily, for both partners. Persistent chronic cervicitis is treated with cryotherapy if antibiotic treatment fails. If the pH of the mucus is low, particularly if this is associated with a low number of active sperm, sperm migration and viability may be improved by advising a gentle douche with sodium bicarbonate (1 tablespoon in a quart of water) 30 minutes before coitus. Poor mucus quality can be treated with a small dose of estrogen from day 7 until ovulation, but intrauterine insemination of washed sperm appears to be more effective.

Uterine-Tubal Factor

Abnormalities of the uterine cavity are seldom the cause of infertility. Large submucosal myomata or endometrial polyps may rarely be associated with infertility but more often are associated with first-trimester spontaneous abortions. The role of intramural myomata is not clear, although myomectomy has been associated with conception in 40 to 50 per cent of couples in uncontrolled series.

Tubal occlusion may occur at three locations: the fimbrial end, the midsegment, or the isthmus-cornu. Fimbrial occlusion is by far the most common. Prior salpingitis and use of the IUD are common causes, although about one half are unassociated with any such history. Midsegment occlusion is almost always secondary to tubal sterilization. Such occlusion in the absence of this history suggests tuberculosis. Isthmic-cornual occlusion can be congenital or due to endometriosis, tubal adenomyosis, or prior infection. In 90 per cent of cases, the occlusion is located in the isthmus near the cornu or may involve the superficial portion of the intramural tubal lumen.

Investigations

Tubal abnormalities may be diagnosed by hysterosalpingography or laparoscopy. To perform an HSG, an occlusive cannula is placed in the cervix, and the instillation of a radiopaque dye is followed under fluoroscopy with image intensification. Selected radiographs are taken for permanent documentation (Fig. 51–2). Anesthesia is generally not required. A water-soluble dye is used initially to confirm tubal patency because of the adverse effects of sequestration of an oil-based dye within the lumen of an occluded tube. If patency is confirmed, an oil-based dye is then instilled because of its prominent therapeutic effect in women with unexplained infertility. If only one tube fills with dye, the HSG should be considered normal, since this finding is usually, although not invariably, due to the dye following the path of least resistance.

Serious infections can result from HSG. A normal pelvic examination, normal erythrocyte sedimentation rate, and prophylactic doxycycline are precautions that should reduce this risk to essentially zero.

If no cause for the infertility is identified, laparoscopy should be delayed for 6 months to see if pregnancy occurs. The couple should be sure to have coitus at least once during each preovulatory period during the following 6 months to achieve the maximum probability of conception.

Rubin's test is an older method for evaluating tubal patency. Carbon dioxide is insufflated through the cervix under controlled pressure, and patency is confirmed by shoulder pain. The test provides little information and little or no therapeutic effect and so should be considered obsolete.

Treatment

In most circumstances, microsurgical tuboplasty is more effective than conventional surgical techniques for reversal of tubal occlusion. About 60 to 80 per cent of patients achieve pregnancy after reversal of sterilization using microsurgical techniques, with a decreasing prognosis for the following types of reanastomoses: isthmic-isthmic, isthmic-cornual, ampullary-isthmic, ampullary-ampullary, and ampullary-cornual. Neosal-

Figure 51–2. *A*, Normal hysterosalpingogram showing free spill of contrast material; *B*, bilateral hydrosalpinges.

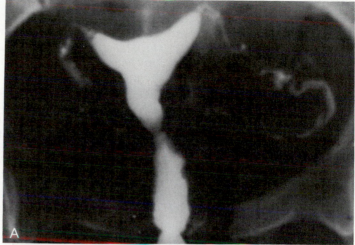

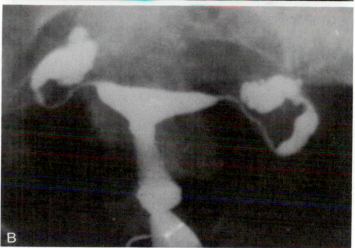

pingostomy, which is required following fimbriectomy, is associated with a success rate of about 40 to 50 per cent. For an isthmic-cornual occlusion caused by disease, clearing of the obstruction with danazol has been reported when the occlusion coexists with peritoneal endometriosis. Selective catheterization has restored patency in the majority of proximal occlusions and should be the first line of therapy. Microsurgical resection and reanastomosis are associated with a 50 to 60 per cent pregnancy rate. If the intramural portion of the tube is occluded, a reimplantation is required, with a new opening being made into the endometrial cavity. A substantially lower rate of success is achieved in this circumstance. Finally, the prognosis with neosalpingostomy for fimbrial occlusion is a 20

to 30 per cent success rate, although it has reached 40 per cent with long-term follow-up.

At least 10 per cent of conceptions following repair of diseased tubes are ectopic in the tube. Reanastomosis of healthy tubes carries an ectopic risk of about 5 per cent. This possibility must always be considered in the management of an early pregnancy following tuboplasty.

Peritoneal Factor

Laparoscopy identifies previously unsuspected pathology in 30 to 50 per cent of women with unexplained infertility. Endometriosis is the most common finding. Periadnexal adhesions may be found that may hold the fimbriae away from the ovarian surface or entrap the released oocyte.

Endometriosis interferes with fertility in a number of ways. It may interfere with tubal motility, cause tubal obstruction, or cause adhesions that directly disturb the pick-up of the oocyte by the fimbriae. The inflammation caused by retrograde menstruation and the ectopic endometrium induces an increased number of peritoneal macrophages, each of which is more active in engulfing sperm, thus reducing the number of sperm available to penetrate the oocyte-cumulus complex. The presence of endometriosis is also associated with an increased incidence of luteinized unruptured follicle syndrome, in which, in spite of the presence of the usual indirect signs of ovulation, the oocyte is not released from the follicle. The presence of ectopic endometrium in the pelvic cavity also induces subtle alterations of luteal function with a delayed and shortened elevation of progesterone. Luteal phase defects may be more common in women with endometriosis. It is controversial whether or not the incidence of spontaneous abortion is increased in the presence of active endometriosis.

Treatment

Treatment of endometriosis depends on its extent and is fully discussed in Chapter 34. If substantial adhesions or endometriomas are present, surgery is preferable, since these generally do not respond to medical management. Intermediate amounts of disease may respond similarly to hormonal or surgical therapy (the latter being slightly more effective), with the choice depending largely on the prejudices of the patient against one or the other modality. With more advanced operative laparoscopic techniques (pelviscopy), most endometriosis can be removed or ablated without laparotomy by using advanced instrumentation, lasers, or thermocoagulation. Danazol, GnRH analogs, or oral medroxyprogesterone acetate is highly effective, with continuous oral contraception therapy being generally inferior. If minimal disease with scattered implants is found, simple cautery at the time of laparoscopy should suffice, particularly since studies have suggested that

minimal to mild degrees of endometriosis may not interfere with fertility.

Periadnexal adhesions may be lysed by operative laparoscopy or may require laparotomy. Microsurgical techniques diminish adhesions. The most effective adjunct in preventing recurrent scarring is the placement of 32 per cent dextran 70 in the pelvic cavity at the end of surgery or covering raw surfaces with an artificial tissue barrier moistened with heparin. Either modality functions to separate the raw surfaces during the early period of healing. An early postoperative laparoscopy may also be helpful, since the immature adhesions are filmy and avascular and can be released readily during the procedure.

UNEXPLAINED INFERTILITY

No cause is found for infertility in 5 to 10 per cent of cases. The problem appears to be primarily one of sperm transport, since intrauterine insemination with washed sperm appears to increase the rate of conception.

In other cases, a defect in the ability of the sperm to fertilize the egg may be present, since some infertile males have sperm that are unable to penetrate zona-free hamster eggs. Also, a lower rate of fertilization is noted in couples with unexplained infertility who undergo IVF compared with those with a tubal cause for their infertility. Another male problem that may not be detected by routine evaluation is the presence of anti-sperm antibodies.

Treatment of idiopathic infertility should start with an HSG with oil-based dye if it has not been done previously. Intrauterine insemination, eventually with ovulation induction and hCG timing, is next employed. The final therapy is IVF or gamete intrafallopian transfer (GIFT).

ASSISTED REPRODUCTIVE TECHNOLOGY

The last resort for infertile couples with any of the aforementioned factors and failure of lesser treatments is the procedure of IVF and embryo transfer (IVF-ET) or, if the tubes are patent and normal, GIFT. In some cases of tubal occlusion in which the rate of success with tubal repair is low (less than 30 per cent), IVF appears to be preferable to surgery because of the more rapid conception rate and the lower ectopic pregnancy rate. In some cases of male infertility or high levels of antisperm antibodies, IVF may be done, followed by tubal embryo transfer. Although still controversial, procedures that allow the conceptus to reside in the fallopian tube for a period of time are probably associated with improved results.

Technique

Clomiphene, hMG, or both are given to induce the maturation of multiple follicles, the growth of which is monitored by serum estradiol levels and pelvic sonography. A GnRH analog can also be used to prevent premature LH release. An injection of hCG is given to induce the resumption of meiosis and to ready the oocytes for fertilization. Thirty-six hours after the hCG injection, multiple oocytes are aspirated under either laparoscopic or ultrasonic guidance. After a further 5 to 8 hours of in vitro maturation, washed sperm are added. Fertilization may be identified 14 to 18 hours after insemination by the visualization of two pronuclei. The conceptuses are then transferred to the uterine cavity or the fallopian tube 2 days after oocyte retrieval by means of a tiny catheter. With GIFT, mature eggs are placed in the fallopian tube at laparoscopy together with washed sperm. Efforts to guide the placement of gametes or embryos into the fallopian tubes transcervically have met with inconsistent results.

Outcome

The pregnancy rate with IVF has been highly variable from center to center, owing to the complexity of the laboratory required, whereas the pregnancy rate with GIFT has been more consistent. The mean live delivery rates with IVF and GIFT in 1989 were 14 and 23 per cent respectively, but individual programs have almost doubled these rates. Ectopic pregnancy occurs in about 5 per cent of pregnancies with both techniques. The rate of fetal abnormalities has not increased.

Egg Donation

It is now possible to achieve pregnancy with IVF-ET using donor eggs, with a rate of success approximately double that of regular IVF-ET. The recipient can be programmed for optimal uterine receptivity by replacement doses of estradiol and progesterone. In addition, the eggs generally come from young fertile women (sisters or anonymous volunteers). Estradiol and progesterone must be continued at increasing levels until the placenta takes over in the late first trimester. The excellent success of egg donation mandates the conservation of the uterus whenever future fertility is desired, even if the ovaries must be removed.

OVERALL SUCCESS OF INFERTILITY THERAPY

Conventional therapies result in conception in 50 to 60 per cent of infertile couples. The application of the new treatments described here should enable most couples who are willing to exhaust all measures to reach their goal.

SUGGESTED READING

Buttram VC, Malinak R, Cleary R, et al (Adhesion study group): Reduction of postoperative pelvic adhesions with intraperitoneal 32 dextran 70: A prospective, randomized clinical trial. Fertil Steril 40:612, 1983.

Daly DC: Endometrial biopsy during treatment of luteal phase defects is predictive of therapeutic outcome. Fertil Steril 40:305, 1983.

Daly DC, Walters CA, Soto-Albors CE, et al: A randomized study of dexamethasone in ovulation induction with clomiphene citrate. Fertil Steril 41:844, 1984.

Dodson WC, Haney AF: Controlled ovarian hyperstimulation and intrauterine insemination for treatment of infertility. Fertil Steril 55:457, 1991.

Federation CECOS, Schwartz D, Mayaux MG: Female fecundity as a function of age. Results of artificial insemination in 2193 multiparous women with azoospermic husbands. N Engl J Med 1:404, 1982.

Guzick DS, Rock JA: A comparison of danazol and conservative surgery for the treatment of infertility due to mild or moderate endometriosis. Fertil Steril 40:580, 1983.

Hammond MG, Halme JK, Talbert LM: Factors affecting the pregnancy rate in clomiphene citrate induction of ovulation. Obstet Gynecol 62:196, 1983.

Hurley DM, Brian RJ, Burger HG: Ovulation induction with subcutaneous pulsatile gonadotropin-releasing hormone: Singleton pregnancies in patients with previous multiple pregnancies after gonadotropin therapy. Fertil Steril 40:575, 1983.

Investigation of the infertile couple: American Fertility Society, Birmingham, Alabama, 1991.

In-vitro fertilization–embryo transfer (IVF-ET) in the United States: 1989 results from the IVF-ET Registry. Fertil Steril 55:14, 1991.

Meldrum DR: Low dose follicle-stimulating hormone therapy for polycystic ovarian disease. Fertil Steril 55:1039, 1991.

Schwabe MG, Shapiro SS, Haning RV: Hysterosalpingography with oil contrast medium enhances fertility in patients with infertility of unknown etiology. Fertil Steril 40:604, 1983.

Shoupe D, Mishell DR, Lacarra M, et al: Correlation of endometrial maturation with four methods of estimating ovulation. Obstet Gynecol 73:88, 1989.

Part 5

Gynecologic Oncology

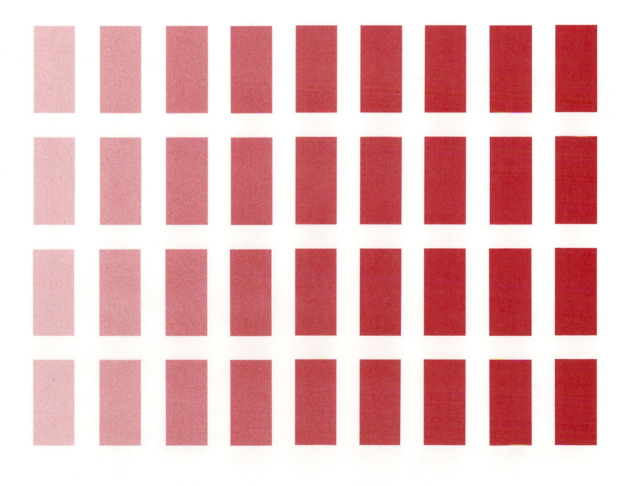

Fifty-two

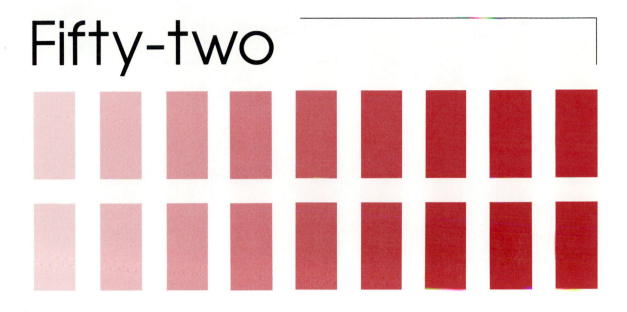

Principles of Cancer Therapy

NEVILLE F. HACKER

The standard modalities for the management of gynecologic cancer are surgery, chemotherapy, radiation therapy, and hormonal therapy. In this chapter, the principles of chemotherapy, radiation therapy, and hormonal manipulation are discussed. Immunotherapy and hyperthermia are currently experimental modalities and are not included.

CHEMOTHERAPY

One of the major advances in medicine since the 1950s has been the successful treatment of certain disseminated malignancies, including choriocarcinoma and some ovarian tumors, with chemotherapy. Prior to reviewing the agents used to treat gynecologic tumors, a brief review of the relevant cellular biology is presented.

Cellular Biology

The characteristic feature of malignant tumor growth is its uncontrolled cellular proliferation, which requires replication of DNA. There are two distinct phases in the life cycle of all cells: mitosis (M phase), during which cellular division occurs, and interphase, the interval between successive mitoses.

Interphase is subdivided into three separate phases (Fig. 52–1). Immediately following mitosis is the G_1 phase, which is of variable duration and is characterized by a diploid content of DNA. DNA synthesis is absent, but RNA and protein synthesis occur. During the shorter S phase, the entire DNA content is duplicated. This is followed by the G_2 phase, which is characterized by a tetraploid DNA content and by continuing RNA and protein synthesis in preparation for cell division. When mitosis occurs, a duplicate set of

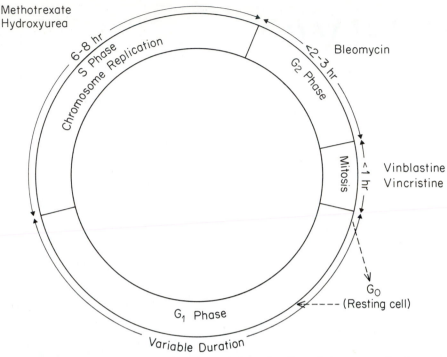

Figure 52–1. Phases of the cell cycle and sites of action of phase-specific drugs.

chromosomal DNA is inherited by each daughter cell, thus restoring the diploid DNA content. Following mitosis, some cells leave the cycle temporarily or permanently and enter the G_0 or resting phase.

The growth fraction of the tumor is the proportion of actively dividing cells. The higher the growth fraction, the fewer the number of cells in the G_0 phase and the faster the tumor doubling time. As tumors enlarge, their vascularity becomes compromised, and there is a progressive decrease in their growth fraction.

Chemotherapeutic agents and radiation kill cells by first-order kinetics, which means that a constant proportion of cells is killed for a given dosage, regardless of the number of cells present. Both modalities of therapy are most effective against actively dividing cells, since cells in the resting (G_0) phase are better able to repair sublethal damage. By surgically removing bulky, hypoxic tumor masses in patients with ovarian cancer, the growth fraction of the residual tumor is increased, thereby rendering it more susceptible to chemotherapy or radiation therapy. Unfortu-

nately, both therapeutic modalities also suppress rapidly dividing normal cells, such as those in the gastrointestinal mucosa, bone marrow, and hair follicles.

Classification of Chemotherapeutic Agents

Chemotherapeutic agents act primarily by disrupting nuclear DNA, thus inhibiting cellular division. They may be subdivided into two categories according to their mode of action relative to the cell cycle:

1. Cycle-specific agents, such as alkylating agents and *cis*-platinum, which exert their damage at any phase of the cell cycle. They may damage resting as well as cycling cells, but the latter are much more sensitive.

2. Phase-specific agents, which exert their lethal effects exclusively or primarily during one phase of the cell cycle. Examples include hydroxyurea and methotrexate, which act primarily during the S phase; bleomycin,

which acts in the G_2 phase; and the vinca alkaloids, which act in the M phase.

Principles of Chemotherapy

Chemotherapeutic agents are selected on the basis of previous experience with particular agents for any given tumor, although much current research is being undertaken to develop an effective assay for in vitro chemotherapy sensitivity testing. The drugs are usually given systemically so that the tumor can be treated regardless of its anatomic location. To increase the local concentration, certain drugs may occasionally be administered topically, by intra-arterial infusion, or by intrathecal or intracavitary instillation (e.g., intraperitoneal therapy for ovarian cancer).

Chemotherapy is generally not administered if the white cell count is less than $3000/mm^3$ or the platelet count less than $100,000/mm^3$. Nadir blood counts are obtained 7 to 14 days following treatment, and subsequent doses may need to be reduced, depending on the degree of myelosuppression. Dosage reduction may also be necessary because of toxicity to other organs, such as the gastrointestinal tract, liver, or kidneys.

Resistance to chemotherapeutic agents may be temporary or permanent. Temporary resistance is related mainly to the poor vascularity of bulky tumors, which results in poor tissue concentrations of the drugs and an increasing proportion of cells in the relatively resistant G_0 phase of the cell cycle. Permanent resistance is mainly due to spontaneous mutation to phenotypic resistance and occurs most commonly in bulky tumors. Permanent resistance may also be acquired by frequent exposure to chemotherapeutic agents. The smaller the tumor burden, the fewer the number of cycles required to eliminate the disease, thereby decreasing the likelihood of acquired chemotherapeutic resistance.

Chemotherapeutic Agents

The common agents used in the management of gynecologic malignancies may be classified as shown in Table 52–1. A summary of the main indications and side effects of these drugs is presented in Table 52–2.

Table 52–1. CHEMOTHERAPEUTIC AGENTS COMMONLY USED IN GYNECOLOGIC ONCOLOGY

Alkylating Agents
  Melphalan (Alkeran)
  Chlorambucil (Leukeran)
  Cyclophosphamide (Cytoxan)

Antimetabolites
  Methotrexate (Methotrexate)
  5-Fluorouracil (Fluorouracil)

Antibiotics
  Actinomycin-D (Cosmegen)
  Doxorubicin (Adriamycin)
  Bleomycin (Blenoxane)

Vinca Alkaloids
  Vinblastine (Velban)
  Vincristine (Oncovin)

Other Drugs
  Cis-diaminodichloroplatinum (Platinol)
  Hexamethylmelamine (Hexamine)
  Epipodophyllotoxins (Etoposide or VP16)

Alkylating Agents. The cytotoxicity of alkylating agents is due to their ability to cause alkylation to DNA, resulting in cross-linkage between DNA strands and prevention of DNA replication. Although not phase-specific, these agents are most effective during the S phase when DNA is being replicated. Nonreplicating cells are able to repair DNA damage enzymatically. There is cross-resistance among the various alkylating agents.

Antimetabolites. Antimetabolites are compounds that closely resemble normal intermediaries, for which they may substitute in biochemical reactions and thereby produce a metabolic block. Methotrexate competitively inhibits the enzyme dihydrofolate reductase, thus preventing the conversion of dihydrofolate to tetrahydrofolate. The latter is required for the methylation reaction necessary for the synthesis of purine and pyrimidine subunits of nucleic acid. 5-Fluorouracil (5-FU) is a fluoridated analog of uracil, one of the two pyrimidine bases in RNA. It may be converted to the nucleotide 5-fluorodeoxyuridine monophosphate (5-FdUMP), which inhibits thymidylate synthetase, an essential enzyme in DNA synthesis.

Table 52–2. INDICATIONS, SIDE EFFECTS, AND PRECAUTIONS FOR COMMONLY USED CHEMOTHERAPEUTIC AGENTS

DRUG	MAIN INDICATIONS	SIDE EFFECTS	PRECAUTIONS
Chlorambucil	Ovarian carcinoma	Bone marrow depression	—
Melphalan	Ovarian and tubal carcinoma	Bone marrow depression, leukemia	Avoid prolonged courses (>12 cycles) to avoid leukemia
Cyclophosphamide	Ovarian carcinoma, germ cell tumors, squamous carcinomas, sarcomas	Bone marrow depression, nausea and vomiting, alopecia, hemorrhagic cystitis, sterility	Maintain adequate fluid intake to avoid cystitis
Methotrexate	Gestational trophoblastic disease	Bone marrow depression, nausea and vomiting, stomatitis, alopecia, liver and renal failure, dermatitis	Ensure normal renal and liver function
5-Fluorouracil	Vaginal and vulvar intraepithelial neoplasia (topical application)	Pain and ulceration	—
Actinomycin-D	Gestational trophoblastic disease	Bone marrow depression, nausea and vomiting, diarrhea, stomatitis, alopecia, dermatitis, local tissue necrosis	Administer through running IV infusion to avoid extravasation
Doxorubicin	Ovarian carcinoma, recurrent endometrial carcinoma, sarcoma	Bone marrow depression, nausea and vomiting, cardiomyopathy, cardiac arrhythmias, alopecia, local tissue necrosis	Administer through running iV infusion; do not exceed total dose of 550 mg/m^2 to avoid cardiac toxicity; avoid if significant heart disease
Bleomycin	Germ cell tumors, squamous carcinomas	Pneumonitis and pulmonary fibrosis, alopecia, stomatitis, cutaneous reactions	Do not exceed total dose of 400 units; monitor pulmonary function with carbon monoxide diffusion capacity
Vinblastine	Germ cell tumors, sarcomas	Bone marrow depression, nausea and vomiting, stomatitis, diarrhea, local tissue necrosis	Administer through running IV infusion
Vincristine	Germ cell tumors, sarcomas	Neurotoxicity, constipation, alopecia, local tissue necrosis, bone marrow depression less marked	Administer through running IV infusion; prophylactic cathartics may be helpful
Etoposide	Germ cell tumors	Bone marrow depression, nausea and vomiting	Administer slowly by IV

Table 52–2. INDICATIONS, SIDE EFFECTS, AND PRECAUTIONS FOR COMMONLY USED CHEMOTHERAPEUTIC AGENTS *Continued*

DRUG	MAIN INDICATIONS	SIDE EFFECTS	PRECAUTIONS
Cis-platinum	Ovarian carcinoma, germ cell tumors, squamous carcinomas	Renal toxicity, ototoxicity, neurotoxicity, severe nausea and vomiting, bone marrow depression less marked, hypokalemia, hypomagnesemia	Administer IV fluids to maintain urinary output of 100 ml/hr during infusion; discontinue if creatinine clearance <35 ml/hr
Carbo-platinum	Ovarian carcinoma, germ cell tumors	Bone marrow depression, less gastrointestinal toxicity, less renal toxicity, less neurotoxicity	Suitable for outpatient therapy because no need for high urinary output
Hexamethylmelamine	Ovarian carcinoma	Bone marrow depression, nausea and vomiting, neurotoxicity, depression	Given orally

Antibiotics. Antibiotics are naturally occurring antitumor agents elaborated by certain species of *Streptomyces*. They have no single clearly defined mechanism of action, but many agents in this group intercalate between strands of the DNA double helix, thereby inhibiting both DNA and RNA synthesis and causing oxygen-dependent strand breaks.

Vinca Alkaloids. The vinca alkaloids are derived from the periwinkle plant. They are spindle toxins that interfere with cellular microtubules and cause metaphase arrest.

Other Drugs. *Cis*-platinum, one of the more important drugs in gynecologic oncology, causes inhibition of DNA synthesis by forming interstrand and intrastrand linkages. *Carbo*-platinum is an analog of *cis*-platinum with a similar mechanism of action and efficacy, but with less gastrointestinal and renal toxicity.

Hexamethylmelamine is an active agent against ovarian cancer, but its mechanism of action has not been elucidated. It does not display cross-resistance with the alkylating agents.

Etoposide (VP16), an abstract from the mandrake plant, appears to act by causing single-strand DNA breaks.

RADIATION THERAPY

Radiation may be defined as the propagation of energy through space or matter.

Types of Radiation

There are two main types of radiation: (1) electromagnetic and (2) particulate.

Electromagnetic Radiation. Examples of electromagnetic radiation include

1. Visible light.
2. Infrared light.
3. Ultraviolet light.
4. X-rays (photons).
5. Gamma rays (photons).

X-rays and gamma rays are identical electromagnetic radiations, differing only in their mode of production. X-rays are produced by bombardment of an anode by a high-speed electron beam; gamma rays result from the decay of radioactive isotopes, such as cobalt-60 (^{60}Co).

X-rays and gamma rays (photons) are differentiated from electromagnetic radiations of longer wavelength by their greater energy, which allows them to penetrate tissues and cause ionization.

Particulate Radiation. Particulate radiation consists of moving particles of matter. Their energy consists of the kinetic energy of the moving particles.

$$Energy = 0.5 \; Mass \times Velocity^2$$

The particles vary greatly in size and include

1. Neutrons (no charge).
2. Protons (positive charge).
3. Electrons (negative charge).

The most commonly used particles are electrons. These may be derived from a linear accelerator, the beam of electrons being directed into the patient without first striking a metal target and producing x-rays. Alternatively, high-energy electrons (called beta particles) may be derived from the radiodecay of an unstable isotope, such as phosphorus-32 (^{32}P). Particulate radiation penetrates tissues less than photons but also produces ionization.

Units of Radiation Measurement

The rad was the most commonly used unit of absorbed dose. One rad is equivalent to an energy absorption of 100 ergs per gram of any material. More recently the Gray has been defined and is equivalent to an absorbed dose of 1 joule/kg (1 Gray = 100 rad). One rad is equivalent to 1 cGy.

Inverse Square Law

The intensity of electromagnetic radiation is inversely proportional to the square of the distance from the source. Thus, the dose of radiation 2 cm from a point source will be 25 per cent of the dose at 1 cm.

Biological Considerations

Ionization of Molecules. Radiation damage is caused by the ionization of molecules in the cell, with the production of free radicals. Because approximately 80 per cent of a mammalian cell is water, most of the cellular radiation damage is mediated by ionization of water and the production of the free radicals H (hydrogen) and OH (hydroxyl). Free radicals may cause irreversible damage to DNA, making it impossible for the cell to continue replication. Minor or sublethal damage to DNA, which the cell is capable of repairing, may also occur. RNA, protein, and other molecules in the cell are also damaged, but these molecules can be more readily repaired or replaced.

Oxygen Effect. In the absence of oxygen, cells show a twofold to threefold increase in their capacity to survive radiation exposure —that is, hypoxic cells are less radiosensitive than fully oxygenated cells. The enhancement of the lethal effects of radiation by oxygen is presumed to occur because the oxygen will combine with the free radicals split from cell targets by the radiation. This prevents the recombination of the free radicals with the targets, which would restore the integrity of the targets.

The effect of oxygen has important clinical implications. First, anemic patients should be transfused before radiation therapy. Second, bulky tumors are usually poorly vascularized and, therefore, are hypoxic, particularly in the center. Such areas are likely to be relatively resistant to radiation so that viable tumor cells may remain in spite of marked shrinkage of the tumor. This principle is used in recommending extrafascial hysterectomy following radiation therapy for bulky stage Ib cervical cancer to decrease the incidence of central recurrence.

Pharmacologic Modification of the Effects of Radiation. A variety of chemical compounds are being developed to enhance the lethal effects of radiation, particularly in hypoxic tissues. The most common of these radiosensitizing compounds are the electron affinic agents, such as metronidazole (Flagyl). These substances act like oxygen in preventing repair of radiation damage, but because they are not metabolized like oxygen, they can penetrate and act in the hypoxic centers of tumors. Chemicals may also interact with radiation by preferentially killing cells more resistant to radiation. For example, cells are most resistant to radiation in the S phase of the cell cycle. Hydroxyurea is an S phase–specific drug, so it acts in conjunction with radiation to achieve maximum cell kill. Radioprotective agents, such as the sulfhydryl-containing compounds and other reducing substances, act in the reverse fashion and tend to make cells more resistant.

Time-Dose Fractionation of Radiation. Successful radiation therapy requires a delicate balance between dosage to the tumor and that to the surrounding normal tissues. A dose of radiation that is too high sterilizes the tumor but results in an unacceptably high complication rate because of the destruction of normal tissues.

Most normal tissues, such as gastrointestinal mucosa and bone marrow, have a remarkable capacity to recover from radiation damage by the division of stem cells as well as by repair of sublethal radiation damage. Tumors, in general, have less ability to repair and repopulate. This difference can be exploited by administering the radiation in multiple fractions, thereby allowing some recovery, particularly of normal cells, between fractions.

If the interval between each fraction increases, the total dose must increase to produce the same biological effect because of the amount of recovery that will occur in the interval. Cells that survive the acute effects of radiation usually repair sublethal damage within 24 hours; therefore, conventionally fractioned radiation is usually given in daily increments.

When treating the pelvis with external radiation, each fraction is usually 180 to 200 cGy. In treating the whole abdomen, fractions are decreased to 100 to 120 cGy because the tolerance of normal tissues decreases as the volume irradiated increases. The exact reason for this phenomenon is unclear. The converse of this principle allows a small radiation field (e.g., one pelvic side wall) to be boosted to a higher dose without significant risk to normal tissues. This may be important in treating a patient found to have fixed, positive lymph nodes on one side of the pelvis. The major factors influencing the outcome of radiation therapy are summarized in Table 52–3.

Modalities of Radiation Therapy

The modalities used to deliver radiation therapy are listed in Table 52–4. In general,

---

Table 52–3. MAJOR FACTORS INFLUENCING THE OUTCOME OF RADIATION THERAPY

Normal tissue tolerance
Malignant cell type
Total volume irradiated
Total dose delivered
Total duration of therapy
Number of fractions
Type of equipment used
Tissue oxygen concentration

---

there are two radiation techniques: teletherapy and brachytherapy. In teletherapy, a device quite removed from the patient is used, as with external beam techniques. In brachytherapy, the radiation source is placed either within or close to the target tissue, as with intracavitary and interstitial techniques. In contrast to external beam therapy, intracavitary and interstitial techniques allow a high dose of radiation to be delivered only to the tumor itself. Dosages to surrounding normal tissues are considerably lower and determined by the inverse square law.

External Beam Therapy. As the energy of the electromagnetic radiation increases, the

---

Table 52–4. MODALITIES OF RADIATION THERAPY

External beams
  Kilovoltage ("orthovoltage") (125–400 kV)
  Cobalt-60 machine (1.25 MeV)
  Linear accelerator (4–35 MeV)
  Betatrons (20–42 MeV)
  Particle accelerators (e.g., electrons, protons, neutrons)

Intracavitary (radium or cesium)
  Rigid applicators (e.g., Ernst)
  Afterloading applicators (e.g., Fletcher-Suit)
  Intraperitoneal (e.g., ^{32}P, ^{198}Au)

Interstitial
  Permanent
    Seeds (e.g., ^{198}Au, ^{125}I)
  Removable
    Ribbons (e.g., ^{192}Ir)
    Needles (e.g., ^{226}R, ^{137}C)

Table 52–5. ADVANTAGES OF MEGAVOLTAGE THERAPY

Skin sparing
Greater dose at deeper depth in tissues
Shorter treatment times
No differential bone absorption (therefore no bone necrosis)
Can treat larger fields easily (e.g., whole abdomen)

penetration of the tissues increases, resulting in a relative sparing of the skin and an increased dosage to deeper tissues. At megavoltage energies (1 million electron volts or greater), there is no differential absorption of energy by bone.

Orthovoltage machines are no longer used except to treat skin cancers. Cobalt machines, developed in the early 1950s, have also been largely replaced by linear accelerators, which have a higher range of energies. The advantages of megavoltage therapy over the earlier orthovoltage machines (1000 electron volts) are listed in Table 52–5.

External radiation allows a uniform dose to be delivered to a given field. The tolerance of the normal tissues (e.g., bowel, bladder, liver, kidneys) limits the total dosage that can be delivered. External radiation is usually used to shrink a large tumor mass prior to brachytherapy. When used alone, it is generally useful only when there is small residual macroscopic or microscopic disease following surgery, such as when whole pelvic radiation is given following total abdominal hysterectomy and bilateral salpingo-oophorectomy for stage I endometrial cancer or when whole abdominal radiation is given following surgical removal of gross disease in stage III ovarian cancer. With highly radiosensitive tumors (e.g., dysgerminoma), external radiation alone may sterilize even bulky disease.

Intracavitary Radiation. Intracavitary therapy is used particularly in the treatment of cervical cancer, stage II endometrial cancer, and vaginal cancer. All applicators now in use should be "afterloaded," which means that they are placed in the patient and their position checked by x-ray before the radioactive radium or cesium is loaded into the applicator. The correct placement of the ap-

plicator is critical if the tumor is to receive the maximum dose and the surrounding tissues the minimum dose. The ability to afterload these devices has improved the accuracy of their placement and spared medical and paramedical personnel from excessive radiation exposure. The Fletcher-Suit afterloading device, used in the treatment of cervical and endometrial cancer, is shown in Figure 52–2. Remote afterloading devices, such as the Selectron, allow the radioactive sources to be removed from the applicators when medical or nursing personnel enter the room, thereby significantly limiting staff exposure to radiation.

Radioactive colloids, such as gold (^{198}Au) and chromic phosphate (^{32}P), may be instilled directly into the peritoneal or pleural cavity to treat malignant effusions or minimal residual disease, particularly in patients with ovarian cancer. To be effective, these agents must achieve a uniform distribution throughout the cavity. Prerequisites for uniform distribution include instillation in an adequate fluid volume, frequent positional change after instillation, and freedom from physical barriers such as adhesions. ^{32}P is a pure beta (electron) emitter, in contrast to ^{198}Au, which also emits the more penetrating gamma rays; therefore, radiation safety is enhanced with the use of ^{32}P.

Interstitial Radiation. Interstitial therapy (in which the radioactive source is placed directly in the tumor) may be delivered by removable implants or permanent implants. Permanent implants are used for inaccessible tumors. They use radioisotopes such as radon (^{222}Rn) or iodine (^{125}I) seeds and are usually placed in an unresectable tumor nodule at the time of laparotomy.

Removable implants are placed in tumors that are accessible (e.g., cervical or vaginal tumors). Interstitial therapy has the theoretic advantage of better dose distribution within the tumor but the disadvantage that it is easier to overdose normal tissues, therefore increasing the complication rate. Interstitial therapy should be performed only by therapists who have had adequate experience with the technique. As with intracavitary devices, afterloading devices are now available for interstitial therapy. Figure 52–3 illustrates the Syed-Nesbit template used for treating pelvic malignancies. The radioisotope of choice for

Figure 52–2. Devices for intracavitary radium or cesium: (1) vaginal cylinder, *A*; (2) components of the Fletcher-Suit afterloading device: uterine tandems, *B*; vaginal colpostats, *C*; afterloading devices for colpostats, *D*; vaginal spacers, *E*.

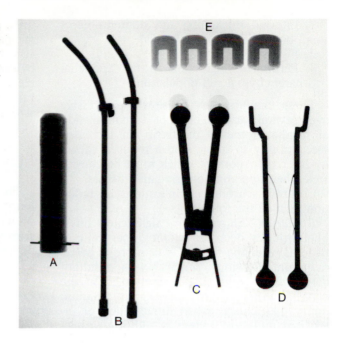

afterloading interstitial implants is iridium (^{192}Ir).

Complications Associated with Radiation

The success of radiation therapy depends on an exploitable gradient of susceptibility to injury in favor of normal tissue. Unfortunately, most malignant tumors are only marginally more sensitive to radiation than normal tissues, so the total dose that can be

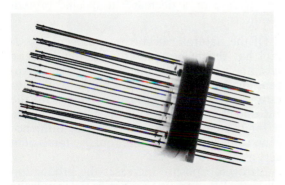

Figure 52–3. Syed-Nesbit template for interstitial radiation with iridium (^{192}Ir). Note that the needles have been loaded into the template.

delivered, and therefore the radiocurability, is limited by the associated complications.

Acute Complications. Acute reactions to radiation include the following pathologic changes:

1. Rapid cessation of mitotic activity.
2. Cellular swelling.
3. Tissue edema.
4. Tissue necrosis.

In the management of gynecologic tumors, these acute reactions may produce the following effects:

1. Acute cystitis, manifested by hematuria, urgency, and frequency.
2. Proctosigmoiditis, manifested by tenesmus, diarrhea, and passage of blood and mucus in the stool.
3. Enteritis, manifested by nausea, vomiting, diarrhea, and colicky abdominal pain.
4. Bone marrow depression, which is uncommon with pelvic radiation but common with pelvic and abdominal radiation, particularly if the patient has had previous cytotoxic chemotherapy.

Chronic Complications. Chronic complications occur 6 to 24 months after completion of radiation and are characterized pathologically by the following changes:

1. Internal thickening and obliteration of small blood vessels (endarteritis).

2. Fibrosis.

3. Permanent reduction in the epithelial and parenchymal cell populations.

These changes may be slowly progressive over several years. The poor vascularization of irradiated tissues results in an increased susceptibility to injury and a reduced capacity for repair, both of which must be considered when operating on irradiated tissues.

Common chronic complications of radiation include the following.

Radiation Enteropathy. Significant intestinal injuries occur in about 5 per cent of patients receiving 5000 cGy or more of pelvic radiation. Previous surgery, with resultant loops of adherent small bowel fixed in the pelvis, predisposes the patient to radiation injury, particularly when intracavitary or interstitial radiation is used in addition to teletherapy.

Large bowel injuries, which are best diagnosed by sigmoidoscopy or colonoscopy, may include

1. Proctosigmoiditis, manifested by pelvic pain, tenesmus, alteration in bowel habits, anorexia, and weight loss.

2. Ulceration, manifested by rectal bleeding.

3. Rectovaginal fistula, manifested by passage of stool through the vagina.

4. Rectal or sigmoid stenosis, manifested by progressive large bowel obstruction.

Small bowel injuries usually present with symptoms of an incomplete small bowel obstruction.

Vaginal Vault Necrosis. This is associated with severe pain and tenderness of the vaginal vault, and hemorrhage may occur. The condition may mimic recurrent cancer, but biopsy other than by fine-needle aspiration cytology should be delayed until the necrosis has cleared, or a fistula may be produced.

Urologic Injuries. These may include

1. Hemorrhagic cystitis, which may necessitate frequent blood transfusions and, occasionally, urinary diversion. Cystoscopy confirms the diagnosis.

2. Vesicovaginal fistula, in which the patient complains of the constant leakage of urine. Methylene blue instilled into the bladder passes immediately into the vagina.

3. Ureterovaginal fistula, also manifested by constant leakage of urine and demonstrable with an intravenous pyelogram.

4. Ureteric stenosis, manifested by progressive hydronephrosis.

HORMONAL THERAPY

The estrogen-receptor (ER) status of primary and metastatic breast cancer has been shown to be of therapeutic and prognostic significance. More recently, research has been directed to the measurement of estrogen and progesterone receptors (PRs) in gynecologic cancers, and the potential significance of this information is being evaluated.

Mechanism of Action of Hormonal Receptors

Most steroid hormones influence their target tissues by the following series of steps:

1. Passive diffusion of the hormone through the cell membrane.

2. Specific binding in the cytoplasm with the hormone receptor.

3. Translocation of the receptor-hormone complex to the nucleus.

4. Binding of the receptor-hormone complex to an "acceptor" site on the chromatin.

5. Transcription of DNA in a manner characteristic of the specific hormone–target cell interaction, resulting eventually in either an increase or a decrease in specific protein synthesis.

Of the naturally occurring estrogens, estradiol has the highest affinity for the estrogen receptor. The synthetic, nonsteroidal estrogen, diethylstilbestrol, also binds readily to estrogen receptors. Tamoxifen binds with the ER and is translocated to the nucleus, where it binds to chromatin. It does not influence gene transcription, so functionally, tamoxifen acts as an antiestrogen.

Estrogen exposure increases the production of both ER and PR, whereas progesterone inhibits production of both ER and PR. This suggests that patients whose tumors are ER-positive should also be PR-positive, which is usually true. It also suggests that tumors should not contain PR in the absence of ER. In practice, however, some such tumors will be found.

Clinical Applications

Since tumor growth in patients who are ER-positive and PR-positive is likely to be stimulated by estrogen exposure, tumor regression should occur if endogenous estrogen production is abolished or if the patient is exposed to a progestin or antiestrogen. In breast cancer, patients whose tumors are ER-positive and PR-positive have an 80 per cent response rate to hormonal manipulation, whereas fewer than 10 per cent of receptor-poor tumors respond. In addition, prognosis in primary, operable cases is better in receptor-rich tumors.

Objective response to progestin therapy occurs in about one third of patients with recurrent or metastatic endometrial carcinoma. It has been known for many years that progestin therapy is more effective among well-differentiated endometrial adenocarcinomas than among more poorly differentiated tumors, and it has been demonstrated that well-differentiated tumors are the ones that are most likely to contain ER and PR. The presence of steroid receptors is a more reliable guide to response to progestin therapy than is histologic grade.

ER and PR have been demonstrated in some ovarian adenocarcinomas, but the therapeutic implications of these findings await further investigation.

SUGGESTED READING

Berek JS, Hacker NF: Practical Gynecologic Oncology. Baltimore, Williams & Wilkins, 1989, pp 3–72 and 589–610.

Ehrlich CE, Young PCM, Cleary RE: Cytoplasmic progesterone and estradiol receptors in normal, hyperplastic, and carcinomatous endometria: Therapeutic implications. Am J Obstet Gynecol 141:539, 1981.

Ehrlich CE, Young PCM, Stehman FB, et al: Steroid receptors and clinical outcome in patients with adenocarcinoma of the endometrium. Am J Obstet Gynecol 158:796, 1988.

Harding M, Cowan S, Hole D, et al: Estrogen and progesterone receptors in ovarian cancer. Cancer 65:486, 1990.

Hoffman PG, Siiteri PK: Sex steroid receptors in gynecologic cancer. Obstet Gynecol 55:648, 1980.

Fifty-three

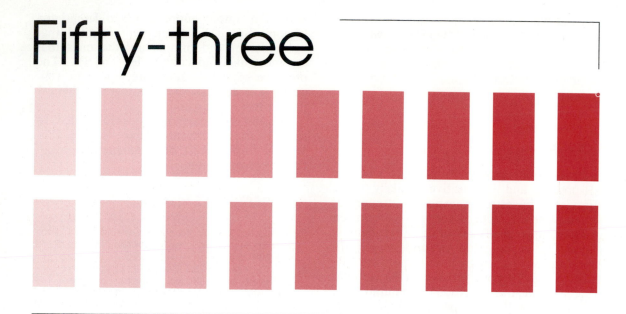

Uterine Corpus Cancer

RONALD S. LEUCHTER and JAMES M. HEAPS

Cancer of the endometrium is the most common gynecologic malignancy, being twice as common as carcinoma of the cervix in the United States. It is the fourth most common malignancy found in American women after breast, colorectal, and lung cancer. There was an increase in the incidence of endometrial cancer in the 1970s that may be related in part to the increased use of unopposed estrogen by postmenopausal women. Since the use of unopposed estrogens has been curtailed, the incidence has fallen back to its original level. The majority of tumors associated with this medication are of low stage and grade, and over the last 30 years, overall mortality rates have fallen.

EPIDEMIOLOGY AND ETIOLOGY

The median age for endometrial cancer is about 60 years. The risk factors associated with the development of carcinoma of the endometrium are listed in Table 53–1. Many of these factors are associated with prolonged stimulation of the endometrium by unopposed estrogen. If the proliferative effects of estrogen are not counteracted by a progestin, endometrial hyperplasia and possibly adenocarcinoma can result (see Chapter 32).

Obesity results in an increased extraovarian aromatization of androstenedione to estrone. Androstenedione is secreted by the adrenal glands, whereas the increased peripheral conversion occurs predominantly in fat depots but also in the liver, kidneys, and skeletal muscles. Granulosa–theca cell tumors of the ovary produce estrogen, and up to 15 per cent of patients with these tumors have an associated endometrial cancer.

Unopposed estrogen stimulation also occurs in premenopausal, anovulatory patients, such as those who have polycystic ovarian syndrome (Stein-Leventhal syndrome), and in

Table 53–1. RISK FACTORS FOR ENDOMETRIAL CANCER

Obesity
Nulliparity
Late menopause
Diabetes mellitus
Hypertension
Gallbladder disease
Breast, colon, or ovarian cancer
Chronic unopposed estrogen stimulation

postmenopausal women taking estrogen replacement without a progestin for menopausal symptoms. In this latter group, the risk of developing cancer appears to be both dose-dependent and duration-dependent. This increased risk varies from twofold to 14-fold compared with nonusers. The addition of an oral progestin during the last 10 to 14 days of the month eliminates this risk. Young women who use oral contraceptives have been shown to have a lower incidence of subsequent endometrial cancer.

SCREENING OF ASYMPTOMATIC WOMEN

Cytologic screening for endometrial cancer in asymptomatic women is less effective than screening for cervical cancer, since only about 40 per cent of cases have adenocarcinoma cells detected on a Papanicolaou smear. Furthermore, routine endometrial sampling of all postmenopausal women has not been shown to be practical or cost-effective. Outpatient techniques for endometrial sampling include use of the Kevorkian curette, Vabra aspirator, Gravlee jet washer, and Pipelle cannula. These techniques have a diagnostic accuracy of about 90 per cent.

Premenopausal patients who have chronic anovulation should have their endometrium periodically sampled to exclude endometrial hyperplasia or carcinoma. Similarly, postmenopausal women receiving unopposed estrogen therapy should ideally have an endometrial biopsy annually. Other high-risk patients, such as those who are obese, nulliparous, hypertensive, diabetic, or who have a strong family history of adenocarcinomas, should also undergo endometrial sampling.

SYMPTOMS

The most common symptom of endometrial cancer is abnormal vaginal bleeding; this is present in 90 per cent of such patients. Postmenopausal bleeding is always abnormal and must be investigated. The most common conditions associated with postmenopausal bleeding are listed in Table 53–2. Although a single episode of vaginal spotting is most likely due to a nonmalignant lesion, the physician must exclude malignancy. The older the patient, the more likely it is that she has cancer. In the premenopausal patient, especially after age 35, menorrhagia or intermenstrual bleeding may signal an endometrial lesion.

SIGNS

General physical examination may reveal obesity, hypertension, and stigmata of diabetes mellitus. Evidence of metastatic disease is unusual at initial presentation, but the chest should be examined for any effusion and the abdomen carefully palpated and percussed to exclude ascites, hepatosplenomegaly, or evidence of upper abdominal masses. Any evidence of general lymphadenopathy should be sought.

On pelvic examination, the external genitalia are usually normal. The vagina and cervix

Table 53–2. ETIOLOGY OF POSTMENOPAUSAL BLEEDING

FACTOR	APPROXIMATE PERCENTAGE
Exogenous estrogens	30
Atrophic endometritis/vaginitis	30
Endometrial cancer	15
Endometrial or cervical polyps	10
Endometrial hyperplasia	5
Miscellaneous (e.g., cervical cancer, uterine sarcoma, urethral caruncle, trauma)	10

are also usually normal but should be carefully inspected and palpated for evidence of involvement. A patulous cervical os or a firm, expanded cervix may indicate extension of disease from the corpus to the cervix. The uterus may be of normal size or enlarged, depending on the extent of the disease and the presence or absence of other uterine conditions, such as adenomyosis or fibroids. The adnexae should be carefully palpated for evidence of extrauterine metastases or an ovarian neoplasm. A granulosa cell tumor or an endometrioid ovarian carcinoma may occasionally coexist with an endometrial cancer.

DIAGNOSIS

Any woman who presents with postmenopausal bleeding should have a Papanicolaou smear, an endocervical curettage, and an endometrial biopsy performed as an outpatient. If the endometrial biopsy reveals endometrial cancer, definitive treatment can be arranged. If the endometrial biopsy is negative or reveals endometrial hyperplasia, a fractional dilatation and curettage should be performed under general anesthesia or an outpatient hysteroscopy arranged. Specimens from the endometrium and endocervix should be submitted separately for histologic evaluation to determine if the tumor has extended to the endocervix. Diagnosis of endometrial cancer in a premenopausal patient requires a high index of suspicion, but in a patient with high-risk factors and abnormal uterine bleeding, a similar work-up should be undertaken. A grossly obvious lesion of the cervix or vagina should be biopsied directly.

STAGING

The International Federation of Gynecologists and Obstetricians (FIGO) has changed from a clinical to a surgical staging system for endometrial cancer. The old clinical staging is shown in Table 53–3, whereas the new surgical staging, based on pathologic confirmation of the extent of spread, is shown in Table 53–4.

PREOPERATIVE INVESTIGATIONS

In addition to a thorough physical examination, blood tests should include a complete blood count, hepatic enzymes, serum electrolytes, blood urea nitrogen, serum creatinine, and a coagulation profile. A routine urinalysis should also be obtained. Radiologic studies include a chest radiograph and bone radiographs if bone pain is present. Additional radiographic tests including an abdominopelvic computed tomographic scan (CT), an intravenous pyelogram (IVP), and a barium enema are performed only if indicated. A stool guaiac examination should be performed to test for occult blood.

PATHOLOGY

Several histologic types of endometrial carcinoma exist. About 75 per cent of the cases are pure adenocarcinomas. When benign squamous elements are present, the tumor is sometimes called an adenoacanthoma. Lesions that contain malignant squamous epithelium are called adenosquamous carcinomas and carry a poorer prognosis. Less often, clear cell, squamous, or papillary serous carcinomas occur in the endometrium. They also carry a worse prognosis.

Invasive adenocarcinoma of the endometrium demonstrates proliferative glandular formation with minimal or no intervening stroma. Tumor grade is determined by the degree of abnormality of the glandular architecture. A lesion that is well differentiated (grade 1) forms a glandular pattern similar to normal endometrial glands (Fig. 53–1). A moderately well-differentiated lesion (grade 2) has glandular structures admixed with papillary, and occasionally solid, areas of tumor. In a poorly differentiated lesion (grade 3), the glandular structures have become predominantly solid with a relative paucity of identifiable endometrial glands (Fig. 53–2).

PATTERN OF SPREAD

Endometrial cancer spreads by (1) direct extension, (2) exfoliation of cells that are shed through the fallopian tubes, (3) lym-

Table 53–3. FIGO* STAGING OF CARCINOMA OF THE CORPUS UTERI

Stage 0	Carcinoma in situ
Stage I	The carcinoma is confined to the corpus
Stage Ia	The length of the uterine cavity is 8 cm or less
Stage Ib	The length of the uterine cavity is more than 8 cm

It is desirable that the stage I cases be subgrouped with regard to the histologic grade of the adenocarcinoma as follows:

G1	Highly differentiated adenomatous carcinoma
G2	Moderately differentiated adenomatous carcinoma with partly solid areas
G3	Predominantly solid or entirely undifferentiated carcinoma
Stage II	The carcinoma has involved the corpus and the cervix but has not extended outside the uterus
Stage III	The carcinoma has extended outside the uterus but not outside the true pelvis
Stage IV	The carcinoma has extended outside the true pelvis or has obviously involved the mucosa of the bladder or rectum. A bullous edema as such does not permit a case to be allotted to stage IV
Stage IVa	Spread of the growth to adjacent organs
Stage IVb	Spread to distant organs

* International Federation of Gynecology and Obstetrics

phatic dissemination, and (4) hematogenous dissemination.

The most common route of spread is direct extension of the tumor to adjacent structures. The tumor may invade through the myometrium and eventually penetrate the serosa. It may also grow downward and involve the cervix. Although very uncommon, progressive direct extension may eventually involve the vagina, parametrium, rectum, or bladder. Exfoliated cells that pass through the fallopian tubes may implant on the ovaries, the visceral or parietal peritoneum, or the omentum.

Lymphatic spread occurs most commonly in patients with significant myometrial penetration. Spread occurs mainly to the pelvic lymph nodes and subsequently to the periaortic lymph nodes. The incidence of lymph node metastases is dependent on the tumor grade and the depth of myometrial invasion. In stage I endometrial cancer, the overall incidence of pelvic lymph node metastases is about 12 per cent, and periaortic lymph node metastases are present in about 8 per cent of cases. In patients with deeply invasive, poorly differentiated stage I adenocarcinomas, however, pelvic lymph node metastases occur in up to 40 per cent. Lymphatic spread is also responsible for vaginal vault recurrences. Hematogenous dissemination is less common, but it results in parenchymal metastases, particularly in the lungs, liver, or both.

TREATMENT

Stage I

Surgery

The primary treatment of stage I endometrial cancer is surgical. In the past, it was common practice to use preoperative intracavitary radiation in an attempt to sterilize the disease before surgical intervention. Currently it is generally considered preferable to operate primarily to allow proper surgical staging (Table 53–5). Adjuvant postoperative therapy can then be given more appropriately.

An exploratory laparotomy with total abdominal hysterectomy and bilateral salpingo-oophorectomy is performed on all patients, unless there are absolute medical contraindications (Fig. 53–3). To prevent potential spillage of cancer cells through the fallopian tubes, the tubes are clamped before performing the operation. On entering the peritoneal cavity, any free fluid is submitted for cytologic evaluation. If there is no free fluid and

Table 53–4. NEW FIGO (1988) STAGING OF ENDOMETRIAL CARCINOMA

Stage Ia	Tumor limited to endometrium
Stage Ib	Invasion through less than one half the myometrium
Stage Ic	Invasion through more than one half the myometrium
Stage IIa	Endocervical glandular involvement only
Stage IIb	Cervical stroma invasion
Stage IIIa	Tumor invades serosa and/or adnexa and/or positive peritoneal cytology
Stage IIIb	Vaginal metastases
Stage IIIc	Metastases to pelvic and/or para-aortic lymph nodes
Stage IVa	Tumor invasion of bladder and/or bowel mucosa
Stage IVb	Distant metastases including extra-abdominal and/or inguinal lymph nodes
Histologic grade—Tumor grade does not change the stage	
Grade 1	Well differentiated
Grade 2	Moderately differentiated
Grade 3	Poorly differentiated

no macroscopic evidence of tumor dissemination, saline washings are taken from the pelvis, paracolic gutters, and subdiaphragmatic areas and sent for cytologic evaluation. Approximately 12 per cent of patients with stage I disease have positive peritoneal cytology. Retroperitoneal spaces should be opened and evaluated, and any enlarged pelvic or periaortic lymph nodes should be resected. If the tumor is poorly differentiated or penetrates beyond the inner half of the myometrium, pelvic and para-aortic lymph node biopsies should be performed, even when there is no macroscopic evidence of spread.

Radiation Therapy

An algorithm summarizing the treatment of stage I endometrial cancer is presented in Figure 53–4. After exploratory laparotomy and an evaluation of the histopathology and peritoneal cytology, adjuvant radiation is given to selected patients. The depth of myo-metrial invasion cannot be readily determined preoperatively, so some patients with only superficial invasion may be spared pelvic radiation if the surgery is done initially.

Most patients who require additional treatment are candidates for external beam pelvic radiation, which is given in an attempt to prevent recurrent disease at the vaginal vault and pelvic side wall. Any patient with a poorly differentiated (grade 3) carcinoma or with invasion beyond the inner one third of the myometrium should receive whole pelvic irradiation postoperatively.

In patients with a superficially invasive, well-differentiated (grade 1) carcinoma, the incidence of recurrent disease is so low that no adjuvant therapy is indicated. If a superficially invasive grade 2 carcinoma is present, intracavitary radiation to the vaginal vault, which carries virtually no serious morbidity, may be given to prevent a vault recurrence.

In patients with periaortic lymph node involvement, extended-field radiation to include the pelvis and periaortic area is indicated. The management of patients who have positive peritoneal cytology is controversial. Whole abdominal radiation or intraperitoneal radioactive phosphorus (^{32}P) has been advocated, although these treatments are associated with significant morbidity, and no randomized prospective study has been done to demonstrate proved benefit.

In patients medically unfit for surgery, radiation therapy without surgery may be employed. A combination of intracavitary plus external beam radiation is used. The overall 5-year survival is about 25 per cent lower than for patients treated with hysterectomy.

Stage II

If the cervix is grossly normal and involvement is detected only on the histologic evaluation of the endocervical curettage material (occult stage II disease), treatment may be the same as for stage I disease (i.e., total abdominal hysterectomy, bilateral salpingo-oophorectomy, surgical staging, and postoperative radiotherapy).

If the cervix is grossly enlarged, preoperative external beam and intracavitary radiation are indicated, followed by total abdominal

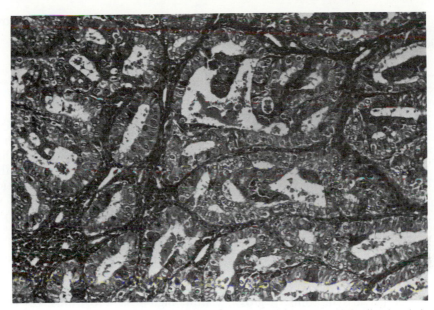

Figure 53–1. Well-differentiated endometrial adenocarcinoma (histology). Note the back to back glands with minimal intervening stroma and the gland within gland formation.

hysterectomy and bilateral salpingo-oophorectomy 6 weeks later. There are two alternative approaches. The first is to use preoperative external radiation only, followed in 6 weeks by a modified radical hysterectomy and bilateral salpingo-oophorectomy. The second is to use primary modified radical hysterectomy, bilateral salpingo-oophorectomy, surgical staging, and postoperative external beam therapy.

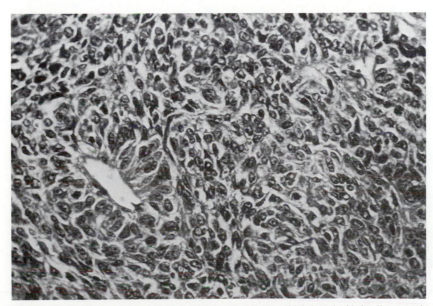

Figure 53–2. Poorly differentiated endometrial adenocarcinoma (histology). Note the predominantly solid nature of the tumor with minimal gland formation.

Table 53–5. HIGH-RISK FACTORS IN STAGE I ENDOMETRIAL CANCER

High tumor grade
Deep myometrial invasion
Pelvic and/or periaortic lymph node metastasis
Occult cervical involvement
Occult adnexal spread
Occult upper abdominal spread
Positive peritoneal cytology

Advanced Stages

For advanced disease, treatment is individualized. The uterus, tubes, and ovaries are best removed, if possible, for palliation of bleeding and other pelvic symptoms. If gross disease is present in the upper abdomen, tumor metastases that are readily removable, such as an omental "cake," should be extirpated in an attempt to improve the patient's quality of life by temporarily decreasing abdominal discomfort and ascites. In addition to preoperative or postoperative radiation, patients with advanced disease also require hormonal therapy, with or without chemotherapy.

Recurrent Disease

Seventy-five per cent of recurrences occur within 2 years of treatment, and a further 10 per cent occur by the end of the third year. If recurrent disease is detected, the patient should undergo a complete physical examination and metastatic work-up. If the disease appears to be limited to the vaginal vault, surgery, radiation, or a combination of the two may be effective, particularly if radiation was not used as part of the primary therapy. Metastases in other sites, such as the upper abdomen, lungs, or liver, are treated initially with high-dose progestins or antiestrogens. Medroxyprogesterone acetate (Provera), 50 mg three times daily; Depo-Provera, 400 mg intramuscularly weekly; or megestrol acetate (Megace), 80 mg twice daily, may be given. If disease progresses on progestins, chemotherapy may be offered. Doxorubicin (Adriamycin) appears to be the most active single agent, but the response rate is only about 35

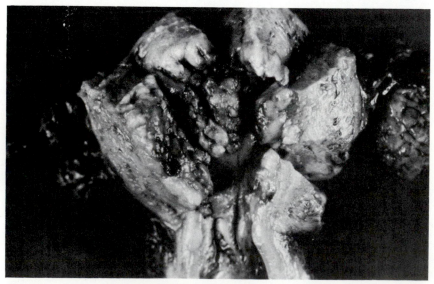

Figure 53–3. Specimen from a total abdominal hysterectomy and bilateral salpingo-oophorectomy. The uterus has been opened to reveal an exophytic carcinoma on the posterior wall of the corpus.

Figure 53–4. Algorithm of the treatment of stage I and occult stage II endometrial cancer.

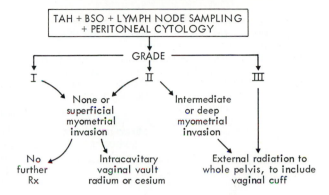

TREATMENT OF ENDOMETRIAL CANCER:

STAGES I + II OCCULT

For positive periaortic node, add periaortic radiation.

per cent, and most responses are partial and of short duration.

Hormone Receptors

About one third of recurrent endometrial carcinomas contain estrogen and progesterone receptors. The frequency of positive receptors is dependent on the grade of the tumor, the more well-differentiated tumors being more likely to be receptor-positive. As with breast cancer, the likelihood of a patient responding to progestin treatment is increased in patients whose tumors are receptor-positive. Approximately 80 per cent of such patients respond to progestin therapy, compared with fewer than 10 per cent of receptor-negative patients.

PROGNOSIS

Prognosis is dependent on several variables, including uterine size, histologic type, grade of tumor, depth of myometrial penetration, status of lymph nodes, status of peritoneal cytology, and presence or absence of occult adnexal or upper abdominal metastases. These factors are generally interrelated. The more poorly differentiated tumors (grade 3) have a greater propensity for deep myometrial invasion and, consequently, an increased

incidence of lymph node metastases. Positive peritoneal cytology also frequently coexists with other poor prognostic factors but may occur as an independent poor prognosticator. About one third of patients with positive washings recur in the peritoneal cavity.

Five-year survivals for each stage of endometrial cancer are presented in Table 53–6. The stages indicated are based on the old clinical staging system. Stage for stage, prognosis is similar to that for cervical cancer.

Table 53–6. CARCINOMA OF THE CORPUS UTERI*

STAGE	PATIENTS TREATED		5-YEAR SURVIVAL	
	No.	%	No.	%
I	11,035	74.0	7876	72.3
II	2014	13.5	1135	56.4
III	921	6.2	290	31.5
IV	409	2.8	43	10.5
No stage	527	3.5	253	47.8
Total	14,906	100.0	9697	65.1

* Distribution by stage and 5-year survival rate in different stages
From the Editorial Office of the Annual Report on the Results of Treatment in Gynecological Cancer. Vol 20. Stockholm, Sweden, 1988, p 80.

Table 53–7. CLASSIFICATION OF UTERINE SARCOMAS

TYPE	HOMOLOGOUS	HETEROLOGOUS
Pure	Leiomyosarcoma Stromal sarcoma Endolymphatic stromal myosis Endometrial stro- mal sarcoma	Rhabdomyosarcoma Chondrosarcoma Osteosarcoma Liposarcoma
Mixed	Carcinosarcoma	Mixed mesodermal sarcoma

Follow-up

Follow-up examinations should be performed every 3 months for 2 years, every 6 months for 3 years, and then annually. An annual chest film may be ordered to exclude lung metastases for the first 3 years of follow-up.

UTERINE SARCOMAS

Uterine sarcomas are rare. They arise from the stromal components of the uterus, either the endometrial stroma or the mesenchymal and myometrial tissues. As a group, sarcomas tend to be more advanced at the time of diagnosis, are more likely to disseminate hematogenously, and have much lower 2- and 5-year survival rates.

Classification

A classification system for uterine sarcomas is presented in Table 53–7. Uterine sarcomas can be classified as either *pure,* in which the only malignant tissue is of mesenchymal origin, or *mixed,* in which malignant mesenchymal and malignant epithelial tissues are present. They may also be classified as *homologous,* implying that the tissue that is malignant is normally present in the uterus (e.g., endometrial stroma, smooth muscle), or *heterologous,* implying that the tissue that is malignant is not normally present in the uterus (e.g., bone or cartilage). The majority of pure uterine sarcomas are leiomyosarcomas and endometrial stromal sarcomas.

Leiomyosarcoma

Leiomyosarcomas may be associated with a benign leiomyoma of the uterus, but the risk of malignant transformation in a benign fibroid is less than 1 per cent. The most important histologic criterion for distinguishing leiomyosarcomas from leiomyomas is the mitotic index. If the tumor's most highly mitotic areas contain 10 or more mitoses per 10 high-power fields (hpf), the lesion is malignant. Lesions with fewer than five mitoses per 10 hpf are generally benign, whereas tumors with five to nine mitoses per 10 hpf can behave in a malignant fashion and may recur.

Clinically, the mean age of patients with a leiomyosarcoma is about 55 years. Patients with this disease may present with menometrorrhagia, postmenopausal bleeding, or a pelvic mass. A vaginal discharge or a sensation of pressure or fullness in the pelvic area may also be noted.

Most cases are not diagnosed preoperatively but are discovered at the time of exploratory surgery for probable uterine myomata. Endometrial curettage material is usually negative. If on pelvic examination the uterus appears to be rapidly enlarging, the suspicion of a uterine malignancy exists.

Leiomyosarcomas tend to spread by local extension as well as by hematogenous and lymphatic dissemination. Isolated pelvic recurrences are uncommon. Most patients die with disease in distant organ parenchyma, particularly the lungs and liver.

The treatment of a uterine leiomyosarcoma is total abdominal hysterectomy and bilateral salpingo-oophorectomy. In the absence of obvious tumor dissemination, peritoneal cytology and selective pelvic and periaortic lymph node biopsies should be obtained, as with an endometrial adenocarcinoma. Following surgery, patients whose tumors are confined to the uterus and contain fewer than five mitoses per 10 hpf require no adjuvant therapy. Patients whose lesions have a high mitotic index should receive adjuvant postoperative radiation—pelvic, extended field, or possibly whole abdominal, depending on the operative findings. Although pelvic radiation does appear to decrease local pelvic recurrence, it does not prolong survival, since most patients develop distant metastases.

The most commonly used chemotherapeutic agents are doxorubicin, *cis*-platinum, cyclophosphamide, vincristine, and actinomycin-D. The most active of these agents appear to be *cis*-platinum and doxorubicin, but objective response rates in patients with metastatic disease are only 25 to 30 per cent. The use of adjuvant chemotherapy in patients with stage I disease has not yet been shown to improve survival.

Endometrial Stromal Sarcoma

There are three types of stromal sarcomas: (1) endometrial stromal nodule, (2) endolymphatic stromal myosis, and (3) endometrial stromal sarcoma. The first of these, the *stromal nodule,* is a rare benign condition. The mitotic index is very low, typically three or fewer per 10 hpf. A hysterectomy is curative.

Endolymphatic stromal myosis is a low-grade sarcoma. Histologically, there is minimal to absent cellular atypism, with usually fewer than five mitoses per 10 hpf. There is always evidence of vascular channel invasion. These patients usually present with abnormal vaginal bleeding and often pelvic pain. This condition is diagnosed at the time of exploratory surgery for presumed benign leiomyomata. About 30 per cent of the tumors have extrauterine extension discovered at laparotomy, which consists of multiple worm-like, rubbery growths in the pelvis.

Most patients are cured with a total abdominal hysterectomy and bilateral salpingo-oophorectomy. With local pelvic extension, a radical or modified radical hysterectomy and bilateral pelvic lymphadenectomy may be necessary to resect all of the disease. Incompletely resected lesions often respond to oral progestin therapy. Local and distant recurrences may occur even 10 to 20 years later and require re-exploration and resection of disease. Metastases may respond to high-dose progesterone therapy. Pelvic disease has also been shown to respond to radiation therapy.

Endometrial stromal sarcoma generally causes menometrorrhagia or postmenopausal bleeding and occasionally pelvic pain. The diagnosis can often be made by endometrial biopsy or by cervical dilatation and curettage of the uterus. Histologically, there are 10 or more mitoses per 10 hpf, and the lesion is composed of rather poorly differentiated stromal cells. Aggressive myometrial invasion occurs, and tumor is commonly seen in lymphatic spaces. About half of the patients present with evidence of metastatic disease, usually to distant organs, particularly the liver or lungs. Recurrence in these sites is high in patients who had disease apparently confined to the uterus at the time of diagnosis.

The treatment of endometrial stromal sarcomas is the same as that for leiomyosarcoma. Postoperative pelvic radiation improves local control but does not improve survival. In patients with metastatic disease, progestogens or chemotherapy should be offered, but response rates are low.

Mixed Müllerian Sarcoma

Mixed müllerian sarcomas account for about 40 per cent of uterine sarcomas. Most patients are postmenopausal and present with vaginal bleeding or discharge. About one third of patients have tumor growing through the cervix into the vagina as a polypoid mass. As opposed to a "fibroid" uterus, these lesions are usually soft to palpation. Up to 50 per cent of patients with this lesion have evidence of metastatic disease at the time of diagnosis.

As with endometrial stromal sarcomas, these tumors aggressively invade the myometrium and disseminate via the lymphatics and the blood stream.

The primary treatment of mixed müllerian sarcoma is the same as that for leiomyosarcoma.

Prognosis

The prognosis for uterine sarcomas is poor, the overall 5-year survival rate being about 35 per cent. Patients with mixed müllerian sarcomas have a poorer overall survival than patients with a leiomyosarcoma or endometrial stromal sarcoma. When compared stage for stage, however, all three uterine sarcomas have the same prognosis. Patients with stage I uterine sarcoma have about a 50 per cent 5-year survival, and patients with disease outside the uterus have a dismal prognosis.

SUGGESTED READING

Aalders J, Abeler V, Kolstad P, Onsrud M: Postoperative external irradiation and prognostic parameters in Stage I endometrial carcinoma: Clinical and histopathologic study of 540 patients. Obstet Gynecol 56:419, 1980.

Berman ML, Ballon SC, Lagasse LD, Watring WG: Prognosis and treatment of endometrial cancer. Am J Obstet Gynecol 136:679, 1980.

Boronow RC, Morrow CP, Creasman WT, et al: Surgical staging in endometrial cancer: Clinical pathologic findings of a prospective study. Obstet Gynecol 63:825, 1984.

Cox JD, Komaki R, Wilson F, Greenberg M: Locally advanced adenocarcinoma of the endometrium: Results of irradiation with and without subsequent hysterectomy. Cancer 45:715, 1980.

Creasman WT, Morrow CP, Bundy BN, et al: Surgical spread patterns of endometrial cancer: A Gynecologic Oncology Group study. Cancer 60:2035, 1987.

DiSaia PJ, Creasman WT, Boronow RC, Blessing JA: Risk factors and recurrent patterns in stage I endometrial cancer. Am J Obstet Gynecol 151:1009, 1985.

Greven K, Olds W: Radiotherapy in the management of endometrial carcinoma with cervical involvement. Cancer 60:1737, 1987.

Hacker NF: Endometrial cancer. In Berek JS, Hacker NF (eds): Practical Gynecologic Oncology. Baltimore, Williams & Wilkins, 1989, p 285.

Koss LG, Schreiber K, Oberlander SG, et al: Detection of endometrial carcinoma and hyperplasia in asymptomatic women. Obstet Gynecol 64:1, 1984.

Marchetti DL, Piver MS, Tsukada Y, Reese P: Prevention of vaginal recurrence of stage I endometrial adenocarcinoma with postoperative vaginal radiation. Obstet Gynecol 67:399, 1986.

Morrow CP, Townsend DE (eds): Synopsis of Gynecologic Oncology. 3rd ed. New York, Churchill Livingstone, 1987, p 159.

Potish RA, Twiggs LB, Adcock LL, et al: Para-aortic lymph node radiotherapy in cancer of the uterine corpus. Obstet Gynecol 65:251, 1985.

Salazar OM, Bontfiglio TA, Pattern SF, et al: Uterine sarcomas: Natural history, treatment and prognosis. Cancer 42:1152, 1978.

Soper JT, Creasman WT, Clarke-Pearson DL, et al: Intraperitoneal chronic phosphate P 32 suspension therapy of malignant peritoneal cytology in endometrial carcinoma. Am J Obstet Gynecol 153:191, 1985.

Zaloudek CJ, Norris HJ: Mesenchymal tumors of the uterus. Prog Surg Pathol 3:1, 1981.

Fifty-four

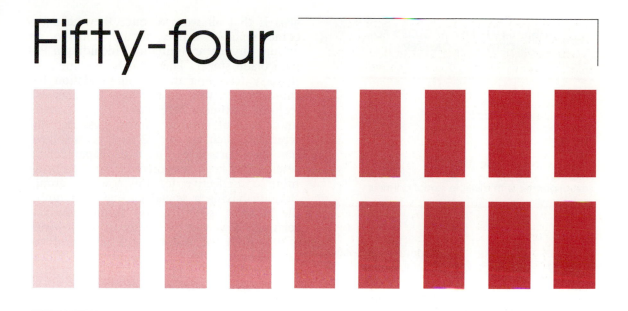

Cervical Dysplasia and Cancer

EDWARD W. SAVAGE, Jr., and GROESBECK P. PARHAM

In the United States, cervical cancer ranks eighth among cancers in women, with 13,500 new cases diagnosed in 1990. The incidence has decreased markedly since the 1930s. Part of the decline in cervical cancer is probably related to the advent of the Papanicolaou smear, which permits detection of preinvasive disease. Therapy for preinvasive disease is usually curative and prevents the subsequent development of invasive cancer. The incidence of preinvasive disease of the cervix has been increasing over the past decade.

ETIOLOGY AND EPIDEMIOLOGY

Cervical cancer and its precursors have been associated with several epidemiologic variables (Table 54–1). Cervical carcinoma is relatively rare before the age of 20 years, the

average age of this occurrence being 47 years. In the lower socioeconomic groups and in some geographic areas, the average age has been reported to be as low as 39 years.

The adolescent cervix is believed to be more susceptible to carcinogenic stimuli because of the active process of squamous metaplasia, which occurs within the transformation zone during that period of development. This squamous metaplasia is normally a physiologic process, but under the influence of a carcinogen, cellular alterations may occur that result in an atypical transformation zone. These atypical changes initiate a process called cervical intraepithelial neoplasia (CIN), which is the preinvasive phase of cervical cancer.

Cervical intraepithelial neoplasia represents a spectrum of disease beginning as a change called mild dysplasia (CIN I), which may

Table 54-1. RISK FACTORS FOR CERVICAL CANCER

Young age at first coitus (under 20 years)
Multiple sexual partners
Young age at marriage
Young age at first pregnancy
High parity
Divorce
Lower socioeconomic status
Smoking
Sexual partner with multiple sexual partners

---

gradually progress to moderate dysplasia (CIN II), and to severe dysplasia and carcinoma in situ (CIN III). This process is not always continuously progressive and may remain in an earlier phase or regress entirely. At least 20 per cent of patients with carcinoma in situ eventually develop invasion beyond the basement membrane, resulting initially in microinvasive carcinoma, then frankly invasive carcinoma.

It is estimated that approximately 10 to 15 per cent of mild to moderate dysplasias progress to invasive cancer if not treated. The length of time for this progression varies, and even a fairly advanced form of dysplasia may require 3 to 20 years to become invasive cancer.

Although herpes type II virus has been implicated as an etiologic agent in the past, more recent studies have documented a stronger link between cervical carcinoma and the human papilloma virus (HPV). HPV can now be "typed" using DNA hybridization techniques. Types 6 and 11 have been frequently associated with cervical condylomata, whereas types 16, 18, 31, 33, and 35 have been associated with noninvasive and invasive cervical neoplasia. Some investigators have related cervical carcinogenesis to contact with human sperm, but these data are controversial.

SCREENING OF ASYMPTOMATIC WOMEN

The current recommendation of the American College of Obstetricians and Gynecolo-gists is that all women, once they have become sexually active, should undergo an annual physical examination, including a Papanicolaou smear. There has been some controversy regarding this recommendation because women who do not have the high-risk features outlined here have a significantly lower rate of cervical cancer. Less rigorous screening, such as every 2 to 5 years following two or three normal Papanicolaou smears, has been proposed by some as being more cost-effective for this low-risk group. Because having a sexual partner with multiple partners is also a risk factor, however, relatively few women belong to the low-risk group. Both the endocervical canal and the ectocervix should be sampled when taking the Papanicolaou smear.

Although cervical cytology generally correlates with the histologic diagnosis, a biopsy is absolutely necessary for the definitive diagnosis prior to therapy. With the Papanicolaou smear, the false-positive rate is less than 1 per cent, whereas the false-negative rate is between 10 and 20 per cent. With simultaneous use of Papanicolaou smears and colposcopically directed biopsies, almost all squamous cervical lesions can be detected on initial evaluation. False-negative Papanicolaou smears, however, have been reported in as many as 40 to 45 per cent of patients ultimately diagnosed as having cervical adenocarcinomas. The latter usually arise in the endocervical canal.

CERVICAL TOPOGRAPHY

To understand the concepts of colposcopy, it is important to understand cervical topography. During early embryonic development, the cervix and upper vagina are covered with columnar epithelium. Progressively, during intrauterine development, the columnar epithelium of the vagina is replaced by squamous epithelium. At birth, the vagina is usually covered with squamous epithelium, and the columnar epithelium is limited to the endocervix and the central portion of the ectocervix. In about 4 per cent of normal female infants and about 30 per cent of those exposed to diethylstilbestrol in utero, the columnar epithelium extends onto the vaginal fornices. Macroscopically, the columnar epi-

Figure 54-1. Schematic representation of the transformation zone.

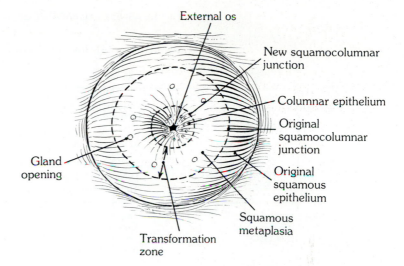

External os

New squamocolumnar junction

Columnar epithelium

Original squamocolumnar junction

Original squamous epithelium

Squamous metaplasia

Transformation zone

Gland opening

thelium has a red appearance because it is only a single cell layer thick, allowing blood vessels in the underlying stroma to show through it.

The squamous and columnar epithelia of infants are designated the original or native squamous and columnar epithelia, respectively. The junction between them is called the original squamocolumnar junction.

Throughout life, but particularly during adolescence and the first pregnancy, metaplastic squamous epithelium covers the columnar epithelium so that a new squamocolumnar junction is formed more proximally. This junction moves progressively closer to the external os, then up the endocervical canal. The transformation zone is the area of metaplastic squamous epithelium located between the original squamocolumnar junction and the new squamocolumnar junction (Fig. 54-1).

EVALUATION OF A PATIENT WITH AN ABNORMAL PAPANICOLAOU SMEAR

Although there is no uniformly accepted system for the classification of Papanicolaou smears, the one shown in Table 54-2 is a reasonable approximation of most that have been devised. In 1988, a consensus meeting was convened by the division of Cancer Control of the National Cancer Institute (NCI) to review existing terminology and to recommend effective methods of cytology reporting. The result of this meeting was what has now come to be known as the Bethesda System, which requires (1) a statement regarding the adequacy of the specimen for diagnosis, (2) diagnostic categorization (normal or other), and (3) a descriptive diagnosis. Any patient with a grossly abnormal cervix should have a punch biopsy performed. The following discussion refers to patients who have an abnormal Papanicolaou smear and a grossly normal-appearing cervix.

An algorithm for the evaluation of patients with abnormal Papanicolaou smears is presented in Figure 54-2. Patients with a class II Papanicolaou smear require evaluation for, and management of, inflammatory conditions (see Chapter 35). Patients with a persistent class II smear and all those with a class III or worse smear require colposcopic evaluation of the cervix. Koilocytosis deserves

Table 54-2. CLASSIFICATION OF ABNORMAL SQUAMOUS CELL CYTOLOGY

Class I	Normal
Class II	Inflammatory atypia
Class III	Dysplasia
Class IV	Carcinoma in situ
Class V	Invasive carcinoma

EVALUATION OF THE ABNORMAL PAPANICOLAOU SMEAR

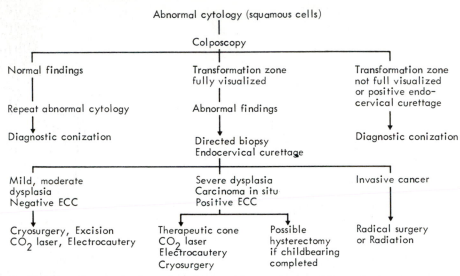

Figure 54–2. Algorithm for evaluation of patients with an abnormal Papanicolaou smear and a grossly normal-appearing cervix.

special attention because of the relationship between HPV and cervical neoplasia. Careful follow-up is mandatory to determine if neoplasia occurs.

Colposcopy

The colposcope is a stereoscopic binocular microscope of low magnification, usually 10 to 40X (Fig. 54–3). Illumination is centered, and the focal length is between 12 and 15 cm.

To perform colposcopy, an appropriately sized speculum is inserted to expose the cervix, which is cleansed with a cotton pledget soaked in 3 per cent acetic acid to remove adherent mucus and cellular debris. It may be necessary to reapply the acetic acid at intervals during a prolonged examination. With direct illumination from the white light, surface features of the cervix can usually be identified. A green filter can be employed to accentuate the vascular changes that frequently accompany pathologic alterations of the cervix. Cameras are available for attachment to colposcopes, and photographs may sometimes by useful to facilitate follow-up when conservative treatment is used.

Colposcopic Findings. The original or native squamous epithelium appears gray and homogeneous. The columnar epithelium is red and grape-like in appearance. The transformation zone can be identified by the presence of gland openings that are not covered by the squamous metaplasia and by the paler color of the metaplastic epithelium compared with the original squamous epithelium. Nabothian follicles may also be seen in the transformation zone. Normal blood vessels are branching like a tree.

The colposcopic hallmark of cervical dysplasia is an area of sharply delineated acetowhite epithelium—that is, epithelium that appears white after the application of acetic acid. It is thought that the acetic acid dehydrates the cells, and there is increased light reflex from areas of increased nuclear density (i.e., areas of CIN). HPV may also produce white epithelium (flat condyloma). These changes are not always easy to distinguish from CIN colposcopically and require biopsy for definitive diagnosis. Within the acetowhite areas, there may or may not be abnormal vascular patterns.

There are two basic changes in the vascular architecture in patients with CIN: punctation and mosaicism. Punctation is caused by sin-

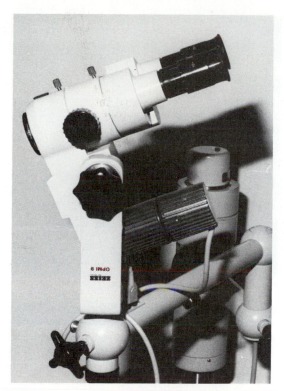

Figure 54–3. A colposcope, used to evaluate patients with an abnormal Papanicolaou smear and a grossly normal cervix.

gle-looped capillaries lying within the subepithelial papillae, seen end-on as a "dot" as they course toward the surface of the epithelium. Mosaicism is due to a fine network of capillaries disposed parallel to the surface in a mosaic pattern. Punctate and mosaic patterns may be seen together within the same area of the cervix.

The more dilated and irregular the punctate and mosaic capillaries and the greater the intercapillary distance, the more atypical is the tissue on histologic examination. Similarly, the whiter the lesion, the more severe the dysplasia. True branching vessels have not been observed in dysplasia or carcinoma in situ.

With microinvasive carcinoma, extremely irregular punctate and mosaic patterns are found as well as small atypical vessels. The irregularity in size, shape, and arrangement of the terminal vessels becomes even more striking in frankly invasive carcinoma, with

exaggerated distortions of the vascular architecture producing comma-shaped, corkscrew-shaped, and dilated, blind-ended vessels.

Directed Biopsy and Endocervical Curettage

If the colposcopic examination is satisfactory, which implies that the entire transformation zone has been visualized, a punch biopsy is taken from the worst area(s), together with an endocervical curettage (ECC). The ECC is not performed in patients who are pregnant.

If the colposcopic examination is unsatisfactory, the endocervical curettings are positive, there is significant discrepancy between the biopsy and Papanicolaou smear, or microinvasion is present on the biopsy, conization should be performed (see Chapter 46).

Schiller's Test

The superficial cells of the normal mature squamous epithelium of the vagina and cervix contain glycogen. Therefore, when a dilute aqueous solution of Lugol's iodine is applied, the epithelium stains brown almost immediately. When no glycogen is present, as is usually the case with carcinoma in situ and cervical dysplasia, the involved area fails to stain. The nonstaining areas are designated Schiller-positive, or iodine-negative. Many benign conditions of the cervix, including ectropions, atrophic epithelium, nonmalignant ulcers, and columnar epithelium, are also Schiller-positive. The test is, therefore, not specific for malignant lesions. In addition, Schiller-negative areas have been described in patients with intraepithelial neoplastic disease. Schiller staining may serve as a complementary technique to colposcopic examination but should never replace it.

SYMPTOMS

Preinvasive disease (dysplasia and carcinoma in situ) does not produce symptoms. The discharge frequently seen in preinvasive disease is most often due to accompanying infection. Clinical symptoms of microinvasive carcinoma are also either nonexistent or nonspecific and, therefore, are of no assistance in making the diagnosis.

The most common symptoms of invasive cervical carcinoma are abnormal bleeding and vaginal discharge. Approximately 80 to 90 per cent of patients experience some abnormal bleeding. The bleeding may be postcoital, abnormal menstrual bleeding, or intermenstrual spotting. Some patients may present with postmenopausal bleeding. The only symptom in some patients may be a vaginal discharge. The character of the discharge may be serous, purulent, or mucoid. It is not necessarily malodorous except with fairly advanced disease. Other symptoms, such as pelvic pain, leg swelling, and urinary frequency, are usually seen only with advanced disease. A minority of patients are completely asymptomatic.

PHYSICAL FINDINGS

Patients with cervical cancer usually have a normal general physical examination. Weight loss occurs late in the disease. With advanced disease, there may be enlarged inguinal or supraclavicular lymph nodes, edema of the legs, ascites, pleural effusion, or hepatomegaly, but these are not commonly seen.

The pelvic examination in early disease may reveal a cervix that appears normal, especially if the lesion is endocervical. Visible disease may take several forms: ulcerative, exophytic, granular, or necrotic. The cervix may be friable and bleed on palpation. There is often an associated serous, purulent, or bloody discharge. The lesion may involve the upper portion of the vagina and extend toward the introitus. The cervix may be distorted or completely replaced by tumor (Fig. 54–4).

The rectovaginal examination is essential to determine the extent of involvement. The degree of cervical expansion and any spread to the parametria are much more easily detected with the rectal finger in this examination, as is extension into the vaginal fornices or uterosacral ligaments. Occasionally, a palpable mass on the pelvic wall representing an enlarged node can be felt.

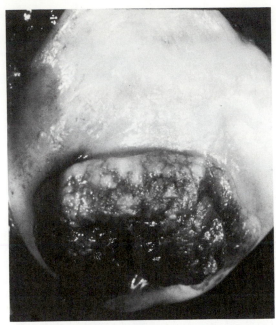

Figure 54–4. Squamous cell carcinoma of the cervix. A granular, nodular lesion that bleeds easily on contact is seen replacing the ectocervix.

PATHOLOGY

Most uterine cervical cancers are squamous in origin. Adenocarcinomas and adenosquamous carcinomas, which appear to be increasing in incidence, account for about 20 per cent of cases. Melanomas and sarcomas occur rarely.

Cervical Intraepithelial Neoplasia

The cellular changes associated with atypia are related to the loss of the normal maturation of the epithelium. There is a tendency for the basal and parabasal cells to proliferate abnormally, with distortion of the normal architecture and lack of the usual differentiation. The severity of the lesion may be judged by the percentage of epithelium involved. Thus, involvement of the inner one third of the epithelium represents CIN I, involvement of the inner one half to two thirds represents CIN II, and full-thickness involvement represents CIN III. In carcinoma in situ, the cells are indistinguishable from

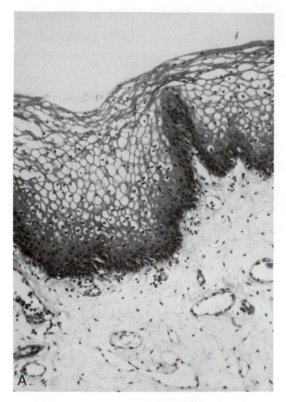

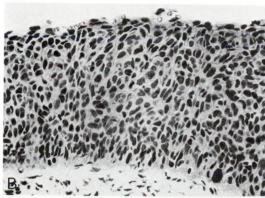

Figure 54–5. Histology of normal cervical squamous epithelium (A) and carcinoma in situ (B) of the cervix. In the normal epithelium, note the orderly maturation from the basal layer to the parabasal cells, glycogenated intermediate cells, and flattened superficial cells. In the carcinoma in situ, the entire thickness of the epithelium is replaced by immature cells that are variable in size and shape and have irregular nuclei. Mitotic figures are seen in the lower two thirds of the epithelium.

those of frankly invasive cancer except that the basement membrane remains intact (Fig. 54–5).

Microinvasive Carcinoma

With progression to microinvasive carcinoma, there is a breakthrough of the basement membrane with malignant cells invading into the cervical stroma. There are no universally accepted criteria for deciding whether a tumor is microinvasive or frankly invasive. Most gynecologic oncologists in the United States accept penetration below the basement membrane to a depth of 3 mm, with no evidence of vascular or lymphatic permeation as the definition for microinvasive carcinoma, and this definition is most commonly used when planning conservative treatment. The International Federation of Gynecology and Obstetrics (FIGO) has issued a different set of criteria (see Table 54–3).

The diagnosis of microinvasive carcinoma can be made only on the basis of a cone biopsy of the cervix, which allows multiple step-sections to be taken at 2-mm intervals. With a punch biopsy, the sampling of the cervix is too limited, and a more frankly invasive focus may be missed. The concept of microinvasive carcinoma should be applied only to squamous cell carcinomas. All invasive adenocarcinomas should be regarded as frankly invasive.

Invasive Carcinoma

Squamous carcinomas, which account for about 75 per cent of all invasive lesions, can be divided into the small cell carcinoma, which is a poorly differentiated lesion, and the better differentiated large cell carcinoma. Large cell carcinomas may be nonkeratinizing or keratinizing. Some pathologists use simpler terminology: poorly differentiated, moderately differentiated, and well differentiated.

About 20 to 25 per cent of invasive cervical cancers are adenocarcinomas or mixed adenosquamous carcinomas. The most poorly differentiated adenosquamous carcinoma is the "glassy cell" carcinoma. Rare cervical lesions, such as melanomas, sarcomas, and lym-

Table 54–3. FIGO* STAGING OF CERVICAL CARCINOMA

PREINVASIVE CARCINOMA

Stage 0	Carcinoma in situ, intraepithelial carcinoma
	Cases of stage 0 should not be included in any therapeutic statistics for invasive carcinoma

INVASIVE CARCINOMA

Stage I	Carcinoma strictly confined to the cervix (extension to the corpus should be disregarded)
Stage Ia	Preclinical carcinomas of the cervix, i.e., those diagnosed only by microscopy
Stage Ia1	Minimal microscopically evident stromal invasion
Stage Ia2	Lesions detected microscopically that can be measured. The upper limit of the measurement should not show a depth of invasion of more than 5 mm taken from the base of the epithelium, either surface or glandular, from which it originates, and a second dimension, the horizontal spread, must not exceed 7 mm. Larger lesions should be staged as Ib
Stage Ib	Lesions of greater dimensions than stage Ia2 whether seen clinically or not. Preformed space involvement should not alter the staging but should be specifically recorded so as to determine whether it should affect treatment decisions in the future
Stage II	Carcinoma extends beyond the cervix, but has not extended onto the pelvic wall. The carcinoma involves the vagina, but not the lower third
Stage IIa	No obvious parametrial involvement
Stage IIb	Obvious parametrial involvement
Stage III	Carcinoma extended to the pelvic wall. On rectal examination there is no cancer-free space between the tumor and the pelvic wall. The tumor involves the lower third of the vagina. All cases with a hydronephrosis or nonfunctioning kidney should be included, unless they are known to be due to another cause
Stage IIIa	No extension onto the pelvic wall
Stage IIIb	Extension onto the pelvic wall and/or hydronephrosis or nonfunctioning kidney
Stage IV	Carcinoma extended beyond the true pelvis or clinically involved the mucosa of the bladder or rectum. Bullous edema of the bladder alone does not permit a case to be allotted to stage IV
Stage IVa	Spread of the growth to adjacent organs
Stage IVb	Spread to distant organs

* International Federation of Gynecology and Obstetrics.

phomas, together account for fewer than 1 per cent of cases.

PREOPERATIVE INVESTIGATIONS FOR INVASIVE CERVICAL CANCER

Clinical Staging

The official FIGO staging for cervical cancer is a clinical staging method based on physical examination and noninvasive testing (Table 54–3).

The studies used for the FIGO staging of cervical cancer include biopsies, cystoscopy, sigmoidoscopy, chest and skeletal radiographs, intravenous pyelography, and liver function tests. Cystoscopy and sigmoidoscopy seldom reveal mucosal invasion, unless the central disease is advanced. Lung metastases are seen in about 5 per cent of patients with advanced disease and almost never in early disease.

Other tests that may be useful, especially in advanced or recurrent disease, include a bipedal lymphangiogram, liver-spleen scan, barium enema, and computed tomographic (CT) scan of the abdomen and pelvis. Results of these latter tests are not used for FIGO staging, but may be helpful in establishing the extent of the disease and in guiding management.

Laboratory studies may reveal abnormalities with advanced disease, the most common being anemia from bleeding, elevated blood urea nitrogen and creatinine levels if the ureters are obstructed, and abnormal liver function tests if there are liver metastases. Ureteral obstruction occurs in about 30 per cent of patients with stage III disease and 50 per cent of patients with stage IV disease. Hypercalcemia may denote advanced disease, sometimes without bone involvement.

Surgical Staging

Less than 2 decades ago, several investigators began to use surgical staging prior to radiation therapy to determine the extent of disease better. The stimulus was the occasional finding of periaortic lymph node metastases at the time of radical hysterectomy for early-stage disease. Many centers now use surgical staging to define the extent of the disease and to plan optimal radiation therapy. The incidence of periaortic lymph node metastases is approximately 20 per cent in stage II disease and 30 per cent in stage III. Approximately 10 per cent of patients with stage II lesions or greater have unsuspected peritoneal, adnexal, or liver metastases diagnosed at surgery. Occasionally patients may be down-staged because of surgical findings that do not represent carcinoma, such as endometriosis. In some series, the incidence of complications following radiation, particularly bowel injuries, has been higher after surgical staging. If a retroperitoneal approach is used rather than a transperitoneal approach, there is no significantly increased incidence of postradiation complications. Periaortic irradiation appears to improve survival in patients whose periaortic metastases are microscopic.

TREATMENT

Intraepithelial Neoplasia

The ability to locate and precisely define the size and distribution of the intraepithelial lesion by colposcopy in most patients has allowed a more conservative approach to the disease. Superficial ablative techniques, such as local excision, cryosurgery, CO_2 laser, or electrocoagulation, may be appropriate. For these more conservative forms of management, the entire transformation zone must be visible and accessible to the method to be employed. The more conservative methods are particularly preferred as long as invasive disease has been excluded, in patients who desire to maintain their childbearing capacity, and may be repeated should failure occur.

Cryosurgery. Cryosurgery is probably most widely used for the treatment of CIN in this country. The advantages of this method are as follows: (1) it is relatively painless, (2) there is minimal or no blood loss, (3) it is inexpensive, (4) it is an outpatient procedure, and (5) it has no appreciable effect on childbearing capacity. The major side effect is a rather copious vaginal discharge that persists for several weeks. Another disadvantage is that the squamocolumnar junction frequently recedes into the endocervical canal, making colposcopic evaluation less valuable in the follow-up of these patients. The failure rate is approximately 10 to 20 per cent but may be higher with gland involvement or with more advanced or larger lesions.

Laser. The CO_2 laser (light amplification by stimulated emission of radiation) is a more recent technique for the treatment of CIN. The technique has the advantages of precision, rapid tissue destruction, and minimal scarring. Treatment without anesthesia may be painful, and cervical bleeding may sometimes occur. The entire transformation zone should be destroyed. Post-treatment surveillance by colposcopy is more likely to be satisfactory because the squamocolumnar junction is not moved into the endocervical canal by treatment. When properly used, failure rates are approximately 5 to 10 per cent. This technique is more expensive than cryotherapy.

Electrocoagulation. Success rates of up to 97 per cent have been reported for electrocoagulation. It causes more discomfort than the other techniques, however, and, therefore, requires general anesthesia. Cervical stenosis may occasionally occur.

Loop Electrodiathermy Excision Procedure. Loop excision of the transformation zone has been used for cervical intraepithelial neoplasia. The equipment is much cheaper than that required for laser ablation, and the other advantage over ablative techniques is that tissue is obtained for histologic evaluation. Hence, occult invasive lesions should be more readily diagnosed.

Cervical Conization. Once widely used for diagnosis, this technique is also sometimes used for treatment. Therapeutic indications for cone biopsy are extension of the lesion into the endocervix and the presence of extensive carcinoma in situ. Provided that the margins of resection are clear, cure rates are as high as with hysterectomy. Compared with simpler techniques, the advantage is that an optimal portion of tissue is submitted for pathologic evaluation. Bleeding, infection, cervical stenosis, and cervical incompetence are the major complications. Colposcopy performed before conization may alter the complication rate by allowing one to target the extent of the lesion and thus limit the amount of tissue removed.

Hysterectomy. Since this method has a high cure rate, it is acceptable to employ it to treat CIN III in patients who have completed childbearing. Hysterectomy is particularly applicable in the following circumstances: (1) when there is a positive margin on the cervical cone, (2) when the lesion is anaplastic, and (3) when there is deep endocervical glandular involvement. It is the preferred technique when sterilization is desired for other reasons or when there is concomitant uterine or adnexal disease.

Persistence or recurrence rates combined are approximately 2 to 3 per cent after hysterectomy. This number should be significantly reduced by using colposcopy and Schiller's staining preoperatively, since it is likely that most of the disease is persistent because of inadequate surgical resection of the vaginal cuff.

Stage Ia (Microinvasive Carcinoma)

Because microinvasive carcinoma has not been well defined, the management remains controversial. The crux of the problem is finding the point in the evolution of this disease from intraepithelial to invasive carcinoma at which the lesion changes its biological behavior and becomes capable of lymphatic metastasis.

Surgery is almost always employed except when medically contraindicated. Intracavitary radium or cesium may be used under such exceptional circumstances. When the depth of invasion on cone biopsy is less than 3 mm and there is no lymphatic or vascular space involvement, an extrafascial abdominal hysterectomy is appropriate treatment. Cervical conization alone may be used in special circumstances in which the patient desires to maintain her childbearing capacity and the cervical cone margins are clear of disease.

Stage Ib

Stage Ib disease may be treated by either radical hysterectomy and bilateral pelvic lymphadenectomy or radiation therapy. The advantage of surgery is that the ovaries may be spared in premenopausal women. There may also be less interference with coital function. Complications involving the rectum, ureters, or bladder are less common following radical hysterectomy than following radiation therapy, and repair is more likely to be successful if injury does occur.

The results of treatment by either method are similar when both the surgeon and the radiotherapist are knowledgeable and skilled. Radiation is usually chosen, however, when the lesion is expanded beyond 4 cm because a more extensive surgical resection is required, which increases the likelihood of postoperative bladder dysfunction. Some patients may require self-catheterization for the rest of their lives after an extensive radical hysterectomy.

A stage Ib barrel-shaped carcinoma of the cervix is one in which the entire length of the cervix is markedly expanded so that the junction between the lower uterine segment and the large cervical lesion cannot be appreciated. Even when these lesions are treated with radiation, it is common practice to perform an extrafascial hysterectomy 6 weeks following completion of radiation to reduce the incidence of central pelvic recurrence.

Radical Hysterectomy. Radical hysterectomy is an operation for the removal of the uterus with adjacent portions of the vagina, cardinal ligaments, uterosacral ligaments, and bladder pillars (see Fig. 46–5). Surgery is easier to perform in thin patients and should be performed in those with colonic diverticular disease or chronic pelvic inflammatory disease, in whom radiation may induce pelvic abscesses. It may also be chosen for patients who have a fear of radiation therapy or in whom rapid treatment is desirable (i.e., psychologically compromised patients).

The most serious complication of radical hysterectomy is ureteric fistula or stricture. These are less common than they once were. In more recent years, the incidence of ureteric complications has declined from 10 to 15 per cent to 1 to 2 per cent. This has occurred because surgeons avoid extensive stripping of the ureter from the parietal peritoneum, as was once the case. There is also general use of suction drainage of the retroperitoneal spaces, which helps minimize infection.

The most common complication of radical hysterectomy is bladder dysfunction. This occurs as a result of interruption of the portion of the autonomic nerve supply traversing the cardinal and uterosacral ligaments. Although normal bladder function is usually restored within 1 to 3 months after surgery, dysfunction can be prolonged and is occasionally permanent. A suprapubic catheter is generally placed at the time of radical hysterectomy and is removed when satisfactory voiding occurs.

A less common but life-threatening complication of radical hysterectomy is deep venous thrombosis with pulmonary embolism. The incidence of pulmonary embolism can probably be reduced with the use of early ambulation, together with prophylactic low-dose subcutaneous heparin or external pneumatic calf compression at the time of surgery and before adequate postoperative mobilization.

Radiation Therapy. For patients with stage Ib disease, radiation may be the only modality of therapy, in which case both external and intracavitary therapy are required. Radiation may be given preoperatively in an attempt to shrink bulky cervical lesions and make them amenable to more limited surgical procedures. Postoperative pelvic radiation may also be used for patients with lymph node metastases or inadequate surgical margins. Radiation therapy is well tolerated by most patients with medical contraindications to surgery.

If radiation alone is to be used, the treatment plan is based primarily on the extent and distribution of the disease. Treatment is directed at the upper vagina, cervix, paracervical tissues, and lymph nodes on the pelvic wall. Therapy usually begins with external radiation in an attempt to shrink the central lesion and improve the dosimetry of the subsequent intracavitary therapy. The relative proportion of external radiation versus intracavitary radium or cesium is determined by the size of the primary tumor, its response to the external therapy, and the capacity of the vagina for the intracavitary applicators. Most patients require a minimum of 4500 to 5000 cGy external radiation to the pelvis.

Stage IIa

In patients with minimal involvement of the vaginal fornix, radical surgery or radiation therapy may be employed the same as for patients with stage Ib lesions. With more extensive upper vaginal involvement, radiation therapy alone is the treatment of choice.

Stage IIb

Most patients with stage IIb lesions are treated with a combination of external beam and intracavitary radiation therapy. Some patients with bulkier lesions may be selected for an adjunctive extrafascial hysterectomy following radiation therapy in an effort to reduce the risk of persistent central disease. If positive periaortic or high common iliac lymph nodes are detected by surgical staging or CT scan–directed fine-needle aspiration cytology, extended-field radiation may be employed to treat all of the periaortic lymph nodes up to the diaphragm.

Stages IIIa and IIIb

These patients are treated almost exclusively with radiation therapy, usually external therapy followed by intracavitary radium or cesium. There are study protocols using combinations of chemotherapy and radiation in an effort to improve the cure rates, since many of these patients have occult distant metastases.

In patients with locally advanced disease, distortion of the cervix and vagina may make intracavitary radiation therapy difficult to apply. Therefore, a higher dose of external therapy, up to 6000 to 7000 cGy, may be necessary. Alternatively, interstitial radiation may be given to get a better dose distribution than would be possible with intracavitary therapy (see Chapter 52).

Stage IVa

Pelvic radiation therapy is used in most of these patients. If radiation therapy results in only partial tumor regression, a "salvage" pelvic exenteration may be performed. Primary pelvic exenteration is performed only rarely, usually when the patient presents with a rectovaginal or vesicovaginal fistula.

Stage IVb

These patients may receive some pelvic radiation therapy to palliate bleeding from the vagina, bladder, or rectum. Because distant metastases are present, however, chemotherapy is often employed but is only palliative.

Recurrent or Metastatic Disease

Chemotherapy. The effectiveness of chemotherapy is limited in the treatment of cervical cancer because most cervical carcinomas are relatively resistant. In addition, many patients have had previous radiation, which decreases the vascularity of the tissues so that optimal tissue levels of the drug are not reached. Some tumors may be bulky, with fairly large necrotic centers that act as pharmacologic sanctuaries. Other factors that may limit the use of chemotherapy are (1) diminished marrow reserve secondary to radiation; (2) ureteral obstruction, which affects excretion of the drug; and (3) sepsis and fistulas, which may occur following administration of the chemotherapy.

Several drugs have been tested and found to be active in up to 35 per cent of cases. Most responses are partial, and the patients soon relapse and die of their disease. The most active agents are *cis*-platinum, bleomycin, mitomycin C, methotrexate, and cyclophosphamide.

Pelvic Exenteration. Pelvic exenteration is generally reserved for those patients who have a central recurrence following pelvic radiation. The operation involves removal of the pelvic viscera, including the uterus, tubes, vagina, ovaries, bladder, and rectum (Fig. 54–6). Depending on the site and extent of the recurrence, the operation may be limited to an anterior exenteration, which spares the rectum, or a posterior exenteration, which spares the bladder.

Following the extirpative surgery, pelvic reconstruction is necessary. If the bladder is removed, the ureters must be implanted into a portion of the small or large bowel that has been isolated from the remainder of the gastrointestinal tract to form a conduit. When the disease is confined to the upper vagina and rectovaginal septum, the lower rectum and anal canal may be preserved and reanastomosed to the sigmoid colon. A temporary colostomy is often required to protect the reanastomosis because of the prior radiation. Vaginal reconstruction can be performed simultaneously using a split-thickness skin graft or bilateral gracilis myocutaneous grafts. This helps to reconstruct the pelvic floor, thereby significantly decreasing the risk of a perineal hernia or an enteroperineal fistula.

Relatively few patients with recurrent cancer of the cervix are suitable for pelvic exenteration because of metastases outside the pelvis or fixation of the tumor to structures that cannot be removed, such as the pelvic side wall. If an extensive metastatic work-up is negative, patients undergo exploratory laparotomy with a view to pelvic exenteration. If the tumor is discovered to have spread to pelvic or periaortic lymph nodes or to intra-abdominal viscera, the procedure is abandoned because of the low likelihood of cure in such circumstances. Palliative exenteration is not advisable.

In selecting patients who may be suitable for pelvic exenteration, the triad of unilateral leg edema, sciatic pain, and ureteral obstruction is ominous and suggests unresectable disease in the pelvis. Obesity, advanced age

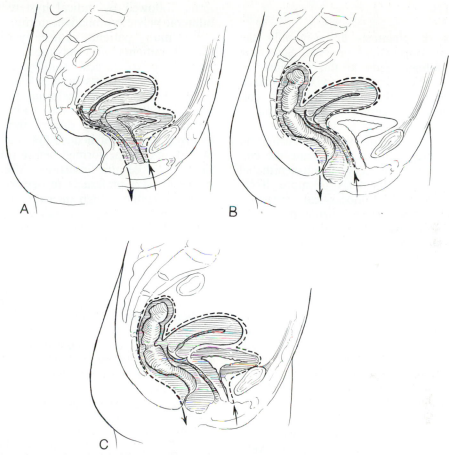

Figure 54–6. Organs removed in anterior exenteration *(A)*, posterior exenteration *(B)*, and total pelvic exenteration *(C)*.

(over 65 years), and systemic disease are relative contraindications, considering the serious morbidity associated with this operation. Some patients may be unsuitable for psychological reasons. A few patients regard the surgery as too mutilating and would prefer to die of disease rather than undergo the procedure.

CERVICAL CARCINOMA IN PREGNANCY

Carcinoma of the cervix associated with pregnancy usually implies diagnosis during pregnancy or within 12 months postpartum. It is relatively uncommon, invasive carcinoma occurring in approximately one out of 2200 pregnancies. The proportion of patients with invasive cancer who are pregnant is about one in 34 cases, and the average age is about 34 years.

Symptoms

The symptoms are similar to those in nonpregnant patients, painless vaginal bleeding being the most common. During pregnancy, this symptom can readily be attributed to conditions such as threatened abortion or placenta previa, so there is often unnecessary delay in diagnosis even though the patients are under regular medical surveillance.

Diagnosis

Methods of diagnosis are generally the same as in nonpregnant patients. Screening cervical cytology leads to the diagnosis in most cases. The pregnant cervix lends itself to colposcopic evaluation because the columnar eversion or gaping of the cervical os that occurs during pregnancy facilitates adequate visualization of the transformation zone. Pregnancy tends to exaggerate the colposcopic features of cervical intraepithelial neoplasia, so overdiagnosis is more likely than the reverse. Endocervical curettage should not be performed during pregnancy because of the risk of rupturing the membranes. Cone biopsy, if required, is best performed during the second trimester to avoid the possibility of induced abortion in the first trimester and severe hemorrhage and premature labor in the third trimester. Unfortunately, about half of the patients are not diagnosed until the postpartum period. The later the diagnosis is made, the more likely is the cancer to be in an advanced stage.

Management

Carcinoma in situ diagnosed during pregnancy should be managed conservatively, with the pregnancy allowed to proceed to term, vaginal delivery anticipated, and appropriate therapy carried out 6 to 8 weeks postpartum. Microinvasive carcinoma of the cervix diagnosed by conization of the cervix during pregnancy may also be managed conservatively, the pregnancy being allowed to continue to term with colposcopic surveillance of the cervix every 6 weeks. At term, either cesarean hysterectomy or vaginal delivery followed by postpartum extrafascial hysterectomy is appropriate.

Frankly invasive cancer requires relatively urgent treatment. After 22 to 26 weeks, it is reasonable to continue the pregnancy until fetal viability, if the patient desires. The general principles of treatment are essentially the same as in the nonpregnant patient. For early lesions, radical hysterectomy may be performed. Before 20 weeks gestation, this is done with the fetus in situ. After that time, hysterotomy through a high incision in the uterine fundus is performed to remove the fetus, followed by radical hysterectomy and bilateral pelvic lymphadenectomy.

For many patients with early disease and for all patients with advanced disease, the alternative to radical surgery is radiation therapy. For patients with disease diagnosed in the first trimester, external irradiation is started to shrink the tumor. Abortion usually occurs spontaneously during the course of external therapy; if it does not, uterine curettage should be performed before intracavitary radium or cesium insertion. After the first trimester, it is preferable to perform a hysterotomy through a high incision in the corpus before instituting radiotherapy.

If a decision is made to await fetal viability, it is important to be certain by ultrasonography that the baby is apparently healthy and to obtain a mature lecithin to sphingomyelin ratio to ensure fetal lung maturity before delivery. Because of the increased risk of hemorrhage and infection likely to be associated with delivery through a cervix containing gross cancer, classic cesarean section is the preferred method of delivery. For patients in whom inadvertent vaginal delivery has occurred, however, there is no evidence to suggest that prognosis is altered.

PROGNOSIS FOR CERVICAL CANCER

Prognosis is related directly to clinical stage (Table 54–4) and the frequency of pelvic and periaortic lymph node metastasis. With higher stage disease, the frequency of nodal metastasis escalates, and the 5-year survival diminishes. Adenocarcinomas and adenosquamous carcinomas have a somewhat lower 5-year survival than squamous carcinomas, stage for stage. This may be because these lesions are more likely to occur in older women and are usually endophytic (the growth initiates from the endocervical canal), so they may not be detected as readily as squamous carcinomas.

Patients with a central recurrence treated by pelvic exenteration have a 5-year survival rate of about 40 to 50 per cent. For cervical cancer in pregnancy, the overall prognosis for all stages of disease is similar to that in nonpregnant women. This is because of the

Table 54–4. CARCINOMA OF THE UTERINE CERVIX DISTRIBUTION BY STAGE AND 5-YEAR SURVIVAL IN THE DIFFERENT STAGES*

STAGE	PATIENTS TREATED		5-YEAR SURVIVAL	
	No.	%	No.	%
I	10,912	34.6	8265	75.7
II	10,765	34.1	5877	54.6
III	8255	26.2	2527	30.6
IV	1386	4.4	101	7.3
No stage	225	0.7	106	47.1
Total	31,543	100.0	16,876	53.5

* Patients treated in 1979–1981.
From the Annual Report on the Results of Treatment in Gynecological Cancer. Vol 20. Stockholm, Sweden, 1988, p 37.

higher proportion of patients with stage I disease during pregnancy. For more advanced disease, pregnancy has an unfavorable effect on prognosis. The reason for this is not clear but may be related to problems associated with radiation dosimetry in pregnancy or interruptions to the radiation therapy necessitated by genital tract sepsis.

SUGGESTED READING

Alvarez RD, Soong S-J, Kinney WK, et al: Identification of prognostic factors and risk groups in patients found to have nodal metastases at the time of radical hysterectomy for early-stage squamous carcinoma of the cervix. Gynecol Oncol 35:130, 1989.

Berek JS, Castaldo TW, Hacker NF, et al: Adenocarcinoma of the uterine cervix. Cancer 48:2734, 1981.

Berman M, Keys N, Creasman W, DiSaia P: Survival and patterns of recurrence in cervical cancer metastatic to paraaortic lymph nodes. Gynecol Oncol 19:8, 1984.

Charles EH, Savage EW: Cryosurgical treatment of cervical intraepithelial neoplasia. Obstet Gynecol Surv 35:539, 1980.

Hacker NF, Berek JS: Surgical staging. In Surwit E, Alberts D (eds): Cervix Cancer. Boston, Martinus Nijhoff, 1987, pp 43–57.

Hacker NF, Berek JS, Lagasse LD, et al: Carcinoma of the cervix associated with pregnancy. Obstet Gynecol 59:735, 1982.

Hatch KD: Cervical cancer. In Berek JS, Hacker NF (eds): Practical Gynecologic Oncology. Baltimore, Williams & Wilkins, 1989, pp 241–283.

Maier RC, Norris HJ: Coexistence of cervical intraepithelial neoplasia with primary adenocarcinoma of the endocervix. Obstet Gynecol 56:361, 1980.

Monaghan JM, Ireland D, Mor-Yosef S, et al: Role of centralization of surgery in stage Ib carcinoma of the cervix: A review of 498 cases. Gynecol Oncol 37:206, 1990.

Piver M, Rutledge F, Smith J: Five classes of extended hysterectomy for women with cervical cancer. Obstet Gynecol 44:265, 1974.

Savage EW: Microinvasive carcinoma of the cervix. Am J Obstet Gynecol 113:708, 1972.

Van Nagell JR Jr, Greenwell N, Powell DF, et al: Microinvasive carcinoma of the cervix. Am J Obstet Gynecol 145:981, 1983.

Wright TC, Richard RM: Role of human papillomavirus in the pathogenesis of genital tract warts and cancer. Gynecol Oncol 37:151, 1990.

Fifty-five

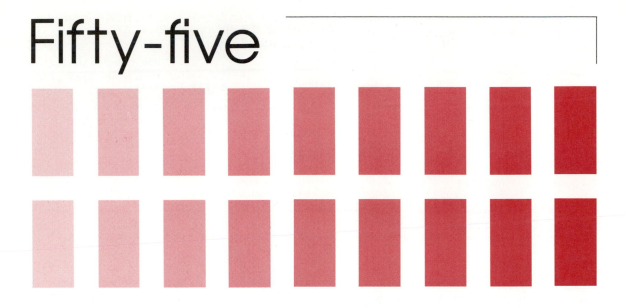

Ovarian Cancer

JONATHAN S. BEREK

Ovarian cancer is the fifth most common cancer among females in the United States, accounting for one fourth of all gynecologic malignancies. It is the leading cause of death from gynecologic cancer because it is difficult to detect before its dissemination. In 1990, there were over 20,000 new cases and over 12,000 deaths from this disease. Most women who develop ovarian cancer are in their fifth or sixth decade of life.

ETIOLOGY AND EPIDEMIOLOGY

The cause of ovarian cancer is unknown. The patient characteristics found to be associated with an increased risk for epithelial ovarian cancer include white race, late age of menopause, family history of cancer of the ovary or endometrium, and prolonged intervals of ovulation uninterrupted by pregnancy. About 1 per cent of epithelial ovarian cancer

is hereditary, in which two or more first-degree relatives have had the disease. In addition, pedigrees of several ovarian cancer families have revealed multiple adenocarcinomas in siblings and offspring. There is an increased prevalence of ovarian cancer in unmarried women, nuns, and nulliparous married women.

The use of oral contraceptives has been found to protect against ovarian cancer, possibly because of suppression of ovulation. It has been postulated that incessant ovulation may predispose to malignant transformation in the ovary. Postmenopausal estrogen use has not been shown to cause ovarian cancer.

It has also been postulated that an etiologic agent could enter the peritoneal cavity through the lower genital tract. For example, the perineal use of asbestos-contaminated talc has been linked to the development of epithelial ovarian cancer. This possibility remains controversial, however. The role of the mumps virus is also controversial, although more recent epidemiologic data suggest that a prior history of infection with this agent probably does predispose the patient to the subsequent development of epithelial ovarian malignancies.

The incidence of ovarian cancer varies in different geographic locations. Western countries, including the United States, have rates three to seven times greater than Japan. Second-generation Japanese immigrants to the United States have an incidence of ovarian cancer similar to that of American women. White Americans develop ovarian cancer about 1½ times more frequently than do black Americans.

CLINICAL FEATURES

Symptoms

Unfortunately, most patients who develop ovarian cancer are relatively asymptomatic before disease dissemination. In early-stage disease, the patient may complain of nonspecific symptoms or irregular menses if she is premenopausal. Symptoms of a mass compressing the bladder or rectum, such as urinary frequency or constipation, may bring the patient to a physician. Sometimes the patient complains of a lower abdominal or pelvic "fullness" or of dyspareunia. Only rarely does a patient present with acute symptoms, such as pain secondary to torsion, rupture, or intracystic hemorrhage.

In advanced-stage disease, patients most often present with abdominal pain or swelling. The latter may be from the tumor itself or from associated ascites. On careful questioning, there has usually been a history of vague abdominal symptoms, such as bloating, constipation, nausea, dyspepsia, anorexia, or early satiety. Premenopausal patients may complain of irregular menses or heavy vaginal bleeding. Postmenopausal bleeding occasionally is a symptom of ovarian neoplasms, particularly functional stromal tumors.

Signs

Pelvic examination is critical to the diagnosis of ovarian cancer. The disease is fre-
quently misdiagnosed for several months because patients with nonspecific abdominal symptoms do not receive a vaginal and rectal examination. A solid, irregular, fixed pelvic mass is very suggestive of ovarian cancer, and if combined with upper abdominal masses, ascites, or both, the diagnosis is almost certain. In a woman 2 or more years postmenopausal, any palpable ovarian mass is suspicious, since the ovaries should then be atrophic and not clinically palpable. This circumstance has been referred to as the *postmenopausal palpable ovary syndrome.*

Preoperative Evaluation

The diagnosis and management of any neoplasm require laparotomy. Routine preoperative hemotologic and biochemical studies should be obtained, as should a chest radiograph and intravenous pyelogram. Extensive preoperative evaluation of the patient, however, with pelvic and abdominal computed tomographic scan, liver-spleen scan, and bone scan is not indicated.

A Papanicolaou smear should be obtained to evaluate the cervix, but this test is of limited value in detecting ovarian cancer. An endometrial biopsy and endocervical curettage are necessary in patients with abnormal vaginal bleeding because concurrent primary tumors occasionally occur in the ovary and endometrium. In the presence of a pelvic mass, it is preferable not to perform abdominal paracentesis for cytologic evaluation of ascitic fluid because seeding of the abdominal wall may occur.

An abdominal radiograph may be useful in a younger patient to locate calcifications associated with a benign cystic teratoma (dermoid cyst), which is the most common neoplasm in patients under 25 years of age. In patients over 45 years of age, a barium enema should be obtained to rule out a primary colon cancer with ovarian metastasis. Similarly, an upper gastrointestinal barium study is important if there are significant gastric symptoms. Breast cancer may also metastasize to the ovaries, so bilateral mammograms should be obtained if there are any suspicious breast masses.

Pelvic ultrasonography may be useful for smaller (less than 8 cm) masses in premenopausal women. Masses that are predominantly solid or multilocular have a higher probability of being neoplastic, whereas unilocular cystic masses are generally functional cysts.

Several tumor markers have been investigated, but none has been consistently reliable. The tumor-associated antigen, CA-125, which can be detected by a murine monoclonal antibody serum assay (OC-125), is present in many women who have documented ovarian cancer. When this assay is elevated, it is useful in monitoring the clinical course of the disease. It is currently being studied for evaluation of its utility in detecting early ovarian cancer.

Differential Diagnosis

Ovarian malignancies must be differentiated from benign neoplasms and functional cysts of the ovaries. In addition, a variety of gynecologic conditions can simulate a neoplastic process, including tubo-ovarian abscess, endometriosis, and pedunculated uterine leiomyoma. Nongynecologic causes for a pelvic tumor must also be excluded, such as inflammatory or neoplastic disease of the colon or a pelvic or horseshoe kidney.

Mode of Spread

Ovarian cancer typically spreads by exfoliating cells that disseminate and implant throughout the peritoneal cavity. The distribution of intraperitoneal metastases tends to follow the circulatory path of peritoneal fluid, so metastases are commonly seen on the posterior cul-de-sac, paracolic gutters, right hemidiaphragm, liver capsule, and omentum. Implants are also common on the bowel serosa and its mesenteries. Generally, they grow around the intestines, encasing them with tumor, without invading the bowel lumen. Widespread bowel metastases can lead to a functional obstruction known as carcinomatous ileus.

Lymphatic dissemination to the pelvic and periaortic nodes is common, particularly with advanced disease. Extensive blockage of the diaphragmatic lymphatics is at least partially responsible for the development of ascites.

Hematogenous metastases are not common, and parenchymal metastases to the liver and lungs are seen in only about 2 to 3 per cent of patients at initial presentation.

Death from ovarian cancer usually results from progressive encasement of abdominal organs leading to anorexia, vomiting, and inanition. The bowel obstruction caused by tumor growth is often incomplete and intermittent and may last for several months before the patient's demise.

STAGING

The standard staging system for ovarian cancer is presented in Table 55–1. It is based on surgical exploration of the patient in addition to the clinical examination. Ovarian cancer is the only gynecologic cancer in which surgery is formally incorporated into the International Federation of Gynecology and Obstetrics (FIGO) staging system.

Even though all microscopic disease may appear to be confined to the ovaries at the time of laparotomy, microscopic spread may have already occurred; thus patients must undergo a thorough "surgical staging." Procedures necessary to stage ovarian cancer are shown in Table 55–2.

CLASSIFICATION

The histogenetic classification of ovarian neoplasms is listed in Table 55–3. These lesions fall into four categories according to their tissue of origin. Most ovarian neoplasms (80 to 85 per cent) are derived from coelomic epithelium and are called epithelial carcinomas. Less common tumors are derived from primitive germ cells, specialized gonadal stroma, or nonspecific mesenchyme. In addition, the ovary can be the site of metastatic carcinomas, most often from the gastrointestinal tract or the breast.

EPITHELIAL OVARIAN CARCINOMAS

Pathology

The main histologic subtypes of epithelial tumors are serous, mucinous, endometrioid,

Table 55–1. FIGO* STAGE FOR PRIMARY CARCINOMA OF THE OVARY

Stage I	Growth limited to the ovaries
Stage Ia	Growth limited to one ovary; no ascites. No tumor on the external surface; capsule intact
Stage Ib	Growth limited to both ovaries; no ascites. No tumor on the external surfaces; capsules intact
Stage Ic	Tumor either stage Ia or Ib but with tumor on the surface of one or both ovaries; or with capsule ruptured; or with ascites present containing malignant cells or with positive peritoneal washings
Stage II	Growth involving one or both ovaries with pelvic extension
Stage IIa	Extension and/or metastases to the uterus and/or tubes
Stage IIb	Extension to other pelvic tissues
Stage IIc	Tumor either stage IIa or IIb but with tumor on the surface of one or both ovaries; or with capsule(s) ruptured; or with ascites present containing malignant cells; or with positive peritoneal washings
Stage III	Tumor involving one or both ovaries with peritoneal implants outside the pelvis and/or positive retroperitoneal or inguinal nodes. Superficial liver metastasis equals stage III. Tumor is limited to the true pelvis, but with histologically proved malignant extension to small bowel or omentum
Stage IIIa	Tumor grossly limited to the true pelvis with negative nodes but with histologically confirmed microscopic seeding of abdominal peritoneal surfaces
Stage IIIb	Tumor of one or both ovaries with histologically confirmed implants of abdominal peritoneal surfaces, none exceeding 2 cm in diameter. Nodes negative
Stage IIIc	Abdominal implants >2 cm in diameter and/or positive retroperitoneal or inguinal nodes
Stage IV	Growth involving one or both ovaries with distant metastasis. If pleural effusion is present, there must be positive cytologic test results to allot a case to stage IV. Parenchymal liver metastasis equals stage IV.

* International Federation of Gynecology and Obstetrics.

clear cell (mesonephroid), Brenner's, and undifferentiated. The relative percentages of these subtypes are listed in Table 55–4. About 70 per cent of serous, 85 per cent of mucinous, and over 95 per cent of Brenner's tumors are benign, whereas almost all endometrioid and clear-cell tumors are malignant.

Serous tumors resemble fallopian tube epithelium histologically (Fig. 55–1). About 30 per cent of patients with stages I and IIa disease have bilateral involvement, whereas if all stages are included, about two thirds of patients have bilateral disease. On gross examination, serous carcinomas have an irregular and multilocular appearance (Fig. 55–2).

Mucinous tumors histologically resemble endocervical epithelium and are often quite large, measuring 20 cm or greater in diameter. They are bilateral in 10 to 20 per cent of patients. Pseudomyxoma peritonei is occasionally associated with a mucinous carcinoma. In this condition, extensive tumor deposits are present throughout the peritoneal cavity, producing a thick mucinous ascites

that ultimately leads to bowel obstruction. A mucocele or carcinoma of the appendix or gallbladder may occasionally be seen in conjunction with these tumors.

Endometrioid tumors closely resemble carcinomas of the endometrium and arise in association with a primary endometrial cancer in about 20 per cent of cases. In early-stage disease, they are bilateral in about 10 per cent of cases. Approximately 10 per cent of endometrioid ovarian carcinomas are associated with endometriosis, although malignant transformation of endometriosis occurs in fewer than 1 per cent of patients.

Clear cell carcinomas of the ovary are uncommon. They have been called mesonephroid carcinomas because their histologic features resemble tumors of mesonephric origin. They are only rarely bilateral, but in about 25 per cent of cases they occur in association with endometriosis.

The Brenner tumor represents only 2 to 3 per cent of all ovarian neoplasms, and fewer than 2 per cent of these are malignant. About

Table 55-2. REQUIREMENTS FOR A "STAGING" OR "SECOND-LOOK" OPERATION*

Multiple cytologic assays
  Free ascitic fluid, if present
  Peritoneal "washings" (50 ml normal saline)
    Pelvic cul-de-sac
    Both paracolic gutters
    Both hemidiaphragms
Multiple intraperitoneal biopsies
  Pelvis
    Cul-de-sac peritoneum
    Bladder peritoneum
    Pedicles of infundibulopelvic ligaments
    Any adhesions
  Abdomen
    Both paracolic gutters
    Bowel serosa and mesenteries
    Omentum
    Any adhesions
Extraperitoneal biopsies
  Pelvic and periaortic lymph nodes

* Procedures performed in patients with no visible evidence of metastatic disease.

10 per cent of Brenner's tumors occur in conjunction with a mucinous cystadenoma or dermoid cyst in the same or the opposite ovary.

Tumors of low malignant potential or borderline histology exist for each histologic type. Approximately 5 to 10 per cent of malignant serous tumors are borderline (Fig. 55-3), whereas 20 per cent of malignant mucinous tumors fall into this category. The endometrioid, clear cell, or Brenner's tumors are only rarely borderline.

Management of Epithelial Ovarian Cancer

The initial approach to all patients with ovarian cancer is surgical exploration of the abdomen and pelvis.

Early-Stage Disease

In patients with no gross evidence of disease beyond the ovary, the standard operation is total abdominal hysterectomy, bilateral salpingo-oophorectomy, infracolic omentectomy, and thorough surgical staging, as shown in Table 55-2. Patients who wish to preserve fertility may have a unilateral salpingo-oophorectomy, unless the tumor is poorly differentiated on frozen section. In patients with grade 1 or 2 tumors confined to one or both ovaries after surgical staging, no further treatment is necessary. Patients with poorly differentiated (grade 3) tumors are subsequently treated with systemic chemotherapy.

Advanced-Stage Disease

In patients with advanced disease, cytoreductive surgery ("debulking") is required. The objectives are to remove the primary tumor and all of the metastases, if possible. If all macroscopic disease cannot be removed, an attempt should be made to reduce individual tumor nodules to 1.5 cm or less in diameter. Patients in whom this goal is achieved are said to have had "optimal" cytoreduction, which can be achieved in about 80 per cent of patients. In addition to a total or subtotal abdominal hysterectomy, bilateral salpingo-oophorectomy, omentectomy, and resection of peritoneal metastases, optimal cytoreduction may necessitate bowel resection; therefore, all patients having surgery for suspected ovarian cancer should have a bowel preparation preoperatively. In retrospective studies, patients whose individual residual tumor nodules are 1.5 cm or less in diameter before the commencement of chemotherapy have been shown to have longer median survivals and more complete responses to therapy. The longest survival is seen in those patients in whom all visible tumor has been removed before treatment.

Following primary cytoreductive surgery, combination chemotherapy is given, most commonly *cis*-platinum and cyclophosphamide. *Cis*-platinum–containing combination chemotherapy has resulted in a greater number of responses and longer median survivals than were previously achieved with single alkylating agent therapy. A newer agent, *carbo*-platinum, is now used frequently instead of *cis*-platinum because it has less renal and neurotoxicity. Its efficacy relative to *cis*-

Table 55–3. HISTOGENETIC CLASSIFICATION OF PRIMARY OVARIAN NEOPLASMS

DERIVATION	TYPE OF TUMOR

Coelomic epithelial origin (80–85%)	"Common" epithelial tumors; benign, borderline, malignant
	  Serous tumor
	  Mucinous tumor
	  Endometrioid tumor
	  Clear cell (mesonephroid) tumor
	  Brenner's tumor
	Undifferentiated carcinoma
	Carcinosarcoma and mixed mesodermal tumors

Germ cell origin (10–15%)	Teratoma
	  Mature teratoma
	    Solid adult teratoma
	    Dermoid cyst
	    Struma ovarii
	    Malignant neoplasms secondarily arising from teratomatous tissues (squamous carcinoma, carcinoid tumor, sarcoma)
	  Immature teratoma
	Dysgerminoma
	Endodermal sinus tumor
	Embryonal carcinoma
	Choriocarcinoma
	Gonadoblastoma*
	Mixed germ cell tumors

Specialized gonadal-stromal origin (3–5%)	Granulosa-theca tumors
	  Granulosa cell tumor
	  Thecoma
	Sertoli-Leydig tumors
	  Arrhenoblastoma
	  Sertoli tumor
	Gynandroblastoma
	Lipid cell tumors

Nonspecific mesenchymal origin (fewer than 1%)	Fibroma, hemangioma, leiomyoma, lipoma Lymphoma Sarcoma

* Combined germ cell and specialized gonadal-stromal elements.
Adapted from Hart WR, Morrow CP: The ovaries. In Romney SL, Gray MJ, Little AO, et al (eds): Gynecology and Obstetrics: The Health Care of Women. 2nd ed. New York, McGraw-Hill, 1981.

platinum, however, is still being studied. Single-agent therapy, typically melphalan (L-phenylalanine mustard [L-PAM]), is still commonly used for frail or elderly patients. It is unclear whether patients with "metastatic" borderline tumors benefit from chemotherapy.

Whole abdominal radiation therapy has been used as primary therapy instead of chemotherapy, but it appears to have its major role in patients who have no gross residual disease following initial surgery. A comparison of combination chemotherapy with whole abdominal radiation as primary treatment in such patients has not been reported.

Second-Look Laparotomy

In patients who are clinically free of disease after completing a prescribed course of chemotherapy (usually about 6 cycles), a "second-look" laparotomy may be performed to determine whether the patient has had a complete response to chemotherapy. Prolonged alkylating agent chemotherapy is asso-

Table 55-4. PERCENTAGE OF EPITHELIAL OVARIAN MALIGNANCIES BY HISTOLOGIC TYPE

TYPE	PER CENT
Serous	35-40
Endometrioid	15-25
Mucinous	6-10
Clear cell	5
Brenner's	<1
Undifferentiated	15-30

Derived from Scully RE: Tumors of the ovary and maldeveloped gonads. In Atlas of Tumor Pathology. 2nd series, fasc. 16. Washington, DC, Armed Forces Institute of Pathology, 1979.

ciated with a significant risk for the subsequent development of acute nonlymphocytic leukemia. Therefore, it is desirable to use briefer, more intensive chemotherapeutic programs whenever feasible and to discontinue therapy when a complete surgical response has been documented. If there is no macroscopic or microscopic evidence of disease at second-look laparotomy, essentially the same procedures as are carried out for surgical staging should be performed (see Table 55-2). If gross disease is present, an attempt should be made to resect persistent disease to facilitate a response to subsequent therapy. It is unclear whether the performance of a second-look laparotomy and the administration of further treatment ultimately prolong survival, so the surgery is discretionary.

Second-Line Therapies

Secondary systemic chemotherapy has been disappointing in patients with ovarian cancer who have failed primary combination therapy. Experimental approaches are currently being tried, including whole-abdominal radiation, intraperitoneal chemotherapy, and intraperitoneal immunotherapy.

Prognosis

Patients with stage I disease have 5-year survival rates of 80 to 95 per cent, depending

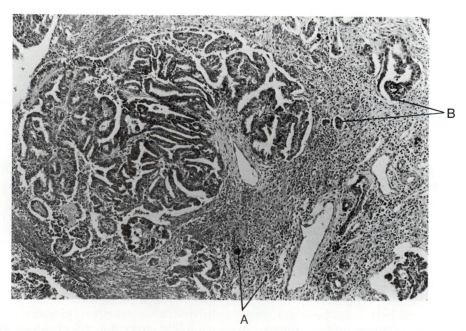

Figure 55-1. Histology of a grade 1 serous adenocarcinoma of the ovary. Note the papillary nature of the tumor and the well-formed glands. Psammoma bodies (calcifications) (A) and stromal invasion (B) are evident (×60).

Figure 55–2. Bilateral serous cystadenocarcinomas. Note the papillary projections from the surface of both ovaries and the implants on the serosal surfaces of the uterus and fallopian tubes.

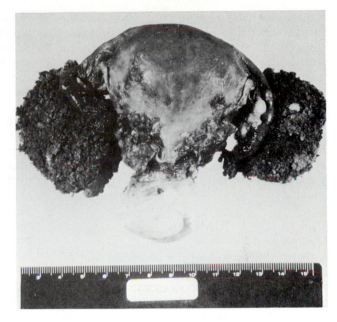

on the histology and grade. Almost all patients with carefully staged stage Ia grade 1 ovarian cancer are cured surgically, whereas the 5-year survival rate of patients with poorly differentiated bilateral lesions is as low as 80 per cent. The 5-year survival rate for patients with stage II disease is about 70 per cent. In spite of aggressive primary surgery and combination chemotherapy, the 5-year survival rate for patients with advanced-stage disease is about 20 per cent. Patients with advanced-stage disease who have a negative second-look laparotomy have a 5-year survival rate of about 60 per cent.

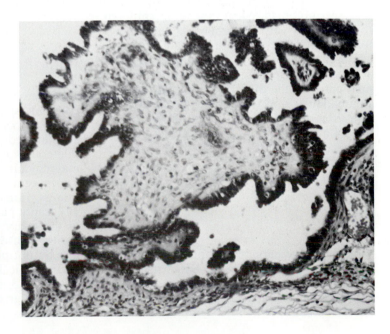

Figure 55–3. Histology of a "borderline" serous cystadenoma of the ovary. Note the multiple, papillary projections lined by pseudostratified columnar epithelium. There is no stromal invasion, as demonstrated by the clear delineation of the epithelium from the underlying stroma (×60).

Patients who have borderline ovarian tumors can be expected to have a prolonged survival. If the disease is confined to the ovary, the vast majority of tumors never recur. Five- and 10-year survival rates are 95 to 100 per cent, but late recurrences may present, and 20-year survival rates are approximately 85 to 90 per cent. Patients who initially present with metastatic disease are most likely to develop subsequent clinical evidence of disease, although the rate of progression is slow; most live at least 5 years.

GERM CELL TUMORS

Germ cell tumors of the ovary account for only about 2 to 3 per cent of all ovarian malignancies. They occur predominantly in young patients and frequently produce either human chorionic gonadotropin (hCG) or alpha-fetoprotein (AFP), which serve as tumor markers. The most common germ cell tumors are the dysgerminoma and immature teratoma. Endodermal sinus tumors, embryonal tumors, and nongestational choriocarcinomas are less common. Mixed germ-cell tumors are not uncommon.

Dysgerminomas

Dysgerminomas occur predominantly in children and young women. About 10 per cent are bilateral. These tumors are occasionally seen in patients with gonadal dysgenesis or the testicular feminization syndrome. In such patients, the dysgerminoma may arise in a gonadoblastoma. In about two thirds of cases, the disease is confined to the ovaries at the time of diagnosis. About 10 per cent of dysgerminomas are associated with other germ cell malignancies. Pure dysgerminomas do not produce the tumor markers hCG or AFP.

Treatment

In most patients, the contralateral ovary and uterus can be preserved. Surgical staging, as outlined earlier in this chapter, is important. Particular attention should be paid to the pelvic and periaortic lymph nodes be-

cause of the propensity of these tumors for lymphatic dissemination. If disease extends beyond one ovary in patients who desire preservation of fertility, the treatment of choice is chemotherapy. The regimen employed for these patients is usually vincristine, actinomycin-D, and cyclophosphamide (VAC); vinblastine, bleomycin, and *cis*-platinum (VBP); or bleomycin, etoposide, and *cis*-platinum (BEP). Alternatively, when fertility is not an issue, postoperative radiation to the pelvis and abdomen can be used after hysterectomy and bilateral salpingo-oophorectomy because dysgerminomas are uniquely radiosensitive. If there are metastases to the periaortic lymph nodes, the radiation field may include the mediastinal and supraclavicular lymph nodes. Recurrence after conservative surgery is also treated with radiation or chemotherapy.

Prognosis

The overall 5-year survival rate for patients with a pure dysgerminoma is approximately 95 per cent for stage I, 80 per cent for stage II, and 60 to 70 per cent for stage III. The 5-year survival rate for patients with stage Ia pure dysgerminoma treated with a unilateral oophorectomy is about 95 per cent. Because of the radiosensitivity of dysgerminomas, recurrences following conservative surgery have at least a 50 per cent 5-year survival rate.

Immature Teratomas

Immature teratomas are the second most common malignant ovarian germ cell tumor. About 75 per cent of malignant teratomas are encountered during the first 2 decades of life. Bilaterality is rare, although the other ovary may contain a benign dermoid cyst in about 5 per cent of cases. Like other germ cell tumors, immature teratomas grow fairly rapidly, cause pain early, and are found confined to the ovary in about two thirds of cases at the time of diagnosis. Pure immature teratomas do not produce hCG or AFP.

Histologically, the tumors can be graded from 1 to 3 according to the degree of differentiation, grade 3 tumors being the least differentiated. Neural elements are most frequently seen, but cartilage and epithelial tissues are also common.

Treatment

The primary tumor should be removed. In young patients, however, the uterus and contralateral ovary should be preserved to maintain fertility. All patients with other than stage Ia, grade 1 immature teratomas should receive postoperative chemotherapy using VAC, VBP, or BEP. Therapy should be given for 4 to 6 cycles. A second-look laparotomy is not considered necessary in patients with stage I disease.

Prognosis

Survival correlates with grade and stage of disease. The 5-year survival rate for patients with grade 1 immature teratomas is about 90 per cent, compared with 80 per cent for grade 2 and 60 to 70 per cent for grade 3.

Other Germ Cell Tumors

The endodermal sinus tumor is a rare malignancy. It is also referred to as a *yolk sac* tumor. Endodermal sinus tumors produce AFP, which can serve as a useful serum marker for this neoplasm. Embryonal carcinomas produce both hCG and AFP, whereas choriocarcinomas produce hCG. All occur in children and young women, and all grow rapidly. Most are confined to one ovary at the time of diagnosis. Bilaterality is rare.

Therapy for these lesions includes surgical resection of the primary tumor followed by systemic combination chemotherapy with VBP or BEP. Prior to the advent of effective chemotherapy, these tumors were usually fatal. The overall 5-year survival rate is now about 60 per cent.

SPECIALIZED GONADAL-STROMAL TUMORS

This group of relatively uncommon tumors is derived from the specialized ovarian stroma. As such, they are often endocrinologically functional, many of them being capable of synthesizing gonadal or adrenal steroid hormones. Since the ovarian stroma is sexually bipotential, hormones that are secreted can be either female or male. Estrogen and progesterone are typically associated with granulosa-theca tumors, whereas testosterone and other androgens may be secreted by many Sertoli-Leydig cell tumors. Rarely, lipid cell tumors, which are usually virilizing, produce adrenal corticoids and a clinical cushingoid syndrome.

Pathology

Granulosa cell tumors are the most common stromal carcinomas. The granulosa tumors have a distinct histologic pattern; small groups of cells called Call-Exner bodies are the hallmark. They may secrete large amounts of estrogen and can be associated with endometrial cancer in adults or sexual pseudoprecosity in children.

Thecomas, which are only one third as common as granulosa cell tumors, are rarely malignant. Mixtures of the two types of tumor exist.

Sertoli-Leydig cell tumors (arrhenoblastomas) contain both Sertoli-type and Leydig-type stromal cells and are classically associated with masculinization. Only 3 to 5 per cent of these tumors are malignant.

Lipid cell tumors are often referred to as hilar cell tumors because they are located in the ovarian hilus. Only a rare lipid tumor, usually larger than 8 cm in diameter, behaves in a malignant fashion.

Treatment

Most stromal tumors occur in postmenopausal women, and a total abdominal hysterectomy and bilateral salpingo-oophorectomy are indicated in such cases. Conservation of the uterus and contralateral ovary is appropriate for carefully staged young patients with stage I disease, provided that the possibility of an associated adenocarcinoma of the endometrium has been excluded by dilatation and curettage. Postoperative radiation therapy to the pelvis is occasionally used in early-stage disease. Effective chemotherapy is not available at this time.

Prognosis

Granulosa cell tumors, which tend to be slow-growing tumors, are usually confined to one ovary at the time of diagnosis. The 5-year survival rate is approximately 90 per cent for stage I cases. Recurrences are usually detected late and may result in death 15 to 20 years after removal of the primary lesion.

METASTATIC CANCERS

About 4 to 8 per cent of ovarian malignancies are metastatic, most commonly from either the gastrointestinal tract or the breast. The Krukenberg tumor is a specific type of metastatic tumor in which "signet-ring" cells are seen in the ovarian stroma histologically. Most Krukenberg's tumors are bilateral and metastatic from the stomach. Rarely, it has not been possible to locate a primary focus, and removal of the ovarian disease has produced apparent cures.

FALLOPIAN TUBE CARCINOMA

Primary carcinoma of the fallopian tube accounts for only 0.1 to 0.5 per cent of gynecologic cancers. Most carcinomas of the fallopian tube are adenocarcinomas, but sarcomas and mixed tumors can also occur. There is no official staging system for fallopian tube carcinoma, but generally it is staged like ovarian cancer because its mode of dissemination is similar. Bilateral carcinomas are seen in 10 to 20 per cent of patients.

Clinical Features

Clinically, patients can present with a vaginal discharge that is typically serous in nature, vaginal bleeding, pelvic pain, or some combination. In postmenopausal patients, the vaginal discharge may be yellow, watery, and similar to the symptoms of a urinary fistula. Physical examination may reveal an adnexal mass. A fallopian tube cancer should be suspected in a postmenopausal patient whose bleeding or abnormal cytology is not explained by an endometrial or endocervical curettage. In most patients, the diagnosis is not made preoperatively.

Treatment

The treatment for fallopian tube carcinoma is total abdominal hysterectomy, bilateral salpingo-oophorectomy, and omentectomy. Surgical staging should be performed in patients whose disease appears to be confined to the pelvis, and cytoreductive surgery is appropriate in patients with metastatic disease. Postoperatively, combination chemotherapy, including *cis*-platinum and cyclophosphamide with or without Adriamycin, is usually used for patients with metastatic disease. Whole-abdominal radiation may be given for patients with completely resected disease.

Prognosis

Prognosis for fallopian tube carcinoma is similar to that for ovarian cancer.

SUGGESTED READING

Berek JS: Epithelial ovarian cancer. In Berek JS, Hacker NF (eds): Practical Gynecologic Oncology. Baltimore, Williams & Wilkins, 1989, pp 327–364.

Berek JS, Hacker NF, Lagasse LD, et al: Second-look laparotomy in Stage III epithelial ovarian cancer: Clinical variables associated with disease status. Obstet Gynecol 64:207, 1984.

Berek JS, Hacker NF, Lagasse LD, et al: Survival following secondary cytoreductive surgery in ovarian cancer. Obstet Gynecol 61:189, 1983.

Dembo AJ, Bush RS, Beole FA, et al: The Princess Margaret Hospital study of ovarian cancer: Stages I, II, and asymptomatic III presentations. Cancer Treat Rep 63:249, 1979.

Gershensen DM, Wharton JT: Malignant germ cell tumors of the ovary. In Albert DS, Surwit EA (eds): Ovarian Cancer. Hingham MA, Martinus Nijhoff, 1985, pp 227–269.

Gordon A, Lipton D, Woodruff JD: Dysgerminoma: A review of 158 cases from the Emil Novak Ovarian Tumor Registry. Obstet Gynecol 58:497, 1981.

Hacker NF, Berek JS, Lagasse LD, et al: Primary cytoreductive surgery for epithelial ovarian cancer. Obstet Gynecol 61:413, 1983.

Nejit JP, ten Bokkel Huinink WW, van der Burg MEL, et al: Randomised trial comparing two combination chemotherapy regimes (CHAP-5 v CP) in advanced ovarian carcinoma. J Clin Oncol 5(8): 1157, 1987.

Scully RE: Tumors of the ovary and maldeveloped gonads. In Atlas of Tumor Pathology. 2nd series, fasc. 16. Washington, DC, Armed Forces Institute of Pathology, 1979.

Young RC, Walton LA, Ellenberg SS, et al: Adjuvant therapy in Stage I and Stage II epithelial ovarian cancer. N Engl J Med 322: 1021, 1990.

Fifty-six

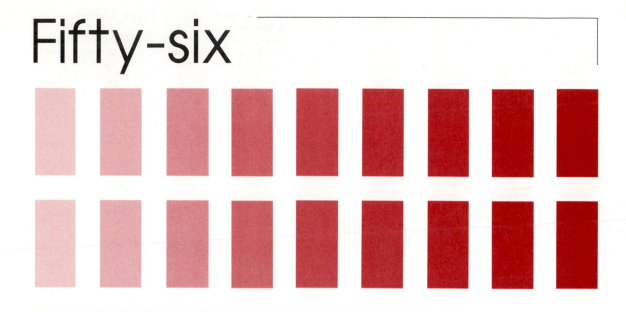

Vulvar and Vaginal Cancer

NEVILLE F. HACKER

VULVAR NEOPLASMS

Malignant tumors of the vulva are uncommon, representing about 3 to 4 per cent of malignancies of the female genital tract. Most tumors are squamous cell carcinomas, with melanomas, adenocarcinomas, basal cell carcinomas, and sarcomas occurring much less frequently.

Squamous cell carcinoma of the vulva occurs mainly in postmenopausal women, and the mean age at diagnosis is 65 years. A history of chronic vulvar itching is common. Vulvar cancer tends to be found more frequently in patients who are obese and in those who have hypertension, diabetes mellitus, or arteriosclerosis. Hidradenomas of the Bartholin gland occasionally are diagnosed erroneously as vulvar carcinoma. Other primary malignancies have been reported in up to 22 per cent of cases, the most common primary site being the cervix.

Epidemiology

No specific etiologic agent has been identified for vulvar cancer. Because of the common association among squamous cancers of the lower genital tract, it has been postulated that a common pathogen may be involved. The human papilloma virus has been regarded as a possible carcinogen. Approximately 5 per cent of vulvar cancers develop within pre-existing genital condylomas, and about 5 per cent of patients have a positive serologic test for syphilis. In the latter group of patients, vulvar cancer occurs at an earlier age and carries a graver prognosis. Although rarely seen in the United States, vulvar cancer also occurs in association with lymphogranuloma venereum and granuloma inguinale.

Vulvar dystrophies that show cellular atypia on biopsy carry a small risk of malignant transformation, particularly if untreated.

With adequate treatment, however, a vulvar dystrophy should not significantly predispose the patient to the development of vulvar cancer. The malignant potential of carcinoma in situ of the vulva is also uncertain but appears to be low except in elderly patients and those who are immunosuppressed.

INTRAEPITHELIAL NEOPLASIA

The International Society for the Study of Vulvar Disease recognizes two varieties of intraepithelial neoplasia: squamous cell carcinoma in situ (Bowen's disease) and Paget's disease.

Squamous Cell Carcinoma In Situ

During the past 2 decades, the incidence of carcinoma in situ of the vulva has increased. Younger patients are being affected, and the mean age is approximately 45 years.

Clinical Features

Itching is the most common symptom, although some patients present with palpable or visible abnormalities of the vulva. Approximately half of the patients are asymptomatic. There is no absolutely diagnostic appearance. Most lesions are elevated, but the color may be white, red, pink, gray, or brown (Fig. 56–1). Approximately 20 per cent of the lesions have a "warty" appearance, and the lesions are multicentric in about two thirds of cases.

Diagnosis

Careful inspection of the vulva in a bright light, with the aid of a magnifying glass, if necessary, is the most useful technique for detecting abnormal areas. In a patient with pruritus vulvae and no gross abnormality, colposcopic examination of the entire vulva after the application of 2 per cent acetic acid is helpful. The toluidine blue dye test (Collin's test) may also help direct biopsies. Because the dye fixes to cell nuclei, false-nega-

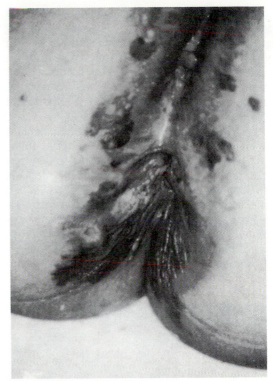

Figure 56–1. Carcinoma in situ of the vulva. Note the pigmented and multicentric nature of the lesions and the extensive perianal involvement in this patient.

tive results may be seen in the presence of hyperkeratosis, and false-positive results may be seen in the presence of excoriations. A liberal number of directed biopsies must be taken to establish the diagnosis and rule out invasive carcinoma.

Management

A number of methods of treatment are used for carcinoma in situ of the vulva. In the past, total vulvectomy was usually performed. It is now clear, however, that the incidence of recurrence following total vulvectomy (about 30 per cent) is not less than that following local excision of the individual lesions. Because of the distressing psychological consequences of vulvectomy, local excision is now considered the mainstay of treatment.

The microscopic disease seldom extends significantly beyond the macroscopic lesion, so that margins of about 5 mm are usually adequate. For extensive lesions involving most of the vulva, a skinning vulvectomy, in which the vulvar skin is removed and replaced by a split-thickness skin graft, may be used. Because the subcutaneous tissues are not excised, the cosmetic result is superior to vulvectomy.

Topical 5-fluorouracil cream is effective in about 50 per cent of cases, but patient tolerance is low because of the painful ulceration that results. Laser therapy is also effective, particularly for multiple small lesions. When large areas of the vulva are treated with laser therapy, postoperative pain is severe and patient tolerance for this procedure is low. Topical chemotherapy and laser therapy offer the optimal cosmetic outcome, but because no specimen is available for histology, a liberal number of biopsies must be taken before treatment to exclude invasive disease.

Bowenoid Papulosis of the Vulva

Bowenoid papulosis is a clinical entity that usually affects younger individuals. It is characterized clinically by multiple reddish brown or violaceous papules on the vulva or penis. Histologically, it is indistinguishable from carcinoma in situ. A viral etiology has been postulated but not proved. Treatment should be by local excision or laser therapy.

Paget's Disease

Paget's disease of the vulva predominantly affects postmenopausal white women.

Clinical Features

Itching and tenderness are common and may be longstanding. The affected area is usually well demarcated and eczematoid in appearance, with the presence of white plaque-like lesions. As growth progresses, extension beyond the vulva to the mons pubis, thighs, and buttocks may occur; rarely, it may extend to involve the mucosa of the rectum, vagina, or urinary tract. In about 20

per cent of cases, Paget's disease is associated with an underlying adenocarcinoma.

Histology

The disease is characterized by large, pale, pathognomonic Paget's cells, which are seen within the epidermis and skin adnexae. They are rich in mucopolysaccharide, a diastase-resistant, PAS-positive substance. The intracytoplasmic mucin may also be demonstrated by Mayer's mucicarmine stain. The histogenesis of this lesion has been controversial, but it is currently believed to be a type of adenocarcinoma in situ. The Paget's cells are typically located adjacent to the basal layer, both in the epidermis and in the adnexal structures.

Management

Unlike Bowen's disease, the histologic extent of Paget's disease is frequently far beyond the visible lesion. Hence, wide local excision is required to clear the lesion, and frozen sections should be obtained on the margins of resection. Recurrences still occur in approximately 30 per cent of cases and may be treated by further excision or laser therapy. If an underlying invasive carcinoma is present, the treatment should be the same as for other invasive vulvar cancers, requiring at least a radical vulvectomy and bilateral inguinofemoral lymphadenectomy.

INVASIVE VULVAR CANCER

Squamous Cell Carcinoma

Squamous cell carcinoma accounts for about 90 per cent of vulvar cancers.

Clinical Features

Patients generally present with a vulvar lump, although longstanding pruritus is common and may be associated with an underlying vulvar dystrophy. Other common presenting symptoms include vulvar pain, bleeding, discharge, or dysuria. The lesions may be raised, ulcerated, pigmented, or warty

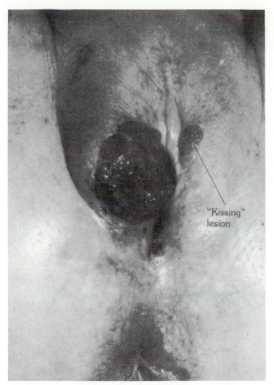

"Kissing" lesion

Figure 56–2. Squamous cell carcinoma of the right labium majus. Note the small "kissing" lesion on the left labium majus.

in appearance (Fig. 56–2), and definitive diagnosis requires biopsy under local anesthesia. Most lesions occur on the labia majora; the labia minora are the next most common sites. Less commonly, the clitoris or the perineum is involved. Approximately 5 per cent of cases are multifocal.

Methods of Spread

Vulvar cancer spreads by direct extension to adjacent structures, such as the vagina, urethra, and anus; by lymphatic embolization to regional lymph nodes; and by hematogenous spread to distant sites, including the lungs, liver, and bone. In most cases, the initial lymphatic metastases are to the inguinal lymph nodes, located between Camper's fascia and the fascia lata. From these superficial nodes, spread occurs to the femoral nodes located along the femoral vessels. Cloquet's node, which is situated be-

neath the inguinal ligament, is the most cephalad of the femoral node group. From the inguinofemoral nodes, spread occurs to the pelvic nodes, particularly the external iliac group (Fig. 56–3). Metastasis to the femoral nodes without involvement of the inguinal nodes has occasionally been reported, but metastasis to pelvic nodes without initial involvement of the groin nodes is rare.

The incidence of lymph node metastases in vulvar cancer is approximately 30 per cent. It is related to lesion size (Table 56–1) and to the stage of the disease (Table 56–2). Approximately 5 per cent of patients have metastases to pelvic lymph nodes. Such patients usually have three or more positive unilateral inguinofemoral lymph nodes. Hematogenous spread usually occurs late in the disease and rarely occurs in the absence of lymphatic metastases.

Staging

For many years, vulvar cancer has been staged clinically, as shown in Table 56–3. Staging was based on an evaluation of the primary tumor and regional lymph nodes and a limited search for distant metastases. Although the clinical assessment of inguinal lymph nodes is helpful, false-positive and false-negative rates of 25 to 30 per cent may be expected. Hence in 1989, the FIGO Cancer Committee introduced a surgical staging system, as shown in Table 56–4. Almost all data currently in the literature are based on the original clinical staging system, however, and this is the system used for reporting results in this chapter.

Management

During the past 40 years, en-bloc radical vulvectomy and bilateral inguinofemoral lymphadenectomy, with or without pelvic lymphadenectomy, has been considered the standard treatment for invasive vulvar cancer. This operation involves removal of the lymph nodes and fatty tissue in the femoral triangle and overlying the inguinal ligament, together with the entire vulva between the labiocrural folds, from the perineal body to the upper

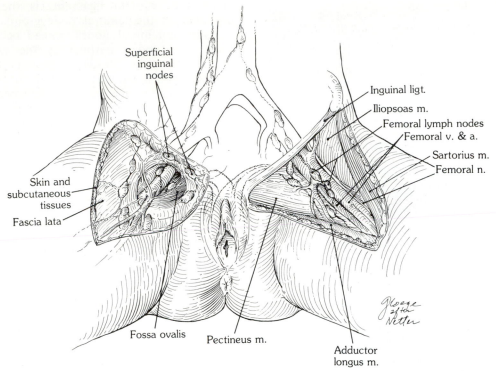

Figure 56–3. Lymphatic drainage of the vulva. Inguinal nodes displayed in the right groin and femoral nodes in the left groin.

margin of the mons pubis. The vulvar dissection is carried down to the level of the fascia overlying the symphysis pubis, which is coplanar with the inferior fascia of the urogenital diaphragm and the fascia lata. If necessary to obtain adequate surgical margins, the distal portions of the urethra and vaginal wall are included in the en-bloc dissection.

With an en-bloc approach, prolonged hospitalization is common because of postoperative wound breakdown. Chronic leg edema also occurs in about 50 per cent of patients. To decrease this postoperative morbidity, separate incisions may be used for the groin dissections. This allows the wounds to be

Table 56–1. INCIDENCE OF LYMPH NODE METASTASES IN RELATION TO LESION SIZE IN VULVAR CANCER

LESION SIZE (cm)	NUMBER	POSITIVE NODES	PER CENT
1	40	2	5
1–2	81	13	16
2–4	33	11	33.3
>4	15	8	53.3

From Hacker NF, et al: Vulvar cancer. In Haskell CM (ed): Cancer Treatment. 2nd ed. Philadelphia, WB Saunders, 1985.

Table 56–2. INCIDENCE OF LYMPH NODE METASTASES IN RELATION TO STAGE OF DISEASE IN VULVAR CANCER

STAGE	NUMBER OF CASES	POSITIVE NODES	PER CENT
I	140	15	10.7
II	145	38	26.2
III	137	88	64.2
IV	18	16	88.9

Combined data from Green TH Jr (Obstet Gynecol 52:462, 1978); Iverson T, et al (Gynecol Oncol 9:271, 1980) and Hacker NF, et al (Obstet Gynecol 61:408, 1983).

Table 56-3. OLD FIGO* CLINICAL STAGING FOR VULVAR CANCER (1969)

FIGO STAGE	CLINICAL FINDINGS
Stage 0	Carcinoma in situ, e.g., VIN 3, noninvasive Paget's disease
Stage I	Tumor confined to the vulva up to 2 cm in diameter, and no suspicious groin nodes
Stage II	Tumor confined to the vulva more than 2 cm in diameter, and no suspicious groin nodes
Stage III	Tumor of any size with adjacent spread to the urethra and/or the vagina, the perineum, and the anus; and/or clinically suspicious lymph nodes in either groin
Stage IV	Tumor of any size infiltrating the bladder mucosa, or the rectal mucosa, or both, including the upper part of the urethral mucosa, and/or; fixed to the bone; and/or other distant metastases

* International Federation of Gynecology and Obstetrics.

closed without tension and significantly improves the incidence of wound breakdown.

In 1986, the Gynecologic Oncology Group reported the results of a phase III study that randomized patients with one or more positive groin nodes between ipsilateral pelvic node dissection and bilateral groin and pelvic radiation. There was a significant survival advantage at 2 years (68 versus 54 per cent; $P = 0.03$) for the group receiving radiation, owing to a significant decrease in the incidence of groin recurrence in the irradiated group. The benefit was seen only for patients with multiple positive nodes or a grossly enlarged node. Postoperative pelvic and groin radiation therapy has therefore become standard treatment for patients with multiple positive groin nodes. Patients with one microscopically involved node require no additional treatment.

Although direct lymphatic channels to the pelvic lymph nodes have been demonstrated from the clitoris and Bartholin's gland, the involvement of pelvic lymph nodes with these tumors is very uncommon in the absence of inguinofemoral lymph node metas-

tases; therefore, tumors in these sites should be managed in the standard way.

Complications

Using the separate incision technique, major wound breakdown in the groins may be reduced from about 45 to about 15 per cent. Anterior thigh anesthesia from injury to the cutaneous branches of the femoral nerve is common in the immediate postoperative period but usually progressively resolves with time. Less common acute complications include groin seromas, cellulitis, thrombophlebitis, and pulmonary embolus. Chronic complications include leg edema, genital prolapse, and urinary stress incontinence. Rarely, introital stenosis, pubic osteomyelitis, femoral hernia, or a rectoperineal fistula may occur.

Early Vulvar Cancer

During the past decade, a significant weight of evidence has suggested that it is possible to modify the standard radical approach to vulvar cancer for selected patients with stage I disease, in an attempt to decrease both physical and psychological morbidity. Modifica-

Table 56-4. FIGO STAGING OF VULVAR CARCINOMA (1989)

STAGE	CLINICAL FINDINGS
Stage 0	Carcinoma in situ, intraepithelial carcinoma
Stage I	Tumor confined to the vulva and/or perineum—2 cm or less in greatest dimension. No nodal metastasis
Stage II	Tumor confined to the vulva and/or perineum—more than 2 cm in greatest dimension. No nodal metastasis
Stage III	Tumor of any size with adjacent spread to the urethra and/or the vagina, or the anus, and/or; unilateral regional lymph node metastasis
Stage IVa	Tumor invades any of the following: upper urethra, bladder mucosa, rectal mucosa, pelvic bone, and/or bilateral regional node metastasis
Stage IVb	Any distant metastasis including pelvic lymph nodes

tions may involve either the lymphadenectomy or the primary tumor.

With respect to the lymphadenectomy, it has become apparent that the only patients without significant risk of lymph node metastases are those in whom the depth of penetration is less than 1 mm from the overlying basement membrane. In this group of patients, groin dissection may be eliminated. For patients with midline lesions, bilateral groin dissection is necessary. If the lesion is situated laterally on the labia, unilateral inguinofemoral lymphadenectomy is an acceptable approach, although there is about a 1 per cent risk of positive contralateral nodes.

With respect to the primary tumor, evidence suggests that a wide and deep local excision (radical local excision) is as effective as radical vulvectomy in preventing local recurrence, provided that the remainder of the vulva is normal. For patients with stage I vulvar cancer, there is about a 10 per cent risk of local recurrence, even with radical vulvectomy, and this incidence appears to be no higher with radical local excision. Surgical margins should be at least 1 cm.

Advanced Vulvar Cancer

The standard management for patients with advanced vulvar cancer involving the proximal urethra, anus, or rectovaginal septum has been pelvic exenteration performed in conjunction with radical vulvectomy and bilateral inguinofemoral lymphadenectomy. Although the 5-year survival rate for such patients approximates 50 per cent, the operative mortality rate is about 10 per cent, and the cure rate is very low if there are any positive lymph nodes. More recently, some centers have been using preoperative radiation to shrink the primary tumor, followed by more conservative surgical excision. Survival does not seem to be compromised by this approach, and most patients can be spared pelvic exenteration.

Prognosis

The overall survival for vulvar carcinoma is about 70 per cent. This reflects the trend toward earlier diagnosis. Survival correlates

Table 56–5. SURVIVAL OF PATIENTS WITH VULVAR CANCER TREATED WITH CURATIVE INTENT VERSUS STAGE OF DISEASE

STAGE	NUMBER	DEAD OF DISEASE	CORRECTED 5-YEAR SURVIVAL RATES (PER CENT)
I	306	25	91.8
II	259	51	80.3
III	215	100	53.5
IV	101	86	14.6
Total	881	262	70.3

From Hacker NF, et al: Vulvar cancer. In Haskell CM (ed): Cancer Treatment. 2nd ed. Philadelphia, WB Saunders, 1985.

with the International Federation of Obstetrics and Gynecology (FIGO) clinical staging, 5-year survival rate ranging from approximately 90 per cent for patients with stage I disease to 15 per cent for patients with stage IV (Table 56–5). Survival also correlates significantly with lymph node status, since patients with positive nodes have a 5-year survival rate of about 50 per cent, whereas those with negative nodes have a 5-year survival rate of about 90 per cent. Patients with one positive node have good prognosis, regardless of stage, whereas those with three or more positive nodes do poorly, regardless of stage.

Malignant Melanoma

Malignant melanoma is the second most common type of vulvar cancer. Melanomas may arise de novo or from a pre-existing junctional or compound nevi. They occur predominantly in postmenopausal white women and most commonly involve the labia minora or clitoris (Fig. 56–4).

Diagnosis and Staging

Any pigmented lesion on the vulva requires excisional biopsy for histologic diagnosis. The staging of vulvar cancer as used for squamous cell carcinomas does not apply well to melanomas, which are usually smaller

Figure 56-4. Malignant melanoma arising from the clitoris.

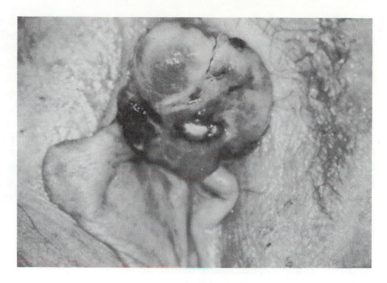

lesions and tend to metastasize earlier. The prognosis correlates more closely with the depth of penetration into the dermis, and those lesions that penetrate to a depth of 1 mm or less from the granular layer of the epidermis rarely metastasize. Clark's levels are not readily applicable to vulvar melanomas.

Management

For the superficial lesions referred to previously, radical local excision is adequate therapy. For more invasive tumors, en-bloc radical vulvectomy and bilateral inguinofemoral lymphadenectomy are usually performed. There has been a trend toward vulvar conservation for melanomas, with radical local excision of the primary tumor being preferred to radical vulvectomy in some centers. Adjuvant therapy with nonspecific immunostimulants or chemotherapeutic agents has been disappointing. Estrogen receptors, however, have been demonstrated in some melanomas, and occasional responses to tamoxifen (Nolvadex) have been reported.

Prognosis

The overall 5-year survival rate for vulvar melanomas is approximately 30 per cent, which is comparable to that for cutaneous melanomas of nongenital origin.

Verrucous Carcinoma

Verrucous carcinoma is a variant of squamous cell carcinoma and was originally described in the oral cavity. The lesions, which are cauliflower-like in nature, may occur in the cervix, vulva, or vagina. Invasion occurs with a broad "pushing" front, and unless the base of the lesion is submitted for histologic examination, these tumors may be difficult to differentiate from a condyloma acuminatum or squamous papilloma. Metastasis to regional lymph nodes is rare, but the tumors are locally aggressive and prone to local recurrence, unless wide surgical margins are obtained. Radiation therapy may induce anaplastic transformation and is contraindicated.

Bartholin's Gland Carcinoma

Adenocarcinomas, squamous cell carcinomas, and, rarely, transitional cell carcinomas may arise from Bartholin's gland. A history of preceding inflammation of Bartholin's gland is present in about 10 per cent of patients, and malignancies may be mistaken for benign cysts or abscesses. Treatment consists of radical vulvectomy and bilateral inguinofemoral lymphadenectomy, with pelvic lymphadenectomy reserved for patients with positive groin nodes. Stage for stage, the prognosis is similar to that for squamous cell carcinoma, although diagnosis is often delayed because of the deep location of the gland.

Basal Cell Carcinoma

Basal cell carcinomas of the vulva are rare. They commonly present as a rolled edge "rodent" ulcer, although nodules and macules may occur. They are locally aggressive but nonmetastasizing, so wide local excision is adequate treatment.

Vulvar Sarcoma

Vulvar sarcomas represent 1 to 2 per cent of vulvar malignancies. Many histologic types have been reported, including leiomyosarcomas, fibrosarcomas, neurofibrosarcomas, liposarcomas, rhabdomyosarcomas, angiosarcomas, and epithelioid sarcomas. Leiomyosarcomas are the most common, and prognosis correlates with lesion size, mitotic activity, and growth patterns. Recurrence is most likely with lesions larger than 5 cm, with infiltrating margins, and with 5 or more mitotic figures per 10 high power fields.

VAGINAL NEOPLASMS

Intraepithelial Neoplasia

Carcinoma in situ of the vagina is much less common than its counterpart in the cervix or vulva. Most lesions occur in the upper third of the vagina, and the patients are usually asymptomatic.

Etiology

The etiology is unknown, but patients with a past history of in situ or invasive carcinoma of the cervix or vulva are at increased risk, suggesting that the squamous epithelium of the lower genital tract may respond to the same carcinogenic factors. Some lesions may occur after irradiation for cervical cancer.

Diagnosis

The diagnosis is usually considered because of an abnormal Papanicolaou smear in a woman who either has had a hysterectomy or has no demonstrable cervical abnormality. Definitive diagnosis requires vaginal biopsy, which should be directed by colposcopy or Lugol's iodine staining. Colposcopic findings are similar to those seen with cervical lesions, although thorough colposcopy of all vaginal walls is technically more difficult. In postmenopausal patients, a 4-week course of topical estrogen before colposcopy is indicated to enhance the colposcopic features and eliminate those patients with Papanicolaou smear abnormalities due to inflammatory atypia.

Management

Surgical excision is the mainstay of therapy, and this usually requires excision of the vaginal apex. At times, extensive disease requires total vaginectomy and creation of a neovagina using a split-thickness skin graft. More recently, laser therapy has increased in popularity. Topical 5-fluorouracil is another alternative to surgical excision.

Squamous Cell Carcinoma of the Vagina

Squamous cell carcinoma of the vagina is uncommon, and the etiology is unknown. The mean age of patients is about 60 years. Symptoms consist of abnormal vaginal bleeding, vaginal discharge, and urinary symptoms. On physical examination, ulcerative, exophytic, and infiltrative growth patterns may be seen. About half of the lesions are in the upper third of the vagina, particularly on the posterior wall. Punch biopsy is required to confirm the diagnosis.

Patterns of Spread

Vaginal cancer spreads by direct invasion as well as by lymphatic and hematogenous dissemination. Direct tumor spread may result in involvement of the bladder, urethra, or rectum, or progressive lateral extension to the pelvic sidewall. The lymphatic drainage from the upper vagina is to the obturator, hypogastric, and external iliac nodes, whereas the lower vagina drains primarily to the in-

Table 56–6. FIGO STAGING OF VAGINAL CANCER

STAGE	DESCRIPTION
Stage I	Carcinoma limited to the vaginal wall
Stage II	Carcinoma has involved the subvaginal tissue but has not extended onto the pelvic sidewall
Stage III	Carcinoma has extended to the pelvic sidewall
Stage IV	Carcinoma has extended beyond the true pelvis or has involved the mucosa of the bladder or rectum
IVa	Spread to bladder or rectum
IVb	Spread to distant organs

guinofemoral nodes. Hematogenous spread is uncommon until the disease is advanced.

Staging

FIGO staging for vaginal cancer is clinical, as shown in Table 56–6. All patients should have at least a chest radiograph, intravenous pyelogram, cystoscopy, and sigmoidoscopy. A pelvic and abdominal computed tomographic scan may be useful to detect lymph node metastases, which can be confirmed by fine needle aspiration, but a finding of positive nodes does not alter the FIGO stage.

Management

Radiotherapy is the main method of treatment for primary vaginal cancer. Initial treatment usually consists of 4500 to 5000 cGy external irradiation to the pelvis to shrink the primary tumor and treat the pelvic lymph nodes and paravaginal tissues. Small tumors may then be treated with intracavitary vaginal applicators, but, in general, interstitial therapy is preferable because of the higher dosages that can be delivered to deeper tissues. When the lower third of the vagina is involved, the groin nodes should be either included in the treatment field or surgically removed.

Radical surgery has a limited role in the management of vaginal cancer. Radical hysterectomy, partial vaginectomy, and pelvic lymphadenectomy may be performed for early lesions in the posterior fornix. Surgery should otherwise be reserved for medically fit patients who develop a central recurrence following radiation. Pelvic exenteration with creation of a neovagina may be appropriate in such patients, provided that there are no lymph node metastases at the time of exploratory laparotomy and adequate surgical margins can be attained.

Prognosis

The overall 5-year survival for vaginal cancer is about 50 per cent. When corrected for death from intercurrent disease, 5-year survival rates should be approximately 85 to 90 per cent for stage I lesions, 55 to 65 per cent for stage II, 30 to 35 per cent for stage III, and 5 to 10 per cent for stage IV.

Rare Vaginal Cancers

Adenocarcinoma

Most adenocarcinomas of the vagina are metastatic, usually from the cervix, endometrium, or ovary, but occasionally from more distant sites, such as the kidney, breast, or colon. Most primary vaginal adenocarcinomas are clear-cell carcinomas in female offspring of women who ingested diethylstilbestrol (DES) during pregnancy (see later in this chapter). Non–DES-related primary adenocarcinomas of the vagina are rare but may arise in residual glands of müllerian (paramesonephric) origin, Gartner's duct (a remnant of the embryonic wolffian or mesonephric duct), or foci of endometriosis.

Malignant Melanoma

Vaginal melanomas account for fewer than 2 per cent of vaginal malignancies. The mean age at diagnosis is 55. The carcinoma usually occurs on the distal anterior wall. Radiation therapy is not effective treatment, so radical surgery is required to achieve the best results. This may require radical hysterectomy and vaginectomy or some type of pelvic exenteration, depending on the location and extent of disease. The prognosis is poor, with an overall 5-year survival rate of 5 to 10 per cent.

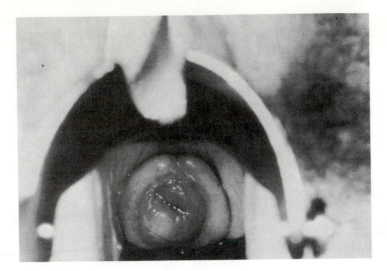

Figure 56–5. A cervical collar in a patient exposed to diethylstilbestrol in utero. (Courtesy of Dr. William Growdon, Department of Obstetrics and Gynecology, UCLA School of Medicine.)

Sarcoma

Vaginal sarcomas are rare. In adults, leiomyosarcomas are most common, whereas in infants and children, sarcoma botryoides predominates. The latter term comes from the Greek *botrys,* a bunch of grapes, which these lesions usually grossly resemble. The mean age at diagnosis of sarcoma botryoides is 2 to 3 years, with a range of 6 months to 16 years. They are usually multicentric, and histologically the tumor is an embryonal rhabdomyosarcoma. Treatment consists of surgical resection of gross disease followed by adjuvant chemotherapy, with or without radiation.

DIETHYLSTILBESTROL EXPOSURE IN UTERO

In 1971, an association between in utero exposure to DES and the later development of clear-cell adenocarcinoma of the vagina was reported. Since that time, numerous non-neoplastic uterine and vaginal anomalies have been reported in young women exposed in utero to DES. Vaginal adenosis (vaginal columnar epithelium) is the most common anomaly and is present in about 30 per cent of exposed females. This tissue behaves similarly to the columnar epithelium of the cervix and is replaced initially by immature metaplastic squamous epithelium. Colposcopically, the latter resembles dysplasia, mainly because of the frequent occurrence of mosaic pattern and punctation. With progressive squamous maturation, complete resolution of this anomaly usually occurs.

Structural changes of the cervix and vagina occur in about 25 per cent of exposed females. Possible changes include a transverse vaginal septum, cervical collar (Fig. 56–5), cockscomb (a raised ridge, usually on the anterior cervix), or cervical hypoplasia. Most of these changes tend to disappear as the individual matures. Pregnancy hastens their maturation. The occurrence of these anomalies is related to the dosage of medication given and the time of first exposure. The risk is insignificant if administration was begun after the twenty-second week.

In addition to these changes in the lower genital tract, upper genital tract anomalies occur in at least half of the patients and may be associated with exposure later in pregnancy. The most common abnormalities are a T-shaped uterus and a small uterine cavity (less than 2.5 cm in length). Exposed individuals have an increased risk of miscarriage, premature delivery, or ectopic pregnancy, but most are able to deliver a viable infant successfully.

Clear-Cell Adenocarcinoma

Since 1971, over 400 cases of clear-cell adenocarcinoma of the cervix or vagina have been reported to the Registry for Research on

Hormonal Transplacental Carcinogenesis in Chicago. The risk for developing clear-cell adenocarcinoma following DES exposure in utero is somewhat less than one in 1000. The tumors are rare before age 14, and the mean age of patients is about 19 years. Very few cases have been reported after 30 years of age. Diagnosis is best made by thorough inspection and palpation of the entire vagina and cervix, with biopsies taken of any abnormal areas. Papanicolaou smears should be obtained from the cervix and vagina, but colposcopy is necessary only for the evaluation of an abnormal Papanicolaou smear. A young woman exposed to DES in utero should be examined at menarche, or at about 14 years of age if menstruation has not occurred. Any vaginal bleeding or discharge in a prepubertal child should be investigated by examination under anesthesia. For early tumors, radical hysterectomy and vaginectomy (with creation of a neovagina) or radiation therapy are effective. Overall, the 5-year survival rate is about 80 per cent, which is considerably better than that for squamous cell cancer of the cervix or vagina.

SUGGESTED READING

Benedet JL, Murphy KJ, Fairey RN, et al: Primary invasive carcinoma of the vagina. Obstet Gynecol 62:715, 1983.

Boronow RC, Hickman BT, Reagan MT, et al: Combined therapy as an alternative to exenteration for locally advanced vulvovaginal cancer II. Results, complications, and dosimetric and surgical considerations. Am J Clin Oncol (CCT) 10(2):171, 1987.

Burke TW, Stringer CA, Gershenson DM, et al: Radical wide excision and selective inguinal node dissection for squamous cell carcinoma of the vulva. Gynecol Oncol 38:328, 1990.

Buscema J, Woodruff JD, Parmley TH, et al: Carcinoma in situ of the vulva. Obstet Gynecol 55:225, 1980.

Chung AF, Woodruff JM, Lewis JL Jr: Malignant melanoma of the vulva. Obstet Gynecol 45:639, 1975.

Creasman WT, Gallager HS, Rutledge F: Paget's disease of the vulva. Gynecol Oncol 3:133, 1975.

Crum CP, Braun LA, Shah KV: Vulvar intraepithelial neoplasia: Correlation of nuclear DNA content and the presence of a human papilloma virus (HPV) structural antigen. Cancer 49:468, 1982.

Hacker NF: Vulvar Cancer. In Berek JS, Hacker NF (eds): Practical Gynecologic Oncology. Baltimore, Williams & Wilkins, 1989, pp 391–424.

Hacker NF, Berek JS, Lagasse LD, et al: Individualization of treatment for Stage I squamous cell vulvar carcinoma. Obstet Gynecol 63:155, 1984.

Hacker NF, Berek JS, Lagasse LD, et al: The management of regional lymph nodes in vulvar cancer and their influence on prognosis. Obstet Gynecol 61:408, 1983.

Heaps JM, Fu YS, Montz FJ, et al: Surgical-pathologic variables predictive of local recurrence in squamous cell carcinoma of the vulva. Gynecol Oncol 38:309, 1990.

Herbst AL, Cole P, Norusis MJ, et al: Epidemiologic aspects and factors related to survival in 384 Registry cases of clear cell adenocarcinoma of the vagina and cervix. Obstet Gynecol 135:876, 1979.

Homesley HD, Bundy BN, Sedlis A, Adcock L: Radiation therapy versus pelvic node resection for carcinoma of the vulva with positive groin nodes. Obstet Gynecol 68:733, 1986.

Leuchter RS, Hacker NF, Voet RL, et al: Primary carcinoma of the Bartholin gland: A report of 14 cases and review of the literature. Obstet Gynecol 60:361, 1982.

Morley GW: Infiltrative carcinoma of the vulva: Results of surgical treatment. Am J Obstet Gynecol 124:874, 1976.

Fifty-seven

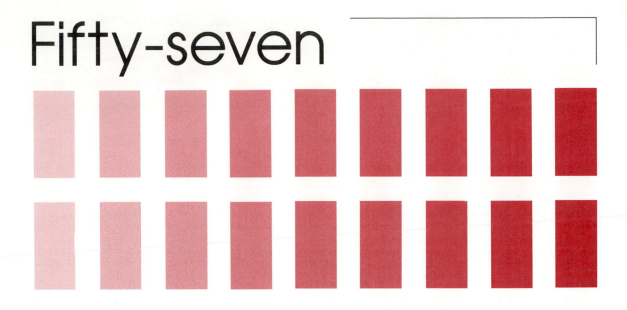

Gestational Trophoblastic Neoplasia

JONATHAN S. BEREK

Gestational trophoblastic neoplasia (GTN) represents a unique spectrum of diseases that includes benign hydatidiform mole; invasive mole (chorioadenoma destruens), which can metastasize; and the frankly malignant variety, choriocarcinoma. About 3000 hydatidiform moles are diagnosed annually in the United States. The majority of patients (80 to 90 per cent) with GTN follow a benign course, with their disease spontaneously remitting. Most patients with metastatic disease can be effectively cured with chemotherapy. This diverse group of diseases has a sensitive tumor marker, the beta subunit of human chorionic gonadotropin (β-hCG), which is secreted by all of these tumors and allows accurate follow-up and assessment of the disease.

EPIDEMIOLOGY AND ETIOLOGY

The incidence of molar pregnancy is about one in every 1500 to 2000 pregnancies among whites in the United States. There is a much higher incidence among Asian women in the United States (one in 800) and an even higher incidence among Asian women in the Far East, for example, Taiwan (one in every 125 to 200 pregnancies). The risk of developing a second molar pregnancy is 1 to 3 per cent, or as much as 40 times greater than that of developing the first.

Although the cause of GTN is unknown, it is known to occur more frequently in women under 20 years and in those older than 40 years. It appears that GTN may result from defective fertilization, a process that is more

626

Figure 57–1. Cytogenetic makeup of hydatidiform mole. *A*, Chromosomal origin of a complete mole. A single sperm fertilizes an "empty egg." Reduplication of its 23 X set gives a completely homozygous diploid genome of 46 XX. A similar result follows fertilization of an empty egg by two sperms with two independently drawn sets of 23 X or 23 Y; note that both karyotypes, 46 XX and 46 XY, can ensue. *B*, Chromosomal origin of the triploid, partial mole. A normal egg with a 23 X haploid set is fertilized by two sperms that can carry either sex chromosome to give a total of 69 chromosomes with a sex chromosome configuration of XXY, XXX, or XYY. A similar result can be obtained by fertilization with a sperm carrying the unreduced paternal genome 46 XY (resulting sex complement, XXY only). (From Szulman AE: Syndromes of hydatidiform moles: Partial vs complete. J Reprod Med 29:789–790, 1984.)

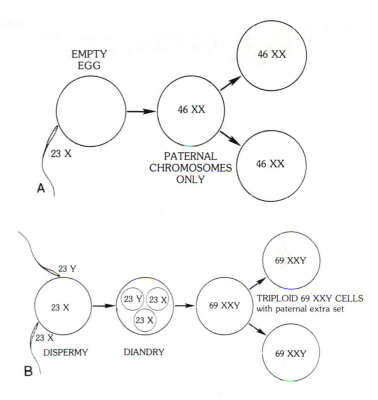

common in both younger and older individuals. Diet may play an etiologic role. The incidence of molar pregnancy has been noted to be higher in geographic areas where people consume less beta-carotene (a retinoid) and folic acid.

Cytogenetics

The cytogenetic analysis of tissue obtained from molar pregnancies offers some clue to the genesis of these lesions. Figure 57–1 illustrates the genetic composition of molar pregnancies. The majority of hydatidiform moles are "complete" moles and have a 46 XX karyotype. Specialized studies indicate that both of the X chromosomes are paternally derived. This androgenic origin probably results from fertilization of an "empty egg" (i.e., an egg without chromosomes) by a haploid sperm (23 X), which then duplicates to restore the diploid chromosomal complement (46 XX). Only a small percentage of lesions are 46 XY. Complete molar pregnancy is only rarely associated with a fetus, and this may represent a form of twinning.

In the "incomplete" or partial mole, the karyotype is usually a triploid, often 69 XXY (80 per cent). The majority of the remaining lesions are 69 XXX or 69 XYY. Occasionally mosaic patterns occur. These lesions, unlike complete moles, often present with a coexistent fetus. The fetus is usually triploid and defective.

Genetic analysis of choriocarcinomas usually reveals aneuploidy or polyploidy, typical for anaplastic carcinomas.

CLASSIFICATION

The term *gestational trophoblastic neoplasia* is of clinical value because often the diagnosis is made and therapy instituted without definitive knowledge of the precise histologic pattern. GTN may be benign or malignant and nonmetastatic or metastatic (Table 57–1).

The benign form of GTN is called hydatidiform mole. Although this entity is usually confined to the uterine cavity, trophoblastic tissue can occasionally embolize to the lungs. The malignant forms of GTN are invasive

Table 57–1. CLASSIFICATION OF GESTATIONAL TROPHOBLASTIC NEOPLASIA (GTN)

Benign
 Hydatidiform mole
  Complete mole
  Incomplete ("partial") mole
Malignant
 Invasive mole ("chorioadenoma destruens")
 Choriocarcinoma
Malignant GTN may be:
 Nonmetastatic
 Metastatic
  Good prognosis
  Poor prognosis

mole and choriocarcinoma. Invasive mole (chorioadenoma destruens) is usually a locally invasive lesion, although it can be associated with metastases. This lesion accounts for the majority of patients who have persistent hCG titers following molar evacuation. Choriocarcinoma is the frankly malignant form of GTN.

Metastatic GTN can be subdivided into "good prognosis" and "poor prognosis" groups, depending on the sites of metastases and other clinical variables (Table 57–2).

PATHOLOGY

Grossly, a hydatidiform mole appears as multiple vesicles that have been classically

Table 57–2. CLINICAL FEATURES OF POOR PROGNOSIS METASTATIC GESTATIONAL TROPHOBLASTIC NEOPLASIA

Urinary hCG titer greater than 100,000 IU/24 hours or serum hCG titer greater than 40,000 IU
Disease present more than 4 months from the antecedent pregnancy
Metastasis to the brain or liver (regardless of hCG titer or duration of disease)
Failure to respond to prior single agent chemotherapy
Choriocarcinoma after a full-term delivery

described as a "bunch of grapes" (Fig. 57–2). The characteristic histopathologic findings associated with a complete molar pregnancy are (1) hydropic villi, (2) absence of fetal blood vessels, and (3) hyperplasia of trophoblastic tissue (Fig. 57–3). Invasive mole differs from hydatidiform mole only in its propensity to invade locally and to metastasize.

A partial mole has some hydropic villi, whereas other villi are essentially normal. Fetal vessels are seen in a partial mole, and the trophoblastic tissue exhibits less striking hyperplasia.

Choriocarcinoma in the uterus appears grossly as a vascular-appearing, irregular, and "beefy" tumor, often growing through the uterine wall. Metastatic lesions appear hemorrhagic and have a consistency of "currant jelly." Histologically, choriocarcinoma consists of sheets of malignant cytotrophoblast and syncytiotrophoblast with no identifiable villi.

HYDATIDIFORM MOLE

Symptoms

Most patients with hydatidiform mole present with irregular or heavy vaginal bleeding during the first or early second trimester of pregnancy (Table 57–3). The bleeding is usually painless, although it can be associated with uterine contractions. In addition, the patient may expel molar "vesicles" from the vagina and occasionally may develop excessive nausea, even "hyperemesis gravidarum." Irritability, dizziness, and photophobia may occur, since some patients develop preeclampsia. Patients may occasionally exhibit symptoms relating to hyperthyroidism, such as nervousness, anorexia, and tremors.

Signs

The patient's vital signs may reveal tachycardia, tachypnea, and hypertension, reflecting the presence of pre-eclampsia or clinical hyperthyroidism. Funduscopic examination may show arteriolar spasm. In the rare case of trophoblastic emboli to the pulmonary system, wheezing and rhonchi may be noted

Figure 57–2. Complete hydatidiform mole. Multiple hydropic villi (vesicles), resembling a "bunch of grapes," are admixed with areas of necrosis (white areas) and hemorrhage. Note the absence of a fetus.

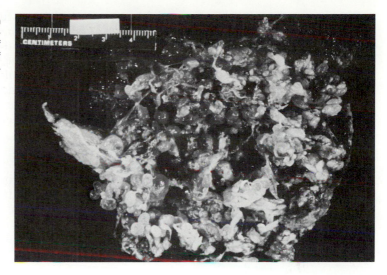

on chest examination. Abdominal examination may reveal an enlarged uterus. Auscultation of the uterus is typically remarkable for the absence of fetal heart sounds.

On pelvic examination, the grape-like vesicles of the mole may be detected in the vagina. Blood clots may be present. About one half of patients with molar pregnancy present with a uterine size that is greater than expected based on their last menstrual period, whereas about one fourth each have a size compatible with or smaller than gestational age. Ovarian enlargement by theca-lutein cysts occurs in about one third of women with molar pregnancies. This may be difficult to detect until the uterus has been evacuated.

Diagnosis

β-hCG titers can be very high for early pregnancy. This should alert the physician that the patient might have GTN or multiple gestation. The condition must also be distinguished from a threatened spontaneous abortion or an ectopic pregnancy.

Definitive diagnosis of hydatidiform mole can usually be made by ultrasonography (Fig. 57–4). The ultrasound test is noninvasive and produces a "snow storm" pattern that is diagnostic. Another test that can be employed is amniography, a procedure in which water-soluble radiopaque dye is introduced into the uterus. It produces an irregular, "moth-

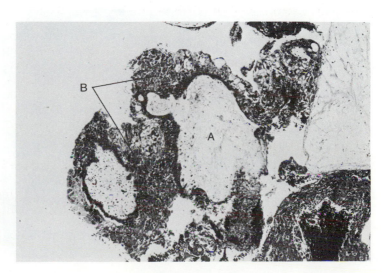

Figure 57–3. Histology of a complete hydatidiform mole. Note the hydropic, avascular villi (A) and increased trophoblastic proliferation (B). In the bottom right corner is an area of hemorrhage and necrosis (×60).

Table 57–3. DIAGNOSIS OF HYDATIDIFORM MOLE

Clinical data
  Bleeding in the first half of pregnancy
  Lower abdominal pain
  Toxemia before 24 weeks gestation
  Hyperemesis gravidarum
  Uterus large for dates (only 50% of cases)
  Absent fetal heart tones and fetal parts
  Expulsion of vesicles
Diagnostic studies
  Ultrasonography
  Chest film
  Serum β-hCG higher than normal pregnancy
    values

eaten" appearance in the absence of a fetus. This test is used only when the diagnosis is in question.

Investigations

Patients who have the presumptive or definitive diagnosis of hydatidiform mole should undergo a complete blood count to exclude anemia, which might require a transfusion. They require an assessment of the platelet count, prothrombin time, partial thromboplastin time, and a fibrinogen level, since an occasional patient may develop disseminated intravascular coagulation. Liver and renal function tests should be obtained. Blood should be typed and cross-matched in the event that excessive bleeding is encountered at the time of evacuation of the mole. A chest film should be obtained and an electrocardiogram (ECG) performed if tachycardia is present or if the patient is over 40 years of age.

Staging

An anatomic staging system for GTN was adopted at a meeting of the International Society for the Study of Trophoblastic Neoplasms in 1979. The staging is shown in Table 57–4.

Treatment

Evacuation

The standard treatment of hydatidiform mole is suction evacuation followed by sharp curettage of the uterus, regardless of the duration of pregnancy. This should be performed in the operating room with general or regional anesthesia. Intravenous oxytocin is given simultaneously to help stimulate uterine contractions and reduce blood loss. This technique is associated with a low incidence of uterine perforation and trophoblastic embolization.

Most patients have an uncomplicated course in the immediate postoperative period.

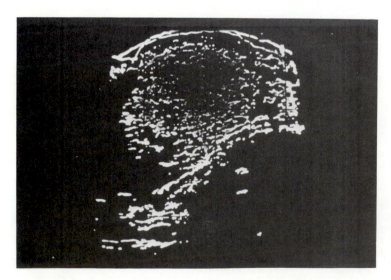

Figure 57–4. An ultrasound study of a hydatidiform mole. Note the "snow storm" pattern without evidence of a fetus.

Table 57-4. STAGING OF GESTATIONAL TROPHOBLASTIC NEOPLASIA	
Stage I	Confined to uterine corpus
Stage II	Metastases to the pelvis and vagina
Stage III	Metastasis to lung
Stage IV	Distant metastasis

Some require transfusion, however, because of excessive blood loss. Abnormal clotting parameters should be treated with fresh frozen plasma and platelet transfusions, as indicated. Rarely, a patient can develop acute respiratory distress from trophoblastic embolization or fluid overload. Such patients may require respiratory support via a ventilator and careful cardiopulmonary monitoring.

Monitoring β-hCG Titers

Following the evacuation of a hydatidiform mole, the patient must be monitored with weekly serum assays of β-hCG. Because the titers drop to a very low level, a nonspecific pregnancy test cannot be used because of cross-reactivity with luteinizing hormone (LH). The radioimmunoassay, sensitive to levels of 1 to 5 mIU/ml, should be used. Following the evacuation, the β-hCG titers should steadily decline to undetectable levels, usually within 12 to 16 weeks. A normal regression curve for β-hCG titers following evacuation of a molar pregnancy is shown in Figure 57-5.

Chemotherapy

Of patients with a molar pregnancy, 90 per cent have spontaneous remissions, so prophylactic chemotherapy is not indicated. If the β-hCG titers plateau or rise at any time, chemotherapy should be initiated. This is discussed later in this chapter.

PARTIAL MOLE

The incomplete or partial mole is usually associated with a developing fetus. Patients with a partial mole display most of the pathologic and clinical features of a complete mole, although usually in a less severe form. Partial moles are usually diagnosed later than complete moles and generally present as a spontaneous or missed abortion.

It is unusual for a partial mole to be detected before the spontaneous termination of a pregnancy. An ultrasound test performed for other indications may indicate possible "molar degeneration" of the placenta associated with the developing fetus. Under these circumstances, an amniocentesis should be performed to determine if the karyotype of the coexisting fetus is normal.

Uterine enlargement is much less common; most patients with partial moles are actually small for dates. When pre-eclampsia occurs with a partial mole, it may be severe, but the condition usually occurs between 17 and 22

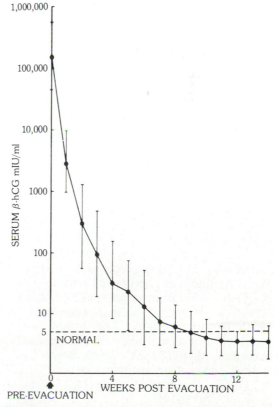

Figure 57-5. Normal regression curve of β-hCG following molar evacuation. (From Morrow CP, et al: Clinical and laboratory correlates of molar pregnancy and trophoblastic disease. Am J Obstet Gynecol 128:428, 1977.)

weeks, about 1 month later than with a complete mole. The most striking difference between partial and complete moles is related to the malignant potential of the two lesions. Partial moles have not been reported to metastasize, and only rarely will there be need for chemotherapy because of plateaued or rising β-hCG titers.

INVASIVE MOLE

Invasive mole is usually a locally invasive tumor. It constitutes about 5 to 10 per cent of all molar pregnancies, representing the majority of those with persistent β-hCG titers following molar evacuation. The lesion may penetrate the entire myometrium, rupture through the uterus, and result in hemorrhage into the broad ligament or peritoneal cavity. Rarely, invasive mole is associated with metastases, particularly to the vagina or lungs, although brain metastases have been documented.

Histologic confirmation of invasive mole is almost always made at the time of hysterectomy. The latter is usually performed in patients with persistent β-hCG titers following evacuation of a molar pregnancy or in those with persistent titers despite chemotherapy, who have no evidence of metastatic disease. The hysterectomy is usually curative.

CHORIOCARCINOMA

The frankly malignant form of GTN is choriocarcinoma. About one half of patients with gestational choriocarcinoma have had a preceding molar pregnancy. In the remaining patients, the disease is preceded by a spontaneous or induced abortion, ectopic pregnancy, or normal pregnancy. Trophoblastic disease following a normal pregnancy is always choriocarcinoma. The tumor has a tendency to disseminate hematogenously, particularly to the lungs, vagina, brain, liver, kidneys, and gastrointestinal tract.

Symptoms

Most patients with choriocarcinoma present with symptoms of metastatic disease.

Vaginal bleeding is a common symptom of uterine choriocarcinoma or vaginal metastasis. Because of the gonadotropin excretion, amenorrhea may develop, simulating early pregnancy. Hemoptysis, cough, or dyspnea may occur as a result of lung metastasis. In the presence of central nervous system metastases, the patient may complain of headaches, dizzy spells, "blacking out," or other symptoms referable to a space-occupying lesion in the brain. Rectal bleeding or "dark stools" could represent disease that has metastasized to the gastrointestinal tract.

Signs

The signs, like the symptoms, are common to many pathologic entities. Uterine enlargement may be present, with blood coming through the os, as seen on speculum examination. A tumor metastatic to the vagina may present with a firm, discolored mass. Occasionally, the patient presents with an acute abdomen because of rupture of the uterus, liver, or theca-lutein cyst. Neurologic signs, such as partial weakness or paralysis, dysphasia, aphasia, or unreactive pupils, indicate probable central nervous system involvement.

Diagnosis

Choriocarcinoma is a great imitator of other diseases, so unless it follows a molar pregnancy, diagnosis may not be suspected. In females of reproductive age, a β-hCG titer to screen for choriocarcinoma should be performed when any unusual symptoms or signs develop.

Investigations

If the β-hCG titer is positive, the work-up of a patient with choriocarcinoma is the same as that for patients with hydatidiform mole but should also include a computed tomographic scan of the abdomen, pelvis, and head. In addition, a lumbar puncture should be performed if the brain computed tomographic scan is negative because simultaneous evaluation of the β-hCG titer in the cerebrospinal fluid and serum may allow detection of very early cerebral metastases. Because the beta subunit does not readily cross the blood–brain barrier, a ratio of serum to cerebrospinal fluid β-hCG levels of less than 40 : 1 suggests central nervous system involvement, with secretion of the β-hCG directly into the cerebrospinal fluid.

TREATMENT OF GESTATIONAL TROPHOBLASTIC NEOPLASIA

If the β-hCG titers plateau or rise, chemotherapy is required. Because of the sensitivity of this tumor marker, chemotherapy is usually initiated without histologic confirmation of disease. Before initiating chemotherapy, a full metastatic work-up must be done to determine whether there is metastatic disease present, and, if so, whether the liver, brain, or both are involved.

Nonmetastatic and Good Prognosis Metastatic Gestational Trophoblastic Neoplasia

The chemotherapy most often employed is either methotrexate or actinomycin-D (Table 57–5). Methotrexate is usually given as a daily dose for 5 consecutive days or every other day for 8 days, alternating with folinic acid (leukovorin). This folinic acid "rescue" regimen is associated with significantly less bone marrow, gastrointestinal, and liver toxicity. Actinomycin-D is given for 5 consecutive days intravenously or every other week as a single dose.

In appropriately selected patients, hysterectomy may be the primary therapy for hydatidiform mole. Women over 40 years of age have an increased incidence of choriocarcinoma developing after molar pregnancy. These patients may decrease their risk of malignant sequelae by undergoing hysterectomy.

Table 57–5. CHEMOTHERAPY FOR MOLAR PREGNANCY

STANDARD CHEMOTHERAPY REGIMENS
Actinomycin-D
  10–12 μg/kg/day IV for 5 days
                    or
Methotrexate
  0.4 mg/kg/day IM or IV for 5 days
Repeat cycle after minimum gap of 7 days if: granulocytes greater than 1500/mm³; platelets greater than 100,000/mm³; stomatitis and gastrointestinal toxicity recovered; SGOT, SGPT, BUN, and bilirubin levels normal
Continue chemotherapy cycles
  One or two courses past normal β-hCG titer (less than 1.0 mIU/ml), or
  Until β-hCG titers plateau or begin rising
Obtain weekly β-hCG values and peripheral blood counts
Before each treatment cycle, obtain SGOT, SGPT, BUN, bilirubin, CBC, and platelet count
Obtain monthly β-hCG titers for 12 mo, then every 2 mo for 12 mo
Continue contraception for 1 yr after remission induction

ALTERNATIVE CHEMOTHERAPY REGIMENS
Actinomycin-D
  1.25 mg/M² IV q 2 wk
                    or
Methotrexate
  1.0 mg/kg/day IM or IV on days 1,3,5,7 followed 24 h later by 0.1 mg/kg/day of folinic acid "rescue" on days 2,4,6,8

SGOT = serum glutamic-oxaloacetic transaminase; SGPT = serum glutamate pyruvate transaminase; BUN = blood urea nitrogen; CBC = complete blood count.

Adapted from Morrow CP, Townsend DE (eds): Gestational trophoblastic neoplasia. In Synopsis of Gynecologic Oncology. 2nd ed. New York, John Wiley & Sons, 1981, p 348.

Poor Prognosis Metastatic Gestational Trophoblastic Neoplasia

For patients with poor prognosis disease, combination chemotherapy is always used. Regimens that have been successfully employed include methotrexate, actinomycin-D, and cyclophosphamide (MAC), or the modified "Bagshawe" regimen (EMA-CO), which is a six-drug chemotherapy regimen. The drugs used include etoposide (VP-16), actinomycin-D, vincristine, cyclophosphamide, methotrexate, and folinic acid. For patients who fail these agents, combinations of *cis*-platinum and etoposide (VP-16) or vinblastine, with or without bleomycin, have been used.

In patients with disease metastatic to the brain or liver, radiation is often employed to these areas in conjunction with chemotherapy. The whole brain tolerates an initial dose of 2000 to 3000 cGy, with fractions of approximately 200 cGy per day. Together with systemic chemotherapy, a 50 per cent cure rate can be expected. Liver metastases are usually treated with about 2000 cGy.

Follow-up Studies

Following three negative β-hCG titers, good prognosis patients should be followed with monthly titers for 1 year. Poor prognosis patients should have monthly titers for 2 or more years. Thereafter, titers should be checked every 3 months until 5 years have elapsed. Patients should be advised not to become pregnant again within the first 9 to 12 months after molar evacuation and should be given a reliable contraceptive. If a patient's titers become "negative" and later are found to be rising, a second metastatic workup must be undertaken before the initiation of secondary therapy.

Prognosis

About 95 to 100 per cent of patients with good prognosis GTN will be cured of their disease. Patients with poor prognostic features can be expected to be cured in only 50 to 70 per cent of cases. The majority of the patients who die develop brain or liver metastasis.

SUGGESTED READING

Bagshawe KD: Risk and prognostic factors in trophoblastic neoplasia. Cancer 38:1373, 1976.

Berkowitz RS, Goldstein DP: Gestational trophoblastic neoplasia. In Berek JS, Hacker NF (eds): Practical Gynecologic Oncology. Baltimore, Williams & Wilkins, 1989.

Berkowitz RS, Goldstein DP, Bernstein MR: Methotrexate with citrovorum factor rescue as primary therapy for gestational trophoblastic disease. Cancer 50:2024, 1982.

Curry SL, Hammond CB, Tyrey L, et al: Hydatidiform mole: Diagnosis, management and long-term follow-up of 347 patients. Obstet Gynecol 45:1, 1975.

Goldstein DP, Berkowitz RS: Gestational Trophoblastic Neoplasms. Philadelphia, WB Saunders, 1982.

Lurain JR, Brewer JI, Torok EE, et al: Natural history of hydatidiform mole after primary evacuation. Am J Obstet Gynecol 145:591, 1983.

McDonald TW, Ruffolo EH: Modern management of gestational trophoblastic disease. Obstet Gynecol Surv 38:67, 1983.

Morrow CP, Kletzky OA, DiSaia PJ, et al: Clinical and laboratory correlates of molar pregnancy and trophoblastic disease. Am J Obstet Gynecol 128:424, 1977.

Surti U, Szulman AE, O'Brien S: Dispermic origin and clinical outcome of three complete hydatidiform moles with 46 XX karyotype. Am J Obstet Gynecol 144:84, 1982.

Surwit EA, Hammond CB: Treatment of metastatic trophoblastic disease with poor prognosis. Obstet Gynecol 55:565, 1980.

Index